Gastrointestinal Infections

Gastroenterology and Hepatology

Executive Editor

J. Thomas LaMont, M.D.

Chief, Division of Gastroenterology
Beth Israel Hospital
Boston, Massachusetts
and
Charlotte F. and Irving W. Rabb Professor of Medicine
Harvard Medical School
Boston, Massachusetts

1. *Crohn's Disease*, edited by Cosimo Prantera and Burton I. Korelitz
2. *Clinical Gastroenterology in the Elderly*, edited by Alvin M. Gelb
3. *Biliary and Pancreatic Ductal Epithelia: Pathobiology and Pathophysiology*, edited by Alphonse E. Sirica and Daniel S. Longnecker
4. *Viral Hepatitis: Diagnosis • Treatment • Prevention*, edited by Richard A. Willson
5. *Gastrointestinal Infections: Diagnosis and Management*, edited by J. Thomas LaMont

ADDITIONAL VOLUMES IN PREPARATION

Gastrointestinal Infections

Diagnosis and Management

edited by

J. Thomas LaMont

Beth Israel Hospital
and Harvard Medical School
Boston, Massachusetts

MARCEL DEKKER

MARCEL DEKKER, INC. NEW YORK • BASEL • HONG KONG

ISBN: 0-8247-0055-4

The publisher offers discounts on this book when ordered in bulk quantities. For more information, write to Special Sales/Professional Marketing at the address below.

This book is printed on acid-free paper.

Marcel Dekker, Inc.
270 Madison Avenue, New York, New York 10016
http://www.dekker.com

Current printing (last digit):
10 9 8 7 6 5 4 3 2 1

Printed in the United States of America

Preface

Gastrointestinal infections comprise one of the fastest growing and most rapidly changing areas in medical practice. Common gastrointestinal infections of today, such as *Helicobacter pylori*, *Clostridium difficile*, and *Cryptosporidia*, were rare, or even unheard of, 10 or 20 years ago. Another example of rapid change is provided by the AIDS epidemic, which has led to tremendous awareness of opportunistic GI and hepatobiliary infections, most of which were not seen prior to the mid-1980s. Another new player is enterohemorrhagic *Escherichia coli* (EHEC). Despite its rarity, this organism has been highly publicized in the lay media. Outbreaks of hemorrhagic colitis and hemolytic–uremic syndrome, secondary to EHEC infection, have received intense media coverage in the United States, Canada, and Japan, and have led to stricter laws in the United States regarding the safe handling of meat products. Knowledge of these emerging pathogens is essential, not only for public health officers and specialists in infectious disease, but for gastroenterologists, primary care internists, and family practitioners.

Gastrointestinal Infections is aimed at just this audience and has as its main goal the presentation of practical information on the most commonly encountered gastrointestinal infections in medical practice. Although each chapter reviews the essential information on bacteriology, virology, and pathophysiology, the main focus is not on basic science topics but on clinical features, diagnosis, and management. Physicians in practice, whether in rural Appalachia or in a Boston teaching hospital, want to know how experts in the field diagnose and manage common GI infections, not only the rare or exotic infections but everyday infectious diarrheas seen daily in medical practice. Our authors are gastroenterologists or infectious disease specialists who hold faculty positions at prestigious medical schools, and all are recognized as experts in their specific area. Each chapter contains the basic features of microbiology, pathology, and mechanisms of disease, followed by a strong focus on patient management in the office or hospital. The biliary tract can be considered either an upward extension of the gastrointestinal tract or a downward extension of the liver. Since the biliary tract is almost always infected by a pathogen originating in the GI tract, we have included biliary-tract infections in this book. Viral infections of the liver are not dealt with here, but are covered in another book in this series, *Viral Hepatitis*, edited by Richard A. Willson.

The chapters are organized vertically—starting with the esophagus and concluding at the opposite terminus of the gastrointestinal tract. Some chapters deal with specific pathogens, while others focus on specific types of patients (e.g., AIDS patients) or infections of a certain organ or organ system that may be caused by various infectious agents (e.g., intra-abdominal abscesses). Again, the guiding principle in organizing the book was to provide clinicians with up-to-date, clinically useful information in a diagnosis-oriented format. Where appropriate, readers will find algorithms that provide an overview of diagnosis or treatment.

Some of the greatest challenges facing medicine today are described in this book. Yet, diseases that seemed almost hopeless a few years ago—chronic wasting diarrhea in end-stage AIDS, for example—are now coming under control. The introduction of new antiviral therapies in the past two years has remarkably improved or stabilized large numbers of AIDS patients. Now that their immunodeficiency is less critical, these patients are less likely to suffer from the scourge of opportunistic GI infections. Our greatest hope is that in 50 years, or perhaps sooner, many of the infections described here will be, like syphilis and polio, a dim memory.

J. Thomas LaMont

Contents

Contributors

David W. K. Acheson, M.D. Assistant Professor of Medicine, Department of Infectious Diseases, New England Medical Center, Boston, Massachusetts

Nezam H. Afdhal, M.D., F.R.C.P.I. Associate Professor of Medicine and Chief of Hepatology, Boston University School of Medicine, Boston, Massachusetts

Laurence S. Bailen, M.D. Senior Resident in Internal Medicine, Department of Medicine, Beth Israel Hospital and Harvard Medical School, Boston, Massachusetts

David H. Balaban, M.D. Senior Fellow, Division of Gastroenterology and Hepatology, University of Virginia, Charlottesville, Virginia

Dorsey M. Bass, M.D. Assistant Professor, Department of Pediatrics, Stanford University School of Medicine, Stanford, California

William R. Bishai, M.D., Ph.D. Department of Molecular Microbiology and Immunology, Johns Hopkins School of Hygiene and Public Health, Baltimore, Maryland

Peter D. Bloom, M.D. Instructor in Gastroenterology, Center for Vaccine Development, Division of Gastroenterology, University of Maryland, Baltimore, Maryland

Edgar C. Boedeker, M.D. Professor of Medicine, Center for Vaccine Development, Division of Gastroenterology, University of Maryland, Baltimore, Maryland

James D. DeMaio, M.D. Fellow in Infectious Diseases, Department of Molecular Microbiology and Immunology, Johns Hopkins School of Hygiene and Public Health, Baltimore, Maryland

Matthew E. Falagas, M.D., M.Sc. Clinical and Research Fellow in Infectious Diseases and Geographic Medicine, Department of Medicine, Tufts University School of Medicine and New England Medical Center, Boston, Massachusetts

Sherwood L. Gorbach, M.D. Professor, Department of Family Medicine and Community Health and Medicine, Tufts University School of Medicine, Boston, Massachusetts

David K. R. Karaolis, Ph.D. Research Associate in Geographic Medicine, Center for Vaccine Development, Division of Gastroenterology, University of Maryland, Baltimore, Maryland

Michael S. Karasik, M.D. Assistant Professor of Medicine and Director, Gastrointestinal Immunodeficiency Clinic, Boston University School of Medicine, Boston, Massachusetts

Dennis L. Kasper, M.D. William Ellery Channing Professor of Medicine, Harvard Medical School; Director, Channing Laboratory; Co-Director, Division of Infectious Diseases; and Executive Vice Chairman, Department of Medicine, Brigham and Women's Hospital, Boston, Massachusetts

Andrew P. Keaveny, M.D. Fellow, Section of Gastroenterology, Boston University School of Medicine, Boston, Massachusetts

Ciaran P. Kelly, M.D., F.R.C.P.I. Assistant Professor of Medicine, Division of Gastroenterology, Beth Israel Deaconess Medical Center and Harvard Medical School, Boston, Massachusetts

Gerald T. Keusch, M.D. Professor of Medicine, Division of Geographic Medicine and Infectious Diseases, Tupper Research Institute, New England Medical Center, Boston, Massachusetts

Karen L. Kotloff, M.D. Associate Professor, Department of Pediatrics, University of Maryland School of Medicine, Baltimore, Maryland

J. Thomas LaMont, M.D. Chief, Division of Gastroenterology, Beth Israel Hospital, and Charlotte F. and Irving W. Rabb Professor of Medicine, Harvard Medical School, Boston, Massachusetts

Myron M. Levine, M.D., D.T.P.H. Professor and Director, Department of Medicine, University of Maryland School of Medicine, Baltimore, Maryland

Joanne K. Linevsky, M.D. Assistant Professor of Medicine, Section of Gastroenterology, Boston University School of Medicine, Boston, Massachusetts

Mark A. Peppercorn, M.D. Associate Professor in Medicine and Director, Center for Inflammatory Bowel Disease, and Division of Gastroenterology, Beth Israel Hospital and Harvard Medical School, Boston, Massachusetts

David A. Peura, M.D. Professor of Medicine and Associate Chief, Division of Gastroenterology and Hepatology, University of Virginia, Charlottesville, Virginia

Stuart Jon Spechler, M.D. Director, Center for Swallowing Disorders, Division of Gastroenterology, Beth Israel Deaconess Medical Center, Boston, Massachusetts

Phillip P. Toskes, M.D. Director, Division of Gastroenterology, Hepatology, and Nutrition, and Professor and Associate Chairman for Clinical Affairs, Department of Medicine, University of Florida, Gainesville, Florida

George Triadafilopoulos, M.D., D.Sc., F.A.C.P., F.A.C.G. Chief, Gastroenterology Section, Palo Alto Veterans Affairs Health Care System, and Associate Professor of Medicine, Stanford University School of Medicine, Stanford, California

Dori F. Zaleznik, M.D. Assistant Professor of Medicine, Harvard Medical School, and Division of Infectious Diseases, Department of Medicine, Beth Israel Deaconess Medical Center, Boston, Massachusetts

Gastrointestinal Infections

1

Infectious Esophagitis

STUART JON SPECHLER
Beth Israel Deaconess Medical Center, Boston, Massachusetts

I. INTRODUCTION

Although the esophagus is susceptible to infection by many fungi, viruses, bacteria, and parasites, most esophageal infections are caused by one or a combination of only three organisms: candida, herpes simplex virus (HSV), and cytomegalovirus (CMV) (1,2). These organisms rarely infect the esophagus of normal individuals, but frequently cause esophagitis in patients whose immune system has been compromised severely by infection with the human immunodeficiency virus (HIV), by advanced malignancy, or by organ transplantation with the administration of potent immunosuppressive drugs. The more subtle immune defects that can accompany diabetes mellitus, alcoholism, and advanced age also may predispose to esophageal infection, especially by candida. Antibiotic therapy that alters the normal microbial flora of the upper gastrointestinal tract, and corticosteroid therapy that suppresses lymphocyte function both can result in candida esophagitis, as can abnormalities that delay the clearance of candida from the esophageal lumen such as progressive systemic sclerosis (scleroderma), achalasia, and esophageal strictures. Some of the risk factors that predispose to infectious esophagitis are listed in Table 1. These predisposing factors should be investigated for any patient found to have infectious esophagitis, particularly when the offending microorganism is anything other than candida or HSV.

Table 1 Risk Factors for Esophageal Infection

Conditions associated with immune defects	Medications
HIV infection	Corticosteroids
Cancer	Immunosuppressive agents
Organ transplantation	Antibiotics
Diabetes mellitus	Acid suppressing agents
Alcoholism	Esophageal abnormalities
Advanced age and debility	Motility disorders (e.g. progressive systemic sclerosis, achalasia)
Cushing syndrome	Strictures
Chronic mucocutaneous candidiasis	Diverticula
	Caustic injuries

II. GENERAL CLINICAL FEATURES OF INFECTIOUS ESOPHAGITIS

Although a number of different microorganisms can infect the esophagus of patients who have a variety of underlying illnesses, the clinical manifestations of the different esophageal infections tend to be remarkably similar. Dysphagia, odynophagia, and persistent chest pain are the most frequent complaints, regardless of the type of pathogen causing the esophagitis (1,2). A recent meta-analysis of reports of esophageal infections found that 59% to 95% of patients complained of dysphagia, odynophagia, or both (1). Other symptoms associated with infectious esophagitis are far less specific for esophageal disease and occur much less frequently. For example, weight loss has been reported in up to 35% of patients with esophageal infections (1). This weight loss may be the result of decreased oral intake due to severe dysphagia and odynophagia, or may be a manifestation of the debilitating illness that often underlies the infectious esophagitis. Unlike candida and HSV infections that commonly involve only the esophagus and oropharynx in the immunocompromised host, CMV esophagitis often is only one part of a widespread CMV infection that may involve the stomach, intestine, and a number of other organs (3). Consequently, some 20% to 40% of patients with CMV esophagitis experience fever, nausea, vomiting, and abdominal pain, whereas these systemic symptoms are much less common in patients with esophageal infections due to candida and HSV (1). In contrast, oral lesions (e.g., thrush, focal ulcerations) are found frequently in patients who have candida and HSV esophagitis, whereas CMV esophagitis is not commonly associated with oral lesions. Despite these occasional differences in the clinical manifestations of the various infectious esophagitides, none of the clinical features are sufficiently distinctive to establish the identity of the offending microorganism reliably. Furthermore, in patients with the acquired immunodeficiency syndrome (AIDS), the esophagus frequently is infected with multiple pathogens simultaneously (4), and a deep esophageal ulceration initially caused by one microorganism may be secondarily infected by another (5). Therefore the establishment of a specific diagnosis of esophageal infection requires the procurement of tissue specimens for histologic and cytologic examination, for culture, or both.

Serious local complications of infectious esophagitis are not common but can develop when the infection causes deep ulcerations of the esophagus. Such deep ulcerations can erode into large blood vessels, which can result in massive hemorrhage (6). Deep, infectious esophageal ulcerations may cause perforation, though rarely (7), or they may penetrate into adjacent organs forming esophago–bronchial or esophago–mediastinal fistulae (8). The onset of coughing with swallowing often heralds the development of an esophago–bronchial fistula. Healing of deep esophageal ulcerations may be accompanied by fibrosis and stricture formation, a process that can cause severe and progressive dysphagia (9).

Although infectious esophagitis can cause debilitating symptoms and life-threatening local complications, a surprising number of esophageal infections are asymptomatic. In published series, for example, approximately one-quarter of all patients with candida esophagitis had the infection discovered incidentally during radiographic or endoscopic examinations performed for the evaluation of extraesophageal symptoms (1). The precise frequency of asymptomatic esophageal infection is not clear because completely asymptomatic individuals rarely have barium swallows or endoscopic examinations.

III. CANDIDA ESOPHAGITIS

Candida, a yeast found in the oropharynx of most normal individuals, is the most frequent cause of esophageal infections in immunocompromised patients (2). The only major exception to this rule is found in bone marrow transplant recipients. In these cases, viral esophagitis predominates in the first several months after transplantation, possibly because prophylactic antifungal therapy may be administered routinely during this period of intense immunosuppression (10). Most candida esophagitis is caused by *Candida albicans*, although other candida species such as *Candida tropicalis* and *Candida glabrata* occasionally infect the esophagus (4). Infection of the esophageal squamous cells appears to follow a variable period of esophageal colonization with candida. The defective lymphocyte function that typifies AIDS frequently allows superficial epithelial infection by candida. Deep invasion and disseminated candidiasis are uncommon in AIDS, however, and generally are seen only in patients who have severe granulocytopenia (11).

Candida esophagitis often causes dysphagia and odynophagia but, as mentioned above, many patients with this infection have no esophageal symptoms whatsoever. Most patients with esophageal infection by candida also have oral thrush, and the combination of oral thrush and esophageal symptoms has a very high positive predictive value for candida esophagitis (12). Thrush however, is absent in approximately 15% of patients with esophageal infection by candida (1). Even in patients who have thrush and esophageal symptoms, candida esophagitis alone is an uncommon cause of nausea, vomiting, abdominal pain, hemorrhage, fever, cough, and diarrhea (1). When the latter symptoms are prominent, the clinician should consider the possibility of infection with an organism other than, or in addition to, candida.

Figure 1 shows the typical endoscopic appearance of candida esophagitis, with innumerable raised, white plaques resembling cottage cheese clinging to the esophageal mucosa. This material cannot be washed away readily, and the friable underlying mucosa frequently bleeds when the adherent plaques are dislodged by contact with the endoscope, cytology brush, or biopsy forceps. On radiographic examination, coating of the raised plaques and their interstices with barium gives the esophageal mucosa a characteristic irregular, shaggy appearance (Figure 2). Although these endoscopic and radiographic abnormalities strongly suggest candida esophagitis, similar findings occasionally are caused by other infections (e.g. HSV, CMV) or by retained ingested material that clings to the wall of the esophagus. Therefore, confirmation of the diagnosis of candida esophagitis requires the demonstration of budding yeast cells, hyphae, or pseudohyphae in brush cytology or biopsy specimens of the esophagus (Figure 3). Culture of these specimens is not recommended routinely,

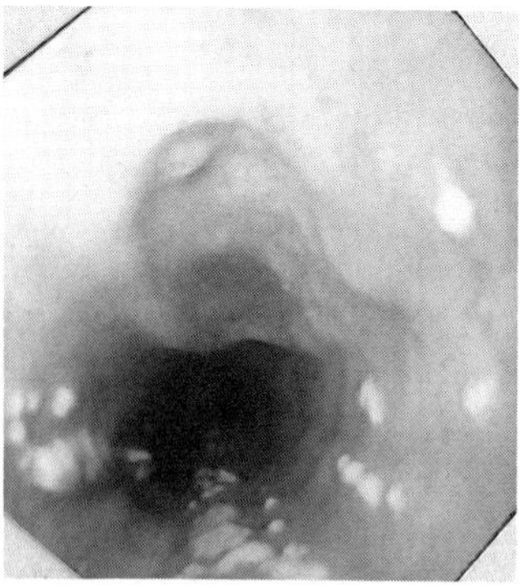

Figure 1 Esophageal infections with multiple organisms are common in patients with AIDS. This endoscopic photograph shows the esophagus of a patient who had both candida and CMV esophagitis. Note the innumerable raised, white candidal plaques resembling cottage cheese clinging to the esophageal mucosa. At the 12 o'clock position, there is a large, shallow ulceration surrounded by a rim of erythematous tissue. Biopsy specimens from the ulcer base revealed CMV esophagitis.

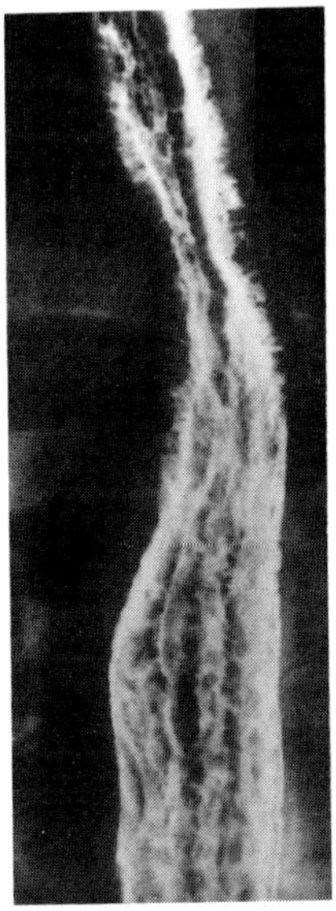

Figure 2 Barium swallow of candida esophagitis. Note how barium coating of the raised plaques and their interstices gives the mucosa an irregular, shaggy appearance. (Reprinted with permission from the Clinical Teaching Project of the American Gastroenterological Association.)

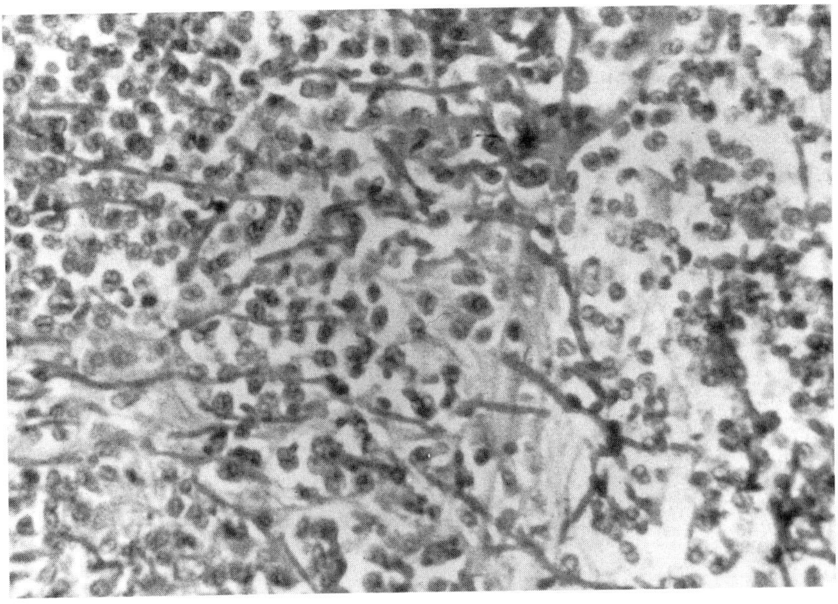

Figure 3 Photomicrograph of an esophageal biopsy specimen revealing intense inflammation and numerous candida pseudohyphae. (Reprinted with permission from the Clinical Teaching Project of the American Gastroenterological Association.)

because a culture positive for candida does not distinguish among esophageal infection, esophageal colonization, and specimen contamination (1). Culture may be advisable, however, for patients who have clinical features that suggest esophageal infection with an unusual or antibiotic-resistant pathogen (e.g. patients initially suspected of having candida esophagitis, but who fail to improve after empiric therapy with antifungal agents).

The medications available for the treatment of candidal infections are summarized in Table 2. For patients with candida esophagitis, the decision regarding which of these antifungal agents to choose should be influenced by two major factors: 1. how severe is the candidal infection and 2. how severely compromised is the patient's immune system? A patient who has a mild esophageal infection and minimal imunocompromise (e.g. a young patient who develops mild candida esophagitis during a limited course of steroid therapy for asthma) often can be treated effectively with a topical antifungal agent such as clotrimazole. In contrast, a patient with moderately severe candida esophagitis and substantial immunocompromise (e.g. a patient with troublesome odynophagia and AIDS) usually requires the oral administration of a systemic antifungal agent such as ketoconazole or fluconazole (2). Patients who have severe infection and profound immunocompromise (e.g. disseminated candidiasis or candida esophagitis in the setting of severe granulocytopenia) generally should be treated with amphotericin B administered intravenously.

For patients who require an orally administered, systemically absorbed medication, the clinician commonly chooses either the imidazole derivative ketoconazole, or the newer triazole compound fluconazole. Both agents have been shown to be effective for the treatment of candida esophagitis (13,14). However, fluconazole has several biological advantages over ketoconazole (15). For example, contact with gastric acid is necessary for efficient absorption of ketoconazole. Consequently, the bioavailability of ketoconazole may be poor in patients who have hypochlorhydria caused by AIDS or by the administration of antisecretory agents such as the histamine H2-receptor blockers (cimetidine, ranitidine, famotidine, nizatidine) and the proton pump inhibitors (omeprazole, lansoprazole). In contrast, hypochlorhydria does not interfere with the absorption of fluconazole. Ketoconazole can suppress cortisol production (an effect that might be dangerous in patients with adrenal insufficiency) (16), whereas important depression of cortisol synthesis appears to be less likely with fluconazole (17). Furthermore, compared to ketoconazole, fluconazole has a longer half-life (22 hours vs. 8 hours), fewer drug–drug interactions, and greater treatment efficacy (15). In a randomized, double-blind trial comparing fluconazole and ketoconazole for patients with AIDS and candida esophagitis, complete endoscopic healing was seen in 91% of patients treated with fluconazole and in only 52% of those given ketoconazole ($p < 0.001$) (15). The major drawback to fluconazole therapy is its high price. When the agents are administered

Table 2 Treatments for Candida Esophagitis

Drug formulation	No or minimal lymphocyte defects and normal granulocytes	Decreased lymphocyte function but normal granulocytes	Decreased granulocyte function
Oral, nonabsorbable drugs			
Nystatin suspension (1,000,000 units/mL)	1–3 MU orally, 4 times daily	N/A	N/A
Amphotericin B lozenge (10 mg) or suspension (100 mg/mL)[a]	1–2 lozenges or 1 mL suspension, 4 times daily	N/A	N/A
Miconazole oral gel (25 mg/mL)	10 mL orally, 4 times daily	N/A	N/A
Clotrimazole troches (10 mg)	**10 mg troche, dissolved in mouth 5 times daily**	N/A	N/A
Clotrimazole vaginal tablets (100 mg)	100 mg tablet, dissolved in mouth 3 times daily	100 mg tablet, dissolved in mouth 3–5 times daily	N/A
Oral, absorbable drugs			
Ketoconazole tablets (200 mg)	200 mg orally, once daily	400–800 mg orally, once daily	400-800 mg orally, once daily
Fluconazole capsules (50 or 100 mg)	50 mg orally, once daily	**100 mg orally, once daily**	100-200 mg orally, once daily
Flucytosine capsules (250 or 500 mg)[b]	N/A	N/A	50-150 $mg \cdot kg^{-1} \cdot day^{-1}$, at 6-h intervals

(continued)

Table 2 Continued

Drug formulation	No or minimal lymphocyte defects and normal granulocytes	Decreased lymphocyte function but normal granulocytes	Decreased granulocyte function
Intravenous drugs			
Amphotericin B for IV use (5 mg/mL)	N/A	0.3 $mg \cdot kg^{-1} \cdot day^{-1}$, IV	**0.5 $mg \cdot kg^{-1} \cdot day^{-1}$, IV**
Fluconazole for IV use (2 mg/mL)[c]	100 mg IV, once daily	100 mg IV, once daily	100–200 mg IV, once daily

Source: Reprinted from Ref. 1.
NOTE. The therapy of choice under each column is given in bold.
N/A = Not applicable.
[a]Not available in the USA.
[b]Not for use as a single agent. See text for discussion of the use of this drug.
[c]When oral route is not available.

in standard dosages, fluconazole therapy for candida esophagitis is approximately three times more expensive than treatment with ketoconazole (1).

Candida esophagitis usually responds well to appropriate antifungal therapy. Unfortunately, the infection often recurs in patients who have persistent immunocompromise. For example, in one recent study of 21 patients with AIDS whose candida esophagitis was treated successfully with antifungal therapy, 19 (90%) developed a recurrent candida infection of the esophagus after a mean period of only 11 weeks (18). Recurrent candida esophagitis also appears to be common in patients who have disorders that delay esophageal clearance such as scleroderma (19). The use of suppressive therapy to prevent recurrent candida esophagitis in these clinical settings has been proposed, but many authorities discourage the practice (18). Chronic antifungal therapy is expensive and potentially hazardous, and its efficacy for patients who have AIDS or esophageal motility disorders has yet to be demonstrated in a controlled clinical trial. Prophylactic antifungal therapy also may predispose to the development of infections with resistant candida species (20). Even when candida esophagitis returns, the recurrent infection usually responds promptly to another acute course of antifungal therapy.

As mentioned above, esophageal dysmotility is a risk factor for candida esophagitis. Caution must be exercised when treating esophageal infections with ketoconazole or fluconazole in patients who are receiving cisapride, a prokinetic agent used frequently in the treatment of gastrointestinal motility disorders. Cisapride is metabolized by the same hepatic cytochrome P450 3A4 isoenzyme that is inhibited by ketoconazole and fluconazole. Consequently the coadministration of these antifungal agents with the prokinetic drug can lead to elevated blood levels of cisapride, a phenomenon that has been associated with lethal cardiac arrhythmias. It may be necessary to discontinue cisapride during the course of antifungal therapy.

IV. HERPES SIMPLEX VIRUS ESOPHAGITIS

Herpes simplex virus (HSV) is a large, enveloped herpesvirus whose genome is comprised of linear, double-stranded DNA. Primary HSV infections of the oropharynx commonly result when oral mucus membranes or breaks in the facial skin are exposed to secretions from an infected individual (1,21). Oropharyngeal infections with HSV type 1 (HSV-1) are highly prevalent in the general population, and asymptomatic salivary secretion of HSV-1 has been found in 2–9% of otherwise healthy adults (21). Primary infections with HSV-1 frequently is acquired in childhood and usually takes the form of a self-limited gingivostomatitis or pharyngitis (21). Primary infection with HSV-2 also may cause an acute oropharyngitis, but HSV-2 more often is a cause of genital infections.

During primary infection with HSV, the virus can enter the peripheral endings of the sensory and autonomic neurons that supply the infected epithelium. Once in the nerve endings, the virus is transported centripetally through the axon to the nerve cell body. From the nerve cell body, the virus can spread centrifugally to all the mucosal and cutaneous surfaces supplied by that neuron. Healing of the primary HSV infection is followed by a variable period of viral latency in the nerve ganglion cells. Within the neurons, the latent virus can be reactivated and can spread to epithelial cells by centrifugal migration through axons. In immunocompetent individuals, HSV reactivation commonly causes "cold sores" of the lips (herpes labialis). However, when reactivation of latent virus occurs in the setting of immunodeficiency, HSV can spread from the infected nerves to involve the squamous epithelium of the oropharynx and esophagus. Less frequently, HSV esophagitis in the immunocompromised host results from contiguous extension of a primary oropharyngeal herpes infection. Uncommonly, HSV esophagitis (caused either by extension of a primary herpes infection or by reactivation of latent HSV within neurons) affects otherwise healthy individuals who have no apparent immune disorders.

The endoscopic and radiographic findings in HSV esophagitis vary with the interval between esophageal infection and esophageal examination. The earliest lesions, seldom observed, are small (1–3 mm) rounded vesicles that usually involve the mid- to distal esophagus. Sloughing of the vesicles results in small, sharply demarcated ulcers that have raised margins and a yellowish base. The mucosa between the ulcerations is often normal in appearance. In more severe cases, the small ulcers coalesce to form large ulcers that can be covered with dense exudates resembling candidal plaques.

HSV infects the squamous epithelial cells of the esophagus. Therefore histologic confirmation of HSV esophagitis is best accomplished by obtaining biopsy and brush cytology specimens from the squamous epithelium at the edges of ulcerated areas. Specimens obtained from the ulcer base often contain only nonspecific granulation tissue and inflammatory exudate and may not show the characteristic histologic signs of HSV esophagitis. Typical histologic changes in HSV infection include multinucleated giant cells and intranuclear (Cowdry type A) inclusion bodies (Figure 4). These findings are not specific for HSV esophagitis because infection with varicella-zoster virus can cause similar histologic changes. However, HSV esophagitis is far more common than varicella-zoster esophagitis, and the demonstration of multinucleated giant cells and intranuclear inclusions strongly supports the diagnosis of esophageal infection by HSV. Viral culture appears to be more sensitive than histologic examination for diagnosing HSV infection of the esophagus (22). Therefore, biopsy and brush cytology specimens should be sent for viral cultures as well as for routine histologic and cytologic evaluation whenever HSV esophagitis is suspected.

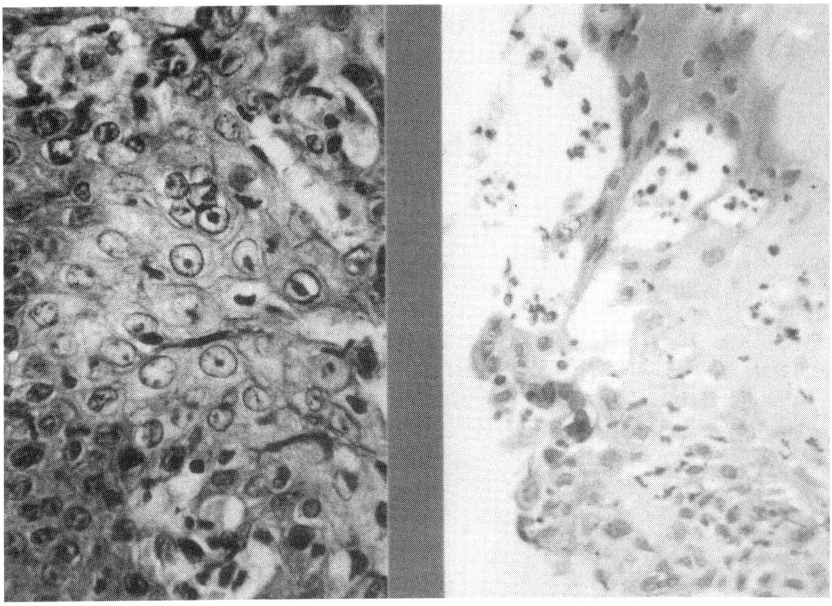

Figure 4 Photomicrograph of esophageal biopsy specimens from a patients with HSV esophagitis. The left panel reveals several intranuclear (Cowdry A) inclusion bodies. The right panel shows a characteristic multinucleated giant cell. (Reprinted with permission from the Clinical Teaching Project of the American Gastroenterological Association.)

In immunocompetent individuals, HSV esophagitis usually is a short-lived illness that may require no therapy other than supportive care and expectant management (23). However, HSV esophagitis often does not resolve spontaneously in immunocompromised patients, and such individuals should receive systemic antiviral therapy. Acyclovir, a nucleoside analogue that inhibits viral DNA polymerase, presently is the drug of choice for treating HSV infections of the esophagus. Although the drug does not eradicate HSV, acyclovir can reduce the severity of HSV esophagitis and may prevent reactivation of the latent virus. Adult patients with HSV esophagitis are treated initially with acyclovir administered intravenously in a dose of 5 mg per kg every 8 hours. Patients who respond well to this treatment within 7 days can be switched to oral preparations of acyclovir given in a dose of 200 mg to 400 mg five times daily. Acyclovir therapy should be continued for at least two weeks. Acute side effects of parenterally administered acyclovir include chemical phlebitis, nephropathy, and encephalopathy. Oral preparations usually are well tolerated, but can cause nausea, vomiting, and headaches. Patients with HSV esophagitis who are allergic to acyclovir or who are infected with an acyclovir-resistant strain of HSV can be treated with foscarnet, another inhibitor of viral DNA polymerase. Foscarnet is administered intravenously in a dose of 60 mg per kg every 8 hours for two to three weeks. Foscarnet is both more expensive and more toxic than acyclovir, often causing renal impairment and alterations in serum electrolytes that can result in seizures.

Prophylactic therapy with acyclovir is recommended for immunosuppressed individuals who are at high risk for reactivation of latent HSV (1). Such individuals include recipients of solid organ and bone marrow transplants who are seropositive for HSV infection, and patients with AIDS who have had multiple bouts of HSV esophagitis. For prophylaxis, acyclovir is administered orally in a dose of 200 to 400 mg four or five times daily, or intravenously in a dose of 5 mg per kg every 12 hours.

V. CYTOMEGALOVIRUS ESOPHAGITIS

Cytomegalovirus (CMV) is a ubiquitous herpesvirus that, like its cousin HSV, has the ability to establish latent infection in otherwise healthy individuals (24). The virus can infect virtually any tissue in the body, and CMV can be found in the saliva, urine, stool, semen, uterine secretions, breast milk, and blood of infected individuals. Commonly, CMV is transmitted from person to person by exposure to infected secretions. Alternatively, the virus can be transmitted through blood transfusions (that carry infected leukocytes) or through the transplantation of infected organs. Infants in developing countries often acquire primary CMV infection at parturition or shortly thereafter. In some developing countries, serologic evidence of CMV exposure has been found in 85% to 95% of children by the age of 5 (25). In the United States, primary CMV infections are common both in preschool children (up to 30% of whom are seropositive for CMV infection by age 5) and in young adults (24,25). Primary CMV infection in normal individuals usually causes few symptoms and often goes unrecognized. Occasionally, primary CMV exposure causes a mononucleosis-type syndrome with fever, fatigue, pharyngitis, and splenomegaly. In immunocompromised patients, primary CMV infection can be a severe systemic disease complicated by retinitis, encephalitis, pneumonitis, hepatitis, adrenal insufficiency, and gastrointestinal ulceration (26). The CMV infection also can cause bone marrow dysfunction with depressed myelopoiesis, a phenomenon that further compromises the immune system (27).

After the primary infection, evidence of latent CMV infection can by found in most organs of the body using in situ hybridization techniques to identify viral DNA (28). With the development of immunodeficiency, the patients latent virus can be reactivated and cause esophagitis (29). Alternatively, immunocompromised patients can develop CMV esophagitis during primary CMV infections acquired through the transfusion of blood or the transplantation of organs that harbor the latent virus. Whether due to primary infection or reactivation, CMV esophagitis is extremely uncommon in immunocompetent individuals (30).

Patients who have CMV esophagitis often have widespread CMV disease that involves a number of extraesophageal organs. Consequently, systemic symptoms such as fever, weight loss, nausea, vomiting, and diarrhea are far more common in patients with CMV esophagitis than in those with candida or HSV esophagitis where the infection usually is confined to the esophagus and oropharynx (1). Although the radiographic and endoscopic appearance of CMV esophagitis can be indistinguishable from that of candida or HSV esophagitis, CMV tends to cause discrete, shallow esophageal ulcerations that are very elongated (up to 15 cm in length) and surrounded by normal-appearing esophageal mucosa (Figure 1) (1). Tissue sampling for histologic examination and culture is necessary to distinguish these giant CMV ulcerations from the giant idiopathic esophageal ulcerations that can be associated with HIV infection.

Histologic examination of fibroblasts and endothelial cells infected with CMV reveals distinctive abnormalities that include cellular enlargement (cytomegaly) and inclusion bodies within the nucleus (31). Unlike cells infected with HSV that have inclusion bodies only within the nucleus, CMV-infected cells exhibit granular inclusion bodies in the cytoplasm as well. Immunohistochemical staining for viral peptides and in situ hybridization and polymerase chain reaction techniques that identify CMV DNA can be used to confirm the histologic diagnosis in equivocal cases. Viral culture appears to be more sensitive than histologic and immunohistochemical tests for CMV, and modern centrifugation culture techniques can identify the organism within 24 to 48 hours (32). Histologic tests and viral cultures for CMV are positive only in the presence of the virus, which is found most often in fibroblasts and endothelial cells. Therefore biopsy specimens for histology and culture should be obtained from the granulation tissue in the base of the esophageal ulcer (where the infected cells are likely to be encountered), rather than from the squamous epithelial cells (that do not harbor the virus) at the edges of the ulcer (31). The clinician should appreciate that no single test for CMV infection is highly sensitive. For example, in a recent study of 14 bone marrow transplant recipients who developed CMV disease, conventional and centrifugation cultures of endoscopic biopsy specimens identified the organism in only 57% of patients. Conventional histologic examination of the specimens revealed characteristic findings in only 30% (32). For patients with negative test results, therefore, repeated diagnostic testing may be necessary if the suspicion for CMV infection is high. Conversely, evidence of CMV infection is not proof of CMV disease. The mere identification of CMV in an inflamed esophagus by any diagnostic test (histology, immunohistochemistry, or viral culture) does not establish that the virus is a pathogen responsible for the esophagitis. In patients with AIDS who have simultaneous infection of the esophagus with both candida and CMV, for example, treatment with antifungal therapy alone results in healing of the esophagitis in the great majority of cases (33). This observation suggests that the CMV infection in these patients is not contributing importantly to the esophageal disease.

Cytomegalovirus disease can respond to treatment with ganciclovir, a nucleoside analogue (closely related to acyclovir) that inhibits viral DNA polymerase (34–36). For CMV esophagitis, ganciclovir is administered intravenously in a dose of 5 mg per kg every 12 hours for 2 weeks. Maintenance therapy with ganciclovir may be indicated for patients who develop recurrent CMV disease, or for those who have a high risk for recurrence (e.g. patients with CMV disease and advanced AIDS). For maintenance, the drug is administered intravenously in a dose of 5 mg per kg each day for at least 5 days of the week. Ganciclovir can induce severe myelosuppression, especially when given concurrently with zidovudine. Patients with preexisting bone marrow dysfunction can be rendered dangerously neutropenic by treatment with ganciclovir. For such patients, or for patients whose CMV disease does not respond to ganciclovir, an alternative antiviral drug is foscarnet given in a dose of 60 mg per kg every 8 hours for 2 weeks. For maintenance therapy, foscarnet is administered intravenously in a dose of 60 mg per kg each day.

Organ transplant recipients are especially likely to develop CMV disease if they are seropositive for CMV infection, or if they receive organs and blood products from seropositive donors. To prevent CMV infection, seronegative hosts should receive organs and blood products from seronegative donors whenever possible. Prophylactic antiviral therapy also is indicated for recipients of solid organ and bone marrow transplants. The prophylactic administration of ganciclovir has been shown to be effective in preventing both CMV infection and disease in transplant recipients (37,38).

VI. HIV INFECTION, AIDS, AND THE ESOPHAGUS

Thirty to forty percent of patients who have AIDS develop symptoms of esophageal disease (39,40). As in immunodeficiency states unrelated to HIV, esophageal symptoms in AIDS usually are caused by infections with candida, HSV, or CMV. Certain features of esophageal disease in patients with HIV infection are unique, however, and warrant special consideration.

A. Esophageal Ulceration in the Acute HIV Seroconversion Syndrome

Within 2 to 3 weeks after primary exposure to HIV, many patients develop a self-limited, infectious mononucleosis-like illness characterized by malaise, fever, myalgias, pharyngitis, and rash (41). These patients are seronegative for antibodies to HIV initially, but HIV antibodies can be demonstrated on subsequent serologic testing when the symptoms have resolved. In some cases, this acute HIV seroconversion syndrome is complicated by the development of esophageal ulcerations that cause odynophagia (42). Endoscopically, the ulcers are often multiple, round, 3 mm to 15 mm in diameter, well-demarcated, and surrounded by normal-appearing esophageal mucosa. Analysis of biopsy specimens obtained from these acute ulcerations has revealed retroviral particles and HIV antigens, findings suggesting that the HIV infection may be directly responsible for the esophageal mucosal damage (42,43). No specific therapy other than supportive care is required for patients with these acute esophageal ulcerations. Typically, the ulcers heal and the symptoms of the acute HIV seroconversion syndrome resolve spontaneously within 2 weeks. Patients then remain asymptomatic for years until the development of AIDS.

B. Idiopathic Esophageal Ulcerations in AIDS

Patients with HIV infection and AIDS can develop large esophageal ulcerations in which no pathogenic microorganism can be identified by culture or by histological and immunohistochemical tests. These HIV-associated idiopathic esophageal ulcerations can be found in approximately 10% of patients with AIDS who complain of esophageal symptoms (4) and in up to 40% of such patients who are found to have discrete esophageal ulcerations on endoscopic examination (44). The precise role of HIV in the pathogenesis of these idiopathic ulcerations is disputed. Although HIV RNA can be demonstrated in lymphocytes and mononuclear cells associated with the ulcers, it is not clear that HIV infection of the esophageal mucosa is directly responsible for the tissue damage that results in ulceration (45,46).

Radiographically and endoscopically, HIV-associated idiopathic ulcerations of the esophagus closely resemble the large esophageal ulcerations caused by CMV disease (Figure 1). As mentioned above, CMV easily can be missed by standard diagnostic tests including culture and histologic examination of esophageal tissue. Undoubtedly, some "idiopathic" esophageal ulcerations are caused by infections with CMV or other microorganisms that have escaped detection by standard diagnostic studies. Esophageal involvement by lymphoma and Kaposi's sarcoma also can be difficult to document using standard mucosal biopsy techniques, and some "idiopathic" ulcerations in fact may be ulcerated neoplasms. These potential diagnostic pitfalls should be considered when managing patients who have HIV infection and esophageal ulceration. Idiopathic ulcerations associated with HIV generally do not respond to therapy with antimicrobial agents (47). Interestingly, patients with these lesions usually experience symptomatic relief and ulcer healing during treatment with systemic corticosteroids (48). In one recent series, prednisone administered in a dose of 40 mg daily and tapered each week by 10 mg (for a total of 4 weeks of corticosteroid therapy) resulted in complete symptomatic relief in 10 of 12 patients (48). Prednisone given in a dose of 40 mg daily for two weeks also was found to be effective for relieving symptoms, but the relapse rate appeared to be higher than that for the 4-week, tapered-dose regimen. Although corticosteroid therapy entails substantial risk for patients who already are profoundly immunosuppressed, the treatment is surprisingly well tolerated in most cases. In the aforementioned study, for example, steroid side effects were observed in only 10 of 36 patients (Table 3). As an alternative to systemic corticosteroid therapy, the perendoscopic injection of methylprednisolone directly into an idiopathic ulceration also has resulted in relief of esophageal symptoms (49). Presently, experience with this technique is limited and its role in the management of idiopathic ulcerations is not clear. Finally, the notorious sedative hypnotic agent thalidomide, which has immunomodulatory effects, has been used successfully to treat idiopathic ulcerations (50). This agent is not readily available in most institutions in the United States, however.

C. Multiple Simultaneous Esophageal Infections in HIV-Positive Patients

Candida is by far the most common cause of esophageal infection in AIDS, and candida esophagitis is found in more than 50% of patients who have HIV infection and esophageal symptoms (51). Although CMV and HSV infections are

Table 3 Complications of Prednisone Therapy in 36 Patients with HIV-Associated Idiopathic Esophageal Ulcerations

Complication	Number of patients
CMV esophagitis	2
CMV retinitis	2
Pneumocystis carinii pneumonia	2
Candida esophagitis	1
Herpes zoster	1
Diabetes mellitus	1
Progression of Kaposi's sarcoma	1

Source: Ref. 48.

also common in such patients, CMV or HSV alone are often not the sole pathogens that can be identified in the inflamed esophagus. Cytomegalovirus usually is discovered in biopsy specimens obtained from an esophagus that is also infected by candida, and simultaneous infections with both CMV and HSV are not rare. For example, Table 4 summarizes the results of one recent study on the causes of esophageal symptoms in 110 patients with HIV infection. Note the frequency of multiple, simultaneous esophageal infections. Although simultaneous esophageal infection with CMV and candida is quite common, the CMV does not appear to contribute importantly to the esophageal inflammation in most of these cases. As mentioned above, most patients with coexistent CMV and candida infection of the esophagus respond well to antifungal therapy alone (33).

Endoscopic examination with procurement of esophageal biopsy specimens is required for a definitive diagnosis of infectious esophagitis. Endoscopy is quite expensive, however, and entails some risk. Noting that candida esophagitis is so common in HIV-infected patients, and that even mixed infections (candida and CMV) usually respond to antifungal therapy alone, authorities have suggested that HIV-positive patients who have esophageal symptoms should be treated empirically with antifungal therapy (4). According to this strategy, endoscopic examination generally is reserved only for patients who fail to respond to empiric treatment. The optimal antifungal agent for empiric therapy is disputed, but a recently published decision analysis suggests that initial empiric therapy with fluconazole is the most cost-effective approach (52). Diagnostic evaluation (with endoscopic examination) is much more expensive than a course of antifungal therapy with any oral agent. Although fluconazole is substantially more expensive than ketoconazole, fluconazole also is significantly more effective than ketoconazole for treating candida esophagitis in patients with

Table 4 Pathogens Identified in 110 Patients with HIV Infection and Esophageal Symptoms

Pathogens	Number of patients
Candida alone	33 (30%)
Candida and virus	24 (22%)
Candida and CMV	22
Candida, CMV, and HSV	2
Virus alone	15 (14%)
CMV	7
HSV	6
CMV and HSV	2
Total patients with pathogen identified	72 (65%)

Source: Ref. 51.

AIDS (15). Since treatment failures require costly diagnostic evaluation, and since fluconazole therapy for candida esophagitis results in far fewer treatment failures than ketoconazole, initial empiric therapy with fluconazole appears to be the preferred management strategy (52).

D. Noninfectious Causes of Esophageal Symptoms in HIV-Positive Patients

Patients with advanced HIV infection are predisposed to develop neoplasms such as lymphoma and Kaposi's sarcoma that, on rare occasions, can involve the esophagus and cause esophageal symptoms (53,54). There are even anecdotal reports of patients with AIDS who developed squamous cell carcinoma of the esophagus (55). Gastroesophageal reflux disease (GERD) is another potential noninfectious cause of esophageal symptoms in patients with HIV infection. Symptomatic GERD appears to be far more common in the general population than in patients with AIDS, however, perhaps because these patients may develop gastric acid hyposecretion (hypochlorhydria) (40,56). Certain pills are caustic to the esophageal mucosa and can cause inflammation with ulceration if they linger in the esophagus. Pill esophagitis has been associated with a variety of medications likely to be taken by patients with AIDS including certain antibiotics, nonsteroidal anti-inflammatory drugs, potassium chloride supplements, and zidovudine (57). To prevent pill esophagitis, patients should be instructed to take their medications while in an upright position with a full glass of water.

VII. MISCELLANEOUS CAUSES OF ESOPHAGEAL INFECTION

A. Fungi Other Than Candida

1. Aspergillus Species

Aspergillus species, a ubiquitous group of molds, occasionally infect the esophageal mucosa of immunocompromised patients (58). Extension of the infection through the esophageal wall can result in the formation of esophago-bronchial and esophago-mediastinal fistulae (59). Both candida and aspergillus species can infect the esophagus simultaneously, and therefore aspergillus coinfection should be considered in patients who have candida esophagitis that does not respond to treatment with ketoconazole or fluconazole (aspergillus species are resistant to these agents) (58). The identification of characteristic septated hyphae and conidiophores on examination of esophageal biopsy and brush cytology specimens strongly suggests the diagnosis of aspergillus infection. The diagnosis is further supported by demonstration of the organism in fungal cultures of esophageal specimens. Such culture results must be interpreted with caution, however, because aspergillus species are common laboratory contaminants. Presently, amphotericin B administered intravenously is the treatment of choice for aspergillus esophagitis. Limited data suggest that itraconazole, a new imidazole agent, also may be useful for treating aspergillus infections of the esophagus (60).

2. *Histoplasma Species*

Histoplasma species do not appear to infect the esophageal mucosa directly. The esophagus usually is involved secondarily when a primary histoplasma infection of the lungs spreads into the mediastinum or when the esophagus is compressed by the mediastinal lymph node enlargement and fibrosis that can complicate histoplasma pulmonary infection (61–63). Esophageal ulcerations due to histoplasma infection are rare and have been described only in severely immunocompromised patients who developed disseminated histoplasmosis (64). Unlike patients with other infectious esophagitides who typically complain primarily of odynophagia (caused by esophageal mucosal erosions and ulcerations), dysphagia (due to extrinsic compression of the esophagus) is usually the primary complaint of patients with histoplasma involvement of the esophagus. In the absence of mucosal disease, endoscopic examination of the esophagus cannot establish a diagnosis of histoplasma infection. Bronchoscopy, mediastinoscopy, or thoracotomy may be necessary to obtain infected tissue for diagnostic tests. Patients ordinarily are treated with amphotericin B administered intravenously, although ketoconazole and other imidazoles have been used successfully in selected cases (65).

3. *Blastomyces Dermatitidis*

Blastomyces dermatitidis is the agent of North American blastomycosis, a chronic infectious disease that primarily involves the lungs, skin, bones, and genitourinary tract. Blastomycosis rarely can involve the esophagus, causing dysphagia and bleeding (66). Biopsy specimens of the inflamed esophagus may contain granulomas, and yeast forms of *B. dermatitidis* can be seen on examination of silver stains of infected tissues. The diagnosis is confirmed by fungal culture of esophageal tissue specimens. Treatment is with amphotericin B administered intravenously.

B. Viruses Other Than HSV, CMV, and HIV

1. *Varicella Zoster Virus*

Varicella zoster virus (VZV) is the ubiquitous herpesvirus that causes chickenpox. Long after healing of the primary infection, latent VZV in neurons can be reactivated and cause shingles. Although primary and recurrent VZV infections can involve the esophagus, symptomatic VZV esophagitis is a very uncommon complication that is seen only in severely ill and immunocompromised patients (67,68). Surprisingly, however, VZV esophagitis occurs rarely, if ever, in patients with AIDS (1). Endoscopically and histologically, VZV esophagitis is virtually indistinguishable from HSV esophagitis. The diagnosis can be established by using immunohistochemical stains with monoclonal antibodies to VZV. Immunosuppressed patients with VZV infection can be treated with acyclovir or foscarnet (69,70).

2. *Epstein–Barr Virus*

Normal individuals infected with the Epstein–Barr virus (EBV) develop infectious mononucleosis that rarely can be complicated by acute esophageal ulcerations (71). In immunocompromised patients, EBV infection can cause oral hairy leukoplakia and, uncommonly, symptomatic esophageal ulcerations that have histologic features indistinguishable from those of the oral lesions of hairy leukoplakia (72,73). Few data are available on the treatment of esophageal infection with EBV. Whereas EBV esophagitis in immunocompromised patients appears to be a variant of oral hairy leukoplakia—a lesion that often responds to treatment with oral acyclovir—protracted therapy with oral acyclovir is recommended for patients with symptomatic esophageal infection by EBV (1,74).

3. *Human Papilloma Virus*

Human papillomavirus (HPV) is a member of the papovavirus family that can infect squamous epithelial cells in the esophagus and other organs. In contrast to the other infectious agents discussed in this chapter, HPV usually infects the esophagus of immunocompetent individuals and typically causes no symptoms (75). The virus has clinical importance because it may contribute to neoplasia, and HPV infections usually are discovered by immunohistochemical analyses of squamous cell tumors. Human papillomavirus infections have been associated with squamous cell carcinomas of the uterine cervix, larynx, and nasopharynx. In the esophagus, HPV infection has been implicated in the development of squamous cell papilloma (a rare benign tumor) and squamous cell carcinoma. For example, one group of investigators recently found HPV DNA in 17 of 72 (22%) squamous cell cancers of the esophagus (76).

C. Bacteria

1. *Mycobacterium Tuberculosis*

Primary infection with *M. tuberculosis* usually is acquired through the inhalation of droplet nuclei that carry the organisms. The inhaled bacilli are phagocytized by macrophages, thus activating cell-mediated immune mechanisms that either destroy or contain the organisms within granulomas. Years later, with the development of immunodeficiency, the latent *M. tuberculosis* infection can be reactivated. Tuberculous mediastinal lymph nodes can enlarge and compress the esophagus, thereby causing dysphagia (77). The tuberculous infection also can spread from mediastinal and hilar lymph directly through the wall of the esophagus, a process that can result in bleeding, esophageal perforation, and the formation of esophago-bronchial fistulae (77,78). Finally, rare cases of primary esophageal infection with *M. tuberculosis* (in the absence of apparent pulmonary or mediastinal infection) have been reported (78). Although tuberculosis can involve the esophagus of immunocompetent individuals, esophageal tuberculosis in the United States is rare and seen almost exclusively in profoundly immunosuppressed patients (1). If the tuberculous infection involves the esophageal mucosa, the diagnosis can be made endoscopically by procuring biopsy specimens for acid fast bacillus (AFB) stain and mycobacterial culture (79). In the absence of esophageal mucosal involvement, bronchoscopy, mediastinoscopy, or thoracotomy may be necessary to obtain infected tissue for diagnostic tests. In immunocompetent individuals, tuberculous esophagitis usually responds well to standard antituberculous therapy, although surgery occasionally is required to repair perforations and fistulae (77). Patients with AIDS frequently are infected with resistant strains of *M. tuberculosis*, and often respond poorly to antituberculous therapy (78,80).

2. *Mycobacterium Avium Complex*

Patients with advanced AIDS often are infected by a group of opportunistic mycobacteria collectively called *Mycobacterium avium* complex (MAC). Uncommonly, disseminated MAC infections involve the esophagus where they cause ulcerations that can burrow into adjacent organs (81). The bacilli sometimes can be seen on examination of AFB stains of tissue specimens, and the diagnosis is established by culture of the specimens. The MAC infections are notoriously difficult to eradicate, although symptoms may be alleviated temporarily by treatment with combination-drug regimens that often involve the administration of three or four antituberculous agents (82).

3. *Oropharyngeal Flora*

Esophageal erosions and ulcerations due to peptic injury, caustic ingestions or pathogenic microorganisms can be infected secondarily by bacteria that normally reside in the oropharynx such as *Staphylococcus aureus, Staphylococcus epidermidis, Streptococcus viridans*, and bacillus species (1). Granulocytopenia is a risk factor for the development of bacterial esophagitis, but even immunocompetent individuals rarely acquire bacterial infections of the esophagus (83). The diagnosis is established when large numbers of bacteria (and no other infectious organisms) are seen invading the subepithelial tissues in Gram's stains of esophageal biopsy specimens (84). Bacterial cultures of esophageal tissue specimens are of limited diagnostic value because it is virtually impossible to prevent contamination by oropharyngeal flora during specimen procurement.

Nevertheless, bacterial culture results may help to identify a predominant organism and to guide antibiotic therapy in some cases.

4. *Other Bacteria*

There are case reports of esophageal infections caused by *Treponema pallidum* (85) (the agent of syphilis) and by *Nocardia* (86).

D. Parasites

With the exception of *Trypanosoma cruzi*, a parasite endemic to South and Central America that attacks neurons in the esophageal wall and causes Chagas's disease in immunocompetent individuals (87), parasitic infections of the esophagus are rare and are seen almost exclusively in patients with AIDS. For example, there are case reports of patients who had AIDS with esophageal involvement by *Pneumocystis carinii* (88), *Cryptosporidium* (89), and leishmaniasis (90). Undoubtedly, as the AIDS epidemic progresses, case reports will accumulate of esophageal infections by other exotic parasites, bacteria, viruses, and fungi that have not been mentioned in this chapter.

REFERENCES

1. Baehr PH, McDonald GB. Esophageal infections: risk factors, presentation, diagnosis, and treatment. Gastroenterology 1994; 106:509–532.
2. Pegram PS. Esophagitis in the immunocompromised host. In: Castell DO, ed. The esophagus. Boston: Little, Brown and Company, 1995:635–657.
3. McDonald GB, Sharma P, Hackman RC, Meyers JD, Thomas ED. Esophageal infections in immunosuppressed patients after marrow transplantation. Gastroenterology 1985; 88:1111–1117.
4. Laine L, Bonacini M. Esophageal disease in human immunodeficiency virus infection. Arch Intern Med 1994; 154:1577–1582.
5. Poles MA, McMeeking AA, Scholes JV, Dieterich DT. Actinomyces infection of a cytomegalovirus esophageal ulcer in two patients with acquired immunodeficiency syndrome. Am J Gastroenterol 1994; 89:1569–1572.
6. Cappell MS, Gupta A. Gastrointestinal hemorrhage due to gastrointestinal mycobacterium avium intracellular or esophageal candidiasis in patients with the acquired immunodeficiency syndrome. Am J Gastroenterol 1992; 87:224–229.
7. Cronstedt JL, Bouchama A, Hainau B, Halim M, Khouqueer F, al Darsouny T. Spontaneous esophageal perforation in herpes simplex esophagitis. Am J Gastroenterol 1992; 87:124–127.
8. De Silva R, Stoopack PM, Raufman JP. Esophageal fistulas associated with mycobacterial infection in patients at risk for AIDS. Radiology 1990; 175:449–453.
9. Agha FP. Candidiasis-induced esophageal strictures. Gastrointest Radiol 1984; 9:283–286.
10. McDonald GB, Sharma P, Hackman RC, Meyers JD, Thomas ED. Esophageal

infections in immunosuppressed patients after marrow transplantation. Gastroenterology 1985; 88:1111–1117.
11. Niedt GW, Schinella RA. Acquired immunodeficiency syndrome. Clinicopahtologic study of 56 autopsies. Arch Pathol Lab Med 1985; 109:727–734.
12. Porro GB, Parrente F, Cernuschi M. The diagnosis of esophageal candidiasis in patients with acquired immune deficiency syndrome: is endoscopy always necessary? Am J Gastroenterol 1989; 84:143–146.
13. Deschamps MM, Pape JW, Verdier RI, DeHovitz J, Thomas F, Johnson WD Jr. Treatment of candida esophagitis in AIDS patients. Am J Gastroenterol 1988; 83:20–21.
14. De Wit S, Urbain D, Rahir F, Weerts D, Clumeck N. Efficacy of oral fluconazole in the treatment of AIDS associated oesophageal candidiasis. Eur J Clin Microbiol Infect Dis 1991; 10:503–505.
15. Laine L, Dretler RH, Conteas CN, Tuazon C, Koster FM, Sattler F, Squires K, Islam MZ. Fluconazole compared with ketoconazole for the treatment of candida esophagitis in AIDS. A randomized trial. Ann Intern Med 1992; 117:655–660.
16. Best TR, Jenkins JK, Murphy FY, Nicks SA, Bussell KL, Vesely DL. Persistent adrenal insufficiency secondary to low-dose ketoconazole therapy. Am J Med 1987; 82:676–680.
17. Michaelis G, Zeiler D, Biscoping J, Fussle R, Hempelmann G. Function of the adrenal cortex during therapy with fluconazole in intensive care patients. Mycoses 1993; 36:117–123.
18. Laine L. The natural history of esophageal candidiasis after successful treatment in patients with AIDS. Gastroenterology 1994; 107:744–746.
19. Hendel L, Svejgaard E, Walsoe I, Kieffer M, Stenderup A. Esophageal candidiasis in progressive systemic sclerosis: occurrence, significance, and treatment with fluconazole. Scand J Gastroenterol 1988; 23:1182–1186.
20. Sanguineti A, Carmichael JK, Campbell K. Fluconazole-resistant Candida albicans after long-term suppressive therapy. Arch Intern Med 1993; 153:1122–1124.
21. Corey L, Spear PG. Infection with herpes simplex virus. N Engl J Med 1986; 314:686–691, 749–757.
22. McBane RD, Gross JB Jr. Herpes esophagitis: clinical syndrome, endoscopic appearance, and diagnosis in 23 patients. Gastrointest Endosc 1991; 37:600–603.
23. Shortsleeve MJ, Levine MS. Herpes esophagitis in otherwise healthy patients: clinical and radiographic findings. Radiology 1992; 182:859–861.
24. Cytomegalovirus infections: epidemiology, diagnosis and treatment strategies. Proceedings of a symposium. Cambridge, Massachusetts. 10–12 November 1988. Rev Infect Dis 1990; 12 (suppl 7):S691–S860.
25. Pass RF. Epidemiology and transmission of cytomegalovirus. J Infect Dis 1985; 152:243–248.
26. Gallant JE, Moore RD, Richman DD, Keruly J, Chaisson RE. Incidence and natural history of cytomegalovirus disease in patients with advanced human immunodeficiency virus diseasee treated with zidovudine. J Infect Dis 1992; 166:1223–1227.
27. Sing GK, Ruscetti FW. Preferential suppression of myelopoiesis in normal human

bone marrow cells after in vitro challenge with human cytomegalovirus. Blood 1990; 75:1965–1973.

28. Myerson D, Hackman RC, Nelson JA, Ward DC, McDougall JK. Widespread presence of histologically occult cytomegalovirus. Hum Pathol 1984; 15:430–439.
29. McDonald GB, Sharma P, Hackman RC, Meyers JD, Thomas ED. Esophageal infections in immunosuppressed patients after marrow transplantation. Gastroenterology 1985; 88:1111–1117.
30. Altman C, Bedossa P, Dussaix E, Buffet C. Cytomegalovirus infection of esophagus in immunocompetent adult. Dig Dis Sci 1995; 40:606–608.
31. Theise ND, Rotterdam H, Dieterich D. Cytomegalovirus esophagitis in AIDS: diagnosis by endoscopic biopsy. Am J Gastroenterol 1991; 86:1123–1126.
32. Hackman RC, Wolford JL, Gleaves CA, Myerson D. Beauchamp MD, Meyers JD, McDonald GB. Recognition and rapid diagnosis of upper gastrointestinal cytomegalovirus infection in marrow transplant recipients. A comparison of seven virologic methods. Transplantation 1994; 57:231–237.
33. Laine L Bonacini M, Sattler F, Young T, Sherrod A. Cytomegalovirus and candida esophagitis in patients with AIDS. J Acquir Immune Defic Syndr 1992; 5:605–609.
34. Meyers JD. Prevention and treatment of cytomegalovirus infection. Ann Rev Med 1991; 42:179–187.
35. Wilcox CM, Diehl DL, Cello JP, Margaretten W, Jacobson MA. Cytomegalovirus esophagitis in patients with AIDS: a clinical, endoscopic, and pathologic correlation. Ann Intern Med 1990; 113:589–593.
36. Chachoua A, Dietrich D, Krasinski K, et al. 9–(1,3 dihydroxy–1–propoxymethyl) guanine (ganciclovir) in the treatment of cytomegalovirus gastrointestinal disease with the acquired immunodeficiency syndrome. Ann Intern Med 1987; 107:133–137.
37. Schmidt GM, Horak DA, Niland JC, Duncan SR, Forman SJ, Zala JA. A randomized, controlled trial of prophylactic ganciclovir for cytomegalovirus pulmonary infection in recipients of allogeneic bone marrow transplants; the City of Hope–Stanford–Syntex CMV Study Group. N Engl J Med 1991; 324:1005–1011.
38. Hibberd PL, Tolkoff–Rubin NE, Conti D, Stuart F, Thistlethwaite JR, Neylan JF, Snydman DR, Freeman R, Lorber MI, Rubin RH. Preemptive ganciclovir therapy to prevent cytomegalovirus disease in cytomegalovirus antibody–positive renal transplant recipients. A randomized controlled trial. Ann Intern Med 1995; 123:18–26.
39. Gelb A, Miller S. AIDS and gastroenterology. Am J Gastroenterol 1986; 81:619–622.
40. Connolly GM, Hawkins D, Harcourt–Webster JN, Parsons PA, Husain OA, Gazzard BG. Oesophageal symptoms, their causes, treatment, and prognosis in patients with the acquired immunodeficiency syndrome. Gut 1989; 30:1033–1039.
41. Kessler HA, Blaauw B, Spear J, Paul DA, Falk LA, Landay A. Diagnosis of human immunodeficiency virus infection in seronegative homosexuals presenting with an acute viral syndrome. JAMA 1987; 258:1196–1199.
42. Rabeneck L, Popovic M, Gartner S, McClean DM, McCleod WA, Read E, Wong

KK, Boyko WJ. Acute HIV infection with painful swallowing and esophageal ulcers. JAMA 1990; 263:2318-2322.
43. Bartelsman JF, Lange JM, van Leeuwen R, van den Tweel JG, Tytgat GN. Acute primary HIV-esophagitis. Endoscopy 1990; 22:184–185.
44. Wilcox CM, Schwartz DA, Clark WS. Esophageal ulceration in human immunodeficiency virus infection. Causes, response to therapy, and long-term outcome. Ann Intern Med 1995; 122:143–149.
45. Kotler DP, Wilson CS, Haroutiounian G, Fox CH. Detection of human immunodeficiency virus-1 by 35S-RNA in situ hybridization in solitary ulcers in two patients with the acquired immune deficiency syndrome. Am J Gastroenterol 1989; 84:313-317.
46. Smith PD, Eisner MS, Manischewitz JF, Fill VJ, Masur H, Fox CF. Esophageal disease in AIDS is associated with pathologic processes rather than mucosal human immunodeficiency virus type 1. J Infect Dis 1993; 167:547–552.
47. Bach MC, Howell DA, Valenti AJ, Smith TJ, Winslow DL. Aphthous ulceration of the gastrointestinal tract in patients with the acquired immunodeficiency syndrome (AIDS). Ann Intern Med 1990; 112:465–467.
48. Wilcox CM, Schwartz DA. Comparison of two corticosteroid regimens for the treatment of HIV-associated idiopathic esophageal ulcer. Am J Gastroenterol 1994; 89:2163-2167.
49. Prego V, Ayataman A, Levendoglu H, Fruchter G. Intralesional steroids are safe and effective therapy in HIV-related aphthous ulcerations of the esophagus. Gastroenterology 1993; 104:A764.
50. Naum SM, Molloy PH, Kania RJ, McGarr J, van Thiel DH. Use of thalidomide in treatment and maintenance of idiopathic esophageal ulcers in HIV+ individuals. Dig Dis Sci 1995; 40:1147–1148.
51. Bonacini M, Young T, Laine L. The causes of esophageal symptoms in human immunodeficiency virus infection. A prospective study of 110 patients. Arch Intern Med 1991; 151:1567–1572.
52. Rabeneck L, Laine L. Esophageal candidiasis in patients infected with the human immunodeficiency virus. A decision analysis to assess cost–effectiveness of alternative management strategies. Arch Intern Med 1994; 154:2705–2710.
53. Pass HI, Potter DA, Macher AM, Reichert C, Shelhammer JH, Masur J, Ognibene F, Gelmann E, Lane HC, Fauci A, et al. Thoracic manifestations of the acquired immune deficiency syndrome. J Thorac Cardiovasc Surg 1984; 88:654–658.
54. Bernal A, del Junco GW. Endoscopic and pathologic features of esophageal lymphoma: a report of four cases in patients with acquired immune deficiency syndrome. Gastrointest Endosc 1986; 32:96–99.
55. Frager DH, Wolf EL, Competiello LS, Frager JD, Klein RS. Beneventano TC. Squamous cell carcinoma of the esophagus in patients with acquired immunodeficiency syndrome. Gastrointest Radiol 1988; 13:358–360.
56. Lake-Bakaar G, Quadros E, Beidas S, Elsakr M, Tom W, Wilson DE, Dincsoy HP, Cohen P, Straus EW. Gastric secretory failure in patients with the acquired immunodeficiency syndrome (AIDS). Ann Intern Med 1988; 109:502–504.

57. Edwards P, Turner J, Gold J, Cooper DA. Esophageal ulceration induced by zidovudine. Ann Intern Med 1990; 112:65–66.
58. Bluhm CS, Bickerstaff CA, Holt S. Refractory esophageal candidiasis in acquired immune deficiency syndrome (AIDS). Am J Gastroenterol 1990; 85:479–480.
59. Obrecht WF Jr, Richter JE, Olympio GA, Gelfand DW. Tracheoesophageal fistula: a serious complication of infectious esophagitis. Gastroenterology 1984; 87:1174–1179.
60. Denning DW, Stevens DA. Antifungal and surgical treatment of invasive aspergillosis: review of 2,121 published cases. Rev Infect Dis 1990; 12:1147–1201.
61. Lee JH, Newman DA, Welsh JD. Disseminated histoplasmosis presenting with esophageal symptomatology. Dig Dis 1977; 22:831–834.
62. Goodwin RA, Nickell JA, des Prez RM. Mediasinal fibrosis complicating healed primary histoplasmosis and tuberculosis. Medicine 1972; 51:227–246.
63. Forsmark CE, Wilcox CM, Darragh TM, Cello JP. Disseminated histoplasmosis in AIDS: an unusual case of esophageal involvement and gastrointestinal bleeding. Gastrointest Endosc 1990; 36:604–605.
64. Marshall JB, Singh R, Demm TL, Bickel JT, Everet ED. Mediastinal histoplasmosis presenting with esophageal involvement and dysphagia: case study. Dysphagia 1995; 10:53–58.
65. Francis P, Walsh TJ. Current approaches to the management of fungal infections in cancer patients: Part 1. Oncology 1992; 6:81–92.
66. McKenzie R, Khakoo R. Blastomycosis of the esophagus presenting with gastrointestinal bleeding. Gastroenterology 1985; 88:1271–1273.
67. Sherman RA, Silva J Jr, Gandour-Edwards R. Fatal varicella in an adult: case report and review of the gastrointestinal complications of chickenpox. Rev Infect Dis 1991; 13:424–427.
68. Gill RA, Gebhard RL, Dozeman RL, Sumner HW. Shingles esophagitis: endoscopic diagnosis in two patients. Gastrointest Endosc 1984; 30:26–27.
69. Shepp DH, Dandliker PS, Meyers JD. Current therapy of varicella zoster virus infection in immunocompromised patients. A comparison of acyclovir and vidarabine. Am J Med 1988; 85(2A):96–98.
70. Safrin S, Berger TG, Gilson I, Wolfe PR, Wofsy CB, Mills J, Biron KK. Foscarnet therapy in five patients with AIDS and acyclovir-resistant varicella-zoster virus infection. Ann Intern Med 1991; 115:19–21.
71. Tilbe KS, Lloyd DA. A case of viral esophagitis. J Clin Gastroenterol 1986; 8:494–495.
72. Kitchen VS, Helbert M, Francis ND, Logan RP, Lewis FA, Boylston AW, Pinching AJ, Harris JR. Epstein-Barr virus associated oesophageal ulcers in AIDS. Gut 1990; 31:1223–1225.
73. Greenspan JS, Greenspan D, Lennette ET, Abrams DI, Conant MA, Petersen V, Freese UK. Replication of Epstein-Barr virus within the epithelial cells of oral “hairy” leukoplakia, an AIDS associated lesion. N Engl J Med 1985; 313:1564–1571.
74. Resnick L, Herbst JS, Ablashi DV, Atherton S, Frank B, Rosen L, Horwitz SN. Regression of oral hairy leukoplakia after orally administered acyclovir therapy. JAMA 1988; 259:384–388.

75. Winkler B, Capo V, Reumann W, Ma A, La Porta R, Reilly S, Green PM, Richart RM, Crum CP. Human papillomavirus infection of the esophagus. A clinicopathologic study with demonstration of papillomavirus anttigen by the immunoperoxidase technique. Cancer 1985; 55:149–155.
76. Togawa K, Jaskiewicz K, Takahashi H, Meltzer SJ, Rustgi AK. Human papillomavirus DNA sequences in esophagus squamous cell carcinoma. Gastroenterology 1994; 107:128–36.
77. Mokoena T, Shama DM, Ngakane H, Bryer JV. Oesophageal tuberculosis: a review of eleven cases. Postgrad Med J 1992; 68:110–115.
78. Eng J, Sabanathan S. Tuberculosis of the esophagus. Dig Dis Sci 1991; 36:536–540.
79. Gordon AH, Marshall JB. Esophageal tuberculosis: definitive diagnosis by endoscopy. Am J Gastroenterol 1990; 85:174–177.
80. Goodman P, Pinero SS, Rance RM, Mansell PW, Uribe-Botero G. Mycobacterial esophagitis in AIDS. Gastrointest Radiol 1989; 14:103–105.
81. de Silva R, Stoopack PM, Raufman JP. Esophageal fistulas asssociated with mycobacterial infection in patients at risk for AIDS. Radiology 1990; 175:449–453.
82. Kemper CA, Meng TC, Nussbaum J, Chiu J, Feigal DF, Bartok AE, Leedom JM, Tilles JG, Deresinski SC, McCutchan JA. Treatment of Mycobacterium avium complex bacteremia in AIDS with a four-drug oral regimen. Rifampin, ethambutol, clofazimine, and ciprofloxacin. The California Collaborative Treatment Group. Ann Intern Med 1992; 116:466–472.
83. McManus JPA, Webb JN. A yeast-like infection of the esophagus caused by Lactobacillus acidophilus. Gastroenterology 1975; 68:583–586.
84. Walsh TJ, Belitsos NJ, Hamilton SR. Bacterial esophagitis in immunocompromised patients. Arch Intern Med 1986; 146:1345-1348.
85. Gaskins RD, Pasquale DN. Granulomatous diseases of the pharynx and esophagus. Otolaryngol Clin North Am 1982; 15:533–538.
86. Kim J, Minamoto GY, Grieco MH. Nocardial infection as a complication of AIDS: report of six cases and review. Rev Infect Dis 1991; 13:624–629.
87. Dantas RO, Godoy RA, Oliveira RB, Meneghelli UG, Troncon LE. Lower esophageal sphincter pressure in Chagas' disease. Dig Dis Sci 1990; 35:508–512.
88. Grimes MM, LaPook JD, Bar MH, Wasserman HS, Dwork A. Disseminated Pneumocystis carinii in a patient with acquired immunodeficiency syndrome. Hum Pathol 1987; 18:307–308.
89. Kazlow PG, Shah K, Benkov KJ, Dische R, LeLeiko NS. Esophageal cryptosporidiosis in a child with acquired immune deficiency syndrome. Gastroenterology 1986; 91:1301–1303.
90. Villaneuva JL, Torre-Cisneros J, Jurado R, Villar A, Montero M, Lopez F, Sanchez-Guijo P, Kindelan JM. Leishmania esophagitis in an AIDS patient: an unusual form of visceral leishmaniasis. Am J Gastroenterol 1994; 89:273–275.

2

Helicobacter pylori-Associated Peptic Ulcer and Gastritis

DAVID H. BALABAN and DAVID A. PEURA
University of Virginia, Charlottesville, Virginia

I. INTRODUCTION

Prior to 1983, the stomach was regarded as a sterile organ whose hostile, acidic environment served as a barrier to invasion by bacteria and other microorganisms. It is no surprise, then, that Warren (1) and Marshall (2) faced widespread skepticism when they reported their discovery of spiral-shaped bacteria living happily beneath the gastric mucus layer of patients with active chronic gastritis. Since then, numerous studies have confirmed the intimate association between *Helicobacter pylori* and peptic diseases (3–6). Confusion remains, however, about the best ways to diagnose and treat this infection. The purpose of this chapter will be to review the essential features of this organism with regard to its microbiology, epidemiology, and pathogenic potential. By understanding the natural history of *Helicobacter pylori* infection, one can establish appropriate guidelines for diagnosis and therapy.

II. A HISTORY OF *HELICOBACTER PYLORI* RESEARCH

Spiral-shaped bacteria were first noted in the stomachs of animals near the turn of the century (7–9). In 1906, Krienitz described similar spiral bacteria in humans with gastric cancer (10). Reporting thirty years later, Doenges found "spriochaetes" in 43% of postmortem gastric specimens in both humans and monkeys, although he could make no definitive claims as to their pathogenicity (11).

Questions remained as to whether these organisms were natural inhabitants of the gastric mucosa or simply postmortem saprophytic invaders. Addressing this issue, Freedburg and Barron examined 35 partial gastrectomy specimens from humans and found spiral bacteria in 37% of the cases (12). Although the prevalence of these unidentified organisms was higher in patients with benign and malignant ulceration, they regarded gastric bacteria as nonpathogenic opportunists.

The investigations of Palmer (13) in the early 1950s hastened the demise of further research exploring the causal association between this new bacterium and human disease. He studied 1180 gastric suction biopsy specimens in adults and found no evidence of bacterial infection. Although he employed no special staining techniques, and most of his specimens were from the fundus rather than the antrum where *H. pylori* resides, he concluded that "spirochetes are not part of the histological picture of the human gastric mucosa in health or prior to the agony in illness (13)." From this point forward, any organisms discovered in the stomach were regarded as contaminants swallowed from the oral cavity.

The advent of fiberoptic endoscopy in the 1970s heralded a new era for the gastrointestinal pathologist who now had access to a wealth of biopsy material. Interest in gastric bacteria was renewed by the study of Steer (14) who examined operative and endoscopic biopsies in patients with gastric ulceration and found gram-negative bacteria residing deep in the gastric mucus layer. Transmission electron micrographs revealed that these bacteria were apposed to mucin-secreting cells and were occasionally seen to be phagocytosed within neutrophils. A second study by Steer and Colin-Jones (15) demonstrated the S-shaped bacteria in 80% of biopsy specimens from patients with gastric ulceration. Importantly, the organism was absent in biopsies from normal controls. These findings suggested that the organism was not a contaminant, but rather a pathogenic bacterium capable of stimulating a local inflammatory response.

Robin Warren, a pathologist at the Royal Perth Hospital, Western Australia, had noted spiral-shaped organisms on gastric biopsy specimens in association with gastritis since 1980 (1). He and Barry Marshall, then a Registrar in Microbiology, systematically examined 135 gastric biopsy specimens and found "small curved and S-shaped bacilli" in close association with the surface epithelium, most commonly in the antrum (1,2). These organisms stained well with the Warthin–Starry silver method and were seen only in association with active chronic gastritis. Marshall was able to culture the organism form antral biopsy specimens using *Campylobacter* isolation techniques (2). Indeed, the organism shared many histological and growth characteristics of the *Campylobacter* species, and it was first named *Campylobacter pyloridis* to signify its characteristic prepyloric location. Later, it would be regrouped into a new genus, *Helicobacter*, based upon unique morphological and biochemical characteristics (16). In his seminal paper, Marshall commented, "If these bacteria are truly associated with antral gastritis, as described by Warren, they may have a part to play in other poorly understood, gastritis-associated diseases (i.e. peptic ulcer and gastric cancer)" (2).

III. TAXONOMY, STRUCTURE, AND MICROBIOLOGY

The genus *Helicobacter* comprises a number of gastric and nongastric bacteria, of which *Helicobacter pylori* is the type species. The human stomach is the natural ecological niche of *H. pylori*, but similar bacteria have been found in other species. These include the ferret gastric bacteria, *Helicobacter mustelae* (17), and *Helicobacter felis* isolated from cats and dogs (18). Unfortunately, an ideal animal model has not been developed for the study of *H. pylori*-induced peptic ulcer disease, although the gnotobiotic piglet and mouse serve as functional experimental hosts (19, 20).

Helicobacter pylori is a curved S- or spiral-shaped, gram-negative bacterium with bluntly rounded ends and four to six unipolar sheathed flagellae with bulbous tips (21) (Figure 1). It measures 0.5 to 1.0 μm in width and 2.5 to 4.0 μm in length. The organism can also assume a coccoidal form when cultured

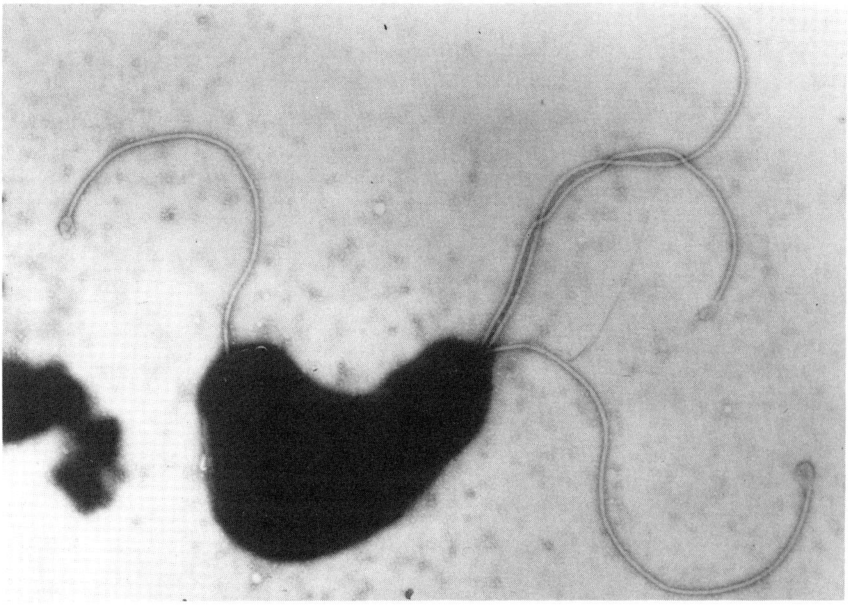

Figure 1 Negative-stained transmission electron micrograph of *Helicobacter pylori*. The coccoidal form shown is often seen in vitro.

on solid media. It has been speculated that this morphology represents *H. pylori* in its dormant state and may serve to protect the bacteria in unfavorable environments (21).

Methods for culturing *H. pylori* have been well described (2, 21). The organism is obligately microaerophilic and requires an atmosphere supplemented with CO_2 (5–10%) for optimal growth. For culture, the biopsy specimen should be transported in a small volume (150–200 μL) of sterile isotonic saline or 20% glucose to ensure that the sample is not too dilute. *H. pylori* grows best on moist chocolate agar, but can be grown on basal media enriched with whole blood or serum (1–5%). The culture plate should be kept at 37°C, and organisms will appear as 1–2 mm colonies in a faint transparent layer within 3–4 days. *H. pylori* is catalase positive, oxidase positive, and urease positive. Its powerful urease activity plays a key role in the bacteria's ability to survive in an acidic environment (22) and forms the basis for the rapid microbiological and noninvasive forms of diagnostic testing to be discussed later.

IV. EPIDEMIOLOGY

A. Prevalence

Based upon its worldwide prevalence and chronicity, *Helicobacter pylori* is estimated to be the most common bacterial infection in humans. The prevalence of *H. pylori* increases dramatically with age in both industrialized (5,23–25) and underdeveloped (26,27) nations. However, *H. pylori* infection and histologic gastritis are evident at a much earlier age in developing countries (Figure 2). In the United States, infection rates increase from 10–15% at age 20 to 50% for those above age 50 (24). In contrast, rates of seroconversion may reach 80% by age 30 in non-Western countries such as Algeria and Vietnam (26). While these data might suggest a steady rate of acquisition of *H. pylori* throughout one's lifetime, epidemiological evidence supports a cohort phenomenon in which infection is acquired in childhood, persists throughout one's lifetime, and may or may not produce gastroduodenal disease based upon bacterial, host, and environmental factors (28). Thus, the prevalence of *H. pylori* seropositivity for any age group reflects the rate of bacterial acquisition during that cohort's childhood years.

B. Risk Factors

The risk of acquiring *H. pylori* is closely tied to one's socioeconomic status in childhood (29–32). Risk factors for infection associated with childhood living conditions include overcrowding (29,30), sharing a bed (29,31), and lack of running water (30). Other environmental factors such as household pets (29), alcohol, nicotine, and nonsteroidal use (24) do not appear to influence infection rates.

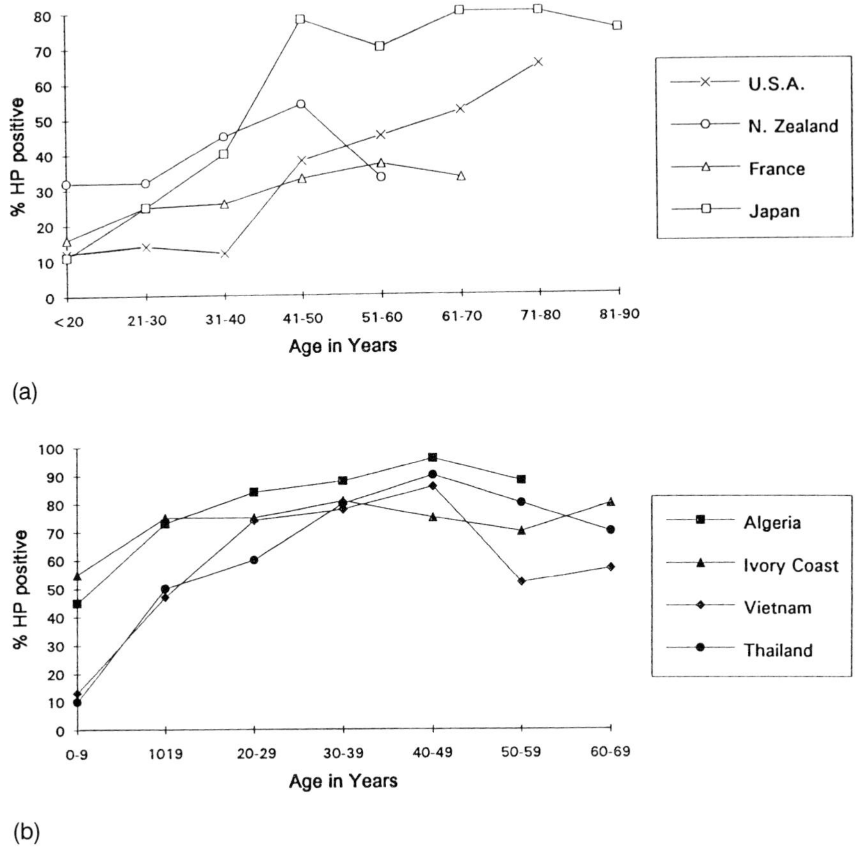

Figure 2 Seroepidemiology of *Helicobacter pylori* infection in (a) developed and (b) underdeveloped countries (From Refs. 23–27).

Seroprevalence rates within a particular country have been noted to change in concert with economic progress. In a seroepidemiological study conducted in Japan (25), prevalence rates of *H. pylori* infection were 70–80% for adults born before 1950 while rates reached only 45% for those born between 1950 and 1960 and fell to 25% for those born between 1960 and 1970. This rapid decline in seroprevalence has been attributed to Japan's post-war modernization, which led to improvements in hygiene and public sanitation.

Like most other infectious diseases, an interplay between host susceptibility and environmental influences leads to acquisition of the organism and development of disease. While a genetic predisposition has not been definitively proven, seroepidemiologic studies suggest that members of certain ethnic and racial groups, including African-Americans (24,32,33) and Hispanics (33), have a higher rate of infection with *H. pylori* than Caucasians. These differences persist after controlling for age and socioeconomic status. Gender does not appear to influence susceptibility to infection (24,32). Further support for a heritable factor influencing susceptibility to *H. pylori* infection comes from a seroepidemiologic twin study conducted in Sweden (34). Monozygotic twins reared apart had a higher concordance rate of *H. pylori* infection than did dizyogotic twins reared apart. However, both monozygotic and dizygotic twins who shared childhood environments demonstrated a higher correlation of infection than those raised separately, strengthening the contention that environmental factors are instrumental in the acquisition of *H. pylori* infection.

C. Transmission

The mode of transmission of *H. pylori* is unknown; however, recent evidence suggests that contaminated water supplies may be an environmental reservoir for *H. pylori* in certain countries. Using highly sensitive PCR assays, Hulten et al. identified *H. pylori* in 50% of water samples tested in Peru (185). Most of the positive samples were from the municipal water supply which could be contaminated by human feces. Several epidemiologic surveys support fecal-oral spread as the most likely route of transmission. *H. pylori* has been cultured from the stool in patients from the United Kingdom with dyspepsia (35) and in children from a village in The Gambia, West Africa (36) where 90% of inhabitants are infected by the age of five (37). Additionally, polymerase chain reaction (PCR) has been employed to detect the organism in the feces of patients with histologic gastritis (38). Infection rates for *H. pylori* have been noted to parallel prevalence curves for viruses known to be transmitted by the fecal-oral route, including Hepatitis A (27).

Indirect evidence supports person-to-person transmission of *H. pylori*. Intrafamilial clustering has been reported in a cohort of infected children (39) and infected adults (40) whose family members, including parents, spouses, and children, were more likely to be seropositive for *H. pylori* than family members of uninfected subjects. In addition, infection of multiple family members with the same strain of *H. pylori* as identified through DNA analysis (41) strongly supports the notion of transmission among persons sharing a close living environment, although a common source exposure cannot be definitively excluded.

Iatrogenic transmission of *H. pylori* has been documented after the use of contaminated gastric biopsy forceps (42) and following sequential upper endoscopy (43) resulting in patient-to-patient transmission of identical bacterial subtypes. Indeed, iatrogenically-transmitted *H. pylori* was identified as the causative agent of epidemic achlorhydria described by Ramsey et al. (44) prior to the discovery of the organism. Despite recent evidence suggesting that current standards for endoscope cleansing are adequate in rendering suction channel washings negative for *H. pylori* by PCR (45), gastroenterologists do appear to be at increased risk for acquiring the infection when compared to age-matched healthy controls (46). Interestingly, although *H. pylori* has been infrequently cultured from dental plaque (47), dentists and oral hygienists do not appear to be at increased risk for infection (48).

D. Natural History

Once acquired, *H. pylori* appears to persist for life unless specifically eradicated by a course of antimicrobial therapy. A study of serial gastric biopsy specimens by restriction endonuclease DNA analysis revealed persistence of the same *H. pylori* isolate for up to two years in untreated patients (49). Xia et al. employed PCR-based DNA fingerprinting to study patients with recurrent *H. pylori* infection following antimicrobial therapy and confirmed that the pre- and post-treatment bacterial isolates were identical (50). Therefore recrudescence rather than reinfection most likely explains recurrent gastritis or ulceration in patients inadequately treated for primary infection.

All current evidence points toward the acquisition of the organism in childhood. The rate of acquisition of *H. pylori* in adulthood appears to be very low. Using banked and fresh sera, a cohort study in a group of epidemiologists demonstrated a rate of new infections at 0.4% per year (51). Similar results were obtained in a seven-year follow-up study of patients with duodenal ulcer rendered *H. pylori* negative by antibiotic therapy (52). The new infection rate in these patients was approximately 1% per year.

Seroprevalence rates rise steadily throughout adulthood, but a close inspection of data from large populations reveals a decreased rate of *H. pylori* positivity in the oldest age groups (see Figure 2). This phenomenon may be due to the increased incidence of gastric atrophy in the elderly (53). As gastric mucosal cells die, *H. pylori* are unable to survive having lost their favored habitat. Antibody levels slowly fall as the immune response wanes. In support of this theory is a study conducted in elderly patients documenting a close correlation between decreasing *H. pylori* seropositivity and low serum pepsinogen I concentrations, a surrogate marker of impaired acid secretion and gastric atrophy (54).

V. PATHOGENESIS

The discovery of *H. pylori* in patients with gastritis and peptic ulcer led to the early hypothesis that this bacteria was the cause of these disorders (2,55). The evidence is now overwhelming that *H. pylori* is the cause of antral, or Type B, gastritis and duodenal ulcers and is a major cause of gastric ulcers in the absence of nonsteroidal use (3–6,56). However, *H. pylori* is not an invasive organism (1,14,15). It must, therefore, exert its cytopathic effects through bacterial toxins, enzymes, and inflammatory mediators that breach the defensive wall of the gastric mucosa rendering it more susceptible to injury (28). *H. pylori* possesses several unique properties that enable it to establish and perpetuate infection in the human stomach.

A. Bacterial Motility

H. pylori is particularly well-suited for life in the stomach. Its spiral configuration and flagellae are common structural features of other bacteria that colonize the gastric mucosa of other species (18) and likely reflect adaptive traits that promote transit through the viscous mucus layer (57,58). Experimental evidence supports the notion that motility itself is a virulence factor. In a study conducted in gnotobiotic piglets, infectivity was directly correlated with the level of motility of various *H. pylori* strains (59). The ability to penetrate the gastric mucus layer quickly and avoid acid injury is critically important if the organism is to establish a foothold in an inhospitable environment.

B. Attachment

H. pylori has an exclusive affinity for gastric mucosa. Following penetration of the gastric mucus layer, *H. pylori* attaches to various phospholipids and glycolipids on the epithelial surface, including phosphatidylethanolamine (60) and GM3 ganglioside (61). In addition, *H. pylori* has been demonstrated to attach to the Lewis^b antigen, a fucosylated blood group antigen that is expressed on epithelial surfaces in humans (62). This may offer an explanation for the early observation that patients with blood group O, who express higher levels of this antigen, are at increased risk for gastric and duodenal ulceration (63).

Ultrastructural and histologic studies in patients with duodenal ulcers demonstrate that *H. pylori* is found only in areas of gastric metaplasia within the duodenal bulb (3,54,64). It is postulated that acid injury initiates cellular metaplasia in the proximal duodenum allowing it to serve as a site for colonization by *H. pylori* (65,66). Once established, the bacteria may cause further injury and metaplasia leading to persistent infection, duodenitis, and, ultimately, duodenal ulceration (67).

C. Urease

H. pylori is a prolific manufacturer of bacterial urease (68), an enzyme that is critical to the organism's pathogenicity. The products of urease are bicarbonate and ammonia; the latter appears necessary for protecting the organism in the acid milieu of the stomach (21,69). In addition, ammonia itself may be toxic to gastric epithelial cells (70). The essential role of urease has been demonstrated experimentally using a urease-deficient mutant strain of *H. pylori*, which was unable to infect the gastric mucosa of an animal host (71). Furthermore, urease may augment gastric epithelial injury by altering the surface charge gradient permitting back-diffusion of hydrogen ions (72). Finally, it has been speculated that *H. pylori* relies upon urease for essential nitrogen-containing nutrients that are liberated from inflammatory cells in response to the enzyme's activity (28).

D. Cytotoxin

The demonstration that broth-culture filtrates of *H. pylori* were able to produce vacuolation in a variety of mammalian cell lines helped to advance our understanding of this organism's pathogenic potential (73). The protein responsible for this activity, vacuolating cytotoxin, has been the subject of intensive investigation.

First, it was noted that only about 50% of strains appeared to produce a cytopathic effect (73) which offered a potential explanation as to why only a small percentage of persons infected with the organism developed gastroduodenal ulcers. Accordingly, it was demonstrated that strains from patients with peptic ulcers had a higher frequency of cytotoxin production (66%) than strains from patients with gastritis alone (30%) (74). The gene responsible for the production of cytotoxin (*vac*A) has been cloned, and its 94-kD protein product has been shown to produce gastric lesions and ulceration in mice (75).

Additional scrutiny has focused upon a 128-kD protein that appears to be associated with cytotoxin production (76,77). This protein has been named CagA for cytotoxin-associated gene A, and its gene (*cag*A) has been cloned and sequenced (76). Covacci et al. used ELISA to detect the serological immune response to this protein in patients with gastroduodenal diseases and found 100% reactivity in those with duodenal ulcer (77). Unfortunately, more recent studies of CagA IgG seropositivity among *H. pylori*-positive subjects with and without gastroduodenal ulceration fail to demonstrate a significant difference between the two groups (78,79). Further investigation is required to delineate the diagnostic utility of these tests in predicting which patients infected with *H. pylori* might be at increased risk for ulcer disease.

E. Mucolytic Enzymes

H. pylori produces several additional enzymes that serve to break down the mucosal defense of its host. Bacterial protease, lipase, and phospholipase A2 are able to degrade key structural components of the gastric mucus layer (80,81). The subsequent decrease in mucus viscosity significantly alters mucosal integrity and may permit back-diffusion of hydrogen ions resulting in cellular injury (80). Phase-contrast dark-field microscopy has revealed depletion of the mucus layer in the gastric body, antrum, and duodenum in *H. pylori*-infected subjects (82).

F. Gastrin, Gastric Acid, and Somatostatin

It has long been recognized that patients with duodenal ulcer disease have higher levels of circulating gastrin, and up to one-third of these patients demonstrate increased basal and stimulated acid output (83,84). It appears that *H. pylori* may be responsible for both of these effects.

Studies of *H. pylori*-positive patients with duodenal ulceration reveal higher levels of both basal (85,86) and stimulated (87,88) gastrin as compared to uninfected controls. Furthermore, eradication of *H. pylori* returns stimulated gastrin release to normal levels, suggesting a direct causal relationship (85,87).

The effects of *H. pylori* on basal and stimulated acid output are more variable (88); however, eradication of the organism has been demonstrated to decrease gastrin-stimulated acid secretion toward normal levels in patients with duodenal ulcers (87). This decrease in acid output lags behind the effects of *H. pylori* eradication on hypergastrinemia. This may reflect persistence of an increased parietal cell mass that occurs in a subset of patients with duodenal ulcer (28,85). While the exact mechanisms by which *H. pylori* influences gastric secretion are not clearly understood, it has been postulated that *H. pylori* enhances gastrin release from the antral mucosa and augments parietal cell responsiveness to gastrin, which results in exaggerated acid output (87).

Based on these findings, one must also hypothesize that the normal inhibitory control of acid on gastrin release is impaired in patients infected with *H. pylori*. In healthy individuals, this action is mediated by somatostatin, a peptide hormone produced in antral D-cells. Moss et al. (89) studied patients with duodenal ulcers and discovered that eradication of *H. pylori* resulted in an increased density of somatostatin-immunoreactive cells and somatostatin mRNA. This suggests that *H. pylori* downregulates production of this gastric hormone. Whether this is a direct effect of the bacteria on gastric antral D-cells or an indirect effect associated with antral inflammation is not yet clear.

G. Cytokines and Inflammatory Mediators

H. pylori engenders both local and systemic immune responses. As will be discussed in the next section, testing for serum IgG antibodies directed against specific bacterial antigens is the best method for noninvasively diagnosing infection with this organism (5,23,39). In addition to its systemic humoral effects, *H. pylori* stimulates a vigorous local inflammatory response. Histologic gastritis is nearly universal in *H. pylori* infection (1,55,90). Typically, there are increased numbers of both acute and chronic inflammatory cells within the lamina propria including polymorphonuclear leukocytes, monocyte/macrophages, eosinophils, plasma cells, and lymphocytes (91). Intracellular invasion of *H. pylori* has only rarely been documented (92).

H. pylori is able to activate neutrophils and monocyte/macrophages via an acid-stabile chemotactic factor (93). Recently, it has been shown that *H. pylori* induces expression of IL-8, a potent neutrophil chemotactic factor, in inflamed gastric mucosa (94). This effect may be strain-specific, as it appears to be correlated with the ability to produce CagA and bacterial cytotoxin, both of which have previously been shown to be associated with gastroduodenal disease (95). By increasing the local presence of neutrophils, *H. pylori* may incite further damage to the gastroduodenal mucosa.

In vitro, human serum is very effective at killing *H. pylori*, and it appears that complement is the specific bactericidal mediator (96). How is the organism able to survive this inflammatory onslaught in vivo? One potential answer is a bacterial product, catalase. This enzyme breaks down H_2O_2 formed in neutrophil phagocytic vacuoles, thus protecting *H. pylori* from the harmful effects of reactive oxygen metabolites (97). Additionally, after prolonged infection the host may downregulate its own inflammatory response as a protective measure (28). The increased presence of T suppressor lymphocytes noted in the gastric epithelium of *H. pylori*-positive patients supports this hypothesis (98).

VI. DIAGNOSIS

The wide variety of diagnostic tests available for *H. pylori* (Table 1) presents today's clinician with both a diagnostic dilemma ("Whom do I test and which test should I use?") and a dilemma of diagnosis ("What do I do with the result?") (99). One must understand that the positive or negative predictive value of a test relies heavily on the prevalence of disease in the population being

Table 1 Diagnostic Tests for *Helicobacter pylori*

Test	Sensitivity	Specificity	Relative cost
Noninvasive			
Serology	88–99%	86–95%	$
Urea breath test	90–97%	90–100%	$$
Invasive			
Rapid urease test	89–98%	93–98%	$$$$[a]
Histology	93–99%	95–99%[b]	$$$$$[a]
Culture	77–92%	100%[b]	$$$$$[a]

Source: Ref. 113.
[a]Includes cost of endoscopy.
[b]Estimated.

tested (Bayes' theorem). Therefore, the decision to diagnose *H. pylori* must be preceded by the following considerations: 1. Is the nature of the patient's symptoms consistent with disease associated with *H. pylori* (i.e., peptic ulcer disease) and 2. What is the likelihood that therapy will be altered by the test result?

Once the decision has been made to test a patient for *H. pylori*, one must determine the most appropriate test to use. Physicians may choose from both invasive and noninvasive methods, each having their own advantages and disadvantages. In the majority of patients, the primary diagnosis of *H. pylori* can be established with a single test.

A. Invasive Tests

Invasive tests require gastroscopy with mucosal biopsy and should be used only in patients who have an a priori indication for an endoscopic procedure. In addition, the cost and risk of the procedure must be borne in mind when comparing these tests to noninvasive diagnostic methods.

1. *Tissue Staining*

Histologic detection of *H. pylori* on the gastric epithelial surface is the most direct means of establishing active infection. Various stains have been used with nearly equal sensitivity, including hematoxylin-eosin (H&E), modified Giemsa, Gram's stain (100), Warthin–Starry (1), carbolfuchsin (101), and acridine orange (102). The most frequently used stains are the H&E stain (Figure 3) and the modified Giemsa stain. The Warthin–Starry silver stain (Figure 4) enhances the appearance of the bacteria, making them appear fatter and deeper black; however, the cost and difficulty of this method limits its routine use (91).

Sensitivities of tissue staining techniques range between 80–100% when compared to bacterial culture (103). Several factors influence the ability to detect *H. pylori* by histological methods. The distribution of bacteria in the stomach may be patchy, thus introducing the possibility of a false negative result due to sampling error (104). Accordingly, several biopsies from different regions of the antrum should be sent for examination. In addition, the experience of the pathologist significantly influences the diagnostic utility of tissue staining (105). *H. pylori* may not be immediately apparent on routine H&E staining; however, the presence of inflammation should alert the pathologist to the possibility of infection. In those instances, special stains may be performed to confirm the presence of *H. pylori*.

2. *Bacterial Culture*

A positive culture for *H. pylori* could be considered the "gold standard" for diagnosis; however, false negatives do occur due to sampling error or improper laboratory technique. Recent antibiotic use may suppress growth of the organism and inhibit culture. Additionally, factors associated with endoscopy have been

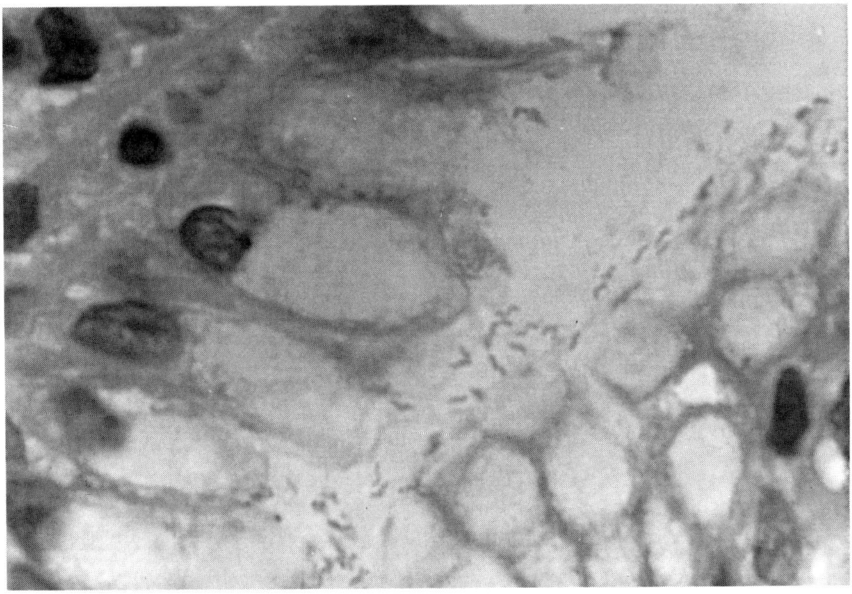

Figure 3 Hematoxylin-eosin stain of gastric mucosa demonstrating *Helicobacter pylori* in close association with the surface epithelium.

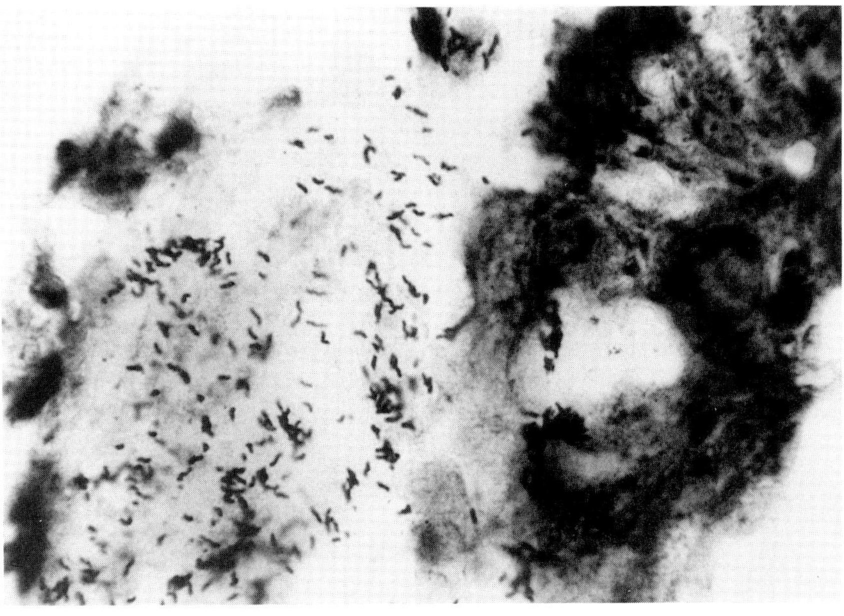

Figure 4 Warthin–Starry silver stain of *Helicobacter pylori*.

demonstrated to hinder growth of *H. pylori*, including ingestion of topical benzocaine (but not lidocaine) (106), simethicone (21), and contamination of biopsy forceps with glutaraldehyde (3).

H. pylori is a fastidious organism requiring special conditions for growth (see Section III, Taxonomy, Structure, and Microbiology). In fact, the first attempts at culturing the organism were unsuccessful until Marshall and his colleagues inadvertantly left a culture plate for six days over a holiday weekend and found numerous colonies of *H. pylori* upon their return (56). Specialized techniques must be implemented for growth, and plates should be incubated for at least 4 days before considering a culture negative. If a local laboratory does not have facilities suitable for culturing *H. pylori*, biopsy specimens can be preserved and shipped to a regional center.

Bacterial culture remains a tedious and expensive method of testing. Its use should be reserved for the determination of antibiotic susceptibility in patients with persistent infection following attempted eradication or for those at high risk for treatment-resistant organisms because of prior antibiotic use.

3. *Rapid Urease Test*

The potent bacterial enzyme, urease, forms the basis for a rapid, simple, inexpensive means of testing for *H. pylori*. Urease hydrolyzes urea to form ammonia and bicarbonate. When biopsy material containing *H. pylori* is placed into Christensen's 2% urea broth with phenol red, a color change occurs due to the liberation of ammonia (107). This test has been modified for use in the endoscopy suite. One example, the CLOtest (Delta West Pty. Ltd, Bently, Australia), employs modified Christensen's agar and a pH indicator embedded in gel on a plastic slide (108). Two antral biopsies are placed in the gel, and the slide is warmed to body temperature. Specimens should be read within 24 hours. A color change will be noted within 20 minutes in 75% of cases (108), thus affording the opportunity to make the diagnosis of *H. pylori* infection prior to a patient's departure from the endoscopy suite.

The rapid urease test is highly sensitive and specific compared to other diagnostic tests and should be considered the endoscopic method of choice (109). While false positives rarely occur (109), false negative urease tests may be due to prior treatment with proton pump inhibitors, such as omeprazole, which suppress the growth of *H. pylori* (110), or recent treatment with antibiotics or bismuth-containing compounds. If infection with *H. pylori* is suspected in these patients, two extra antral biopsies should be placed in formalin and sent for histological examination if the urease test is negative (99).

B. Noninvasive Tests

Noninvasive tests are less expensive than invasive tests that require upper endoscopy. They can be used for the primary diagnosis of *H. pylori* or, with certain limitations, for the confirmation of bacterial eradication following antibiotic therapy. Newer tests offer the practicing physician the ability to diagnose *H. pylori* infection in the office setting.

1. *Urea Breath Test*

The enzymatic activity of urease can be employed to detect *H. pylori* noninvasively. In this test, urea labeled with either the stable isotope, ^{13}C (111), or the radioactive isotope ^{14}C (112), is given to the patient orally. If *H. pylori* is present, the urea will be hydrolyzed, liberating ammonia and labeled bicarbonate. The bicarbonate is then absorbed through the gastric mucosa and expired through the lungs as labeled CO_2. Breath samples are collected at frequent intervals (up to one hour) and are measured either by mass spectrometry (^{13}C) or by a liquid scintillation counter (^{14}C). Both methods are highly reliable and compare favorably with other diagnostic tests (109,113).

The ^{14}C method is more rapid than tests using ^{13}C, requiring only 20 minutes for breath sampling and yielding results which are 97% sensitive and 100% specific for *H. pylori* (114,186). It can be performed either on fasting or nonfasting patients in contrast to the ^{13}C test, which requires a test meal to slow gastric emptying (115). In addition, scintillation counters to measure ^{14}C are present in most nuclear medicine facilities while gas isotope ratio mass spectrometers are usually not available. Alternatively, nonradioactive ^{13}C breath samples may be collected and sent by mail to central laboratory facilities for analysis. Although the radioactive dose of the 1-μCi ^{14}C urea breath test is small, it should not be used in children, pregnant women, or in patients requiring multiple tests (114).

The urea breath test is ideally suited for confirming eradication of *H. pylori* following treatment (116). It is noninvasive, rapid, and less costly than endoscopy with biopsy. Much like the rapid urease test, however, bacterial suppression can lead to false negative results. Therefore, breath testing should be performed at least 4 weeks after cessation of antibiotic therapy. Proton pump inhibitors should be stopped one week prior to testing. Currently, only the ^{13}C urea breath test is FDA-approved for the diagnosis of *H. pylori* infection. Approval for the ^{14}C breath test should be forthcoming.

2. *Serologic Methods*

Serologic tests for the detection of *H. pylori* include indirect immunofluorescence (117), hemagglutination (118), and complement fixation (119). However, these tests have been largely supplanted by ELISA as the most efficient, accurate means of serologic testing (120). The commercially available tests rely upon a wide array of substrate antigens, including formalin-treated whole organisms from single or pooled strains (with or without sonication), acid-extracted proteins, membrane proteins, bacterial lipopolysaccharides, and urease (120). Overall, sensitivities exceeding 90% for the diagnosis of primary infection should be expected from most of the serologic kits.

Serum IgG and IgA antibodies are detectable in patients infected with *H. pylori* (121). When directly compared, it appears that IgA serology has the lowest combination of sensitivity and specificity among commonly available diagnostic tests (109). IgM antibody levels do not differ between infected and uninfected persons (121,122). Therefore, most serologic tests for *H. pylori* rely exclusively on IgG levels.

In untreated individuals, antibody levels remain elevated over time suggesting persistent induction of an immune response (121). As mentioned previously, systemic and mucosal antibodies are unable to clear the organism. Therefore, a positive serology in an untreated patient suggests current infection. Following successful eradication, IgG antibodies can be detected for up to 3 years, but the antibody levels slowly fall (123). Several studies have documented a 50% reduction in titers 6 to 12 months following antimicrobial therapy (123,124). However, these studies utilized standardized serologic tests with serum samples often run in parallel. Therefore, serologic assays should not be relied upon to confirm eradication of *H. pylori* unless pretreatment and posttreatment samples are tested simultaneously (99).

Given its accuracy and low cost, serology should be considered the noninvasive method of choice for establishing a primary diagnosis of *H. pylori* infection. Newer, office-based immunochromatographic serum and whole blood test kits have been developed that allow diagnosis of *H. pylori* infection within minutes from a drop of the patient's serum. Initial studies using the Flex-Sure HP test (SmithKline Diagnostics, USA) and QuickVue test (Quidel) demonstrate 88%–96% sensitivity and 74%–88% specificity when compared with other invasive and noninvasive diagnostic techniques (125,187). The low cost, accuracy, and simplicity of these office test kits make them an attractive option for the rapid diagnosis of *H. pylori* infection.

VII. ASSOCIATION OF *H. PYLORI* WITH DISEASE

Prior to the discovery of *H. pylori*, several observations concerning ulcer disease remained unexplained. It was known that gastritis predisposed to gastric ulceration; furthermore, gastritis had been noted to persist or worsen after medical or surgical therapy for the ulcer (126). The high rate of ulcer relapse following treatment was felt to reflect an inherent derangement in the balance between mucosal protectors and aggressors. The observation in 1981 that patients treated with bismuth had lower rates of duodenal ulcer recurrence than those treated with H_2 blockers was not adequately explained at the time (127).

These earlier findings can now be understood within a framework wherein peptic ulcer disease is considered an infectious disease caused by *H. pylori*. We know that most people infected with *H. pylori* will never develop peptic ulceration. Therefore, the continuum from infection to gastritis to ulceration and, possibly, to gastric cancer must be modified by both host and environmental factors and by strain-specific features of the bacteria. The role of *H. pylori* in nonulcer dyspepsia is less well defined. Each of these disease entities is discussed below.

A. Gastritis

Gastritis is a histologic diagnosis defined as an increase in the number of mononuclear cells and neutrophils within the gastric epithelium (91). It should not be confused with endoscopically visualized lesions (e.g. erosions and submucosal hemorrhages) nor with chronic or recurrent upper abdominal discomfort (dyspepsia). Two forms of nonspecific, nonerosive gastritis have been identified: Type A, or autoimmune gastritis, and Type B, or antral gastritis. Only Type B gastritis is closely associated with *H. pylori* infection and gastroduodenal ulceration.

H. pylori has been detected in 86-99% of patients with chronic superficial gastritis (5,39,90). Conversely, nearly all *H. pylori*-positive patients show evidence of antral inflammation (1,5,55,90). Because of the known lack of correlation between endoscopic and histologic findings, a normal endoscopy does not exclude the presence of *H. pylori*-associated gastritis (3). Other forms of gastritis, such as eosinophilic gastroenteritis, Crohn's gastritis, and Menetrier's disease, are not associated with *H. pylori* (128).

Experimental evidence supports a causal relationship between *H. pylori* and gastritis. Two reports of volunteer ingestion of *H. pylori* organisms document the prompt onset of dyspeptic symptoms with hallmark histopathologic changes occurring within one week of infection (129,130). Symptoms included epigastric pain, vomiting, headache, irritability, and "putrid breath" (129). In one of these cases, an acute inflammatory lesion progressed to asymptomatic chronic gastritis that ultimately healed with antibiotics (131). Additional treatment trials corroborate the reversal of chronic superficial gastritis following eradication of *H. pylori* (89,132), further supporting the causal relationship between infection and gastritis.

B. Duodenal Ulcer

The prevalence of *H. pylori* infection in patients with duodenal ulcers ranges between 90–100% (3,55,90,133). When Marshall carefully examined the case histories of seven *H. pylori*-negative duodenal ulcer patients, he found two taking nonsteroidal agents, one with pancreatic cancer, one chronic alcohol user, and one patient treated with bismuth in the past (3). The absence of *H. pylori* in the setting of duodenal ulcer disease is uncommon and should suggest another diagnosis, such as Zollinger–Ellison syndrome (134) or nonsteroidal-induced ulceration.

The strongest evidence implicating *H. pylori* in the pathogenesis of duodenal ulcer disease is the marked reduction in the rate of ulcer relapse following eradication of the organism (Figure 5). In patients who are persistently *H. pylori*-positive, duodenal ulcer relapse rates may approach 80% at one year (4,6), while recurrence rates for patients rendered *H. pylori*-negative by antimicrobial therapy range between 0–12% (6,137,138). The protective effect of antimicrobial therapy appears to be prolonged. Forbes et al. documented an ulcer recurrence rate of only 3% in duodenal ulcer patients followed for seven years after *H. pylori* eradication (52). In addition, duodenal ulcers heal faster when treated with antibiotics and H_2 blockers as compared to acid suppression alone (138).

Eradication of *H. pylori* also appears to decrease the risk of rebleeding from duodenal ulcers. Two prospective, randomized, controlled trials confirm that antimicrobial therapy with omeprazole and amoxicillin in patients presenting with duodenal ulcers and a prior history of bleeding significantly decreases the rebleeding rate at one year when compared to omeprazole alone (139,140).

Based upon the available data, all patients with *H. pylori*-related duodenal ulceration should receive a course of antibiotic therapy aimed at eradicating the organism. *H. pylori*-positive patients with a healed ulcer on maintenance H_2-blocker therapy are also candidates for eradication therapy to prevent ulcer recurrence.

While most patients who clear their infection will be free of peptic disease, one should be cautious when using the term "cure" in relation to this infection.

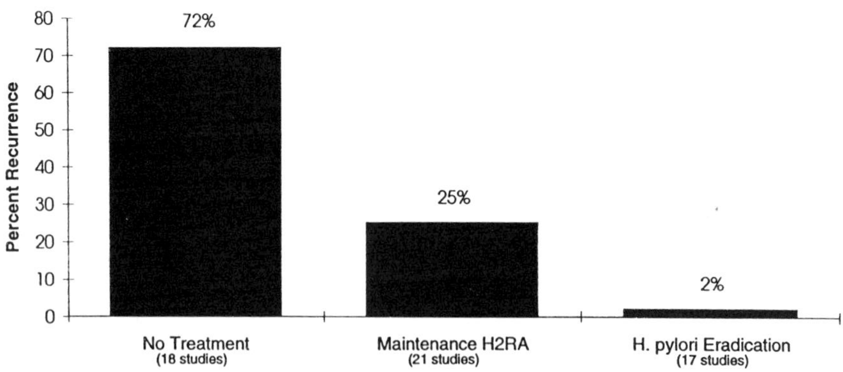

Figure 5 Rationale for eradication of *H. pylori* in duodenal ulcer disease. Six- to twelve-month ulcer recurrence rates are shown. H2RA = histamine-2 receptor antagonists. (From Refs. 135 and 136.)

H. pylori possesses an extraordinary ability to resist pharmacologic means of elimination. It appears that some patients initially thought to be cured of *H. pylori* may be at risk for recrudescence of the infection and recurrent ulceration. In a study of 190 patients undergoing one of five treatment regimens for *H. pylori* eradication (confirmed by single-biopsy urease test, histology, and culture at 4 weeks post-therapy), Xia et al. found that 19% of subjects developed recurrent infection when followed for a mean of 14.2 months (141). Of patients with recurrent infection, 53% experienced recurrent duodenal ulceration compared to 3% in patients free of *H. pylori* at follow-up. These findings contrast with those of other authors who have reported a very low rate of recurrent infection following successfully eradication (50,137), perhaps reflecting the relative sensitivities or timing of diagnostic tests used to document the elimination of the organism.

Thus, in patients at high risk for recurrent ulcer disease (e.g., the elderly, those with a history of a bleeding ulcer), it may be adviseable to confirm eradication with a urea breath test (where available) or endoscopic biopsy for a rapid urease test and/or histology four to six weeks post-therapy. If *H. pylori* is still present, the patient should be treated with an alternative course of antibiotics.

C. Gastric Ulcer

H. pylori is detected in approximately 70% to 80% of patients with gastric ulcer (3,56,109,133). Although the data are more limited than with duodenal ulcer disease, several treatment trials confirm a lower recurrence rate of gastric ulcer following eradication of *H. pylori* (137,142). It is therefore prudent to test patients with gastric ulcer for *H. pylori* and to treat the infection if it is found.

The majority of *H. pylori*-negative gastric ulcers occur in patients using NSAIDs (3, 133). While *H. pylori* and NSAID's appear to be independent risk factors for gastric ulceration (5,24,143), many authors advocate eradicating *H. pylori* when it is discovered in the setting of presumed nonsteroidal-induced gastropathy. The utility of this approach in preventing ulcer complications and recurrence awaits further investigation.

D. Nonulcer Dyspepsia

It remains unclear whether dyspeptic symptoms are directly related to infection with *H. pylori*. Up to 37% of asymptomatic adults examined by endoscopic biopsy have been found to have *H. pylori*-induced gastritis (5). Furthermore, only 50% on patients in Western societies with functional dyspepsia are *H. pylori* positive (144), a number that approximates the overall prevalence of infection in adults. Thus, as Talley has stated, "dyspepsia can occur in the absence of infection and infection can occur in the absence of symptoms (145)."

Therapeutic trials in patients with *H. pylori*-positive functional dyspepsia have produced conflicting results. In a review of 16 treatment trials in the world literature, Talley found 8 that supported the efficacy of antimicrobial therapy in relieving dyspeptic symptoms and 8 that failed to demonstrate improvement (144). While some patients may benefit from eradication of *H. pylori*, no study has conclusively identified any clinical or histologic parameters that predict therapeutic success.

At the present time, patients presenting to a physicians's office with complaints of dyspepsia should be treated conservatively with H_2 blockers. If there is no clinical response, a noninvasive test, such as serology, should be performed to exclude *H. pylori*. If the test is positive, patients should undergo endoscopy or a barium study to diagnose ulcer disease. Only if an ulcer is present should antimicrobial therapy be prescribed in an effort to eradicate *H. pylori*. Until further data are available regarding clinical features that predict improvement in patients with nonulcer dyspepsia, routine antibiotic therapy without a diagnosis of gastric or duodenal ulceration cannot be advocated. However, a course of antibiotics may be reasonable for the highly motivated patient with nonulcer dyspepsia who strongly desires therapy or has a significant family history of gastric malignancy.

E. Gastric Cancer

Epidemiological studies suggest a link between *H. pylori* and various gastric neoplasms, including gastric adenocarcinoma, mucosa-associated lymphoid tissue (MALT), and non-Hodgkin's lymphoma. Three prospective, case-control studies from different geographical regions document an increased prevalence of *H. pylori* infection preceding the development of adenocarcinoma of the distal stomach (146,147,148). *H. pylori* infection is not associated with carcinomas of the gastroesophageal junction or gastric cardia, which behave more like tumors of esophageal origin (147,148).

H. pylori has also been detected in over 90% of cases of gastric MALT lymphoma or MALToma, an uncommon neoplasm with an indolent course (149). Roggero et al. documented the disappearance of near-total regression of these tumors in 60% of patients in whom *H. pylori* was successfully eradicated (150), suggesting a causal association. In a nested case-control study using banked sera, Parsonnet et al. found significantly higher rates of *H. pylori* infection among subjects with primary gastric non-Hodgkin's lymphoma than matched controls (151). The sera collection predated the onset of malignancy by a median of 14 years, and no association was found with nongastric lymphomas. Taken together, these studies point toward *H. pylori* as a causative agent in lymphomatous neoplasms of the stomach.

The mechanisms whereby *H. pylori* may induce neoplastic transformation of gastric epithelial cells in unknown. As with peptic ulcer disease, a small minority of patients with infection will develop gastric cancer. Certainly, host factors, strain variation, and environmental cofactors must play a role (151). Recent data suggest that strains possessing the *cag*A gene are more likely to be associated with gastric adenocarcinoma of the distal stomach than *cag*A-negative strains (152). Identifying specific risk factors for the development of gastric cancer in *H. pylori*-positive patients is critical if the progression from infection to neoplasia is to be halted.

Recent data suggest that *H. pylori*-infected patients receiving long-term omeprazole therapy for reflux esophagitis are at higher risk for the development of atrophic gastritits, a precursor to gastric cancer (188). An increase in corpus gastritis has been demonstrated in *H. pylori*-infected patients during acid suppressive therapy (189). Theoretically, omeprazole may hasten the onset of gastric atrophy by intensifying the gastritis associated with bacterial infection. However, corroboration of these findings by other investigators is necessary before recommending the eradication of *H. pylori* in all patients requiring chronic acid suppressive therapy.

At the present time, treatment of asymptomatic individuals with *H. pylori* is not advocated (153). Patients with gastric MALT lymphoma should receive antibiotic therapy and undergo repeat endoscopy and mucosal biopsy to document eradication following treatment. Further research is necessary to identify a subset of asymptomatic infected patients who may benefit from antimicrobial therapy in an effort to prevent the development of gastric cancer.

Current recommendations for the treatment of *Helicobacter pylori* in different patient populations are shown in Table 2. While the decision to offer a course of therapy to a patient with *H. pylori* should be individualized, a general algorithm for the evaluation and treatment of symptomatic patients has been provided in Figure 6.

VIII. ERADICATION OF *HELICOBACTER PYLORI*

A. General Considerations

H. pylori is highly susceptible in vitro (MIC90 $\leq$ 1 mg/L) to most antibiotics except trimethoprim, sulfonamides, vancomycin, and nalidixic acid (155). Unfortunately, these in vitro data do not translate into comparable efficacy in vivo. Several plausible theories may account for this discrepancy.

H. pylori lives within a protected environment beneath the mucus layer in the stomach. Luminally-active antibiotics, such as bismuth, may be less effective in this setting due to their failure to penetrate deep to the mucus-secreting

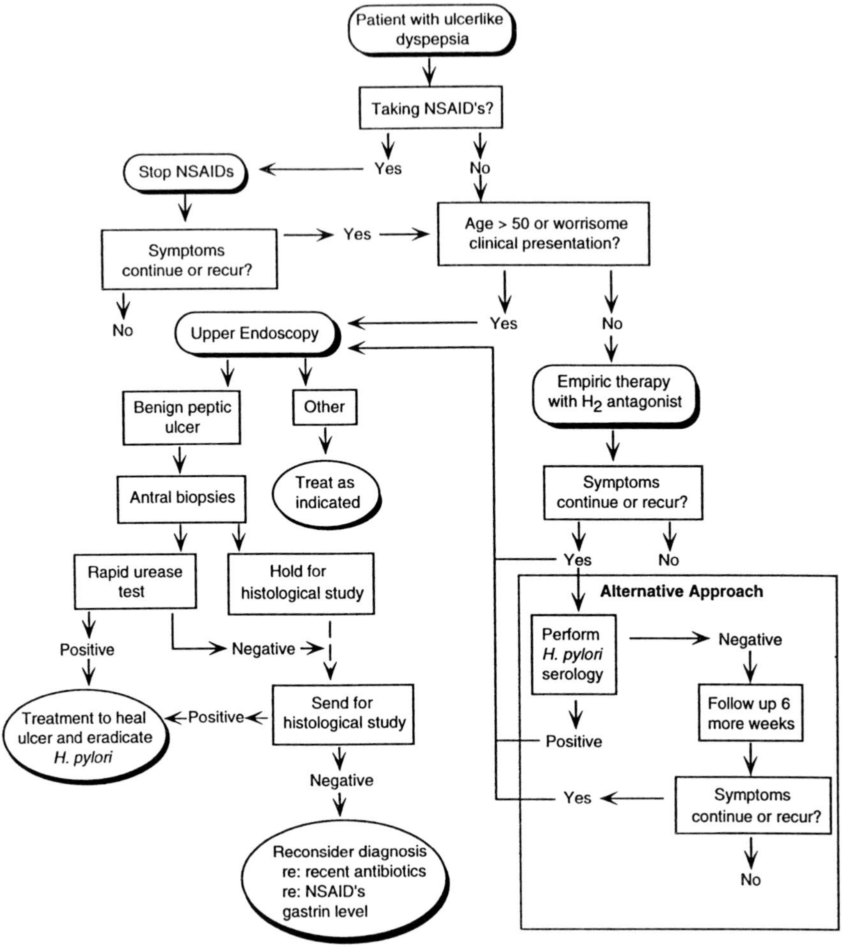

Figure 6 Algorithm for the approach to a patient with dyspeptic symptoms. (From Ref. 154).

glands where *H. pylori* resides (155,156). Systemically active agents, such as erythromycin, may be deactivated by gastric acid (157). In addition, up to 40% of *H. pylori* isolates have been found to contain plasmids that encode for antibiotic resistance (158).

In vitro studies confirm that *H. pylori* can acquire resistance to a variety of antibiotics by plasmid-mediated natural transformation (159). Metronidazole resistance is a significant factor impeding *H. pylori* eradication, especially in

Table 2 Recommendations for Treatment of *Helicobacter pylori*-positive Patients

Proven benefit	Possible benefit	No benefit
Gastric ulcer	First-degree relatives of patients with gastric cancer	Asymptomatic patients without risk factors for gastric malignancy
Duodenal ulcer	Immigrants from nations with a high prevalence of gastric cancer	
MALT lymphoma	Nonulcer dyspepsia patients who request therapy[a]	

[a]Inform patient that treatment may not relieve symptoms.

regions of the world where nitroimidazoles are used frequently. One multicenter study in Europe found metronidazole resistance in 27.5% of strains (160). The rate of resistance was high among women, Africans, and other non-Caucasians, populations who were more likely to have taken nitroimidazoles in the past for gynecologic infections or diarrhea. Immigrants from nations where nitroimidazoles are available over the counter are more likely to harbor resistant strains. In a study conducted in the United Kingdom, an astoundingly high 90% of *H. pylori* strains cultured from Bangladesian immigrants to East London were metronidazole-resistant compared to 37% of strains from persons born in the United Kingdom (161). Again, prior nitroimidazole exposure conferred an increased risk of drug resistance in both immigrants and native subjects. The varying prevalence of antibiotic resistance in different regions of the world may help to explain the discordant eradication rates of nitroimidazole-based regimens observed in studies from different countries (162).

Patient compliance appears to be the single most important factor predicting success of eradication using standardized triple antibiotic therapy (163,164). The dosing frequency (*tid* or *qid*) and pill totals (12 to 16 per day) required by this regimen are daunting and may be too complex for some patients. Therefore, reported eradication rates for different antimicrobial regimens may not be representative of their "real world" efficacy in certain patient populations.

Currently, there are three FDA-approved regimens for *H. pylori*: omeprazole and clarithromycin, ranitidine bismuth citrate and clarithromycin, and bismuth-based triple therapy. However, the clinician may choose from a variety of therapeutic regimens that differ in their simplicity, efficacy, and side-effect profiles. Table 3 lists several of the most widely used regimens for eradicating *H. pylori*. The following sections provide details concerning each mode of therapy.

Table 3 Recommended Therapies for the Eradication of *Helicobacter Pylori*

Regimen	Medications	Duration	Cure rate	Cost	Comments
I. Triple Therapy					
	Bismuth 2 tabs *qid* Metronidazole 250 mg *qid* Tetracycline 500 mg *qid*	14d	90%	+	cost effective; reliable; FDA-approved; side effects in up to 30%; Bismuth is Pepto Bismol™ in U.S.
substitute for tetracycline in allergic patients:					
	Amoxicillin 500 mg *qid*	14d	80%	+	less effective than regimen with tetracycline
substitute for metronidazole in suspected antibiotic resistance:					
	Clarithromycin 500 mg *tid*	14d	90%	++	cure rate highest with tetracycline rather than amoxicillin as part of triple therapy
II. Dual Therapy					
	Omeprazole 40 mg *qd* Clarithromycin 500 mg *tid*	14d	80%	+++	FDA-approved; continue omeprazole 20 mg once daily for 14d after antibiotic course
	Ranitidine bismuth citrate 400 mg *bid* Clarithromycin 500 mg *tid*	14d	80%	+++	FDA-approved; continue ranitidine bismuth citrate 400 mg *bid* for 14d after antibiotic course

III. Short-Course Therapy				
Metronidazole 500 mg *bid* Omeprazole 20 mg *bid*[a] Clarithromycin 500 mg *bid*	7–10d	90%	++	well tolerated; short course decreases cost
Amoxicillin 500 mg *bid* Omeprazole 20 mg *bid* Clarithromycin 500 mg *bid*	7–10d	90%	++	alternative for metronidazole-intolerant patients
Bismuth 2 tabs *qid* Metronidazole 250 mg *qid* Tetracycline 500 mg *qid* Omeprazole 20 mg *bid*	7–10d	95%	++	highly effective; 18–26 pills/day; side effects common, but low dropout rate in largest study

[a]May substitute lansoprazole 30 mg *bid* for omeprazole.

B. Monotherapy

Efforts to simplify the treatment of *H. pylori* have been limited by the lack of an antibiotic that is effective as a single agent. Pooled data from 27 therapeutic trials worldwide reveal an overall eradication rate of 18.6% for monotherapy (165). Clarithromycin appears to be the most effective drug when used alone with a reported eradication rate of 54%, given in a dosage of 500 mg *qid* (166). However, the high level of primary (12%) and secondary (21%) drug resistance reported in this study make clarithromycin an unacceptable option as monotherapy.

C. Dual Therapy

The combination of an antibiotic and a proton pump inhibitor may be the most tolerable regimen for patients. While omeprazole alone is ineffective in permanently eliminating *H. pylori* (110), its use with an antibiotic produces significantly higher eradication rates than those observed with monotherapy (167). The mechanisms whereby acid inhibition enhances the bactericidal activity of antibiotics directed against *H. pylori* are not completely understood. Acid-labile antibiotics may function more effectively in an environment rendered pH neutral by omeprazole (168). In addition, the use of a proton pump inhibitor may prevent the denaturation of *H. pylori*-specific immunoglobulin by gastric acid, thus augmenting host defense mechanisms (169). Finally, proton pump inhibitors may block the bacterial P-type ATPase found in *H. pylori* which appears to protect the organism from excessive cytoplasmic accumulation of toxic ammonium ion liberated by urease (170).

Two-week regimens of omeprazole plus amoxicillin (171,172,173) and omeprazole plus clarithromycin (174,175) have been used widely for *H. pylori*, with the latter combination achieving superior eradication rates of approximately 80%. Omeprazole should be given in a dose of 20 mg twice daily, as the eradication rates with this schedule are better than those observed with 40 mg once daily (162). Higher doses of omeprazole may improve the efficacy of dual therapy with amoxicillin (176).

Because omeprazole suppresses *H. pylori* growth (110), its use prior to the initiation of antibiotic therapy may render *H. pylori* less susceptible to antibiotics (173). Thus, the proton pump inhibitor and the antibiotic should be started together. If a patient is already on omeprazole, an alternative regimen should be selected.

Side effects with omeprazole-based dual therapy are unusual, and these regimens appear to be better tolerated than triple therapy (155,162). In addition, omeprazole/antibiotic combinations may offer more prompt symptom relief in patients with duodenal ulcer disease than standard triple therapy plus H_2 blockade (172). Dual therapy is an appropriate alternative for patients unable to comply with the complex dosing schedule required by triple agent regimens. Eventually, with the emergence of new drugs and treatment schemes, a proton pump inhibitor and a single antibiotic may dethrone triple therapy as the treatment of choice for *H. pylori* infection.

D. Triple Therapy

Treatment with three antibiotics to eradicate *H. pylori* remains the "gold standard" by which all other treatment regimens should be judged. The principle of triple therapy is to attack *H. pylori* with both luminally active and systemically active agents in an effort to overcome the limitations of each (156). Additionally, resistance to medications such as metronidazole may be prevented by the addition of a second antimicrobial drug (177). Unfortunately, this effort comes at the expense of a significant side-effect profile, which results in cessation of therapy in 3% to 7% of patients (162).

Eradication rates with bismuth, metronidazole, and either amoxicillin or tetracycline for two weeks range between 75% to 95% in most trials (162,165). Regimens containing tetracycline appear to be more effective than triple therapy using amoxicillin, achieving an average eradication rate of 94.1% (165). Clarithromycin may be substituted for metronidazole in patients suspected of harboring a resistant organism (178).

Side effects occur in approximately 30% of patients treated with triple therapy (162,165). Common symptoms include nausea, headache, soreness of the mouth, taste disturbance, diarrhea, and darkening of the stools. More severe reactions include allergic rashes, *Candida* infection, and *Clostridium difficile* colitis.

Triple therapy may be offered as first-line treatment for patients with *H. pylori*-related gastroduodenal ulcer disease. An H_2 blocker is frequently added to this regimen for the first 4-to-6 weeks in patients with acute gastric or duodenal ulceration to speed symptomatic recovery. As mentioned previously, medical compliance and the regional prevalence of metronidazole-resistant isolates will affect the expected eradication rates for any particular patient. Therefore, treatment should be individualized and modified to ensure the greatest chance of cure.

E. Short-Course Therapy

Several studies indicate that short course therapy may be as effective as standard two-week regimens. A randomized trial of one-week versus two-week quadruple therapy with bismuth, metronidazole, and tetracycline plus an H_2 blocker for *H. pylori*-related ulcer disease produced equivalent eradication rates of approximately 95% in each group (179). Data from the same institution also revealed an extremely high eradication rate of 98.1% among 54 study subjects receiving bismuth, metronidazole, and tetracycline plus omeprazole (20 mg *bid*) compared with an eradication rate of 83.3% in those receiving one-week of standard triple therapy (180). Both of these studies documented a 70% to 80% incidence of side effects with the various regimens. However, only 3 patients out of 164 (1.8%) receiving one-week courses in these two trials stopped therapy.

Other antibiotic combinations have been tried with varying success. One short-course combination that shows promise is metronidazole, omeprazole, and amoxicillin. In a comparative study of 436 patients given one of three different dosing schemes of this triple therapy combination, a 7-day course of metronidazole (400 mg *tid*) plus omeprazole (40 mg *qd*) plus amoxicillin (500 mg *tid*) emerged as the most efficacious regimen, eradicating *H. pylori* in 91.1% of subjects (181). The incidence of side effects was 33%, but no patients in this group withdrew from the trial.

Recent studies on other short course regimens, including metronidazole, omeprazole, and clarithromycin (MOC therapy) (182), are promising. Ultimately, one-week regimens should afford the clinician the ability to eradicate *H. pylori* in greater than 90% of cases without compromising patient compliance or tolerability profiles.

IX. THE FUTURE FOR *H. PYLORI* RESEARCH

An explosion of intensive research in the past decade has markedly improved our understanding of the role played by *H. pylori* in the pathogenesis of upper gastrointestinal disease, but there is still much to be learned. Future studies should address the bacterial, host, and environmental factors that influence the development of gastroduodenal disease in infected patients. Epidemiologic studies should advance our knowledge regarding the environmental source and mode of transmission of *H. pylori*. Outcomes research should be directed at defining cost-effective strategies of combating this bacterium.

By understanding which patients are at risk for clinical disease, we may be better able to define the patient populations that benefit most from treatment. In geographic regions where *H. pylori* is endemic in children, immunization may be the only therapeutic option. Currently, vaccine development is in its infancy (183,184). Our goals should be to expand these avenues of investigation and to determine if vaccination of children or treatment of asymptomatic infected individuals can lessen the risk of gastroduodenal ulceration and gastric cancer.

If the future scientific exploration of *H. pylori* uncovers as much information as the recent past, physicians will possess a formidable armamentarium to eradicate this bacterium and possibly prevent most upper gastrointestinal disease.

REFERENCES

1. Warren JR. Unidentified curved bacilli on gastric epithelium in active chronic gastritis. Lancet 1983; 1:1273.
2. Marshall BJ. Unidentified curved bacilli on gastric epithelium in active chronic gastritis. Lancet 1983; 1:1273–5.
3. Marshall BJ, McGechie DB, Rogers PA, Glancy RJ. Pyloric campylobacter infection and gastroduodenal disease. Med J Aust 1985; 142:439–44.
4. Coghlan JG, Gilligan D, Humphries H, McKenna D, Dooley C, Sweeney E, Keane C, O'Morain C. *Campylobacter pylori* and recurrence of duodenal ulcers–A 12 month follow-up study. Lancet 1987; ii:1109–11.
5. Dooley CP, Cohen H, Fitzgibbons PL, Bauer M, Appelman MD, Perez-Perez GI, Blaser JH. Prevalence of *Helicobacter pylori* infection and histologic gastritis in asymptomatic persons. N Engl J Med 1989; 321:1562–6.
6. Rauws EAJ, Tytgat GNJ. Cure of duodenal ulcer associated with eradication of *Helicobacter pylori*. Lancet 1990; 335:1233–5.
7. Bottcher. Dorpater Medizinishe Zettschrift. 1874; 5:148.
8. Bizzozero G. Ueber die Schlauchfoermigen Druesen des Magendarmkanals und die Beziehungen ihres Epithels zu dem Oberflaechenepithel der Schleimhaut. Arch Mikr Anat 1893; 42:82–152.
9. Salomon H. Ueber das Spirillum des Saugettermangens und sein Verhalten zu den Belegzellen. Centralbl Bakt Parasit Infekt 1896; 19:433–42.
10. Krienitz W. Ueber das Auftreten von Spirochaeten Verschiedener form in Mageninhalt bei Carcinoma Ventriculi. Dtsch Med Wochenschr 1906; 28:872.
11. Doenges JL. Spirchetes in the gastric glands of *Macacus rhesus* and humans without definite history of related disease. Proc Soc Exp Med Biol 1938; 38:536–8.
12. Freedburg AS, Barron LE. The presence of spirochaetes in human gastric mucosa. Am J Dig Dis 1940; 7:443–5.
13. Palmer E.D. Investigation of the gastric spirochaetes of the human. Gastroenterology 1954; 27:218–20.
14. Steer HW. Ultrastructure of cell migration through the gastric epithelium and its relationship to bacteria. J Clin Pathol 1975; 28:639–46.
15. Steer HW, Colin-Jones DG. Mucosal changes in gastric ulceration and their response to carbenoxalone sodium. Gut 1975; 16:590–7.
16. Goodwin CS, Armstrong JA, Chilvers T, et al. Transfer of *Campylobacter pylori* and *Campylobacter mustelae* to *Helicobacter* gen. nov. as *Helicobacter pylori* comb. nov. and *Helicobacter mustelae* comb. nov., respectively. Int J Syst Bacteriol 1989; 39:397–405.
17. Fox JG, Edrise BM, Cabot EB, Beaucage C, Murphy JC, Prostak KS. Campylobacter-like organisms isolated from gastric mucosa of ferrets. Am J Vet Res 1986; 47:236–9.
18. Paster BJ, Lee A, Fox JG, Dewhirst FE, Tardoff LA, Fraser GJ, O'Rourke JL, Taylor NS, Ferrerro R. The phylogeny of *Helicobacter felis*, sp. nov., *Helicobacter mustelae,* and related bacteria. Int J Syst Bacteriol 1991; 41:31–8.
19. Krakowka S, Morgan D, Kraft W, Leunk RD. Establishment of gastric

Campylobacter pylori infection in the neonatal gnotobiotic piglet. Infect Immun 1987; 55:2789–96.

20. Marchetti M, Aricó B, Bumoni D, Figura N, Rappuoli R, Ghiara P. Development of a mouse model of *Helicobacter pylori* infection that mimics human disease. Science 1995; 267:1655–8.
21. Goodwin CS, Worsley BW. Microbiology of *Helicobacter pylori*. Gastroenterol Clin Nor Am 1993; 22:5–19.
22. Goodwin CS, Armstrong JA, Marshall BJ. *Campylobacter pyloridis*, gastritis, and peptic ulceration. J Clin Pathol 1986; 39:353–65.
23. Morris A, Nicholson G, Lloyd G, Haines D, Rogers A, Taylor D. Seroepidemiology of *Campylobacter pyloridis*. NZ Med J 1986; 99:657–9.
24. Graham DY, Malaty HM, Evans DG, Evans DJ, Klein PD, Adam E. Epidemiology of *Helicobacter pylori* in an asymptomatic population in the United States. Gastroenterology 1991; 100:1495–501.
25. Asaka M, Kimura T, Kudo M, Takeda H, Mitani S, Miyazaki T, Miki K, Graham DY. Relationship of *Helicobacter pylori* to serum pepsinogens in an asymptomatic Japanese population. Gastroenterology 1992; 102:760–6.
26. Mégraud F, Brassens-Rabbé MP, Denis F, Belbouri A, Hoa DQ. Seroepidemiology of *Campylobacter pylori* infection in various populations. J Clin Microbiol 1989; 27:1870–3.
27. Perez-Perez GI, Taylor DN, Bodhidatta L, Wongsrichanalai J, Baze WB, Dunn BE, Echeverria PD. Seroprevalence of *Helicobacter pylori* infections in Thailand. J Infect Dis 1990; 161:1237–41.
28. Blaser MJ. Hypothesis on the pathogenesis and natural history of *Helicobacter pylori*-induced inflammation. Gastroenterology 1992; 102:720–7.
29. Webb PM, Knight T, Greaves S, Wilson A, Newell DG, Elder J, Forman D. Relation between infection with *Helicobacter pylori* and living conditions in childhood: evidence for person to person transmission in early life. Br Med J 1994; 308:750–3.
30. Mendall MA, Goggin PM, Molineaux N, Levy J, Toosy T, Strachan D, Northfield TC. Childhood living conditions and *Helicobacter pylori* seropositivity in adult life. Lancet 1992; 339:896–7.
31. Galpin OP, Whitaker CJ, Dubiel AJ. *Helicobacter pylori* infection and overcrowding in childhood. Lancet 1992; 339:619.
32. Fiedorek SC, Evans DG, Evans DJ, Malaty HM, Pumphrey CL, Casteel HB, Graham DY. *Helicobacter pylori* infection epidemiology in children: importance of socioeconomic status, age, gender and race. Gastroenterology 1990; 98:A44.
33. Smoak BL, Kelley PW, Taylor DN. Seroprevalence of *Helicobacter pylori* infections in a cohort of US Army recruits. Am J Epidem 1994; 139:513–9.
34. Malaty HM, Engstrand L, Pedersen NL, Graham DY. *Helicobacter pylori* infection: genetic and environmental influences. A study of twins. Ann Intern Med 1994; 120:982–6.
35. Kelly SM, Pitcher MCL, Farmery SM, Gibson GR. Isolcation of *Helicobacter pylori* from feces of patients with dyspepsia in the United Kingdom. Gastroenterology 1994; 107:1671–4.

36. Thomas JE, Gibson GR, Darboe MK, Dale A, Weaver LT. Isolation of *Helicobacter pylori* from human faeces. Lancet 1992; 340:1194–5.
37. Thomas JE, Downes RB, Lunn PG, Northrup–Clewes CA, Weaver LT. Seroepidemiology of *Helicobacter pylori* infection in early childhood. Gut 1991; 32:A1231.
38. Mapstone NP, Lynch DAF, Lewis FA, Axon ATR, Tompkins DS, Dixon MF, Quirke P. PCR identification of *Helicobacter pylori* in faeces from gastritis patients. Lancet 1993; 341:447.
39. Drumm B, Perez–Perez GI, Blaser MJ, Sherman PM. Intrafamilial clustering of *Helicobacter pylori* infection. N Engl J Med 1990; 322:359–63.
40. Malaty HM, Graham DY, Klein PD, Evans DG, Adam E, Evans DJ. Transmission of *Helicobacter pylori* infection. Studies in families of healthy individuals. Scand J Gastroenterol 1991; 26:927–32.
41. Rauws EAJ, Langenberg W, Oudbier J, Mulder CJJ, Tytgat GNJ. Familial clustering of peptic ulcer disease colonized with *C. pylori* of the same DNA composition. Gastroenterology 1989; 96:A409.
42. Graham DY, Alpert LC, Smith JL, Yoshimura HH. Iatrogenic *Campylobacter pylori* is a cause of epidemic achlorhydria. Am J Gastroenterol 1988; 974–80.
43. Langenberg W, Rauws EAJ, Oudbier JH, Tytgat GNJ. Patient–to–patient transmission of *Campylobacter pylori* infection by fiberoptic gastroduodenoscopy and biopsy. J Infect Dis 1990; 161:507–11.
44. Ramsey EJ, Carey KV, Peterson WL, Jackson JJ, Murphy FK, Read NW, Taylor KB, Trier JS, Fordtran JS. Epidemic gastritis with hypochlorhydria. Gastroenterology 1979; 76:1449–57.
45. Fanty GF, Zheng Q–X, James SP. Conventional cleaning and disinfection techniques eliminate the risk of endoscopic transmission of *Helicobacter pylori*. Am J Gastroenterol 1995; 90:227–32.
46. Chong J, Marshall BJ, Barkin JS, McCallum RW, Reiner DK, Hoffman SR, O'Phelan C. Occupational exposure to *Helicobacter pylori* for the endoscopy professional: A sera epidemiological study. Am J Gastroenterol 1994; 89:1987–91.
47. Krajden S, Fuksa M, Anderson J, Kempston J, Bocchia A, Petrea C, Babiola C, Karmali M, Penner JL. Examination of human stomach biopsies, saliva, and dental plaque for *Campylobacter pylori*. J Clin Microbiol 1989; 27:1397–8.
48. Malaty HM, Evans DJ, Abramovitch K, Evans DG, Graham DY. *Helicobacter pylori* infection in dental workers: A seroepidemiological study. Am J Gastroenterol 1992; 87:1728–31.
49. Langenberg W, Rauws EAJ, Widjojokusumo A, Tytgat GNJ, Zanen HC. Identification of *Campylobacter pyloridis* isolates by restriction endonuclease DNA analysis. J Clin Microbiol 1986; 24:414–7.
50. Xia HX, Windle HJ, Marshall DG, Smyth CJ, Keane CT, O'Morain Ca. Recrudescence of *H. pylori* after apparently successful eradication: novel application of randomly amplified polymorphic DNA fingerprinting. Gut 1995; 37:30–4.
51. Parsonnet J, Blaser MJ, Perez–Perez GI, Hargrett–Bean N, Tauxe RV. Symp-

toms and risk factors of *Helicobacter pylori* infection in a cohort of epidemiologists. Gastroenterology 1992; 102:41–6.

52. Forbes GM, Glaser ME, Cullen DJE, Warren JR, Christiansen KJ, Marshall BJ, Collins BJ. Duodenal ulcer treated with *Helicobacter pylori* eradication: seven-year follow-up. Lancet 1994; 343:258–60.
53. Mégraud F. Epidemiology of *Helicobacter pylori* infection. Gastroenterol Clin Nor Am 1993; 22:73–88.
54. Faisal MA, Russel RM, Samloff IM, Holt PR. *Helicobacter pylori* infection and atrophic gastritis in the elderly. Gastroenterology 1990; 99:1543–4.
55. Steer HW. Surface morphology of the gastroduodenal mucosa in duodenal ulceration. Gut 1984; 25:1203–10.
56. Marshall BJ, Warren JR. Unidentified curved bacilli in the stomach of patients with gastritis and peptic ulceration. Lancet 1984; 1:1311–5.
57. Hazell SL, Lee A, Brady L, Henressy W. *Campylobacter pyloridis* and gastritis: association with intercellular spaces and adaptation to an environment of mucus as important factors in colonization of the gastric epithelium. J Inf Dis 1986; 153:658–63.
58. Hazell SL. Microbiology and taxonomy of *Helicobacter pylori* and related bacteria. In: Marshall BJ, McCallum RW, Guerrant RL, eds. *Helicobacter pylori* in peptic ulceration and gastritis. Boston: Blackwell Scientific Publications, 1991; 1:19–33.
59. Eaton KA, Morgan DR, Krakowka S. *Campylobacter pylori* virulence factors in gnotobiotic piglets. Infect Immun 1989; 57:1119–25.
60. Gold BD, Huesca M, Sherman PM, Longwood CA. *Helicobacter mustelae* and *Helicobacter pylori* bind to common lipid receptors in vitro. Infect Immun 1993; 61:2632–8.
61. Slomiany BL, Piotrowski J, Samanta A, Van Horn K, Murtry VL, Slomiany A. *Campylobacter pylori* colonization factor shows specificity for lactosylceramide sulfate and GM3 ganglioside. Biochem Internat 1989; 19:929–36.
62. Borén T, Falk P, Roth KA, Larson G, Normark S. Attachment of *Helicobacter pylori* to human gastric epithelium mediated by blood group antigens. Science 1993; 262:1892–5.
63. Clarke CA, et al. Relationship of ABO blood groups to duodenal and gastric ulceration. Br Med J 1955; 2:643–6.
64. Phillips AD, Hine KR, Holmes GKT, Woodings DF. Gastric spiral bacteria. Lancet 1984; ii:100–1.
65. Wyatt JI, Rathbone BJ, Dixon MF, Heatley RV. *Campylobacter pyloridis* and acid induced gastric metaplasia in the pathogenesis of duodenitis. J Clin Pathol 1987; 40:841–8.
66. Wyatt JI, Rathbone BJ, Sobala GM, Shallcross T, Heatley RV, Axon ATR, Dixon MF. Gastric epithelium in the duodenum: Its association with *Helicobacter pylori* and inflammation. J Clin Pathol 1990; 43:981–6.
67. Goodwin CS. Duodenal ulcer, *Campylobacter pylori*, and the "leaking roof" concept. Lancet 1988; 2:1467–9.

68. Langenberg ML, Tytgat GNJ, Schipper MEI, Rietra PJGM, Zanen HC. Campylobacter–like organisms in the stomach of patients and healthy individuals. Lancet 1984; i:1348.
69. Marshall BJ, Barrett LJ, Prakash C, McCallum RW, Guerrant RL. Urea protects *Helicobacter (Campylobacter) pylori* from the bactericidal effect of acid. Gastroenterology 1990; 99:697–702.
70. Triebling AT, Korsten MA, Dlugosz JW, Paronetto F. Lieber CS. Severity of *Helicobacter*-induced gastric injury correlates with gastric juice ammonia. Dig Dis Sci 1991; 36:1089–96.
71. Eaton KA, Brooks CL, Morgan DR, Krakowka S. Essential role of urease in pathogenesis of gastritis induced by *Helicobacter pylori* in gnotobiotic piglets. Infect Imun 1991; 59:2470–5.
72. Hazell SL, Lee A. *Campylobacter pyloridis*, urease, hydrogen ion back diffusion, and gastric ulcers. Lancet 1986; ii:15–7.
73. Leunk RD, Johnson PT, David BC, Kraft WG, Morgan DR. Cytotoxic activity in broth–culture-filtrates of *Campylobacter pylori*. J Med Microbiol 1988; 26:93–9.
74. Figura N, Guglielmetti P, Rossolini A, Barberi A, Cusi G, Musmanno RA, Russi M, Quaranta S. Cytotoxin production by *Campylobacter pylori* strains isolated from patients with peptic ulcers and from patients with chronic gastritis only. J Clin Microbiol 1989; 27:225–6.
75. Telford JL, Ghiara P, Dell'Orco M, Comanducci M, Burroni D, Bugnoli M, Tecce MF, Censini S, Covacci A, Xiang Z, Papini E, Montecucco C, Parente L, Rapouli R. Gene structure of the *Helicobacter pylori* cytotoxin and evidence of its key role in gastric disease. J Exp Med 1994; 179:1653–8.
76. Tummuru MKR, Cover TL, Blaser MJ. Cloning and expression of a high-molecular-mass major antigen of *Helicobacter pylori*: Evidence of linkage to cytotoxin production. Infect Immun 1992; 61:1799–1809.
77. Covaci A, Censini S, Bugnoli M, Petraca R, Burroni D, Macchia M, Massone A, Papini E, Xiang Z, Figura N, Rappuoli R. Molecular characterization of the 128–kDa immunodominant antigen of *Helicobacter pylori* associated with cytotoxicity and duodenal ulcer. Proc Natl Acad Sci USA 1993; 90:5791–5.
78. Crabtree JE, Eyre D, Covacci A, Rappuoli R, Graham Dy. Systemic CagA IgG antibodies in gastric and duodenal ulceration: Comparison with asymptomatic individuals. The VIIth Workshop on Gastroduodenal Pathology and *Helicobacter pylori*. Houston, Texas, September-October, 1994, Abstract 151.
79. Labigne A, Lamouliatte H, Birac C, Sedallian A, Mégraud F. Distribution of the *cag*A gene among *Helicobacter pylori* strains associated with peptic ulcer. The VIIth Workshop on Gastroduodenal Pathology and Helicobacter pylori. Houston, Texas, September–October, 1994, Abstract 166.
80. Sarosiek J, Slomiany A, Slomiany BL. Evidence for weakening of gastric mucus integrity by *Campylobacter pylori*. Scand J Gastroenterol 1988; 23:585–90.
81. Slomiany BL, Nishikawa H, Piotrowski J, Okazaki K, Slomiany A. Lipolytic activity of *Campylobacter pylori*. Effect of sofalcone. Digestion 1989; 43:33–40.

82. Sarosiek J, Marshall BJ, Peura DA, Hoffman S, Feng T, McCallum RW. Gastroduodenal mucus gel thickness in patients with *Helicobacter pylori*: A method for assessment in biopsy specimens. Am J Gastroenterol 1991; 86:729–34.
83. McGuigan JE, Trudeau Wl. Difference in rates of gastrin release in normal persons and patients with duodenal ulcer disease. N Engl J Med 1973; 288:64–6.
84. Blair AJ, Feldman M, Barnett C, Walsh JH, Richardson CT. Detailed comparison of basal and food-stimulated gastric acid secretion rates and serum gastrin concentrations in duodenal ulcer patients and normal subjects. J Clin Invest 1987; 79:582-7.
85. Graham DY, Opekun A, Lew G, Klein PD, Walsh JH, *Helicobacter pylori*-associated exaggerated gastrin release in duodenal ulcer patients. The effect of bombesin infusion and urea ingestion. Gastroenterology 1991; 100:1571–5.
86. Prewett EJ, Smith JT, Nwokolo CU, Hudson M, Sawyerr AM, Pounder RE. Eradication of *Helicobacter pylori* abolishes 24-hour hypergastrinaemia: A prospective study in healthy subjects. Alimen Pharmacol Therap 1991; 5:283–90.
87. el-Omar E, Penman I, Dorrian Ca, Ardill JES, McColl KEL. Eradicating *Helicobacter pylori* infection lowers gastrin mediated acid secretion by two thirds in patients with duodenal ulcer. Gut 1993; 34:1060–5.
88. Rademaker JW, Hunt RH. *Helicobacter pylori* and gastric acid secretion: The ulcer link? Scand J Gastroenterol 1991; 26(suppl 187):71–7.
89. Moss SF, Legon S, Bishop AE, Polak JM, Culane J. Effect of *Helicobacter pylori* on gastric somatostatin in duodenal ulcer disease. Lancet 1992; 340:930–2.
90. Rauws EAJ, Langenberg W, Houthoff HJ, Zanen HC, Tytgat GNJ. *Camolybacter pyloridis*-associated chronic active antral gastritis. A prospective study of its prevalence and the effect of antibacterial and antiulcer treatment. Gastroenterology 1988; 94:33–40.
91. Robert ME, Weinstein WM. *Helicobacter pylori* associated gastric pathology. Gastroenterol Clin Nor Am 1993; 59–72.
92. Meiselman MS, Miller-Catchpole R, Christ M, Randall E. *Campylobacter pylori* gastritis in the acquired immunodeficiency syndrome. Gastroenterology 1988; 95:209–12.
93. Craig PM, Territo MC, Karnes WE, Walsh JH. *Helicobacter pylori* secretes a chemotactic factor for monocytes and neutrophils. Gut 1993; 33:1020–3.
94. Crabtree JE, Wyatt JI, Trejdosiewicz LK, Peichl P, Nichols PH, Ramsay N, Primrose JN, Lindley IJ. Interleukin-8 expression in *Helicobacter pylori* infected, normal, and neoplastic gastroduodenal mucosa. J Clin Pathol 1994; 47:61–6.
95. Crabtree JE, Farmery SM, Linley IJ, Figura N, Peichl P, Tompkins DS. CagA/ cytotoxic strains of *Helicobacter pylori* and interleukin-8 in gastric epithelial cell lines. J Clin Path 1994; 47:945–50.
96. McKinley AW, Young A, Russell RJ, Gemmell CG. Opsonic requirements of *Helicobacter pylori*. J Med Microbiol 1993; 38:209–15.
97. Hazell SL, Evans KJ, Graham DY. *Helicobacter pylori* catalase. J Gen Microbiol 1991; 137:57–61.
98. Fan XJ, Chua A, Shabi CN, McDewitt J, Keeling PWN, Kelleher D. Gastric T

lymphocyte responses to *Helicobacter pylori* in patients with *H. pylori* colonisation. Gut 1994; 35:1379–84.

99. Peura DA. *Helicobacter pylori*: A diagnostic dilemma and a dilemma of diagnosis. Gastroenterology 1995; 109:313–5.
100. Montgomery EA, Martin DF, Peura DA. Rapid diagnosis of *Campylobacter pylori* by Gram's stain. Am J Clin Pathol 1988; 90:606–9.
101. Rocha GA, Queiroz DM, Mendes EN, Lage AP, Barbosa AJ. Simple carbolfuchsin staining for showing *C. pylori* and other spiral bacteria in gastric mucosa [letter]. J Clin Pathol 1989; 42:1004–5.
102. Walters LL, Budin RE, Paull G. Acridine-orange to identify *Campylobacter pyloridis* in formalin fixed paraffin-imbedded gastric biopsies [letter]. Lancet 1986; i:42.
103. Madan E, Kemp J, Westblom TU, Subik M, Sexton S, Cook J. Evaluation of staining methods for identifying *Campylobacter pylori*. Am J Clin Pathol 1988; 90:450–3.
104. Hazell SL, Hennessy WB, Borody TJ, Carrick J, Ralston M, Brady L, Lee A. *Campylobacter pyloridis* gastritis II: Distribution of bacteria and associated inflammation in the gastroduodenal environment. Am J Gastroenterol 1987; 82:297–301.
105. Kolts BE, Joseph B, Achem SR, Bianchi T, Monteiro C. *Helicobacter pylori* detection: a quality and cost analysis. Am J Gastroenterol 1993; 88:650–5.
106. Carr H, Estrin H, Hupertz V, Czinn S. Inhibitory effects of topical anesthetic agents on *Campylobacter pyloridis* culture results. Gastroenterology 1987; 92:A1338.
107. McNulty CAM, Wise R. Rapid diagnosis of campylobacter-associated gastrits. Lancet 1985; i:1443–4.
108. Marshall BJ, Warren JR, Francis GJ, Langton SR, Goodwin CS, Blincow ED. Rapid urease test in the management of *Campylobacter pyloridis*-associated gastritis. Am J Gastroenterol 1987; 82:200–10.
109. Cutler AF, Havstad S, Ma CK, Blaser MJ, Perez-Perez GI, Schubert TT. Accuracy of invasive and noninvasive tests to diagnose *Helicobacter pylori* infection. Gastroenterology 1995; 109:136–41.
110. Weil J, Bell GD, Powell K, Morden A, Harrison G, Gant PW, Jones PH, Trowell JE. Omeprazole and *Helicobacter pylori*: Temporary suppression rather than true eradication. Aliment Pharmacol Ther 1991; 5:309–13.
111. Graham DY, Klein PD, Evans DJ, Evand DG, Alpert LC. Opekun AR, Boutton TW. *Campylobacter pylori* detected noninvasively byu the 13C -urea breath test. Lancet 1987; i:1174–7.
112. Bell GD, Weil J, Harrison G, Morden A, Jones PH, Gant PW, Trowell JE, Yoong AK, Daneshmend TK, Logan RFA. 14C-Urea breath test analysis, a non-invasive test for *Campylobacter pylori* in the stomach. Lancet 1987; i:1367–8.
113. Brown KE, Peura DS. Diagnosis of *Helicobacter pylori* infection. Gastro Clin Nor Am 1993; 22:105–15.

114. Marshall BJ, Plankey MW, Hoffman SR, Boyd Cl, Dye KR, Frierson HR, Guerrant RL, McCallum RW. A 20-minute breath test for *Helicobacter pylori*. Am J Gastroenterol 1991; 86:438–45.
115. Duckworth C, Locke C, Peura D. Does the C14 urea breath test need to be done fasting? Gastroenterology 1995; 108:A85.
116. Slomianski A, Schubert T, Cutler Af. {^{13}C}urea breath test to confirm eradication of *Helicobacter pylori*. Am J Gastroenterol 1995; 90:22426.
117. Rocha GA, Queiroz DM, Mendes EN, de Carvalho AS, de Oliveira AM, de Moura SB. Serodiagnosis of *Helicobacter pylori* infection in children by an indirect immunofluorescence test. J Ped Gastroenterol Nutr 1993; 16:247–51.
118. Marshall BJ, McGechie DB, Francis GJ, Utley PJ. Pyloric campylobacter serology [letter]. Lancet 1984; ii:281.
119. Goossens H, Glupczynski Y, Burette A, Van den Borre C, DePrez C, Bodenmann J, Keller A, Butzler JP. Evaluation of a commercially available complement fixation test for diagnosis of Helicobacter pylori infection and for follow-up after antimicrobial therapy. J Clin Microbiol 1992; 30:3230–3.
120. Jones DM, Eldridge J, Fox AJ, Sethi P, Whorwell PJ. Antibody to the gastric campylobacter-like organism (*"Campylobacter pyloridis"*)-clinical correlations and distribution in the normal population. J Med Microbiol 1986; 22:57-62.
121. Perez-Perez, GI, Dworkin BM, Chodos JE, Blaser MJ. *Campylobacter pylori* antibodies in humans. Ann Intern Med 1988; 109:11–7.
122. Rathbone BJ, Wyatt JI, Worsely BW, Shires SE, Trejdosiewicz LK, Heatley RV, Losowsky MS. Systemic and local antibody responses to gastric *Campylobacter pyloridis* in non-ulcer dyspepsia. Gut 1986; 27:642–7.
123. Hirschl Am, Brandstätter G, Dragosics B, Hentschel E, Kundi M, Rotter ML, Schütze K, Taufer M. Kinetics of specific IgG antibodies for monitoring the effect of anti-*Helicobacter pylori* chemotherapy. J Infect Dis 1993; 168:763–6.
124. Kosunen TR, Seppälä K, Sarna S, Sipponen P. Diagnostic value of decreasing IgG, IgA, and IgM antibody titers after eradication of *Helicobacter pylori*. Lancet 1992; 339:893–5.
125. Cognein P, Costa A, Giacosa A. Serodiagnosis of *Helicobacter pylori*: evaluation of a rapid, miniaturized immunochromatographic test. Eur J Cancer Prev 1994; 3:457–63.
126. Gear MWL, Truelove SC, Whitehead R. Gastric ulcer and gastritis. Gut 1971; 12:639–45.
127. Martin DF, Hollanders D, May SJ, Ravenscroft MM, Tweedle DEF, Miller JP. Difference in relapse rates of duodenal ulcer after healing with cimetidine or tripotassium dicitrate bismuthate. Lancet 1981; i:7–10.
128. Ormand JE, Talley NJ, Shorter RG, Conley CR, Carpenter HA, Fich A, Wilson WR, Phillips SF. Prevalence of *Helicobacter pylori* in specific forms of gastritis. Further evidence supporting a pathogenic role for *H. pylori* in chronic nonspecific gastritis. Dig Dis Sci 1991; 36:142–5.
129. Marshall BF, Armstrong JA, McGechie DB, Glancy RJ. Attempt to fulfill Koch's postulates for pyloric campylobacter. Med J Aust 1985; 142:436–9.

130. Morris A, Nicholson G. Ingestion of *Campylobacter pyloridis* causes gastritis and raised fasting gastric pH. Am J Gastroenterol 1987; 82:192–9.
131. Morris AJ, Ali MR, Nicholson GI, Perez-Perez GI, Blaser MJ. Long term follow-up of voluntary ingestion of *Helicobacter pylori*. Ann Intern Med 1991; 114;662–3.
132. McNulty CAM, Gearty JC, Crump B, Davis M, Donovan IA, Melikian V, Lister DM, Wise R. *Campylobacter pyloridis* and associated gastritis: Investigator blind, placebo controlled trial of bismuth salicylate and erythromycin ethylsuccinate. BMJ 1986; 293:645–9.
133. Martin DF, Montgomery E, Dobek AS, Patrissi GA, Peura DA. *Campylobacter pylori*, NSAIDs, and smoking: risk factors for peptic ulcer disease. Am J Gastroenterol 1989; 84:1268–72.
134. Sonnenberg A, Townsend WF. Testing for *Helicobacter pylori* in the diagnosis of Zollinger-Ellison syndrome. Am J Gastroenterol 1991; 86:606–8.
135. Tytgat GNJ, Noach LA, Rauws EAJ. *Helicobacter pylori* infection and duodenal ulcer disease. Gastro Clin Nor Am 1993; 22:127–39.
136. Freston JW. H_2 receptor antagonists and duodenal ulcer recurrence: analysis of efficacy and commentary on safety, costs, and patient selection. Am J Gastroenterol 1987; 82:1242–9.
137. Graham DY, Lew GM, Klein PD, Evans DG, Evans DJ, Saeed ZA, Malaty HM. Effect of treatment of *Helicobacter pylori* infection on the long-term recurrence of gastric or duodenal ulcer. Ann Intern Med 1992; 116:705–8.
138. Hentschel E, Brandstätter G, Dragosics B, Hirschl AM, Nemec H, Schütze K, Taufer M, Wurzer H. Effect of ranitidine and amoxicillin plus metronidazole on the eradication of *Helicobacter pylori* and the recurrence of duodenal ulcer. N Engl J Med 1993; 328:308–12.
139. Rokkas T, Karameris A, Mavrogeorgis A, Rallis E, Giannikos N. Eradication of *Helicobacter pylori* reduces the possibility of rebleeding in peptic ulcer disease. Gastrointest Endosc 1995; 41:1–4.
140. Jaspersen D, Koerner T, Schorr W, Brennenstuhl M, Raschka C, Hammar C-H. *Helicobacter pylori* eradication reduces the rate of rebleeding in ulcer hemorrhage. Gastrointest Endosc 1995; 41:5–7.
141. Xia H-X, Gilvarry J, Beattie S, Hamilton H, Keane CT, Sweeney EC, O'Morain CA. Recrudescence of *Helicobacter pylori* infection in patients with healed duodenal ulcer after treatment with different regimens. Am J Gastroenterol 1995; 90:1221–5.
142. Bayerdörffer E, Mannes GA, Höchter W, Weingart J, Sommer A, Klann H, Heldwein W, Hatz R, Simon T, Eimiller A, Bolle F, Miehlke S, Bastlein E, Ruckdeschel G, Lehn N, Stolte M. Antibacterial treatment of gastric ulcers—German gastric ulcer study. Gastroenterology 1993; 104:A40.
143. Graham DY, Lidsky MD, Cox AM, Evans DJ, Evans DG, Alpert L, Klein PD, Sessoms SL, Michaletz PA, Saeed ZA. Long term nonsteroidal antiinflammatory drug use and *Helicobacter pylori* infection. Gastroenterology 1991; 100:1653–7.
144. Talley NJ. A critique of therapeutic trials in *Helicobacter pylori*-positive functional dyspepsia. Gastroenterology 1994; 106:1174–83.

145. Talley NJ. The role of *Helicobacter pylori* in nonulcer dyspepsia. A debate—against. Gastroenterol Clin Nor Am 1993; 22:153–67.
146. Forman D, Newell DG, Fullerton F, Yarnell JW, Stacey AR, Wald N, Sitas F. Association between infection with *Helicobacter pylori* and risk of gastric cancer: evidence from a prospective investigation. Br Med J 1991; 302:1302–5.
147. Parsonnet J, Friedman GD, Vandersteen DP, Chang Y, Vogelman JH, Orentreich N, Sibley RK. *Helicobacter pylori* infection and the risk of gastric carcinoma. N Engl J Med. 1991; 325:1127–31.
148. Nomura A, Stemmermann GN, Chyou PH, Kato I, Perez–Perez GI, Blaser MJ. *Helicobacter pylori* infection and gastric carcinoma among Japanese Americans in Hawaii. N Engl J Med 1991; 325:1132–6.
149. Wotherspoon C, Ortiz–Hidalgo C, Falzon MR, Isaacson PG. *Helicobacter pylori*–associated gastritis and primary B–cell gastric lymphoma. Lancet 1991; 338:1175–6.
150. Roggero E, Zucca E, Pinotti G, Pascarella A, Capella C, Savio A, Pedrinis E, Paterlini A, Venco A, Cavalli F. Eradication of *Helicobacter pylori* infection in primary low–grade gastric lymphoma of mucosa–associated lymphoid tissue. Ann Intern Med 1995; 122:767–9.
151. Parsonnet J, Hansen S, Rodriguez L, Gelb AB, Warnke RA, Jellum E, Orentreich N, Vogelman JH, Friedman GD. *Helicobacter pylori* infection and gastric lymphoma. N Engl J Med 1994; 330:1267–71.
152. Blaser MJ, Perez-Perez GI, Kleanthous H, Cover TL, Peek RM, Chyou PH, Stemmemann GN, Nomura A. Infection with *Helicobacter pylori* strains possessing cagA is associated with an increased risk of developing adenocarcinoma of the stomach. Cancer Research 1995; 55:2111–5.
153. *Helicobacter pylori* in peptic ulcer disease. NIH Consens Statement 1994; 12:1–22.
154. Petersen WL. Recurrent ulcers revisited: When to eradicate *Helicobacter pylori*. Gastrointestinal Diseases Today 1993; 2:8.
155. Tytgat GNJ. Review article: treatments that impact favourably upon the eradication of *Helicobacter pylori* and ulcer recurrence. Aliment Pharmacol Ther 1994; 8:359–68.
156. Marshall BJ. Treatment strategies for *Helicobacter pylori* infection. Gastro Clin Nor Am 1993; 22:183–98.
157. McNulty CAM, Gearty JC, Crump B, Davis M, Donovan IA, Melikian V, Lister DM, Wise R. *Campylobacter pyloridis* and associated gastritis: Investigator–blind placebo–controlled trial of bismuth salicylate and erythromycin ethylsuccinate. Br Med J 1986; 293:645–9.
158. Goodwin CS, Armstrong JA. Microbiological aspects of *Helicobacter pylori* (*Campylobacter pylori*). Eur J Clin Microbiol Infect Dis 1990; 9:1–13.
159. Wang Y, Roos KP, Taylor DE. Transformation of *Helicobacter pylori* by chromosomal metronidazole resistance and by a plasmid with a selectable chloramphenicol resistance marker. J Gen Microbiol 1993; 139:2485–93.

160. European Study Group on Antibiotic Susceptibility of *Helicobacter pylori*. Results of a multicentre European survey in 1991 of metronidazole resistance in *Helicobacter pylori*. Eur J Clin Microbiol Infect Dis 1992; 11:777–81.
161. Banatvala N, Davies GR, Abdi Y, Clements L, Rampton DS, Hardie JM, Feldman RA. High prevalence of *Helicobacter pylori* metronidazole resistance in migrants to east London: relation with previous nitroimidazole exposure and gastroduodenal disease. Gut 1994; 35:1562–6.
162. Penston JG. Review article: *Helicobacter pylori* eradication-understandable caution but no excuse for inertia. Aliment Pharmacol Ther 194; 8:369–89.
163. Graham DY, Lew GM, Malaty HM, Evans DG, Evans DJ, Klein PD, Alpert CC, Genta RM. Factors influencing the eradication of *Helicobacter pylori* with triple therapy. Gastroenterology 1992; 102:493–6.
164. Cutler AF, Schubert TT. Patient factors affecting *Helicobacter pylori* eradication with triple therapy. Am J Gastroenterol 1993; 88:505–9.
165. Chiba N, Rao BV, Rademaker JW, Hunt RH. Meta-analysis of the efficacy of antibiotic therapy in eradicating *Helicobacter pylori*. Am J Gastroenterol 1992; 87:1716–27.
166. Peterson WL, Graham DY, Marshall BJ, Blaser MJ, Genta RM, Klein PD, Stratton CW, Dmec J, Prokocimer P, Siepman N. Clarithromycin as monotherapy for eradication of *Helicobacter pylori*: A randomized, double-blind trial. Am J Gastro 1993; 88:1860–4.
167. Unge P, Gad A, Gnarpe H, Olsson J. Does omeprazole improve antimicrobial therapy directed towards gastric *Campylobacter pylori* in patients with antral gastritis? A pilot study. Scand J Gastroenterol 1989; 24(suppl 167):49-54.
168. Axon ATR. The role of acid inhibition in the treatment of *Helicobacter pylori* infection. Scand J Gastroenterol 1994; 29(Suppl 201):16–23.
169. Hunt RH. pH and HP—Gastric acid suppression and *Helicobacter pylori*: Implications for ulcer healing and eradication of the organism. Am J Gastroenterol 1993; 88:481–3.
170. Melchers K, Weitzenegger T, Steinhiller W, Sachs G, Schäfer KP. A novel P type ATPase cloned from *Helicobacter pylori*. Gastroenterology 1994; 109:A165.
171. Bayerdörffer E, Mannes GA, Sommer A, Höchter W, Weingart J, Hatz R, Lehn N, Ruckdeschel G, Dirschedl P, Stolte M. Long–term follow–up after eradication of *Helicobacter pylori* with combination of omeprazole and amoxycillin. Scand J Gastroenterol 1993; S196:19-25.
172. Labenz J, Gyenes E, Ruhl GH, Börsch G. Amoxicillin plus omeprazole *versus* triple therapy for eradication of *Helicobacter pylori* in duodenal ulcer disease: a prospective, randomized, and controlled study. Gut 1993; 34:1167–70.
173. Labenz J, Gyenes E, Ruhl GH, Borsch G. Omeprazole plus amoxicillin: efficacy of various treatment regimens to eradicate *Helicobacter pylori*. Am J Gastroenterol 1993; 88:491–5.
174. Logan RPH, Gummett PA, Hegarty BT, Walker MM, Baron JH, Misiewicz JJ. Clarithromycin and omeprazole for *Helicobacter pylori* [Letter]. Lancet 1992; 340:239.

175. Logan RPH, Gummett PA, Schaufelberger HD, Greaves RRFH, Mendelson GM, Walker MM, Thomas PH, Baron JH, Misiewicz JJ. Eradication of *Helicobacter pylori* with clarithromycin and omeprazole. Gut 1994; 34:323–6.
176. Bayerdörffer E, Miehlke S, Mannes GA, Sommer A, Höchter W, Weingart J, Heldwein W, Klann H, Simon T, Schmit W, Bästlein E, Eimiller A, Hatz R, Lehn N, Dischedl P, Stolte M. Double-blind trial of omeprazole and amoxicillin to cure *Helicobacter pylori* infection in patients with duodenal ulcers. Gastroenterology 1995; 108:1412–7.
177. Goodwin CS, Marshall BJ, Blincow ED, Wilson DH, Blackbourn S, Phillips M. Prevention of nitroimidazole resistance in *Campylobacter pylori* by co-administration of colloidal bismuth subcitrate: Clinical and in vitro studies. J Clin Pathol 1988; 41:207–10.
178. al Assi MT, Ramirez FC, Lew GM, Genta RM, Graham DY. Clarithromycin, tetracycline, and bismuth: a new non-metronidazole therapy for *Helicobacter pylori* infection. Am J Gastroenterol 1994; 84:1203–5.
179. de Boer WA, Driessen WM, Potters HVPJ, Tytgat GNJ. Randomized study comparing 1 with 2 weeks of quadruple therapy for eradicating *Helicobacter pylori*. Am J Gastroenterol 1994; 89:1993–7.
180. de Boer W, Driessen W, Jansz A, Tytgat G. Effect of acid suppression on efficacy of treatment for *Helicobacter pylori* infection. Lancet 1995; 345:817–20.
181. Bell GD, Powell KU, Burridge SM, Bowden AF, Atoyebi W, Bolton GH, Jones PH, Brown C. Rapid eradication of *Helicobacter pylori* infection. Aliment Pharmacol Ther 1995; 9:41–6.
182. Labenz J, Stolte M, Ruhl GH, Becker T. Tillenburg B, Sollbohmer M, Borsch G. One-week low-dose triple therapy for the eradication of *Helicobacter pylori* infection. Eur J Gastroenterol Hepatol 1995; 7:9–11.
183. Doidge C, Gust I, Lee A, Buck F, Hazell S, Manne U. Therapeutic immunisation against Helicobacter infection. Lancet 1994; i:914–5.
184. Michetti P, Corthesy–Theulaz I, Davin C, Haas R, Vaney AC, Heitz M, Bille J, Kraehenbuhl JP, Saraga E, Blum AL. Immunization of BALB/c mice against Helicobacter felis infection with Helicobacter pylori urease. Gastroenterology 1994; 107:1002–11.
185. Hulten K, Han SW, Enroth H, Klein PD, Opekun AR, Gilman RH, Evans DG, Engstrang L, Graham DY, El-Zaatari FAK. *Helicobacter pylori* in the drinking water in Peru. Gastroenterology 1996; 110:1031–1035.
186. Peura DA, pambianco DJ, Dye KR, Lind C, Frierson HF, Hoffman SR, Combs MJ, Guilfoyle E, Marshall BJ. Microdose ^{14}C-urea breath test offers diagnosis of *Helicobacter pylori* in 10 minutes. Am J Gastroenterol 1996; 91:233–8.
187. Graham DY, Evans DJ, Peacock J, Baker JT, Schrier WH. Comparison of rapid serological tests (FlexSureHP and QuickVue) with conventional ELISA for detection of *Helicobacter pylori* infection. Am J Gastroenterol 1996; 91:942–8.
188. Kuipers EJ, Lundell L, Klinkenberg-Knol EC, Havu N, Festen HPM, Leidman B, Lamers CBHW, Jansen JB, Dalenbäck J, Snel P, Nelis GF, Meuwissen SGM. Atrophic gastritis and *Helicobacter pylori* infection in patients with reflux esoph-

agitis treated with omeprazole or fundoplication. N Engl J Med 1996; 334:1018–22.

189. Kuipers EJ, Uyterlinde AM, Peña AS, et al. Increase of *Helicobacter pylori*-associated corpus gastritis during acid suppressive therapy: implications for long-term safety. Am J Gastroenterol 1995; 90:1401–6.

3

Viral Gastroenteritis

DORSEY M. BASS
Stanford University School of Medicine, Stanford, California

I. INTRODUCTION

As the largest mucosal surface and the largest lymphoid organ in the body, the intestinal tract is fertile ground for viral replication. Fortunately, most enteric viruses fail to cause significant disease in the intestine. Some such as polio virus and other enteroviruses replicate locally but disseminate to cause disease in other organs; others such as reoviruses and perhaps picobirnaviruses do not cause any known human pathology. This chapter describes viruses which do cause local pathology and result in gastroenteritis in humans.

Viral gastroenteritis is a major health problem in both developing and developed countries. A large 10-year study of illnesses in Cleveland showed that the number of physician visits for nonbacterial gastroenteritis was second only to the common cold (1). In the United States, each year rotavirus alone accounts for 3.5 million infections, 100 thousand hospitalizations, and a total economic cost of nearly 1 billion dollars (2). In the developing world, figures for cost and hospitalization have less meaning, but rotavirus accounts for 130 million infections and nearly 1 million deaths each year (2).

A great deal has been learned about these ubiquitous and important pathogens over the past two decades. Although viral agents of diarrhea had long been suspected, the tissue culture methods of isolating viruses pioneered by Enders and other failed to isolate any true gastroenteritis viruses. The first positive identification of an agent of viral gastroenteritis was the observation of Norwalk virus particles ins tool by electron microscopy in 1972 (3). Soon thereafter, rotavirus was observed by Bishop et al. in duodenal biopsies of children with acute gastroenteritis (4). A number of observers confirmed, with electron microscopy, that large numbers of rotavirus particles were present in stools of young children with gastroenteritis. Later, the use of appropriate cell lines and the inclusion of trypsin in tissue culture media led to the successful cultivation of rotavirus, enteric adenoviruses, and astrovirus. Some important human agents of viral gastroenteritis such as Norwalk virus and related caliciviruses have proven extremely fastidious and have not yet been cultivated in tissue culture. The advent of newer techniques such as monoclonal antibodies, molecular cloning , and molecular expression systems have led to an explosion in our knowledge about all of the gastroenteritis viruses. Four major groups of viruses cause diarrheal disease in humans: rotaviruses, astroviruses, enteric adenoviruses (serotypes 40 and 41), and caliciviruses including Norwalk virus.

II. AGENTS (TABLE 1)

A. Rotavirus

Rotaviruses are the single most common cause of severe dehydrating diarrhea in infants and young children throughout the world. Virtually all children are infected in the first few years of life.

1. Structure

The rotavirus virion is an icosahedron made up of 3 layers of protein that enclose a double-stranded, segmented RNA genome. The particle is about 100 nm in diameter when examined in a hydrated state by cryoelectron microscopy (5). Older reports using traditional heavy-metal negative staining techniques reported the diameter to be approximately 70–80 nm. The technique of cryoelectron microscopy has been used in conjunction with computer image enhancement to provide strikingly detailed topographic views of rotavirus particles (Figure 1) (5). The outer capsid is made up of two proteins. The glycoprotein, VP7, is the more abundant of the two and is responsible for the smooth outer surface of the virion. The spike-like projections from the smooth surface are multimers of VP4. Also evident in these enhanced cryoelectron micrographs are surface pores that extend through all three capsid layers and may be the pathway for viral mRNA to exit the transcriptional complex. Both viral outer capsid proteins, VP4 and VP7, elicit neutralizing antibodies. The protein VP4 is the viral hemagglutinin and is probably the viral protein that mediates viral attachment to intestinal epithelial cells. Cleavage of VP4 by trypsin into two smaller peptides, VP5* and VP8*, is essential for efficient entry of rotavirus into cells.

Table 1 Important Agents of Viral Gastroenteritis

Virus	Virologic Features	Clinical and Epidemiology	Diagnostic Tests
Group A Rotavirus	80 nm, segmented double-stranded RNA genome, grows in tissue culture	Major cause dehydrating diarrhea in infants throughout the world.	EIA (commercial EM Polyacrylamide gel electrophoresis
Astrovirus	34 nm, single-stranded RNA genome, grows in tissue culture	Common cause of milder diarrhea, mainly in infants.	EIA (research) EM
Norwalk and related caliciviruses	27–32 nm, single-stranded RNA, does not grow in tissue culture	Acute vomiting and diarrhea for 1–2 days, often in outbreaks in older children and adults. May also cause infantile diarrhea.	EIA (research for Norwalk genogroup) Immuno-electron microscopy
Enteric adenovirus	80 nm, double-stranded DNA, grows in tissue culture	Prolonged diarrhea (6–12 days) in infants and young children.	EIA (commercial) EM

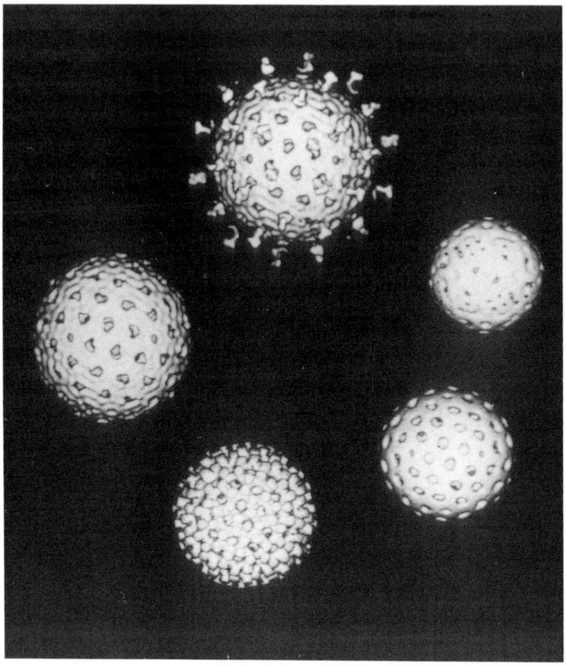

Figure 1 Three-dimensional structure of rhesus monkey rotavirus by cryoelectron microscopy. The structures are from the top, counter-clockwise (a) complete double-shelled, infectious particle with 60 surface spikes consisting of VP4; (b) the smooth outer surface made up of VP7 with the perforating channels that extend to the core; (c) the inner capsid made up of VP6 trimers; d) the base of the VP6 trimers perforated by the channels in register with the outer shell; (e) the innermost protein shell, the core, consisting of VP1, VP2, and VP3, which contains the RNA genome (courtesy Dr. M. Yeager).

The VP7 protein is the determinant of the traditional serotype although more recently an additional serotyping system for VP4 has been proposed.

The inner capsid of rotavirus consists of multimeric VP6, the group and subgroup antigen that is detected in many rotavirus stool-detection immunoassays.

The core of rotavirus particles consists of VP1, VP2, and VP3 as well as 11 segments of double-stranded RNA. Each segment of RNA encodes one viral protein with the exception of segment 11, which encodes two peptides. Because of the segmented genome, rotaviruses reassort readily in cells infected with different viral parents. This phenomena may allow rapid "shifts" in antigenicity of rotaviruses and has been exploited by virologists for the study of functional assessment of viral genes. Reassortment has also been employed in vaccine development (see below). The segmented genome also provides a tool for diagnosis and epidemiologic study in that each strain of rotavirus has its own pattern of genomic RNA migration on acrylamide electrophoresis.

2. *Epidemiology*

Group A rotavirus accounts for the vast majority of human disease although outbreaks and sporadic cases of Group B and C disease are reported. It should be noted that the commonly used immunoassays detect only Group A. Rotavirus strains are further classified by subgroup and by serotype. While more than 10 human serotypes have been described, serotypes 1–4 account for the bulk of human disease.

While rotavirus infection may occur at any age, serious disease occurs mainly in children aged 3 to 24 months. Disease in older patients can occur after intense exposure (household contacts), in travelers, and after exposure to unusual strains such as Group B viruses. The primary infection in infancy is often severe, while subsequent infections tend to be mild or inapparent. Transmission of rotavirus infection is by the fecal-oral route. The efficiency of rotavirus spread through populations (including those with high sanitary standards) is probably due to the very low infectious dose (perhaps as low as a single virion) and the impressive environmental stability of the virus particle. Viable virus can be recovered from contaminated surfaces for months to years.

In temperate climates, the peak incidence of rotavirus disease occurs during the winter (6). In the United States, the peak incidence of rotavirus spreads from the Southwest in November to the Northeast in March (7). This is not due to a single dominant strain as is seen with influenza.

Rotavirus strains vary considerably from community to community and year to year. Usually several minor strains co-circulate with one dominant strain. All of the serotypes are equally virulent. Rotaviruses are host-specific, thus animal strains are avirulent in humans. This fact has been exploited in the so-called "Jennerian" approach to rotavirus vaccine development (8).

3. *Pathophysiology and Pathology*

Rotaviruses enter the host via the fecal-oral route. Stomach acid and pepsin are capable of greatly reducing the infectivity of rotaviruses (9). In the small intestine trypsin cleaves the outer capsid "spike" protein, VP4, which facilitates viral penetration. The virus binds and enters the cytoplasm of mature villus enterocytes where the low calcium concentration leads to the loss of the outer capsid (10,11). Transcription, translation, and replication proceed leading to cell death in 10–14 hours with release of thousands of progeny virions. These are in turn activated by intestinal lumenal trypsin and rapidly infect more mature villus enterocytes. Meanwhile crypt cells rapidly proliferate so that immature transitional-type epithelial cells cover the villi.

The resultant histopathological picture consists of shortened villi, intact crypts, and a mild round-cell infiltration in the lamina propria (12–14). The immature villus epithelial cells may appear cuboidal with poorly developed microvilli. The pathologic changes tend to progress distally from the duodenum so that duodenal biopsies taken later in the process may be normal. Animal studies suggest that clinical symptoms do not begin until the histologic changes are fairly well advanced. In one human study, histopathology of the proximal intestine bore no relation to severity of disease (15).

The biochemical correlates of these changes in the intestinal epithelium include decreased dissacharidase levels (particularly lactase), decreased sodium–potassium ATPase, decreased alkaline phosphotase, and an increase in markers for immature cells such as thymidine kinase (12,16).

Rotaviruses cause diarrhea as a result of their rather strict tissue tropism. They replicate only in villus enterocytes in the small intestine, sparing crypt enterocytes and under normal conditions, not disseminating to other organs. Diarrhea in rotavirus infection is probably multifactorial. The selective loss of mature absorptive villus enterocytes and the preservation of secretory crypt cells leads to net secretion of water and solute. Loss of disacharidases such as lactase leads to an osmotic drag of fluid into the intestinal lumen. Other factors such as cytokines could play a role in the pathophysiology of this disease. One report associated systemic interferon levels with vomiting in rotavirus gastroenteritis (17) while another found elevated prostaglandin levels in stool and blood (18).

4. Clinical Manifestations

The incubation period for rotavirus disease is 2 to 3 days. This is followed by the onset of fever, vomiting, and diarrhea. Fever and vomiting usually subside after the initial 24–48 hours but diarrhea commonly persists for four to eight days. When compared with other diarrheal illnesses, rotavirus gastroenteritis was more likely to be associated with vomiting and dehydration (19). Although most cases cause mild to moderate dehydration, rotavirus gastroenteritis can be fulminant with rapid dehydration and shock. Laboratory manifestations of rotavirus infection include metabolic acidosis, elevation of blood urea nitrogen, and mild transient elevation of transaminases. In immunologically intact individuals, subsequent infections tend to have much milder clinical manifestations.

Persistent disease can occur in immunocompromised patients with dissemination to liver and kidney (20,21). Some reports have linked nursery rotavirus outbreaks to epidemics of necrotizing enterocolitis.

B. Astrovirus

Astroviruses were originally characterized by their distinct appearance under the electron microscope. They contain a five- or six-pointed star. Until fairly recently, electron microscopy was the only method of diagnosing astrovirus.

1. Structure

The viral particles are small, approximately 33 nm icosahedral virions containing a single-stranded RNA genome of about 7.8 kb. The viral genome has been completely sequenced (22,23) and based on the genomic structure, astroviruses have been assigned their own family, Astroviridiae. The viral capsid consists of at least three proteins that are cleavage products of a 90 kd precursor. There are currently 7 human serotypes and all have been adapted to tissue culture using rather high amounts of trypsin (5–10 μg/mL).

2. Epidemiology

With the recent development of convenient enzyme immunoassays (24) it has become clear that throughout the world astrovirus is a very common agent of viral gastroenteritis, particularly among infants and young children (25). After rotavirus, it is probably the second most common pediatric gastroenteritis virus. Nosocomial and daycare outbreaks are common. Like rotavirus, astrovirus gastroenteritis occurs more commonly in the colder months in temperate climates. Outbreaks have also been described among elderly nursing home residents (26). In recent studies astrovirus was found in the stools of HIV infected adults (27) and in bone marrow transplant recipients (28) with diarrhea. Some large outbreaks among older children and young adults, reminiscent of Norwalk virus outbreaks, have also been recently reported (29).

3. Pathology and Pathogenesis

Pathogenesis of astrovirus in humans is not well studied. In lamb astrovirus, infection leads to a histologic picture similar to rotavirus, featuring loss of mature villus cells, crypt hypertrophy, and mild round-cell infiltration (30). Immunohistochemical studies show viral antigen to be present only in upper villus enterocytes. In ducklings, astrovirus causes a severe hepatitis.

4. Clinical Manifestations

Astrovirus diarrhea seems to be similar to but somewhat milder than rotavirus diarrhea. Thus hospital-based studies find lower incidences than do outpatient studies. After a 24–72 hour incubation the illness begins with vomiting, mild watery diarrhea, and low-grade fever. Illness typically lasts 3–4 days in normal individuals but may lead to lactose intolerance for several weeks.

C. *Norwalk Virus and Other Caliciviruses*

Norwalk virus was first discovered by Kapikian et al. by examining stools by electron microscopy from a gastroenteritis outbreak in an elementary school in Norwalk , Ohio (3). This outbreak involved 50% of students and teachers and spread to 32% of the victim's household contacts. A number of similar agents were subsequently described and usually named for the geographic local of the initial outbreaks (Snow Mountain agent, Hawaii agent, Southhampton agent). Some of these appeared to be related antigenically to Norwalk and others did not. Description and classification of Norwalk and related small round viruses was extremely tedious initially because diagnostic reagents consisted of stools and sera from infected volunteers. These viruses have never been cultivated in tissue culture.

In 1990 Jiang and co-workers molecularly cloned the genome of Norwalk virus from volunteer-study stools (31). This led to the development of expression of the Norwalk capsid protein via a baculovirus vector in insect cells (32). The recombinant protein self-assembles into capsid-like particles that now form the basis for a number of assays for Norwalk antigen in stools and Norwalk antibodies in sera. The cloning of the Norwalk genome also allowed Norwalk to be classified as a caliciviruses and allowed a number of other small round viruses to be molecularly categorized using polymerase chain reaction (PCR) amplification from Norwalk-derived primers.

1. *Structure*

Norwalk virus is a 28-nm small round virus that often has rather indistinct morphology when stool samples are examined by electron microscopy. The genome is approximately 7.6 kb, positive-sense single-stranded RNA with three predicted open reading frames. The capsid consists of a single polypeptide with molecular weight of 34 kd. Recombinant-expressed capsids have clear icosahedral symmetry with cuplike surface morphology as seen in nonhuman caliciviruses. The human enteric caliciviruses, including Norwalk virus, have recently been subclassified into 3 genogroups based on predicted amino acid sequence of viral polymerase. The present Enzyme Immunoassay (EIA) test, based on recombinant Norwalk capsid, detects only human caliciviruses that are in the Norwalk genogroup (33).

2. *Epidemiology*

Human caliciviruses are best known for causing water- or food-based explosive outbreaks of vomiting and diarrhea such as the original Norwalk outbreak. Outbreaks occur throughout the year and typically involve school age children and adults. Outbreaks often occur in closed settings such as schools, cruise ships, military bases, camps, and hospitals. Implicated foodstuffs include ice, water, shellfish, cake frosting, salads, and melons. Disease in infancy from non-Norwalk caliciviruses may be more important than previously recognized (34). Further study using PCR and recombinant-expressed proteins will help delineate the true burden of calcivirus gastroenteritis.

3. *Clinical Syndrome*

After an incubation of approximately 48 hours, the typical illness consists of the rapid onset of vomiting and/or diarrhea. Norwalk seems to be associated with vomiting more than the other viral enteritides although histopathologic exam of the stomachs of volunteers shows no abnormalities (35). The illness is relatively mild, intravenous fluids are rarely required, and the duration is typically 24–48 hours. The diarrheal stools are watery and without blood or white blood cells. Recent studies using improved reagents have shown that virus is shed for up to one week after resolution of symptoms and that many volunteers without clinical symptoms shed viral antigen (36).

4. *Pathology and Pathogenesis*

Pathologic studies of volunteers have shown normal gastric and colonic morphology with shortened villi in the proximal small bowel similar to that observed in other viral enteritides (Figure 2).

D. Enteric Adenoviruses

Two serotypes of adenovirus, types 40 and 41, have been associated with gastroenteritis in young children. Although other adenovirus serotypes are commonly identified in stool specimens, only types 40 and 41 are consistently associated with diarrheal illness. These two serotypes do not grow well in tissue-culture systems used for other adenovirus types and have been termed fastidious although they have been propagated in several cell lines such as Graham 293 cells.

1. *Structure*

The virus particles are icosahedral structures with an 80-nm diameter containing a double-stranded DNA genome. Like rotavirus, the adenovirus particles can easily be seen by negative-staining electron microscopy. More than 10^{11} particles per gram stool have been observed in diarrheal stools.

2. *Epidemiology*

Enteric adenoviruses cause diarrhea in young infants throughout the world. More than 90% of symptomatic infections occur in children less than two years of age. There appears to be little seasonal variation in the incidence of adenovirus diarrheas, but there is considerable year-to-year variation (37). For example in an eight-year survey in Washington, DC, the annual percentage of infant diarrheal stools positive for adenovirus ranged from 1.4 to 10.7% (38).

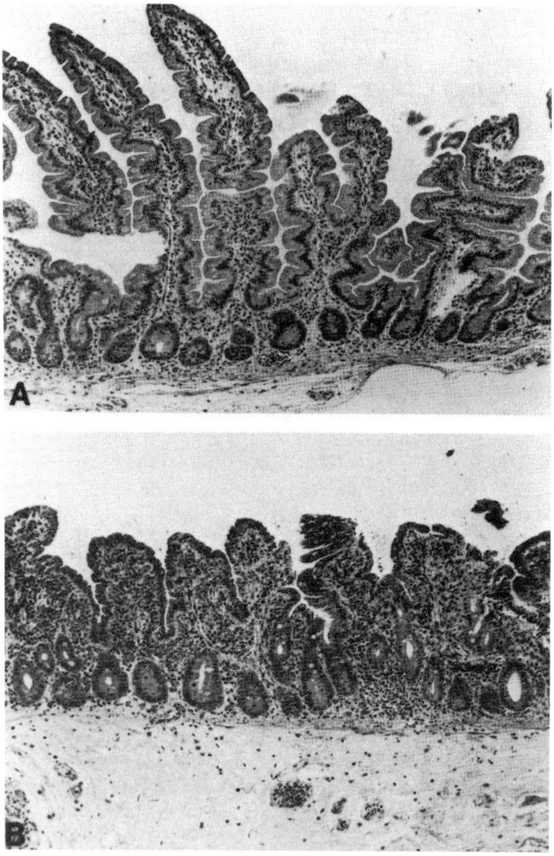

Figure 2 (a) Normal jejunal biopsy from a volunteer prior to experimental infection with Norwalk virus (×100). (b) Jejunal biopsy from the same volunteer after Norwalk infection (×100). (From Ref. 35.)

Enteric adenoviruses cause two the three percent of infantile diarrheal disease in the developing world (25). Adenoviruses of all serotypes are frequently isolated from the stools of patients with acquired immune deficiency syndrome, but the role of these viruses, if any, in diarrheal symptoms is unclear (39).

3. Clinical Manifestations

The clinical illness associated with enteric adenovirus infection is similar to that of rotavirus with two significant exceptions. Fever is less common in adenovirus than rotavirus gastroenteritis. Second, adenovirus causes a longer illness, typically 10–14 days compared to the 5–7 days with rotavirus.

4. *Pathogenesis and Pathology*

Like other agents of viral gastroenteritis, enteric adenoviruses infect epithelial cells of the small intestine. Adenovirus replication is intranuclear in contrast to the cytoplasmic replication of rotavirus, astrovirus, and caliciviruses.

E. Other Putative Agents

A variety of viruses can be found in stools from healthy as well as diseased subects. Enteroviruses such as coxsackie viruses, echo viruses, and polio viruses are not associated with gastroenteritis. Many small particles observed by electron microscopy may be bacteriophage fragments. Coronaviruses are a definite cause of gastroenteritis in animals but their role in human intestinal disease is poorly defined. Picobirnaviruses have been reported in human diarrheal stools (27) but a recent study suggests that they are equally common in healthy controls (40). Toroviruses have also been postulated to be agents of human gastroenteritis (41). It would not be surprising if several more agents of human viral gastroenteritis were described in the next decade.

III. DIAGNOSIS AND DIFFERENTIAL DIAGNOSIS

The vast majority of case of viral gastroenteritis are relatively mild, brief illnesses that can be diagnosed clinically based on history and physical exam. Negative results of stool tests for white blood cells and blood can offer some confirmatory evidence in favor of a viral process. Specific diagnostic tests for viral agents of diarrhea are very important in determining the epidemiology and disease burden of the various agents, in detecting and controlling outbreaks of disease, and in making positive diagnoses in more seriously ill patients. The differential diagnosis of patients with acute diarrhea syndromes includes a large variety of bacterial, parasitic, and toxic agents. Diagnostic tests for viral agents include enzyme-linked immunoassays (EIAs), examination of stools by electron microscopy, isolation of viruses in tissue culture, and stool tests using detection of specific nucleic acid structures or sequences.

A. Electron Microscopy (EM)

For years this was the only method available. It requires expensive equipment and experienced technical personnel. The sensitivity of EM for viruses is poor compared to antibody or nucleic-acid based technology but it can detect novel agents. Sensitivity can be increased by using specific antibody capture methods.

B. Tissue Culture

Stool viruses that grow in tissue culture systems used in hospital diagnostic virology laboratories do not cause diarrhea. Specialized research laboratories can isolate rotaviruses, astroviruses, and enteric adenoviruses from stool specimens but this is again a tedious and expensive process.

C. EIA

Enzyme immunoassays in various formats are generally simple, convenient, and amenable to handling large numbers of samples for large epidemiologic studies. A number of commercial EIAs are available for group A rotaviruses and for enteric adenovirus. They offer approximately 90% sensitivity and specificity and can be performed in a variety of laboratory settings. Enzyme immunoassays for astrovirus (all serotypes) and Norwalk-genogroup caliciviruses are in widespread use for epidemiologic research.

D. Nucleic Acid Detection

The simplest form of a nucleic acid detection system is polyacrylamide electrophoresis of crude extracts of stool to look for double-stranded RNA. Simple protocols usable in field studies int he developing world have been used to detect and categorize rotavirus by segment mobility patterns. Non-group-A rotavirus infections not detectable by EIA and picobirnavirus infections may be detected by this methodology.

The polymerase chain reaction (PCR) and related techniques have revolutionized the detection of viruses in both biologic and environmental samples. Exquisite sensitivity may be obtained in detecting viruses present in very low concentrations or with poorly understood antigenic structure. These analyses are very susceptible to minute contamination and are performed in reference or research laboratories with adequate positive and negative controls. Improving technologies for detecting amplified products will lead to increased clinical use of this technique.

IV. TREATMENT

Generally viral gastroenteritis is a self-limited and mild disease that requires little in the way of specific therapy. The notable exception is rotavirus infection in young children, which can lead to life-threatening dehydration. The goals of therapy of viral enteritis include prevention and treatment of dehydration and the prevention of severe nutritional compromise. Rehydration can usually be achieved using balanced glucose–salt oral rehydration solutions (ORS). These solutions have been shown to be safe and effective alternatives to intravenous fluids in a variety of ages and conditions. While traditional therapy of diarrheal disease has consisted of withholding foods, the ensuing malnutrition actually delays recovery. Current recommendations are for beginning regular feedings as soon as rehydration is complete (usually 6–8 hours). Although biochemical disaccharidase deficiencies are common, most infants do well with their regular diet, including lactose. Breast feeding should be continued during the illness. If an infant is already formula fed, a change to a lactose-free formula in selected cases may be helpful. Restriction of fats or the use of "BRAT" or "ABC" diets have no known benefit.

Drug therapy for viral gastroenteritis in children is ill advised. Opiates and loperimide are generally ineffective and may cause ileus and drowsiness. Likewise phenothiazine antiemetics are generally more likely to cause side effects than benefits in small children and are labeled by their manufacturers as specifically not indicated for children less than three years of age. Pectin-like and psyllium drugs may occasional help the cosmetic appearance of stool but do not change the actual water loss. Lactobacilli, yeast preparations, and bismuth compounds have minor effects on the clinical course of rotavirus disease but do not appear to cause serious side effects.

Some immunocompromised patients with chronic symptomatic rotavirus disease have benefited from enteral administration of immunoglobulin as either commercial intravenous preparations or colostrum with high titers of anti-rotavirus activity (42).

V. PREVENTION

Rotavirus is by far the most clinically important agent of viral gastroenteritis and has been the subject of considerable vaccine development efforts. The most advanced candidate vaccines are animal rotaviruses, which have been reassorted with human strains to express human rotavirus surface proteins (2). These vaccines have been given to hundreds of infants and children and appear to be reasonably safe (43). They require multiple doses and in U.S. trials offered approximately 50% protection for all rotavirus disease and 70% protection from severe disease. One or both of these vaccines could be available within a few years. Unfortunately, most vaccine trials in the developing world, site of the worst morbidity and mortality for rotavirus disease, have been less encouraging.

REFERENCES

1. Dingle JH, Badger FG, Jordan WS. In: Illness in the Home: A Study of 25,000 Illnesses in a Group of Cleveland Families. Cleveland, Ohio: Case Western Reserve University Press, 1964:19–32.

2. Glass RI, Gentsch J, Smith JC. Rotavirus vaccines: success by reassortment? Science 1994; 265:1389–1391.
3. Kapikian AZ, Wyatt Rg, Dolin R, et al. Visualization by immune electron microscopy of a 27 nm particle associated with acute infectious non-bacterial gastroenteritis. J Virol 1972; 1075–1081.
4. Bishop RF, Davidson GP, Holmes IH, Ruck BJ. Virus particles in epithelial cells of duodenal mucosa from children with viral gastroenteritis. Lancet 1973; 1281–1283.
5. Yeager M, Dryden KA, Olson NH, et al. Three-dimensional structure of rhesus rotavirus by cryoelectron microscopy and image reconstruction. J Cell Biol 1990; 110:2133–2144.
6. Brandt CD, Kim HW, Rodriguez WJ, et al. Pediatric viral gastroenteritis during eight years of study. J Clin Microbiol 1983; 18:71–78.
7. Ho MS, Glass RI, Pinsky PF, Anderson LJ. Rotavirus as a cause of diarrheal morbidity and mortality in the United States. J Infect Dis 1988; 158:1112-1116.
8. Glass RI, Gentsch J, Smith JC. Rotavirus vaccines: success by reassortment? Science 1994; 265:1389–1391.
9. Bass DM, Baylor M, Broome R, Greenberg HB. Molecular basis of age-dependent gastric inactivation of rhesus rotavirus in the mouse. J Clin Invest 1992; 89:1741–1745.
10. Bass DM, Mackow ER, Greenberg HB. Identification and partial characterization of a rhesus rotavirus binding glycoprotein on murine enterocytes. Virology 1991; 183:602–610.
11. Bass DM, Baylor MR, Chen C, et al. Liposome-mediated transfection of intact viral particles reveals that plasma membrane penetration determines permissivity of tissue culture cells to rotavirus. J Clin Invest 1992; 90:2313–2320.
12. Davidson GP, Barnes GL. Structural and functional abnormalities of the small intestine in infants and children with rotavirus enteritis. Acta Ped Scand 1979; 181–188.
13. Mebus CA, Wyatt RG, Kapikian AZ. Pathology of diarrhea in gnotobiotic calves induced by the human reovirus-like agent infantile gastroenteritis. Vet Path 1977; 273–282.
14. Osborne MP, Haddon SJ, Spencer AJ, et al. An electron microscopic investigation of time-related changes in the intestine of neonatal mice infected with murine rotavirus. J Pediatr Gastroenterol Nutr 1988; 7:236–248.
15. Kohler T, Erben U, Wiedersberg H, Bannert N. Histological findings of the small intestinal mucosa in rotavirus infections in infants and young children. Kinderarztl Prax 1990; 58:323–7.
16. Graham DY, Sackman JW, Estes MK. Pathogenesis of rotavirus-induced diarrhea. Preliminary studies in miniature swine piglet. Dig Dis Sci 1984; 29:1028–1035.
17. Boissieu DD, Lebon P, Badoual J, et al. Rotavirus induces alpha-interferon release in children with gastroenteritis. J Pediatr Gastroenterol Nutr 1993; 16:29–32.
18. Yamashire Y, Shimizu T, Oguchi S, Sato M. Prostaglandins in the plasma and stool of children with rotavirus gastroenteritis. J Pediatr Gastroenterol Nutr 1989; 9:322–327.

19. Rodriguez WJ, Kim HW, Brandt CD, et al. Longitudinal study of rotavirus infection and gastroenteritis in families served by a pediatric medical practice: clinical and epidemiologic observations. Pediatr Infect Dis J 1987; 6:170–176.
20. Eiden J, Losonsky GA, Johnson J, Yolken RH. Rotavirus RNA variation during chronic infection of immunocompromised children. Pediatr Infect Dis 1985; 4:632–637.
21. Gilger MA, Matson DO, Conner ME, et al. Extraintestinal rotavirus infections in children with immunodeficiency. J Pediatr 1992; 120:912–917.
22. Willcocks MM, Brown TD, Madeley CR, Carter MJ. The complete sequence of a human astrovirus. J Gen Virol 1994; 75:1785–1788.
23. Lewis TL, Greenberg HB, Herrmann JE, et al. Analysis of astrovirus serotype 1 RNA, identification of the viral RNA-dependent RNA polymerase motif, and expression of a viral structural protein. J Virol 1994; 68:77–83.
24. Herrmann JE, Nowak NA, Perron-Henry DM, et al. Diagnosis of astrovirus gastroenteritis by antigen detection with monoclonal antibodies. J Infect Dis 1990; 161:226–229.
25. Herrmann JE, Taylor DN, Echeverria P, Blacklow NR. Astroviruses as a cause of gastroenteritis in children. N Engl J Med 1991; 324:1757–1760.
26. Midthun K, Greenberg HB, Kurtz JB, et al. Characterization and seroepidemiology of a type 5 astrovirus associated with an outbreak of gastroenteritis in Marin County, California. J Clin Microbiol 1993; 31:955–962.
27. Grohmann GS, Glass RI, Pereira HG, et al. Enteric viruses and diarrhea in HIV-infected patients. Enteric Opportunistic Infection Working Group. N Engl J Med 1993; 329:14–20.
28. Cox GJ, Matsui SM, Lo RS, et al. Etiology and outcome of diarrhea after marrow transplantation: a prospective study. Gastroenterology 1994; 107:1398–1407.
29. Oishi I, Yamazaki K, Kimoto T, et al. A large outbreak of acute gastroenteritis associated with astrovirus among students and teachers in Osaka, Japan. J Infect Dis 1994; 170:439–443.
30. Gray EW, Angus KW, Snodgrass DR. Ultrastructure of the small intestine in astrovirus-infected lambs. J Gen Virol 1980; 49:79–82.
31. Jiang X, Rraham DY, Wang K, Estes MK. Norwalk virus genome cloning and characterization. Science 1990; 250:1580–1583.
32. Jiang X, Wang M, Graham DY, Estes MK. Expression, self-assembly, and antigenicity of the Norwalk virus capsid protein. J Virol 1992; 66:6527–6532.
33. Wang J, Jiang X, Madore HP, et al. Sequence diversity of small, round-structured viruses in the Norwalk virus group. J Virol 1994; 68:5982–5990.
34. Lew JF, Petric M, Kapikian AZ, et al. Identification of minireovirus as a Norwalk-like virus in pediatric patients with gastroenteritis. J Virol 1994; 68:3391–3396.
35. Agus SG, Dolin R, Wyatt RG, et al. Acute infectious nonbacterial gastroenteritis: intestinal histopathology. Histologic and enzymatic alterations during illness prodfuced by the Norwalk agent in man. Ann Intern Med 1973; 79:18–25.
36. Graham DY, Jiang X, Tanaka T, et al. Norwalk virus infection of volunteers: new insights based on improved assays. J Infect Dis 1994; 170:34–43.
37. Grimwood K, Carzino R, Barnes GL, Bishop RF. Patients with enteric adenovi-

rus gastroenteritis admitted to an Australian pediatric teaching hospital form 1981 to 1992. J Clin Microbiol 1995; 33:131–136.
38. Brandt CD, Kim HW, Rodriguez WJ, et al. Pediatric viral gastroenteritis during eight years of study. J Clin Microbiol 1983; 18:71–78.
39. Durepaire N, Ranger-Rogez S, Gandji JA, et al. Enteric prevalence of adenovirus in human immunodeficiency virus seropositive patients. J Med Virol 1995; 45:56–60.
40. Gallimore CI, Appleton H, Lewis D, et al. Detection and characterisation of bisegmented double-stranded RNA viruses (picobirnaviruses) in human faecal specimens. J Med Virol 1995; 45:135–140.
41. Koopmans M, Petric M, Glass RI, Monroe SS. Enzyme linked immunoassay reactivity of rotovirus-like particles in fecal specimens from humans with diarrhea. J Clin Microbiol 1993; 31:2738–2744.
42. Losonsky GA, Johnson JP, Winkelstein JA, Yolken RH. Oral administration of human serum immunoglobulin in immunodeficient patients with viral gastroenteritis. A pharmacokinetic and functional analysis. J Clin Invest 1985; 76:2362–2367.
43. Bernstein DI, Glass RI, Rodgers G, et al. Evaluation of rhesus rotavirus monovalent and tetravalent reassortant vaccines in US children. US Rotavirus Vaccine Efficacy Group. JAMA 1995; 273:1191–1196.

4

Food Poisoning

JAMES D. DEMAIO and WILLIAM R. BISHAI
Johns Hopkins School of Hygiene and Public Health, Baltimore, Maryland

I. INTRODUCTION

Food-borne illness is a significant cause of morbidity and mortality worldwide. In the United States, 91,678 cases representing 2397 outbreaks were reported to the Centers for Disease Control (CDC) between 1983 and 1987 (1). However, the mild nature of most cases and the difficulty in identifying certain causative organisms lead to marked underreporting. As many as 24 to 81 million cases of food-borne illness may occur each year in the United States at an estimated cost of over $7.5 billion (2-4). In emerging economies, where the threat of hunger outweighs the fear of food-borne illness, incidence rates are much higher. Diarrheal diseases alone kill 4.6 to 6 million children each year outside of Europe and North America (5,6).

II. EPIDEMIOLOGY AND PREVENTION

A. General Principles

Three separate factors are required for a case of food poisoning to occur: a susceptible human host, a pathogenic organism or toxin, and inadequate food-handling techniques. Careful attention to these factors can help reduce the considerable morbidity associated with food-borne illness.

The susceptibility of the human host may be modified by the development of immunity. For example, in developing countries, childhood diarrhea secondary to enterotoxigenic *Escherichia coli* and *Campylobacter* spp. is very common; however, adults are rarely affected. Maintenance of immunity to food-borne pathogens frequently requires continued exposure to the organism. In the case of Norwalk virus, immunity appears to be lost within 1 to 2 years after the primary infection (7). Reinfection boosts subsequent resistance. Some causes of food-borne disease, most notably toxins from *Staphylococcus aureus* and *Bacillus cereus*, produce no immunity from further illness.

Certain hosts may possess special intrinsic risk factors that increase the likelihood of developing gastroenteritis or disease complications (see Table 1). Patients with achlorhydria are more susceptible to bacterial pathogens, such as *Salmonella*, due to the loss of the stomach's protective acidic barrier. Iron-overload states, such as hemochromatosis and thalassemia, are major risk factors for severe *Yersinia enterocolitica* and noncholera *Vibrio* infections. *Listeria* has been associated with cell-mediated immune defects and pregnancy. Patients with malignancies, liver disease, and diabetes more frequently develop bacteremia due to *Campylobacter* (8).

Human immunodeficiency virus (HIV) infection is an increasingly common cause of severe immunosuppression. Individuals infected with HIV have markedly higher incidences of nontyphoidal *Salmonella* (100 fold) (9), *Salmonella typhi* (60 fold) (10), *Listeria* (280 fold) (11), and *Campylobacter* (35 fold) (12) infection. Disease in this population may not be limited to simple gastroenteritis; focal extraintestinal infections, bacteremia, and chronic infection are very common.

The second factor involved in food-borne outbreaks is the presence of a pathogenic organism or toxin in food. The likelihood of a specific agent being present depends on the particular food source (see Table 2), season of the

Table 1 Host Risk Factors Associated with Foodborne Illnesses

Organism	Associated Risk Factors
Salmonella spp.	HIV infection, achlorhydria, antacid use, diabetes, gastrectomy, lymphoproliferative diseases
Shigella spp.	Age < 5 years
Campylobacter spp.	HIV infection, lymphoproliferative diseases
Yersinia enterocolitica	Iron-overload states including hemochromatosis and thalassemia, desferoxamine use
Listeria monocytogenes	Cell-mediated immune defects, HIV infection, pregnancy, steroid use, elderly

Table 2 Foodborne Infectious Agents and Their Associated Food Sources

Infectious Agent	Food Source
Staphylococcus aureus	Proteinaceous foods, prepared meats, cream-filled desserts, potato salads
Bacillus cereus (emetic)	Starchy foods, rice, pasta, dried spices
Norwalk virus	Shellfish
Clostridium perfringens (Type A)	Prepared meats
B. cereus (diarrheal)	Meat products, vegetables, salads
Giardia lamblia	Salads
Salmonella spp.	Egg, poultry, meats, milk products
Campylobacter spp.	Poultry, milk
Shigella spp.	Prepared foods, soups, salads, vegetables
Vibrio parahemolyticus	Shellfish
Yersinia enterocolitica	Pork products
Escherichia coli O157:H7	Beef products, milk
Clostridium botulinum	Home-canned foods, garlic in oil, improperly smoked meat or fish
Listeria monocytogenes	Unpasteurized milk, soft cheeses, meat products

year, and geographic location. A detailed food history is a critical component in the patient workup, as well as in the epidemiological study of outbreaks.

There is significant seasonal variation for some food-borne diseases. Salmonellosis and *Vibrio* infections are much more common in the summer, whereas the winter holidays bring an increase in *Yersinia* infections. Geographic location is perhaps the least reliable indicator of the type of infection due to the frequent transport of meat, fish, and produce many miles from their site of origin.

The final factor leading to food-borne illness is inadequate food handling. Certain foods, such as dried breads and properly canned products, are intrinsically safe due to processing techniques. However, raw meats, eggs, seafood, and fresh vegetables pose a substantial risk if improperly prepared. Raw meat and eggs should be stored and handled separately from vegetables and previously cooked foods. After handling uncooked foods, kitchen surfaces, cutting boards, knives and hands should be washed thoroughly with soapy water. Heating of meat and egg products to obtain core temperatures of $>160°C$ will eliminate all pathogens except spore forming organisms, such as *Clostridium perfringens*. The consumption of raw meats (e.g., steak tartare), eggs (e.g., Caesar salads), or unpasteurized milk products should be avoided. Patients at increased risk of food-borne illness, including pregnant women and individuals with HIV infection, may need to take special precautions, such as avoiding raw seafood, soft cheeses, and leftover foods.

B. Recent Trends

The epidemiology of food-borne illness is highly dynamic and has changed over the last two decades in response to changes in food preparation practices, transportation, and dietary choices. Large-scale food processing has created the opportunity for scattered outbreaks that may be difficult for local authorities to recognize. Multistate outbreaks of *Salmonella* (13) and *E. coli* 0157:H7 (14) illustrate the potential impact of improper food handling techniques by large-scale manufacturers. The rapid transport of food items has introduced exotic syndromes into new geographic locations. Scombroid fish poisoning has been seen in Tennessee (15), *Vibrio parahemolyticus* has been diagnosed in Missouri (16), and cholera has occurred in Maryland (17). The demand for fresh fruits and vegetables has led to the importation of these items from subtropical areas, in particular Central America, during the winter months. These imports pose a minor, but real, risk for the introduction of foreign pathogens. The need for careful clinical and epidemiological observation in a rapidly changing world is underscored by the emergence of new food-borne illness syndromes, such as enterohemorrhagic *E. coli* and eosinophilia-myalgia syndrome in the last two decades (18).

III. AN APPROACH TO DIAGNOSIS

Food-borne illness may be categorized by a variety of different schemes, such as by type of food, by specific etiological agents, or by the general pathogenic mechanism. However, the most clinically relevant approach is to classify food-borne illnesses based on the predominant symptoms that they produce. The four symptom categories that we will use are nausea/vomiting, noninflammatory diarrhea, inflammatory diarrhea, and gastrointestinal disease with systemic complaints. Although the old adage that "common diseases may present in uncommon ways" certainly holds true for food-borne illness, a symptom-based classification system provides an excellent initial framework for evaluating patients.

Eliciting the patient's symptoms is only the first step in a complete work-up. Further valuable information may be gained from the food history, past medical history, season of the year, and possibly the geographic location of the case. Determination of the exact etiology frequently requires use of the clinical laboratory.

IV. SYNDROMES CHARACTERIZED BY NAUSEA AND VOMITING

In this category of food-borne illness, nausea, and vomiting are the predominant symptoms. Fever is rare. Nearly all of these syndromes are associated with both a short incubation period and a short duration of illness (see Table 3). The most common etiology is intoxication by the preformed protein toxins of either *Staphylococcus aureus* or *Bacillus cereus*.

A. *Staphylococcus Aureus* Intoxication

Staphylococcal food poisoning is due to ingestion of preformed toxins (19). Patients present with severe nausea (73–90%), vomiting (82%), and abdominal cramps (64–74%) (20-22). Although diarrhea occurs in a significant proportion of patients (41-88%), it is always accompanied by nausea and vomiting. Fever and systemic symptoms are rare.

Outbreaks have been associated with a variety of proteinaceous foods. Ham, cream-filled desserts, and macaroni salads have all been implicated. The use of salt and sugar as a preservative may promote the growth of *S. aureus* by inhibiting the growth of competing environmental organisms. In most outbreaks, previously cooked products have been contaminated by a food handler during further preparation. The food handler may either have skin lesions infected with *S. aureus* or simply be a nasal carrier.

Five antigenically distinct enterotoxins (A to E) are responsible for *S. aureus* food poisoning. A sixth enterotoxin, enterotoxin F, has been associated with toxic-shock syndrome, but has not been implicated in food-borne disease. The food-borne *S. aureus* enterotoxins are all heat stable, single polypeptide chain proteins of low molecular weight (28 to 35 kDa). Although reheating contaminated foods will kill the staphylococci, the toxins will remain intact. The exact mechanism of action of the enterotoxins is unknown. In animal models, diarrhea is secondary to net secretion of water and electrolytes from the gut

Table 3 Food Poisoning Syndromes Presenting with Nausea and Vomiting

Syndrome	Incubation	Duration	Treatment
Staphylococcus aureus	1–6 hour	< 24 hours	Supportive care only
Bacillus cereus	1–6 hour	< 24 hours	Supportive care only
Heavy metal ingestion	5–120 minute	< 24 hours	Supportive care only
Anisakiasis	12 hr–2 weeks	Variable	Endoscopic removal of parasites

Source: Bishai WR, Sears CL. Food Poisoning Syndromes. Gastroenterol Clin NA 1993; 3:579–602.

(23). The enterotoxins induce vomiting by direct stimulation of enteric autonomic sensory nerves (24). The *S. aureus* enterotoxins are not absorbed and do not induce a protective immunity to subsequent exposure.

Definitive diagnosis can be made by culturing the implicated food or the stools or vomitus of the patient. *S. aureus* strains responsible for outbreaks are usually from bacteriophage group III. Latex agglutination tests and ELISA are available for the direct detection of enterotoxins in food sources (25,26). Although rarely of value in isolated cases, these tests may help define the epidemiology of large outbreaks. Specific antibiotic therapy directed against *S. aureus* is unnecessary and therefore treatment is entirely supportive.

B. *Bacillus cereus* Emetic Syndrome

Bacillus cereus, an aerobic, spore-forming, gram-positive rod, causes two distinct clinical syndromes: a noninflammatory diarrheal syndrome (see Section V,C) and an acute emetic syndrome (27,28). The acute emetic syndrome has a clinical presentation, incubation period, and duration of illness nearly identical to *S. aureus* food poisoning. Outbreaks have been associated with starchy or dry foods, such as rice, pasta, and spices (29,30). The classic outbreak follows the ingestion of fried rice, often obtained from Chinese restaurants or takeout establishments. The spores of *B. cereus* are extremely hardy and may survive short-term boiling. If large quantities of cooked rice are subsequently held at room temperature (to prevent clumping), unkilled spores may germinate. During vegetative growth, most strains of *B. cereus* are able to form several toxins (31). A low-molecular-weight (10 kDa) protein is responsible for the acute emetic syndrome. Further heating or flash frying does not destroy the emetic toxin, which can withstand temperatures of 121°C for up to 90 minutes.

The diagnosis of *B. cereus* emetic syndrome is based on cultures of the implicated food or the stool or vomitus of the patient. Heat shock or alcohol shock of specimens may reduce contamination with other microorganisms and aid in diagnosis. Asymptomatic fecal carriage of *B. cereus* (14–43%) and the frequent presence of this organism in food makes a definitive diagnosis difficult (32,33). *B. cereus* may be clearly implicated only if the organism is grown in large numbers from both the patient and the food source ($>10^5$ cfu/g) and if strains isolated from both sources have identical serotypes or phage types. Although cell-culture based tests for toxin production have been developed, a positive result provides only circumstantial evidence because many strains are capable of expressing emetic toxin (34,35). Treatment of *B. cereus* intoxication is supportive. Specific antibiotic treatment of the organism is not necessary because further toxin production does not occur in the intestinal tract.

C. Miscellaneous Emetic Syndrome

Bacillus spp. other than *B. cereus* have been associated with nausea and vomiting syndromes. Between 1975 and 1986, 49 outbreaks of an emetic syndrome were associated with toxin-producing *Bacillus subtilis* in the United Kingdom (36). The symptoms and incubation period are nearly identical to those induced by *B. cereus* emetic toxin.

Heavy metal poisoning with cadmium, copper, zinc, iron, or tin may also lead to the acute onset of nausea and vomiting. Metal poisoning is most often associated with the prolonged storage of acidic or carbonated beverages in galvanized metal containers or the use of copper tubing to transfer liquids (37). Although nausea and vomiting are the predominant symptoms, cramps, diarrhea, and a metallic taste may also be noted. Cadmium and zinc are associated with myalgias and increased salivation, respectively. The incubation period (<1 hour) and duration of illness (several hours) are both short. Definitive diagnosis relies on assaying the suspected beverage for metal content.

Anisakiasis is a zoonotic infection with larvae of the genus *Anisakis, Phocaenema*, and others whose usual definitive hosts are marine mammals. Transmission requires the ingestion of raw or pickled fish, such as salmon and herring. The larval worms may penetrate the gastrointestinal tract in either the stomach or ileum. Stomach infections generally produce nausea and vomiting within 48 hours of ingestion. Ileal disease presents with severe abdominal pain and sometimes obstruction. Diagnosis may be made endoscopically. Symptoms are generally self-limited, although some investigators recommend removal of the worms at endoscopy.

V. NONINFLAMMATORY DIARRHEAL SYNDROMES

These syndromes are characterized by profuse watery diarrhea. Although occasional fecal leukocytes may be present, large numbers of fecal leukocytes, blood, and mucus are absent. Low-grade fevers and abdominal pain occur commonly, but vomiting is unusual (see Table 4). The pathophysiology of the viral syndromes discussed here is poorly understood. However, all of the bacterial pathogens in this section multiply in the intestinal tract and produce enterotoxins that lead to an imbalance in intestinal fluid secretion/absorption. Invasion of the intestinal mucosa does not occur. The primary risk to the patient is from dehydration.

A. Viral Gastroenteritis

Viruses from the families Adenoviridae, Astroviridae, Calciviridae, and Reoviridae (rotaviruses) are causative agents of gastroenteritis (38–40). Although

Table 4 Food Poisoning Syndromes Presenting with Noninflammatory Diarrhea

Syndrome	Incubation	Duration	Treatment
Clostridium perfringens (Type A)	8–18 hours	24 hours	Rehydration; antimotility agents
Bacillus cereus	8–18 hours	24–36 hours	Rehydration; antimotility agents
Norwalk virus	24–48 hours	24–48 hours	Rehydration; antimotility agents
Enterotoxigenic *Escherichia coli*	16–72 hours	5–10 days	Rehydration; antimotility agents; fluoroquinolones[a], trimethoprim-sulfamethoxazole
Vibrio cholerae	16–72 hours	5–7 days	Rehydration; tetracycline
Giardia lamblia	2 weeks	days–months	Rehydration; metronidazole

[a]Fluoroquinolones are contraindicated for pregnant women and children under 17 years old.
Source: Bishai WR, Sears CL. Food Poisoning Syndromes. Gastroenterol Clin NA 1993; 3:579–602.

fecal-oral contamination is presumed to be the primary mode of transmission, food-borne illness due to Norwalk and Norwalk-like agents (family calciviridae) has been clearly documented (41,42). Most cases have been associated with raw or improperly cooked shellfish (43,44). In a recent multistate outbreak due to contaminated oysters, molecular biological techniques were used to unravel the epidemiology (45). The point source of this outbreak appears to have been a single oyster boat that discharged fecal waste over an oyster bed.

Norwalk virus infection has an incubation period of 24 to 48 hours. Patients present with abdominal cramps, nausea, and diarrhea. Unlike the bacterial syndromes in this section, Norwalk virus is strongly associated with severe vomiting and low-grade fever (50%). Secondary cases frequently occur and may be an important epidemiological clue to the etiology (46).

The pathogenesis of Norwalk virus gastroenteritis is unknown. Studies have been hindered by the inability to culture the agent. Recently, the entire genome of the Norwalk virus and complete or partial genomes of Norwalk-like agents have been sequenced (47–49). Genetic studies are currently helping to clarify how these viruses are related, as well as providing new tools for epidemiological studies (50).

Infection induces a rise in specific serum IgM and IgG, as well as local IgA production (51,52). However, immunity is transient, with many individuals susceptible to reinfection within less than 1 year.

Diagnosis was originally based on electron microscopic visualization of viral particles. More recently, ELISAs and the polymerase chain reaction (PCR) have been successfully used to identify virus-specific antibodies and viral nucleic acids, respectively (53–55). However, the short duration of viral shedding (< 72 hrs) frequently makes these tests impractical during the analysis of an outbreak. Looking for rises in antibody titers is more suitable to epidemiologic investigations. Although major advancements have been made in the diagnosis of Norwalk virus over the last decade, diagnostic tests are available only as research tools. Most cases are self-limited and treatment is solely supportive.

B. *Clostridium perfringens*

Clostridium perfringens, an anaerobic, spore-forming, gram-positive rod, is responsible for two food-poisoning syndrome. Type C organisms, which are associated with a life-threatening necrotizing enterocolitis seen almost exclusively in developing countries, will not be discussed. Type A organisms cause a noninflammatory diarrheal syndrome of short duration (< 24 hours).

Most cases of *C. perfringens* Type A diarrhea are associated with prepared meat or poultry products that have been allowed to remain between 15° and 60°C for more than 2 hours (56,57). Under these conditions, clostridial spores readily germinate and begin vegetative growth. Ingestion of large numbers of vegetative organisms ($>10^5$ organisms/gram of food) overwhelms the acid barrier of the stomach and leads to transient intestinal colonization. The responsible enterotoxin must be produced within the GI tract to cause illness. Ingestion of spores alone or enterotoxin alone does not produce symptoms. Although *C. perfringens* has generally been associated with large outbreaks, a recent study from England showed the organism to be responsible for 7% of sporadic diarrheal cases (58).

Patients develop symptoms within 6 to 14 hours, with the vast majority reporting diarrhea (92%) and epigastric pain (81%). Nausea (25%), vomiting (9%), and fever are relatively uncommon (59). Symptoms resolve within 24 hours. Treatment is supportive only; antibiotic therapy is unnecessary.

C. perfringens Type A food poisoning is thought to be caused be a 35 kDa heat-labile polypeptide (60). Although the exact mechanism of action is unknown, the enterotoxin causes a net secretion of sodium ions and blocks chloride ion and glucose absorption. In animal models, such as the rabbit ileal loop, the toxin causes fluid accumulation (61). This finding is consistent with the secretory diarrhea seen in humans.

Diagnosis of *C. perfringens* food poisoning is complicated by the frequent presence of this organism in both asymptomatic individuals and also many food products (62). Ideally, the diagnosis should be confirmed by culturing $>10^5$ organisms/gram of food and $>10^6$ organism of the same serotype per gram of stool from symptomatic patients. Alternatively, ELISA or latex agglutination tests may be used to directly detect the enterotoxin in stool (63,64). Recently, DNA hybridization techniques and PCR have been applied to the identification of enterotoxigenic strains in both stool and pure cultures (65,66). Further studies will be required to determine the role of these molecular biological tests in epidemiological investigations.

C. *Bacillus cereus*

Bacilli cereus is responsible for a syndrome of noninflammatory diarrhea, as well as the emetic syndrome described in Section IV B. Epidemiologically and clinically, the diarrheal syndrome is nearly identical to *C. perfringens* Type-A food poisoning. Most cases are associated with prepared foods, such as meats, vegetables, and milk products, that have been held at room temperature for extended periods (67,68). Illness is secondary to the ingestion of large numbers of vegetative organisms that produce an enterotoxin within the GI tract. The incubation period, symptoms, and duration of illness are indistinguishable from disease due to *C. perfringens* Type A. The diarrheal toxin is a 50 kDa heat-labile protein that stimulates fluid secretion throughout the intestinal tract, possibly via a cAMP-dependent mechanism (69). A definitive diagnosis may be made by culturing suspected food products and stool specimens. Organisms of the same serotype should be present in large numbers ($> 10^5$/gram) from both sources. Because symptoms are self-limited, only supportive therapy is required.

D. Enterotoxigenic *Escherichia coli*

Enterotoxigenic *E. coli* (ETEC) are a major cause of traveler's diarrhea. However, outbreaks are uncommon in industrialized countries and account for $<1\%$ of reported cases in the United States (70). Residents of developing countries experience illness as children, but develop immunity over time, presumably secondary to mucosal antibody production, which blocks adhesion (71). Nonimmune travelers become ill when they consume fecally contaminated water, ice, or uncooked foods, such as salads and fruits.

After an incubation period of 24 to 48 hours, patients present with bloating, nausea, and watery diarrhea. Vomiting and fever are uncommon. Symptoms last for only 72 to 96 hours.

Either one of two toxins may be produced by ETEC within the GI tract (72). Heat-stable toxin (ST) is a low-molecular-weight polypeptide that alters intestinal secretion via a cGMP-dependent mechanism. Heat-labile toxin (LT) is a large, multimeric protein composed of one A subunit and five B subunits. The B subunits are responsible for specific binding to intestinal glycoproteins. The subsequent entry of A subunits into the cell leads to adenylate cyclase activation, an increase in cAMP, and, ultimately, fluid and water secretion. It is unclear why LT and cholera toxin produce diseases of different severity, given their close similarity in both structure and function.

Diagnosis is usually made on clinical grounds. A specific bacteriological diagnosis is complicated by the lack of selective media for enterotoxigenic strains. Both antimotility agents and antibiotics, such as ciprofloxacin, may be used in conjunction with fluid repletion in order to decrease the duration of symptoms.

E. Miscellaneous Noninflammatory Diarrheal Syndromes

Giardia lamblia and *Vibrio cholerae* are usually considered water-borne pathogens. However, illness may also occur when food products are contaminated either directly with fecal material or with nonpotable water. *G. lamblia* is most commonly associated with uncooked foods, such as salads (73). The organism is highly contagious; as few as 10 cysts can cause infection. Patients classically present with bloating, diarrhea, nausea, and flatulence, but milder and asymptomatic cases are common. Diagnosis may be made by direct inspection of stools for trophozoites. Therapy with metronidazole is highly effective.

Vibrio cholerae is a major cause of illness in economically emerging countries. Rare cases in the United States have been traced to contaminated food products, such as crab meat and coconut milk (17,74). The diagnosis should be considered in patients with a syndrome of profuse watery diarrhea (>4 liters/day) and exposure to food products imported from endemic areas.

VI. INFLAMMATORY DIARRHEAL SYNDROMES

These syndromes are caused by potentially invasive pathogens, such as *Salmonella, Shigella, Campylobacter,* and *Yersinia* (see Table 5). Classically, patients report fever, abdominal cramps, and blood/mucus-stained stools. Stool examination typically reveals sheets of leukocytes. However, a significant proportion of cases (60%) may experience only watery diarrhea with fever and abdominal pain (75). Treatment decisions, particularly whether antibiotics should be started, must be based on the severity and circumstances of the individual case.

A. Salmonellosis

Salmonellosis is the most commonly reported food-borne disease in the United States. Nontyphoidal *Salmonella* spp. are common components of the intestinal flora of a wide range of animals. Consequently, most food-borne outbreaks can be traced to improperly handled animal products. Currently, raw or partially cooked eggs account for 92% of all cases (76). Eggs with hairline cracks may become contaminated with chicken feces; in addition, uncracked eggs may be transovarially infected (77,78). Incompletely cooked poultry, beef, and pork are also significant sources (79). Pasteurized milk and vegetables may pose a risk if they are fecally contaminated (80). Contamination may occur either from contact with animal products/feces or from food handlers who are chronic carriers of the organism.

Salmonella infections are most common in the late summer and early fall. Risk factors include an age of less than 5 years, achlorhydria, HIV infection, antacid use, gastrectomy, altered intestinal flora, lymphoproliferative disease, and diabetes. Although the infectious inoculum has usually been stated to be between 10^6 and 10^9 organisms, 10^3 or fewer bacteria are probably sufficient to cause gastroenteritis (81). After an incubation period of 6 to 48 hours, patients present with fever, chills, cramps, and diarrhea. Nausea and vomiting are common. Moderate numbers of white and red cells are usually seen on Wright-stained stool smears, but grossly bloody stools are unusual. In the normal host diarrhea generally clears in less than 7 days. However, patients with lymphoproliferative diseases or HIV infection are at increased risk of complications, such as bacteremia and extraintestinal infection (82).

Table 5 Food Poisoning Syndromes Presenting with Inflammatory Diarrhea

Syndrome	Incubation	Duration	Treatment
Nontyphoidal *Salmonella* spp.	6–48 hours	< 7 days	Rehydration; avoid antibiotics in uncomplicated cases; treat bacteremia, focal infections, or high risk hosts[a] with fluoroquinolones[b] or a third generation cephalosporin
Shigella spp.	16–72 hours	1–30 days	Rehydration; fluoroquinolones[b]
Campylobacter spp.	16–48 hours	2–7 days	Rehydration; fluoroquinolones[b], erythromycin, or doxycycline
Vibrio parahemolyticus	5–24 hours	2–7 days	Rehydration; fluoroquinolones[b], doxycycline, or trimethoprim-sulfamethoxazole
Yersinia enterocolitica	16–48 hours	1–3 weeks	Rehydration; +/– third generation cephalosporin plus an aminoglycoside, doxycycline[c]
Escherichia coli O157:H7	1–8 days	3–6 days	Rehydration; supportive care

[a]High risk groups include patients with HIV infection and lymphoproliferative diseases.
[b]Fluoroquinolones are contraindicated for pregnant women and children under 17 years old.
[c]Antibiotics listed are effective in vitro. The clinical efficacy of antibiotic treatment for this organism has not been documented in placebo controlled trials.
Source: Bishai WR, Sears CL. Food Poisoning Syndromes Gastroenterol Clin NA 1993; 3:579–602.

The pathogenesis of *Salmonella* gastroenteritis is poorly understood. The principle pathogenic mechanism appears to be bacterial adherence to intestinal epithelial cells with subsequent intracellular invasion, rather than enterotoxin production (83). The invasive potential of *Salmonella* spp. appears to be a complex trait that is due to the carefully regulated expression of numerous gene products (84).

Diagnosis is made by culturing *Salmonella* from stool or blood. Uncomplicated cases should receive supportive care only, with volume repletion being the primary objective. The routine use of antibiotics in uncomplicated cases is strongly discouraged for two reasons. First, there is increasing antibiotic resistance among *Salmonella* to most commonly used agents, such as beta-lactams and trimethoprim-sulfa. This resistance may be secondary to the use of subtherapeutic doses of antibiotics in animal feeds (85). The spread of resistant strains from antibiotic-fed animals to humans has clearly been demonstrated by molecular epidemiological techniques (86). Second, antibiotic therapy may prolong fecal shedding of the organism and contribute to relapses (87).

Patients with complications of *Salmonella* gastroenteritis, such as bacteremia or extraintestinal disease, should receive antibiotic therapy. If *Salmonella* is suspected, antibiotics should also be given immediately to patients at increased risk for complications including neonates, the elderly, and patients with sickle cell disease, HIV infection, and cancer. Fluoroquinolones (adults) or third-generation cephalosporins (adults or children) are good initial choices until sensitivity results are available.

B. Shigellosis

Shigellosis is one of the most common causes of food-borne disease in the United States with 22,796 cases reported in 1988 (88). The majority of isolates in North America are *Shigella sonnei; S. flexneri* accounts for a small proportion of cases. Disease due to *S. dysenteriae* is very rare in the United States. Although direct fecal-oral trnasmission is the most common means of transmission, particularly among children, food-borne spread also occurs. In most outbreaks, food items such as soups, salads, and sandwiches, have been fecally contaminated after preparation (89–92). Improper handwashing and inadequate toilet facilities are almost always implicated.

Patients classically present with dysentery and fevers 18 to 72 hours after ingesting the organism. Only a minority of patients (<20%) will have grossly bloody stools (89).

Illness results from two pathogenic properties of the organism: enteroinvasion and the elaboration of Shiga toxin (93,94). Enteroinvasion is orchestrated by multiple genes located both on plasmids and on the chromosome. *Shigella* induce phagocytosis by colonic epithelial cells, multiply intracellularly, and then invade adjacent cells. Shiga toxin consists of one A subunit and five B subunits. The B subunits bind to glycolipids on colonic cells and allow entry of the A subunit into the cytoplasm. The A subunit cleaves mammalian 28S rRNA, effectively halting protein synthesis and killing the cell.

Diagnosis is made by culturing the organism from stool or blood. Fluoroquinolones are the treatment of choice in adults; third-generation cephalosporins should be used in children. Drug resistance, in particular to trimethoprim, sulfa, and ampicillin, is a major problem in the developing world. Recent outbreaks in Burundi were complicated by the presence of nearly panresistant strains (95).

C. Campylobacteriosis

Campylobacter spp. are motile, microaerophilic, curved, gram-negative rods widespread in nature as commensals of wild and domestic animals. The most common species infecting humans are *C. fetus* and *C. jejuni*. Campylobacteriosis is the leading cause of acute infectious diarrhea in England (96) and may be a more significant problem than recognized in the United States (97).

Campylobacter food-borne illness is associated with consuming undercooked poultry or raw milk (98). The spectrum of illness is broad. Symptoms typically begin after an incubation period of 16 to 48 hours. Most patients note abdominal pain (63–79%) and secretory diarrhea (54%) (99,100). However, a significant proportion present with bloody diarrhea (46%), nausea (43%), and fever (42–74%). Symptoms usually resolve within 5 to 7 days, although relapses and persistent cases are well documented (100).

Gastroenteritis due to *Campylobacter* has been associated with the secondary development of Henoch Schonlein purpura (101), reactive arthritis (102,103), Reiter's syndrome, and Guillain–Barre syndrome (GBS) (104–106). Recent studies suggest that structural similarities between *C. jejuni* lipopolysaccharide and human gangliosides (GM1) lead to autoimmunity and the symptoms of GBS (107,108).

Diagnosis is made by culturing the organism from stool. Because *Camplylobacter* spp. grow more slowly than the normal enteric flora, special techniques must be used for isolation. The highest yields are obtained using special media, such as Skirrow's or Campy-BAP under microaerophilic conditions.

As in all cases of diarrhea, dehydration should be aggressively treated with fluid repletion. The use of antimotility agents in *Campylobacter* gastroenteritis has been associated with increased severity of disease and should be used with caution (109). The antibiotic of choice is erythromycin for 5 to 7 days. Although contraindicated in pregnant women and children, quinolones and tetracycline are reasonable alternative agents for nonpregnant adults. Therapy must be started within several days of the onset of symptoms to be useful (110). In general, antibiotics should be reserved for patients with bacteremia, bloody diarrhea, fever, or persistent symptoms. Recently, there has been a growing concern about the increasing resistance of *Campylobacter* spp. to commonly used antibiotics, such as erythromycin and quinolones (111,112). Further surveillance of isolates will be essential to ensure that recommended treatment regimens are adequate.

D. Vibrio parahemolyticus

Vibrio parahemolyticus gastroenteritis is associated with the consumption of shellfish, such as crabs, shrimp and oysters (113,114). Cases are most commonly seen during the summer months in coastal regions. This organism accounts for <0.1% of all food-borne illness in the United States. However, in some areas, such as Japan, it is responsible for 60% of all food-borne bacterial disease (115).

Symptoms vary over a wide range of severity. After an incubation period of 12 to 24 hours, the majority of patients present with a secretory diarrhea, nausea, vomiting, and cramps; fever and chills occur in one-quarter of cases. A minority of patients experience bloody dysentery and colonic ulceration. Patients with underlying illness appear to be at increased risk for complications, sepsis, and death (113).

Although *V. parahemolyticus* is widespread in coastal waters, only a small proportion of strains are pathogenic for humans. Pathogenicity has been correlated with the presence of a thermostable direct hemolysin, which causes hemolysis on Wagatsuma blood agar plates (the Kanagawa phenomenon) (116). However, recent evidence suggest that additional factors are also involved in pathogenicity (117).

E. Yersinia enterocolitica

Yersinia enterocolitica is a commensal organism of many wild and domestic animal species including dogs, cattle, and pigs. Although traditionally viewed as a rare cause of human food poisoning, two recent studies observed *Y. enterocolitica* to be a common cause of illness in children, with seasonal (winter) incidences rivaling *Salmonella* and *Campylobacter* (118,119).

Human illness is associated with a limited number of serotypes (0:3, 0:8, and 0:9) (120). Improperly cooked pork products and milk are the most frequently implicated foods (121,122). Because *Y. enterocolitica* readily grows at 4°C, refrigerated meats may develop a high bacterial burden (123). The preparation of homemade pork dishes, such as chitterlings, may pose a particular risk by meat-to-hand contamination and subsequent accidental ingestion of organisms (124–126). It is believed that ingestion of $>10^8$ organisms is required to establish infection.

Patients may present with either enterocolitis or mesenteric adenitis. Enterocolitis, which is more common in children, is characterized by either watery or bloody diarrhea, abdominal pain, and fever. Adolescents and adults are more likely to report symptoms of mesenteric adenitis, such as abdominal pain and fever (127). Mesenteric adenitis is frequently confused with appendicitis and may result in unnecessary laparotomy. Approximately 30% of adults will develop secondary complications of *Yersinia* infection including reactive polyarthritis, ankylosing spondylitis, Reiter's syndrome, and possibly vasculitis (128–130). Complications are more common in individuals with the HLA-B27 haplotype (130,131).

Y. enterocolitica possesses several virulence factors (132). Two chromosomal genes, designated *ail* and *inv*, facilitate yersinial invasion into intestinal epithelial cells and subsequent migration to local lymph nodes (133). Other, less well understood, virulence genes are located on plasmids (134). *Y. enterocolitica* does not produce siderophores and is, therefore, dependent on either the siderophores of other bacteria or free iron. Patients with iron overload states, such as hemochromatosis or thalassemia, as well as patients undergoing iron chelation therapy with desferoxamine, are at increased for severe and disseminated disease (125,135–137).

The diagnosis may be established by stool culture. Although cold enrichment of specimens may increase the sensitivity of culture, this has been shown not to be cost-effective (138). Most cases are self-limited and specific therapy is of uncertain value. However, patients with severe symptoms, evidence of septicemia, or risk factors for dissemination should be treated with a third-generation cephalosporin plus an aminoglycoside.

F. Enterohemorrhagic *E. coli*

Enterohemmorrhagic *E. coli* (EHEC) causes a distinctive hemorrhagic colitis that was initially recognized in 1982 (139). *E. coli* serotype O157:H7 has been implicated in nearly all food-borne outbreaks. However isolated cases may be due to a variety of other strains, such as O26:H11 and O111:NM (140,141).

Outbreaks of *E. coli* 0157:H7 have been associated with contaminated beef products (14,142,143), dairy products (144), and apple cider (145). Asymptomatic dairy cattle appear to be a major reservoir (146). Other meats, such as lamb, poultry, and pork, may also be contaminated (147). Secondary transmission during outbreaks has been clearly documented (148).

After an incubation period of 3 to 9 days, patients present with abdominal pain, nausea (60%), and grossly bloody diarrhea (60–100%) (139,142, 148,149). A smaller proportion of patients may note watery diarrhea without blood. Fever is less common (6–25%). The hemolytic-uremic syndrome (HUS) develops in a variable proportion of patients and is a significant cause of morbidity and mortality (149). Less commonly patients develop full-blown thrombotic thrombocytopenic purpura.

Enterohemorrhagic *E. coli* are capable of attaching to and effacing the colonic epithelium; they are not believed to invade into the submucosa. All EHEC strains produce protein cytotoxins that are closely related to Shiga toxin and inactivate human 28S rRNA. Two slightly different cytotoxins have been discovered, Shiga-like toxin I and II (SLT-I and SLT-II) (97). The EHEC are believed to trigger the HUS by secreting SLT-I or SLT-II into the lamina propria and causing local endothelial damage, microangiopathic hemolysis, and renal damage due to hemolysis.

When EHEC is suspected, stools may be screened by plating on sorbitol MacConkey agar. Sorbitol-negative *E. coli* isolates should then be serotyped. Assays for Shiga-like toxin activity in stool, as well as assays for antibody titers to O-specific antigen or Shiga-like toxins, have been developed, but are limited to research settings (97). Antibiotics have not been shown to be effective in reducing symptoms or the risk of complications. Supportive care is the mainstay of therapy.

VII. SYSTEMIC SYNDROMES

Many food-borne pathogens and toxins primarily cause systemic, rather than gastrointestinal, symptoms (see Table 6). In botulism, ciguatera, scombroid fish poisoning, and shellfish poisoning, neurological symptoms predominate. Listeria and brucellosis may cause both a sepsis syndrome and focal infections, such as meningitis. Chemical intoxicants are responsible for a bewildering list of different syndromes. Careful attention to the patient's food history is essential for diagnosing most of the agents described below.

A. Botulism

Three syndromes of *C. botulinum* intoxication have been described: food-borne botulism, infant botulism (150), and wound botulism. Food-borne illness accounts for about one half of the botulism seen in the United States. Most food-borne outbreaks are related to the consumption of improperly prepared home-preserved vegetables or meats (151,152). However, commercially prepared foods, such as chopped garlic or eggplant in oil and salted fish, have occasionally been implicated (153,154).

Botulism classically presents as a symmetric descending paralysis with minimal sensory or CNS symptoms (151,153). Patients may note blurred vision and photophobia (90%), dysphagia (70%), generalized weakness (58%), and dysphonia (55%). Gastrointestinal symptoms, such as vomiting and diarrhea (40%) may precede the neurological symptoms and lead to confusion as to the diag-

Table 6 Food Poisoning Syndromes Presenting with Systemic Symptoms

Syndrome	Incubation	Duration	Treatment
Botulism	12–36 hours	weeks–months	Respiratory support; trivalent equine antitoxin (Types A, B, and E)
Ciguatera fish poisoning	1–30 hours	days–months	Respiratory support; IV Mannitol, amitryptiline
Scombroid fish poisoning	10–180 minutes	4–6 days	H1 and H2 antagonists
Paralytic shellfish poisoning	5–240 minutes	hours–days	Respiratory support
Neurotoxic shellfish poisoning	5–240 minutes	hours–days	Supportive care; ?Beta agonists
Listeria monocytogenes	1–70 days	variable	Ampicillin plus an aminoglycoside
Trichinella spiralis	1–2 weeks	3 weeks	Mebendazole; corticosteroids in severe cases
Group A streptococcus	2–4 days	3–5 days	Penicillin or erythromycin for 10 days
Brucellosis	1–8 weeks	weeks–months	Doxycycline plus either gentamicin or rifampin

Source: Bishai WR, Sears CL. Food Poisoning Syndromes. Gastroenterol Clin NA 1993; 3:579–602.

nosis (151,153). As the neurological symptoms progress, most patients develop constipation. Physical signs include a dry mouth, respiratory impairment, ptosis, dilated/unreactive pupils, and postural hypotension. Symptoms may persist and even intensify over weeks to months. Illness is more likely to be severe when there is a short incubation period and with the ingestion of type A toxin (155,156).

Infant botulism is due to the colonization of the infant's GI tract with *C. botulinum* and subsequent in vivo toxin production. Illness has been associated with the feeding of honey to infants less than 1 year old. Infants present with hypotonia, constipation, decreased sucking reflex, and eventually respiratory failure.

Botulinum toxins are among the most lethal substances known (human LD_{50} = 100 ng). Seven distinct serological types (A–G) are recognized. Type A predominates in the western United States, type B in the eastern United States, and type E in Alaska. Serotypes C, D, and F have only rarely caused human disease. The mechanism of action of botulinum toxins is well understood at the molecular level and has recently been reviewed (157).

Suspected botulism cases should be reported immediately to the CDC and the local state health department. Diagnosis can be made within the first 3 days after ingestion by identifying botulinum toxin in the patient's stool or serum with a mouse bioassay. After 3 days, special anaerobic stool cultures for *C. botulinum* may be necessary. Electromyography may be valuable in distinguishing botulism from Guillain–Barre syndrome and the Eaton–Lambert variety of myasthenia gravis.

Patients with botulism should be treated with trivalent equine antitoxin (types A, B, and E) to prevent further paralysis; the antitoxin does not reverse preexisting paralysis. The use of guanidine hydrochloride or aminopyridine to increase neurotransmitter release remains controversial. Intensive-care unit management for respiratory failure is frequently necessary. However, with good supportive care, mortality should be less than 5%.

B. Ciguatera

Ciguatera fish poisoning is due to the ingestion of a marine neurotoxin. The toxin originates in dinoflagellates, such as *Gambierdiscus toxicus*, and accumulates up the aquatic food chain in the flesh of fish. Most cases are associated with the consumption of large carnivorous or bottom-dwelling reef fish, such as barracuda, grouper, red snapper, or amberjack (158). Affected fish are found between 35°N latitude and 35°S latitude. Although most cases in the United States occur in Florida and Hawaii (158–160), the transport of fish products has led to outbreaks in northern states, such as Rhode Island (161).

The incubation period of ciguatera intoxication ranges from 5 minutes to 30 hours (mean = 5 hours). Patients present with both gastrointestinal and neurological symptoms including nausea, vomiting, watery diarrhea, paresthesias, ataxia, vertigo, blurred vision, and photophobia (158,162). The most distinctive feature is a reversal of hot and cold temperature sensation reported in 97% of cases (162). A minority of patients develop cranial nerve palsies (10%) or respiratory paralysis. The mean duration of illness is 8.5 days but in some cases neurological disturbances remain for years (162,163). Symptoms may be increasingly severe with subsequent ingestions of the toxin (164).

A variety of specific ciguatoxins have been identified. Ciguatoxin-1 is an 1100 molecular weight, heat-resistant, polyether that opens voltage-dependent sodium channels (165). Maiatoxin is a water-soluble molecule that alters calcium channels.

Although a specific diagnosis is possible using immunoassays or mouse bioassays, the initial diagnosis must be based on clinical grounds alone (166–168). No specific antidote is available; however, intravenous mannitol appears to lessen acute and chronic symptoms (169). Whether mannitol assists in toxin elimination or indirectly affects nerve tissue is currently unknown. Anecdotally, amitriptyline has been felt to alleviate symptoms (170).

C. Scombroid Fish Poisoning

Scombroid poisoning (scombrotoxicosis) occurs after the ingestion of spoiled fish. Classically, illness is due to fish species from the families Scombridae or Scomberesocidae, such as tuna and mackerel. However, a wide variety of other fish including mahi-mahi and herring have been associated with outbreaks (171–173). The tainted fish may be noted to have a peppery or metallic taste.

Symptoms begin 10 minutes to 3 hours after ingestion and include nausea, vomiting, diarrhea, flushing, headache, and oral burning. Occasionally, patients will experience respiratory distress or severe hypotension. Most cases resolve spontaneously within 4 to 6 hours.

The precise etiology of scombrotoxicosis is unclear. Symptoms resemble those of histamine toxicity, and high levels of histamine have been measured in both patients and implicated fish samples (15). Histamine is presumably formed by the bacterial decarboxylation of histidine present in fish flesh. However, histamine is not well absorbed from the GI tract, and volunteer studies with histamine-laced fish fillets have failed to produce symptoms (174,175). A second agent that either increases histamine absorption or leads to basophil degranulation has been proposed (174). Patients frequently respond to treatment with H1 and H2 antagonists, such as diphenhydramine and cimetidine, respectively (176).

D. Shellfish Poisonings

Three types of shellfish poisoning have been described: paralytic shellfish poisoning (PSP), neurotoxic shellfish poisoning (NSP), and toxic-encephalopathic shellfish poisoning (TESP) (177–180). All three are due to toxins produced by dinoflagellates ("red tides") that become concentrated in bivalved mollusks.

Paralytic shellfish poisoning is due to saxitoxin, a sodium channel toxin produced by *Protogonylaux* spp. Cases occur from May to October above 30°N latitude and below 30°S latitude. Patients present within 1 hour of ingestion with nausea, vomiting, and facial paresthesias (181). In severe cases, respiratory failure and paralysis can occur (182).

Neurotoxic shellfish poisoning is due to brevitoxin, a lipophilic, heat-stable neurotoxin that stimulates postganglionic cholinergic neurons (183,184). *Ptychodisucs brevis*, the responsible dinoflagellate, is found along the Gulf of Mexico in the winter months. Symptoms occur within about 3 hours of ingestion and include nausea, vomiting, paresthesias, reversal of hot/cold sensation and ataxia (185). Paralysis does not occur and symptoms are generally milder than those seen in PSP.

Toxic-encephalopathic shellfish poisoning was initially identified during a 1987 outbreak of food poisoning due to toxic mussels from Prince Edward Island (186). Patients developed vomiting (76%), diarrhea (42%), severe headache (43%), and permanent memory deficits (25%) (187). The mussels were subsequently shown to be contaminated with domoic acid, a toxin produce by the diatom *Nitschia pungens* (188). No further outbreaks have been reported, but shellfish samples in Canada are now tested by high pressure liquid chromatography.

E. *Listeria monocytogenes* (189,190)

Listeria monocytogenes, a motile, gram-positive rod, is responsible for approximately 1700 cases of meningitis and bacteremia each year in the United States. In nearly all cases, the GI tract is the presumed portal (191). Neonates, the elderly, pregnant women, and patients with cell-mediated immune defects, such as those with HIV infection or on steroid therapy, appear to be at increased risk of systemic spread (192). Outbreaks have been associated with a wide range of food products including pasteurized milk, soft cheeses, shellfish, raw vegetables, and meat products, such as hotdogs (189,193–195). Food-borne listeriosis is no doubt facilitated by the organism's unique ability to grow at refrigeration temperatures.

The organism may be visualized in CSF gram stain or cultured from the CSF or blood. Gram-stain interpretation is complicated by the morphological and staining variability of the organism. Growth in culture may be slow and delay diagnosis. Although cold enrichment techniques have been developed to enhance recovery, definitive results may require weeks and are of limited use in the treatment of an individual patient. Hopefully, the development of alternative tests, such as DNA probes or PCR-based assays, will overcome the current difficulties in diagnosis (196). Treatment should consist of ampicillin or penicillin plus gentamicin for 3 to 6 weeks.

F. Miscellaneous Infections

During the 1980s fewer than 35 cases of trichinosis were reported in the United States each year (197). The decreasing incidence of *Trichinella spiralis* infection is presumably secondary to a greater emphasis on thoroughly cooking pork products, as well as laws prohibiting the feeding of uncooked meat or garbage to pigs. Patients ingesting large numbers of cysts may present with myositis, periorbital edema, and eosinophilia. Asymptomatic infection is common when only a few cysts are consumed. Diagnosis can be made serologically. Acute trichinosis may be treated with mebendazole; corticosteroids are indicated for severe cases.

Brucella spp. cause human illness with protean manifestations. Patients may develop only flu-like symptoms or meningitis, osteomyelitis, endocarditis, or even severe sepsis. Cases of food-borne brucellosis usually result from the consumption of improperly cooked meat or unpasteurized milk or cheese. During the last decade the proportion of brucellosis cases in the United States from food sources has increased with a corresponding decrease in occupationally acquired illness (198).

Although group-A streptococcal pharyngitis is usually transmitted from person to person by close contact, food-borne spread is also possible. Prior to pasteurization, dairy products were the most common food source. Recent outbreaks have resulted from contaminated macaroni and cheese and cabbage salad (199,200).

Hepatitis A may be spread by fecal contamination of water or food. Most food-borne cases are caused by clams, oysters, and mussels harvested from waters with high coliform counts. A wide range of other food products pose a hepatitis-A risk if contaminated by unpurified water or an infected food handler.

G. Chemical Poisonings

Ingestion of numerous naturally occurring toxins, as well as synthetic chemicals, can lead to gastrointestinal and/or systemic symptoms. The most commonly identified intoxicants are heavy metals (Section IV C.), mushrooms, and

Table 7 Common Food-borne Chemical Intoxicants

Food Substance	Chemical	Symptoms/Syndrome	Onset	Reference
Meats				
Quail meat	Unknown	Myopathy	Hours	201
Fruits and vegetables				
Ackee fruit (Jamaica)	Hypoglycin A	Hypoglycemia, vomiting	4–10 h	202
Bitter cucumber	Curcurbitacin E	Cramps, diarrhea, collapse	1–2 h	203
Brussell sprouts, cabbage	5-vinyloxazolidine-2-thione	Iodine-irreversible goiter	Weeks	203
Cassava root, lima beans, apple seeds	Hydrogen cyanide	Dyspnea, coma, death	Minutes	203
Castor beans	Lectin hemagglutinin	Nausea, vomiting	1–7 h	204
Fava beans	Vicine, covicine	Hemoglobinuria (G6PD-deficient patients)	1–30 h	203
Licorice root	Glycyrrhizic acid	Hypermineralocorticoidism	Weeks	205
Seaweed (Guam)	Palytoxin	Gastroenteritis, numbness	12–24 h	206

Mushrooms				
Amanita muscaria, *A. panterina*	Ibotenic acid, muscimol	Delirium, restlessness	2 h	207
Inocybe spp., *Clitocybe* spp.	Muscarine	Parasympathetic hyperactivity	2 h	207
Psilocybe spp.	Psilocybin	Hallucinations, acute psychosis	2 h	207
Coprinus atramentarius	Unknown	Disulfiram-like reaction	2 h	207
Amanita phalloides, *Galerina* spp.	Amatoxins	Hepatorenal syndrome	6–24 h	207
Gyromitra spp.	Gyromitrin	Hepatic failure, death	6–24 h	207
Mycotoxins				
Aspergillus flavus, *A. parasiticus*	Aflatoxins	Cancer	Years	203
Aspergillus ochraceus	Ochratoxin A	Nephropathy	Months	203
Fusaria spp.	Trichothecenes	Anemia, leukopenia	Days 203	
Contaminants				
Pesticides	Organophosphates	Diplopia, paralysis, seizures	Minutes	208
	Organochlorines	Nausea, seizures	1 h	209
Tryptophan	Unknown	Eosinophilia-myalgia syndrome	Days	210

Source:Bishai WR, Sears CL. Food Poisoning Syndromes. Gastroenterol Clin NA 1993; 3:579–602.

monosodium glutamate (MSG). Mushroom poisoning can present with at least six different syndromes depending on the exact species eaten. A commonly used flavor enhancer, MSG causes flushing, headache, and nausea in susceptible individuals. An exhaustive list of all known chemical intoxicants is beyond the scope of this chapter. However, Table 7 summarizes some of the more commonly encountered chemicals, their sources, and their corresponding syndromes.

VIII. CONCLUSION

Food-borne illness remains a major public health problem throughout the world. Traditional pathogens, such as *Salmonella, Shigella*, and the Norwalk virus, continue to cause significant morbidity and mortality. Emerging pathogens and an ever-increasing population of immunosuppressed patients have created new challenges for clinicians, while changes in food transportation and processing have demanded increased vigilance from public health authorities. Although the complete eradication of food-poisoning syndromes is impossible, significant advances can be made through the sensible regulation of the food-processing industry, as well as through better education of consumers in appropriate food-handling practices.

REFERENCES

1. Bean NH, Griffin PM, Goulding JS, et al. Foodborne disease outbreaks, 5-year summary, 1983–1987. Morb Mortal Wkly Rep 1990; 39:15–57.
2. Todd E. Epidemiology of foodborne illness: North America. Lancet 1990; 336:788–790.
3. Archer DL, Kvenberg JE. Incidence and cost of foodborne diarrheal disease in the United States. J Food Protect 1985; 48:887-894.
4. Kvenberg JE, Archer DL. Economic impact of colonization control on foodborne disease. Food Technol 1987; 41:77–98.
5. Guerrant RL, Bobak DA. Bacterial and protozoal gastroenteritis. NEJM 1991; 325:327-240.
6. Waites WM, Arbuthnott JP. Foodborne illness: An overview. Lancet 1990; 336:722–725.
7. Parrino TA, Schreiber DS, Trier JS, et al. Clinical immunity in acute gastroenteritis caused by Norwalk agent. N Engl J Med 1977; 297:86–89.
8. Guerant RL, Lahita RG, Winn EC Jr, et al. Campylobacteriosis in man: Pathogenic mechanisms and review of 91 bloodstream infections. Am J Med 1978; 65:484.
9. Celum CL, Chaisson RE, Rutherford GW, et al. Incidence of salmonellosis in patients with AIDS. J Infect Dis 1987; 156:998–1002.
10. Gotuzzo E, Frisancho O, Sanchez J, et al. Association between the acquired

immunodeficiency syndrome and infection with *Salmonella typhi* or *Salmonella paratyphi* in an endemic typhoid area. Arch Int Med 1991; 381–382.
11. Rideway EJ, Brown JM. *Listeria monocytogenes* meningitis in the acquired immunodeficiency syndrome—limitations of conventional typing methods in tracing of a foodborne source. J Infect Dis 1989; 19:167–171.
12. Sorvillo FJ, Lieb LE, Waterman SH, et al. Incidence of campylobacteriosis among patients with AIDS in Los Angeles County. J Acquir Immune Defic Syndr 1991; 4:598–602.
13. Hedberg CW, Korlath JA, D'Aoust JY, et al. A multistate outbreak of *Salmonella javiana* and *Salmonella oranienburg* infections due to consumption of contaminated cheese. JAMA 1992; 268:3202–3207.
14. CDC. Update: Multistate outbreak of *Escherichia coli* 0157:H7 infections from hamburger—Western United States. Morb Mortal Wkly Rep 1993; 258–263.
15. Morrow JD, Margolies GR, Rowland J, et al. Evidence that histamine is the causative toxin of scombroid-fish poisoning. N Engl J Med 1991; 324:716–720.
16. Hoff G, Giedinghagen DH, Thomas MC. Vibrio infections in Kansas City. Mo Med 1990; 87:881–883.
17. CDC. Cholera associated with imported frozen coconut milk—Maryland, 1991. Morb Mortal Wkly Rep 1991; 40:844–845.
18. Belongia JN, Hedberg CW, Gleich GJ, et al. An investigation of the cause of the eosinophilia-myalgia syndrome associated with tryptophan use. N Engl J Med 1990; 323:358–365.
19. Tranter HS. Foodborne staphylococcal illness. Lancet 1990; 336:1044–1046.
20. Richards MS, Tittman M, Gilbert TT, et al. Investigation of a staphylococcal food poisoning outbreak in a centralized school lunch program. Publ Health Rep 1993; 108:765–771.
21. Eisenberg MS, Gaarslev K, Brown W, et al. Staphyloccocal food poisoning aboard a commercial aircraft. Lancet 1975; 595–600.
22. Holmberg SD, Blake PA. Staphylococcal food poisoning in the United States: New facts and old misconceptions. JAMA 1984; 251:487–489.
23. Liu CT, DuFault BR. Effects of intestinal infusion of staphylococcal enterotoxin B (SEB) on water and electrolyte fluxes: Possible mechanisms of diarrhea. Physiologist 1977; 20:57.
24. Elwell MR, Liu CT, Spertzel, et al. Mechanisms of oral staphylococcal enterotoxin B-induced emesis in the monkey. Proc Soc Exp Biol Med 1975; 148:424–427.
25. Kraatz-Wadsack G, Ahrens W, von Stuckrad J. ELISA screening of staphylococcal enterotoxins by means of a specially developed test kit. Int J Food Microbiol 1991; 13:265–272.
26. Wieneke AA. Comparison of four kits for the detection of staphylococcal enterotoxin in foods from outbreaks of food poisoning. Int J Food Microbiol 1991; 14:305–312.
27. Drobniewski FA. *Bacillus cereus* and related species. Clin Microbiol Rev 1993; 6:324–338.

28. Lund BM. Foodborne disease due to *Bacillus* and *Clostridium* species. Lancet 1990; 336:982–986.
29. Mortimer R, McCann G. Food poisoning episodes associated with *Bacillus cereus* in fried rice. Lancet 1974 i; 1043–1045.
30. CDC. *Bacillus cereus* food poisoning associated with fried rice at two child day care centers—Virginia, 1993. Morb Mortal Wkly Rep 1994; 43:177–178.
31. Granum PE. *Bacillus cereus* and its toxins. Soc Appl Bacteriol Symp Ser 1994; 23:61S–66S.
32. Ghosh AC. Prevalence of *Bacillus cereus* in the faeces of healthy adults. J Hyg 1978; 80:233–236.
33. Turnbull PC, Kramer JM. Intestinal carriage of *Bacillus cereus*: Faecal isolation studies in three population groups. J Hyg 1985; 95:629–638.
34. Szabo RA, Speirs JI, Akhtar M. Cell culture detection and conditions for production of *Bacillus cereus* heat-stable toxin. J Food Prot 1991; 54:272–276.
35. Mikami T, Horikawa T, Murakami T, et al. An improved method for detecting cytostatic toxin (emetic toxin) of *Bacillus cereus* and its application to food samples. FEMS Microbiol Lett 1994; 119:53–57.
36. Kramer JM, Gilbert RJ. *Bacillus cereus* and other *Bacillus* species In: Doyle MP, ed. Foodborne bacterial pathogens. New York: Marcel Dekker, 1989:21–70
37. Hughes JM, Horowitz MA, Merson MH, et al. Foodborne disease outbreaks of chemical etiology in the United States, 1970–1974. Am J Epidemiol 1977; 105:233–244.
38. Taterka JA, Cuff CF, Rubin DH. Viral gastrointestinal infections. Gastroenterol Clin North Am 1992; 21:303–330.
39. CDC. Viral agents of gastroenteritis: Public health importance and outbreak management. Morb Mortal Wkly Rep 1990; 39:1–21.
40. Kapikian AZ. Viral gastroenteritis. JAMA 1993; 269:627–630.
41. Hedberg CW, Osterholm MT. Outbreaks of food-borne and waterborne viral gastroenteritis. Clin Microbiol Rev; 1993; 6:199–210.
42. Warner RD, Carr RW, McCleskey FK, et al. A large nontypical outbreak of Norwalk virus. Arch Int Med 1991; 151:2419–2424.
43. Morse DL, Guzewich JJ, Hanrahan JP, et al. Widespread outbreaks of clam and oyster associated gastroenteritis: Role of Norwalk virus. N Engl J Med 1986; 314:678–681.
44. CDC. Viral gastroenteritis associated with consumption of raw oysters—Florida, 1993. Morb Mortal Wkly Rep 1994; 43:446–448.
45. CDC. Multistate outbreak of viral gastroenteritis related to consumption of oysters—Louisiana, Maryland, Mississippi and North Carolina, 1993. Morb Mortal Wkly Rep 1993; 42:945–948.
46. Gordon SM, Oshiro LS, Jarvis WR, et al. Food borne Snow Mountain agent gastroenteritis with secondary person-to-person spread in a retirement community. Am J Epidemiol 1990; 131:702–710.
47. Jiang X, Graham DY, Wang K, et al. Norwalk virus genome cloning and characterization. Science 1990; 250:1580–1583.

48. Lew JF, Kapikian AZ, Valdesuso J, et al. Molecular characterization of Hawaii virus and other Norwalk-like viruses: Evidence for genetic polymorphism among human calciviruses. J Infect Dis 1994; 170:535-542.
49. Lambden PR, Caul EO, Ashley CR, et al. Sequence and genome organization of a human small round-structured (Norwalk-like) virus. Science 1993; 259:516-518.
50. Wang J, Jiang X, Madore HP, et al. Sequence diversity of small, round-structured viruses in the Norwalk virus group. J Virol 1994; 68:5982-5990.
51. Agus S, Falchuk ZM, Sessoms CS, et al. Increased jejunal IgA synthesis in vitro during acute infectious nonbacterial gastroenteritis. Am J Dig Dis 1974; 17:127-131.
52. Okhuysen P, Jiang X, Tenjaria G, et al. Detection of Norwalk specific fecal IgA in challenged volunteers utilizing ELISA with baculovirus expressed Norwalk particles as coating antigens. 32nd Interscience Conference on Antimicrobial Agents and Chemotherapy, Anaheim, CA, 1992.
53. Monroe SS, Stine SE, Jiang X, et al. Detection of antibody to recombinant Norwalk virus antigen in specimens from outbreaks of gastroenteritis. J Clin Microbiol 1993; 31:2866-2872.
54. Madore HP, Treanor JJ, Pray KA, et al. Enzyme-linked immunosorbent assays for Snow Mountain and Norwalk agents of viral gastroenteritis. J Virol Methods 1988; 22:207-214.
55. Moe CL, Gentsch J, Ando T, et al. Application of PCR to detect Norwalk virus in fecal specimens from outbreaks of gastroenteritis. J Clin Microbiol 1994; 32:642-648.
56. Pollock AM, Whitty PM. Outbreak of *Clostridium perfringens* food poisoning. J Hosp Infect 1991; 17:179-186.
57. Roach RL, Sienko DG. *Clostridium perfringens* outbreak associated with minestrone soup. Am J Epidemiol 1992; 136:1288-1291.
58. Brett MM, Rodhouse JC, Donovan TJ, et al. Detection of *Clostridium perfringens* and its enterotoxin in cases of sporadic diarrhoea. J Clin Pathol 1992; 45:609-611.
59. Shandera WX, Tacket CO, Blake PA. Food poisoning due to *Clostridium perfringens* in the United States. J Infect Dis 1983; 147:167-170.
60. Granum PE. *Clostridium perfringens* toxins involved in food poisoning. Int J Food Microbiol 1990; 10:101-111.
61. Stark RL, Duncan CL. Biological characteristics of *Clostridium perfringens* Type A enterotoxin. Infect Immun 1971; 4:89-96.
62. Akama K, Otani S. *Clostridium perfringens* as the flora in the intestine in healthy persons. Jpn J Med Sci Biol 1970; 23:161.
63. Harmon SM, Kautter DA. Evaluation of a reversed passive latex agglutination test kit for *Clostridium perfringens* enterotoxin. J Food Protection 1986; 49:523-525.
64. McClane BA, Strouse RJ. Rapid detection of *Clostridium perfringens* type A enterotoxin by enzyme-linked immunosorbent assay. J Clin Microbiol 1984; 19:112-115.

65. Van Damme-Jongsten M, Rodhouse J, Gilbert RJ, et al. Synthetic DNA probes for detection of enterotoxigenic Clostridium perfringens strains isolated from outbreaks of food poisoning. J Clin Microbiol 1990; 28:131–133.
66. Saito M, Matsumoto M, Funabashi M. Detection of *Clostridium perfringens* enterotoxin gene by the polymerase chain reaction amplification procedure. Int J Food Microbiol 1992; 17:47–55.
67. Luby S, Jones J, Dowda H, et al. A large outbreak of gastroenteritis caused by diarrheal toxin-producing *Bacillus cereus*. J Infect Dis 1993; 167:1452–1455.
68. Slaten DD, Oropeza RI, Werner SB. An outbreak of *Bacillus cereus* food poisoning - Are caterers supervised sufficiently. Publ Health Rep 1992; 107:477–480.
69. Turnbull PC, Kramer JM, Jorgensen K, et al. Properties and production characteristics of vomiting, diarrheal, and necrotizing toxins of *Bacillus cereus*. Am J Clin Nutr 1979; 32:219–228.
70. CDC. Foodborne outbreaks of enterotoxigenic *Escherichia coli*—Rhode Island and New Hampshire, 1993. Morb Mortal Wkly Rep 1994; 43:81–89.
71. Levine MM, Kaper JB, Black RE. New knowledge in the pathogenesis of bacterial enteric infections as applied to vaccine development. Microbiol Rev 1983; 47:510–550.
72. Blanco J, Blanco M, Garabal JI, et al. Enterotoxins, colonization factors and serotypes of enterotoxigenic *Escherichia coli* from humans and animals. Microbiologia 1991; 7:57–73.
73. Mintz ED, Hudson-Wragg M, Mshar P, et al. Foodborne giardiasis in a corporate office setting. J Infect Dis 1993; 167:250–253.
74. CDC. Importation of cholera from Peru. Morb Mortal Wkly Rep 1991; 40:258–259.
75. Blaser MJ, Wells JG, Feldman RA, et al. Campylobacter enteritis in the United States: A multicenter study. Ann Int Med 1983; 98:360–365.
76. Mishu B, Koehler J, Lee LA, et al. Outbreaks of *Salmonella enteritidis* infections in the United States, 1985–1991. J Infect Dis 1994; 169:547–552.
77. Mishu B, Griffin PM, Tauxe RV, et al. *Salmonella enteriitidis* gastroenteritis transmitted by intact chicken eggs. Ann Int Med 1991; 115:190–194.
78. Morse DL, Birkhead GS, Guardino J, et al. Outbreak and sporadic egg-associated cases of *Salmonella enteritidis*: New York's experience. Am J Publ Health 1994; 84:859–860.
79. Luby SP, Jones JL, Horan JM. A large salmonellosis outbreak associated with a frequently penalized restaurant. Epidemiol Infect 1993; 110:31–39.
80. CDC. Multistate outbreak of *Salmonella poona* infections - United States and Canada, 1991. Morb Mortal Wkly Rep 1991; 40:549–552.
81. Blaser MJ, Newman LS. A review of human salmonellosis : I. Infective dose. Rev Infect Dis 1982; 4:1096–1106.
82. Roberts FJ. Nontyphoidal, nonparatyphoidal Salmonell septicemia in adults. Eur J Clin Microbiol Infect Dis 1993; 12:205–208.
83. Salyers AA, Whitt DD. Salmonella infections. In: Salyers AA, Whitt DD, eds. Bacterial Pathogenesis: A Molecular Approach. Washington, DC: American Society for Microbiology Press, 1994:229–243.

84. Galan JE, Ginocchio C. The molecular genetic bases of *Salmonella* entry into mammalian cells. Biochem Soc Trans 1994; 22:301–306.
85. Holmberg SD, Osterholm MT, Senger KA, et al. Drug-resistant salmonella from animals fed antimicrobials. N Engl J Med 1984; 311:617–622.
86. Spika JS, Waterman SH, Soo Hoo GW, et al. Chloramphenicol-resistant *Salmonella newport* traced through hamburger to dairy farms. N Engl J Med 1987; 316:565–570.
87. Aserkoff B, Bennett JV. Effect of antibiotic therapy in acute samonellosis on the fecal excretion of Salmonellae. N Engl J Med 1969; 281:636–640.
88. Lee LA, Shapiro CN, Hargrett-Bean, et al. Hyperendemic shigellosis in the United States: A review of surveillance data for 1967–1988. J Infect Dis 1991; 164:894–900.
89. Lee LA, Ostroff SM, McGee HB, et al. An outbreak of shigellosis at an outdoor music festival. Am J Epidemiol 1991; 133:608–615.
90. Gessner BD, Beller M. Moose soup shigellosis in Alaska. West J Med 1994; 160:430–433.
91. Hedberg CW, Leving WC, White KE, et al. An international foodborne outbreak of shigellosis associated with a commercial airline. JAMA 1992; 268:3208–3212.
92. Lew JF, Swerdlow DL, Dance ME, et al. An outbreak of shigellosis aboard a cruise ship caused by a multiple-antibiotic-resistant strain of *Shigella flexneri*. Am J Epidemiol 1991; 134:413–420.
93. O'Brien AD, Holmes RK. Shig and shiga-like toxins. Microbiol Rev 1987; 51:206–220.
94. Hale TL. Genetic bases of virulence in *Shigella* species. Microbiol Rev 1991; 55:206–224.
95. Ries AA, Wells JG, Olivola D, et al. Epidemic *Shigella dysenteriae* type 1 in Burundi: panresistance and implications for prevention. J infect Dis 1994; 169:1035–1041.
96. Skirrow MB. Campylobacter perspectives. PHLS Microbiol Dig 1989; 6:113–117.
97. Riley LW, Finch MJ. Results of the first year of surveillance of Campylobacter infections in the United States. J Infect Dis 1985; 151:956–959.
98. Altekruse SF, Hunt JM, TollefsonLk, et al. Food and animal sources of human *Campylobacter jejuni* infection. J Am Vet Med Assoc 1994; 204:57–61.
99. Melby K, Dahl OP, Crisp L, et al. Clinical and serological manifestations in patients during a waterborne epidemic due to *Campylobacter jejuni*. J Infect 1990; 21:309–316.
100. Blaser MJ, Wells JG, Feldman RA, et al. Campylobacter enteritis in the United States. Ann Int Med 1983; 98:360–365.
101. Lind KM, Gaub J, Pedersen RS. Henoch-Schonlein purpura associated with *Campylobacter jejuni* enteritis. Scand J Urol Nephrol 1994; 28:179–181.
102. Peterson MC. Rheumatic manifestation of *Campylobacter jejuni* and *C. fetus* infections in adults. Scand J Rheumatol 1994; 23:167–170.
103. Bremell T, Bjelle A, Svedhem. Rheumatic symptoms following an outbreak of campylobacter enteritis: A five year follow up. Ann Rheum Dis 1991; 50:934–938.

104. von Wulffen H, Hartard C, Scharein E. Seroreactivity to *Campylobacter jejuni* and gangliosides in patients with Guillain-Barre syndrome. J Infect Dis 1994; 170:828–833.
105. Rees JH, Gregson NA, Griffiths PL, et al. *Campylobacter jejuni* and Guillain Barre syndrome. Q J Med 1993; 86:623–634.
106. Mishu B, Blaser MJ. Role of infection due to *Campylobacter jejuni* in the initiation of Guillain-Barre syndrome. Clin Infect Dis 1993; 17:104–108.
107. Aspinall GO, Fujimoto S, McDonald AG, et al. Lipopolysaccharides from *Campylobacter jejuni* associated with Guillain-Barre syndrome patients mimic human gangliosides in structure. Infect Immun 1994; 62:2122–2125.
108. Aspinall GO, McDonald AG, Pang H, et al. Lipopolysaccharides of *Campylobacter jejuni* serotype 0:19: Structures of core oligosaccharide regions from the serostrain and two bacterial isolates from patients with the Guillain-Barre syndrome. Biochemistry 1994; 33:241–249.
109. Smith GS, Blaser MJ. Fatalities associated with *Campylobacter jejuni* infections. JAMA 1985; 253:2873.
110. Anders BJ, Lauer BA, Paisley JW, et al. Double-blind placebo controlled trial of erythromycin for treatment of *Campylobacter* enteritis. Lancet 1982; i:131.
111. Zaman R. *Campylobacter* enteritis in Saudi Arabia. Epidemiol Infect 1992; 108:51–58.
112. Rautelin H, Renkonen OV, Kosunen TU. Emergence of fluoroquinolone resistance in *Campylobacter jejuni* and *Campylobacter coli* in subjects from Finland. Antimicrob Agents Chemother 1991; 35:2065–2069.
113. Levine WC, Griffin PM, et al. Vibrio infections on the Gulf Coast: Results of first year of regional surveillance. J Infect Dis 1993; 167:479–483.
114. Haddock RL, Cabanero AF. The origin of non-outbreak *Vibrio parahemolyticus* infections on Guam. Trop Geogr Med 1994; 46:42–43.
115. Doyle MP. Pathogenic *Escherichia coli, Yersinia enterocolitica,* and *Vibrio parahemolyticus*. Lancet 1990; 336:1111–1115.
116. Nishibuchi M, Fasano A, Russell TG, et al. Enterotoxigenicity of *Vibrio parehemolyticus* with and without genes encoding thermostable direct hemolysin. Infect Immun 1992; 60:3539–3545.
117. Hoashi K, Ogata K, Taniguchi H, et al. Pathogenesis of *Vibrio parahemolyticus*: intraperitoneal and orogastric challenge experiments in mice. Microbiol Immuno 1990; 34:355–366.
118. Metchock B, Lonsway DR, Carter GP, et al. *Yersinia enterocolitica*: a frequent seasonal stool isolate from children at an urban hospital in the southeast United States. J Clin Microbiol 1991; 29:2868–2869.
119. Naqvi SH, Swirkosz EM, Gerard J, et al. Presentation of *Yersinia enterocolitica* enteritis in children. Pediatr Infect Dis J 1993; 12:386–389.
120. Kapperud G. *Yersinia enterocolitica* in food hygiene. Int J Food Microbiol 1991; 12:53–65.
121. Case records of the Massachusetts General Hospital. A 50-year old man with the onset of fever and diarrhea in Morocco. N Engl J Med 1993; 329:561–568.
122. Lee LA, Taylor J, Carter GP, et al. *Yersinia enterocolitica* 0:3 An emerging

cause of pediatric gastroenteritis in the United States. J Infect Dis 1991; 163:660–663.

123. Hanna MO, Stewart JC, Zink DL, et al. Development of *Yersinia enterocolitica* on raw and cooked beef and pork at different termperatures. J Food Protection 1977; 42:1180.
124. Lee LA, Gerber AR, Lonsway DR, et al. *Yersinia enterocolitica* 0:3 infections in infants and children, associated with the household preparation of chitterlings. N Engl J Med 1990; 322:984–987.
125. Stoddard JJ, Wechsler DS, Nataro JP, et al. *Yersinia enterocolitica* infection in a patient with sickle cell disease after exposure to chitterlings. Am J Pediatr Hematol Oncol 1994; 16:153–155.
126. CDC. *Yersinia enterocolitica* infections during the holidays in black families—Georgia. Morb Mortal Wkly Rep 1990; 39:819–820.
127. Marks MI, Pai CH, LaFleur L, et al. *Yersinia enterocolitica* gastorenteritis: A prospective study of clinical, bacteriologic, and epidemiologic features. J Pediatr 1980; 96:26–31.
128. Borg AA, Gray J, Dawes PT. Yersinia-related arthritis in the United Kingdom. A report of 12 cases and review of the literature. Q J Med 1992; 84:575–582.
129. Ostroff SM, Kapperud G, Lassen J, et al. Clinical features of sporadic *Yersinia enterocolitica* infections In Norway. J Infect Dis 1992; 166:812–817.
130. Pile K, Kwong T, Fryer J, et al. Polyarteritis associated with *Yersinia enterocolitica* infection. Ann Rhem Dis 1992; 51:678–680.
131. Lindholm H, Visakorpi R. Late complications after a *Yersinia enterocolitica* epidemic: a follow up study. Ann Rheum Dis 1991; 50:694–696.
132. O'Loughlin EV, Gall DG, Pai CH. *Yersinia enterocolitica*: Mechanism of microbial pathogenesis and pathophysiology of diarrhoea. J Gastroenterol Hepatol 1990; 5:173–179.
133. Miller VL, Flakow S. Evidence for two genetic loci in *Yersinia enterocolitica* that can promote invasion of epithelial cells. Infect Immun 1988; 56:1242–1248.
134. Portnoy DA, Moseley SL, Falkow S. Characterization of plasmids and plasmid-associated determinants of *Yersinia enterocolitica* pathogenesis. Infect Immun 1981; 31:775–782.
135. Cantinieaux B, Boelaert J, Hariga C, et al. Impaired neutrophil defense against *Yersinia enterocolitica* in patients with iron overload who are undergoing dialysis. J Lab Clin Med 1988; 111:524–528.
136. Monno R, Valenza MA, Quarto M, et al. *Yersinia enterocolitica* infection in a boy with beta thalassemia major. Pediatr Infect Dis J 1994; 13:233–234.
137. Vadillo M, Corbella X, Pac V, et al. Multiple liver abscesses due to *Yersinia enterocolitica* discloses primary hemochromatosis: three case reports and review. Clin Infect Dis 1994; 18:938–941.
138. Kachoris M, Ruoff KL, Welch K, et al. Routine culture of stool specimens for *Yersinia enterocolitica* is not a cost-effective procedure. J Clin Microbiol 1988; 26:582–583.
139. Riley LW, Remis RS, Helgerson SD, et al. Hemorrhagic colitis associated with a rare *Escherichia coli* serotype. N Engl J Med 1983; 308:681–685.

140. Whipp SC, Rasmussen MA, Cray WC. Animals as a source of *Escherichia coli* pathogenic for human beings. J Am Vet Assoc 1994; 204:1168–1175.
141. Griffin PM, Tauxe RV. The epidemiology of infections caused by O157:H7, other enterohemorrhagic *E. coli*, and the associated hemolytic uremic syndrome. Epidemiol Rev 1991; 13:60–98.
142. Belongia EA, MacDonald KL, Parham GL, et al. An outbreak of *Escherichia coli* O157:H7 colitis associated with consumption of precooked meat patties. J Infect Dis 1991; 164:338–343.
143. Ostroff SM, Griffin PM, Tauxe RV, et al. A statewide outbreak of *Escherichia coli* O157:H7 infections in Washington state. Am J Epidemiol 1990; 132:239–247.
144. Anonymous. Outbreak of gastrointestinal disease in Sarnia, Ontario. Ontario Dis Surveill Rep 1986; 7:604–611.
145. Besser RE, Lett Sm, Weber JT, et al. An outbreak of diarrhea and hemolytic uremic syndrome from Escherichia coli O157:H7 in fresh-pressed apple cider. JAMA 1993; 269:2217–2220.
146. Wells JG, Shipman LD, Greene KD, et al. Isolation of *Escherichia coli* serotype O157:H7 and other shiga-like-toxin-producing *E. coli* from dairy cattle. J Clin Microbiol 1991; 29:985–989.
147. Doyle MP, Schoeni JL. Isolation of *Escherichia coli* O157:H7 from retail fresh meats and poultry. Appl Environ Microbiol 1987; 53:2394–2396.
148. Borczyk AA, Carlson JA, Carter AO, et al. A severe outbreak of *Escherichia coli* O157:H7-associated hemorrhagic colitis in a nursing home. N Engl J Med 1987; 317:1496–1500.
149. Pavia AT, Nichols CR, Green DP, et al. Hemolytic-uremic syndrome during an outbreak of *Escherichia coli* O157:H7 infections in institutions for mentally retarded persons: Clinical and epidemiologic observations. J Pediatr 1990; 116:544–551.
150. Wigginton JM, Thill P. Infant botulism. A review of the literature. Clin Pediatr 1993; 32:669–674.
151. Lecour H, Ramos MH, Almeida B, et al. Food-borne botulism: A review of 13 outbreaks. Arch Int Med 1988; 148:578–580.
152. Roblot P, Roblot F, Fauchere JL, et al. Retrospective study of 108 cases of botulism in Poitiers, France. J Med Microbiol 1994; 40:379–384.
153. St. Louis ME, Peck SH, Bowering D, et al. Botulism from chopped garlic: Delayed recognition of a major outbreak. Ann Int Med 1988; 108:363–368.
154. CDC. Outbreak of type E botulism associated with an uneviscerated, salt-cured fish product—New Jersey, 1992. Morb Mortal Wkly Rep 1992; 41:521–522.
155. Woodruff BA, Griffin PM, McCroskey LM, et al. Clinical and laboratory comparison of botulism from toxin types A, B, and E in the United States, 1975–1988. J Infect Dis 1992; 166:1281–1286.
156. Tacket CO, Shandera WX, Mann JM, et al. Equine antitoxin use and other factors that predict outcome in type A botulism. Am J Medd 1984; 76:794–798.
157. Niemann H, Blasi J, Jahn R. Clostridial neurotoxins: new tools for dissecting exocytosis. Trends Cell Biol 1994; 4:179–185.

158. Lawrence DN, Enriquez MB, Lumish RM, et al. Ciguatera fish posoning in Miami. JAMA 1980; 244:254–258.
159. Katz AR, Terrell-Perica S, Sasaki DM. Ciguatera on Kauai: investigation of factors associated with severity of illness. Am J Trop Med Hyg 1993; 49:448–454.
160. CDC. Ciguatera fish poisoning—Florida, 1991. Morb Mortal Wkly Rep 1993; 42:417–418.
161. DeFusco DJ, O'Dowd P, Hokama Y, et al. Coma due to ciguatera poisoning in Rhode Island. Am J Med 1993; 95:240–243.
162. Bagnis R, Kuberski T, Laugier S. Clinical observations on 3,009 cases of ciguatera (fish poisoning) in the South Pacific. Am J Trop Med 1979; 28:1067–1073.
163. Gillespie NC, Lewis RJ, Pearn JH, et al. Ciguatera in Australia: occurrence, clinical features, pathophysiology and management. Med J Aust 1986; 145:584–590.
164. Glaziou P, Martin PM. Study of factors that influence the clinical response to ciguatera fish poisoning. Toxicon 1993; 31:1151–1154.
165. Bidard JN, Vijverberg HP, Frelin C, et al. Ciguatoxin is a novel type of Na channel toxin. J Biol Chem 1984; 259:8353–8357.
166. Hokama Y. A rapid, simplified enzyme immunoassay stick test for the detection of ciguatoxin and related polyethers from fish tissues. Toxicon 1985; 23:939–946.
167. Hoffman PA, Granade HR, McMillan JP. The mouse ciguatoxin bioassay: A dose-response curve and symptomatology analysis. Toxicon 1983; 21:363–369.
168. Hokama Y. Simplified solid-phase immunobead assay for detection of ciguatoxin and related polyethers. J Clin Lab Anal 1990; 4:213–217.
169. Blythe DG, DeSylva DP, Fleming LE, et al. Clinical experience with IV mannitol in the treatment of ciguatera. Bull Soc Pathol Exot 1992; 85:425–426.
170. Davis RT, Villar LA. Symptomatic improvement with amitriptyline in ciguatera fish poisoning. N Engl J Med 1986; 315:65.
171. Hughes JM, Merson MH. Fish and shellfish poisoning. N Engl J Med 1976; 295:1117–1120.
172. Smart DR. Scombroid poisoning. A report of seven cases involving the Western Australian salmon, *Arripis truttaceus*. Med J Austr 1992; 157:748–751.
173. Muller GJ, Lamprecht JH, Barnes JM, et al. Scombroid poisoning. Case series of 10 incidents involving 22 patients. S Afr Med J 1992; 81:427–430.
174. Christman BW. Scombroid-fish poisoning. N Engl J Med 1991; 325:515.
175. Clifford MN, Walker R, Wright J, et al. Studies with volunteers on the role of histamine in suspected scombrotoxicosis. J Sci Food Agric 1989; 47:365–375.
176. Blakesley ML. Scombroid poisoning: Prompt resolution of symptoms with cimetidine. Ann Emerg Med 1983; 12:104–106.
177. Sakamoto Y, Lockey RF, Krznowski JJ, et al. Shellfish and fish poisoning related to the toxic dinoflagellates. South Med J 1987; 80:866–872.
178. Eastaugh J, Shepherd S. Infectious and toxic syndromes from fish and shellfish consumption. Arch Int Med 1989; 149:1735–1740.

179. Underman AE, Leedom JM. Fish and shellfish poisoning. Curr Clin Top Infect Dis 1993; 13:203–225.
180. Rheinstein PH, Klontz KC. Shellfish-borne illness. Am Fam Physician 1993; 47:1837–1840.
181. Morris PD, Campbell DS, Taylor TJ, et al. Clinical and epidemiological features of neurotoxic shellfish poisoning in North Carolina. Am J Publ Health 1991; 81:471–474.
182. CDC. Paralytic shellfish poisoning—Massachusetts and Alaska, 1990. Morb Mortal Wkly Rep 1991; 40:157–161.
183. Grunfeld Y, Spiegelstein MY. Effects of *Gymnodinium breve* toxin on the smooth muscle preparation of guinea pig ileum. Br J Pharmacol 1974; 51:67–72.
184. Morgan MR, Fenwick GR. Natural foodborne intoxicants. Lancet 1990; 336:1492–1495.
185. Music SI, Howell JT, Brumback CL. Red tide, its public health implications. J Fla Med Assoc 1973; 60:27.
186. Perl TM, Bedard L, Kosatsky T, et al. An outbreak of toxic encephalopathy caused by eating mussels contaminated with domoic acid. N Engl J Med 1990; 322:1775–1780.
187. Teitelbaum JS, Zatorre RJ, Carpenter S, et al. Neurologic sequelae of domoic acid intoxication due to the ingestion of contaminated mussels. N Engl J Med 1990; 322:1781–1787.
188. Wright JL, Boyd RK, de Freitas AS, et al. Identification of domoic acid, a neuroexcitatory amino acid, in toxic mussels from eastern Prince Edward Island. Can J Chem 1989; 67:481–490.
189. Jones D. Foodborne listeriosis. Lancet 1990; 336:1171–1174.
190. Schuchat A, Swaminathan B, Broome CV. Epidemiology of human listeriosis. Clin Microbiol Rev 1991; 4:169–183.
191. Pinner RW, Schuchat A, Swaminathan B, et al. Role of foods in sporadic listeriosis: II. Microbiologic and epidemiologic investigation. JAMA 1992; 267:2046–2050.
192. CDC. Update: Foodborne listeriosis—United States, 1988–1990. Morb Mortal Wkly Rep 1992; 41:251–257.
193. Fleming DW, Cochi SL, MacDonald KL, et al. Pasteurized milk as a vehicle of infection in an outbreak of listeriosis. N Engl J Med 1985; 312:404–407.
194. Linnan MJ, Mascola L, Lou XD, et al. Epidemic listeriosis associated with mexican-style cheese. N Engl J Med 1988; 319:823–828.
195. Schwartz B, Cieselski CA, Broome CV, et al. Association of sporadic listeriosis with consumption of uncooked hot dogs and undercooked chicken. Lancet 1988; ii:779–782.
196. King W, Raposa S, Warshaw J, et al. A new colorimetric nucleic acid hybridization assay for Listeria in foods. Int J Food Microbiol 1989; 8:225–232.
197. McAuley JB, Michelson, MK, Schantz PM. Trichinosis surveillance, United States, 1987-1990. Morb Mortal Wkly Rep 1991; 40:35–42.
198. Chomel BB, DeBess EE, Mangeamele DM, et al. Changing trends in the epidemiology of human brucellosis in California from 1973 to 1992: a shift toward foodborne transmission. J Infect Dis 1994; 170:1216–1223.

199. Farley TA, Wilson SA, Mahoney F, et al. Direct inoculation of food as the cause of an outbreak of Group A streptococcal pharyngitis. J Infect Dis 1993; 167:1232–1235.
200. Shemesh E, Fischel T, Goldstein N, et al. An outbreak of foodborne streptococcal throat infection. Isr J Med 1994; 30:275–278.
201. Papetropoulos T, Hadziyannis S, Ouzonellis T. On the pathogenetic mechanism of quail myopathy. JAMA 1980; 244:2263–2264.
202. CDC. Toxic hypoglycemic syndrome—Jamaica, 1989–1991. Morb Mortal Wkly Rep 1992; 41:53–55.
203. Morgan MRA, Fenwick GR. Natural foodborne intoxicants. Lancet 1990; 336:1494–1495.
204. Rodhouse JC, Haugh CA, Roberts D, et al. Red kidney bean poisoning in the UK: An analysis of 50 suspected incidents between 1976 and 1989. Epidemiol Infect 1990; 105:485–491.
205. Farese RV, Biglieri EG, Shackleton CHL, et al. Licorice-induced hypermineralocorticoidism. N Eng J Med 1991; 325:1223–1227.
206. Haddock RL, Cruz OL. Foodborne intoxication associated with seaweed. Lancet 1991; 338:195–196.
207. Hanrahan JP, Gordon MA. Mushroom poisoning: Case reports and a review of therapy. JAMA 1984; 251:1057–1061.
208. Stephens T. Organophosphate pesticides: Neurotoxins threaten farm workers. J of NIH Research 1991; 3:21–24.
209. CDC. Endrin poisoning associated with taquito ingestion—California. Morb Mortal Wkly Rep 1989; 38:345–347.
210. Slutsker L, Hoesly FC, Miller L, et al. Eosinophilia-myalgia syndrome associated with exposure to tryptophan from a single manufacturer. JAMA 1990; 264:2213–217.

5

Traveler's Diarrhea

MATTHEW E. FALAGAS
Tufts University School of Medicine and New England Medical Center, Boston, Massachusetts

SHERWOOD L. GORBACH
Tufts University School of Medicine, Boston, Massachusetts

I. INTRODUCTION

Diarrheal diseases, including traveler's diarrhea (TD), were reported in Hippocractic writings and the Bible. Travelers throughout the ages have described episodes of intestinal indisposition in their journals. It is not surprising that no other disease has attracted so many colorful monikers as TD (Table 1). Several prospective studies have shown that TD is common: approximately 40% of the 20 million people traveling each year from industrialized countries to developing countries experience this condition (1, 2).

Although almost nobody dies from TD and fewer than 1% are admitted to a hospital, every third person stricken with TD is confined to bed, usually for 1–2 days, and 40% change their itinerary (3). Whether the trip is for business or pleasure, TD is an important concern of the traveler because several days can be wasted by unrelenting calls to stool. Since the reputation of TD is sometimes enough to discourage tourists from traveling to a high-risk area, TD has a major impact on international tourism by lost revenues, particularly for developing countries. In terms of frequency and economic impact, TD is the number one health-related problem in international tourism (4, 5).

Table 1 Traveler's Diarrhea: A Disease with Numerous Monikers

Aden gut
Aztec two-step
Backdoor sprint
Bali Bali
Basra belly
Canary disease
Casablanca crud
Coeliac flux
Delhi belly
Emporiatic entritis
GI's
Greek gallop
Gyppy (Egyptian) tummy
Ho Chi Minhs
Hong Kong dog
Maladie de la Mer Rouge
Malta dog
Montezuma's revenge
Passion
Poonah pooh
Rangoon runs
Rome runs
San Fanciscitis
Squitter
Summer complaint
Tokyo trots
Tourist trot
Trotsky's
Traveler's diarrhea
Turista
Turkey trots
Zermattitis

II. DEFINITION

Several definitions have been proposed for TD. Most recent studies define TD as the passage of either four or more unformed stools in a 24-hour period or three or more unformed stools in an 8-hour period with at least one of the following symptoms or signs of enteric disease: nausea, vomiting, abdominal cramps, fever, fecal urgency, or the passage of bloody or mucoid stools (6, 7).

III. ETIOLOGY

Several etiologies have been proposed for TD including spicy foods, too much noonday sun, change in the water, inhaled sand particles, and the general vicissitudes of travel. However, scientific investigations during the last 50 years have established that infectious agents acquired from food and drinks are the causes of TD in the overwhelming majority of cases. Early studies suggested the development of some immunity to TD. In 1943, Bulmer observed in a military hospital in Egypt that the incidence of all diarrheal diseases declined with increasing length of service (8). Later, Ben Kean and his collaborators undertook a classic series of investigations of students traveling to Mexico and Europe. Besides describing the clinical and epidemiologic features of the illness, they showed, in a placebo-controlled trial, that antimicrobial drugs provide protection against TD (9–13). This seminal observation inspired further research that led to the discovery of enterotoxigenic *Escherichia coli* (ETEC) as the major cause of TD (14–18). Several studies have shown that the incidence and the etiologic agents of TD are similar to those of diarrhea in local children, with the possible exception of diarrhea caused by rotavirus, which is more common in children (19, 20).

Since 1974, more than 20 etiologic studies of TD have been published concerning travelers to Mexico, other countries of Latin America, Asia, and Africa. While an array of pathogens have been implicated in TD, it is apparent that the leading causes of TD are various forms of *E. coli*, particularly ETEC. Other etiologic agents include pathogenic bacteria, protozoa, and viruses (Table 2). These studies have shown there is geographic variability among the causes of TD. In Latin America, for example, the median isolation rate of ETEC is about 40% (range 17% to 72%) whereas only 16% of TD in Asia (range 6% to 37%) is due to ETEC (21). An investigation of the etiology of TD in Thailand found ETEC to be in third place (6%) after *Campylobacter* (41%) and *Salmonella* (18%) (22). In addition, there is seasonal variability among the causes of TD. Among Finnish travelers to Morocco, ETEC was the leading cause of TD during the fall, responsible for 56% of the cases, but *Camplyobacter jejuni* was the leading cause of TD during the winter (46% of the bacteriologically confirmed cases), followed by *Salmonella* (16%), and ETEC (14%) (23). Besides *C. jejuni*, rotavirus diarrhea is more common in winter. About 15% of travelers developed TD in the winter, compared to about one-third of travelers in the fall.

Vibrio cholerae is not an important cause in TD, and there are only a few descriptions of cholera as a cause of diarrhea in travelers (24). Other vibrios, e.g. *V. parahaemolyticus* and *V. vulnificus*, can cause a serious form of TD, especially in high-risk groups. Several patients with liver disease died in Florida after eating raw oysters contaminated by *V. vulnificus* (25).

Table 2 Microbial Pathogens in Travelers' Diarrhea

Etiology	Approximate frequency of isolation[a] (%)
Bacteria	
Escherichia coli	30–60
Enterotoxigenic (ETEC)	20–50
Enteroadhesive	10
Enteroinvasive	10
Enteroaggregative	?
Campylobacter spp.	2–15
Salmonella spp	2–10
Shigella	2–15
Aeromonas	2–5
Plesiomonas	2–5
Vibrios	0–5
Other	0–5
Protozoa	
Giardia lamblia	0–5
Entamoeba histolytica	0–5
Cryptosporidium spp.	0–5
Cyclospora cayetanensis	0–2
Viruses	
Rotavirus	2–10
Norwalk	0–5
Calicivirus	0–5
Enteroviruses	0–5
>1 pathogen isolated	35
No pathogen isolated	20

[a]There is wide variability in frequency of isolation of various etiologic agents of TD among the etiologic studies of TD. The differences are partially explained by the geographic and seasonal variability in the etiology of TD (see text).

Traveler's diarrhea caused by *Shigella* tends to be more severe than the usual form of TD. In a report from Cancun, Mexico, some cases of TD due to *Shigella dysenteriae* type I, the most virulent strain of *Shigella*, were associated with hemolytic-uremic syndrome. In addition, many of these strains were resistant to trimethoprim-sulfamethoxazole (26).

Enteric pathogens other than bacteria are less common causes of TD. However, in some parts of the world protozoa, such as *Giardia, Cryptosporidia,* or *Cyclospora* species are responsible for a considerable portion of TD cases (27–32). *Giardia lamblia* is an important cause of diarrhea among travelers to St. Petersburg in the former Soviet Union and mountainous areas of North

America. In addition to bacteria and protozoa, viruses such as rotavirus and Norwalk virus are sometimes the cause of TD, particularly during epidemic seasons (33).

Several studies have reported that a considerable proportion of TD (about 20%) is caused by mixed infections (34). Also, no pathogen has been identified in about 35% of TD despite careful laboratory methodology. It is postulated that infectious agents that escape detection by the available laboratory techniques are the cause of most of these undiagnosed cases of TD. The proportion of culture-negative cases of TD should diminish with the advent of improved laboratory techniques such as the polymerase chain reaction (PCR), which has been used to increase by two-fold the isolation rate of *Shigella* in cases of TD (35).

Some patients with TD develop protracted illness lasting weeks or even months. The differential diagnosis is broad and includes infectious diseases and postinfectious disorders. Among the infectious agents, protozoa—such as *Giardia lamblia, Cryptosporidium,* or *Cyclospora*—tend to cause long-standing diarrhea. In patients with diarrhea of 1–3 weeks duration, an invasive enteric pathogen such as *Shigella, Salmonella*, or *Campylobacter* may be the cause. Among the postinfectious disorders, disaccharidase deficiency caused by bowel mucosa injury or small-bowel bacterial overgrowth syndrome caused by small-bowel stasis are causes of long-standing diarrhea in travelers. Chronic diarrhea known as Brainerd diarrhea (after the outbreak in Brainerd, Minnesota) has been associated with consumption of raw milk or untreated surface water (36, 37). This condition is thought to have an infectious etiology, although the responsible agent has not been identified. Most of the patients with prolonged TD (duration over a month) have a benign outcome (38).

IV. EPIDEMIOLOGY

The risk factors for TD have been investigated in only a few populations. Most data are derived from studies of U.S. visitors to Mexico and, to a lesser extent, other countries. Finnish, Swiss, German, Austrian, and British travelers have been studied most extensively (39). These studies have shown that the major determinants of the risk of TD are the country of destination, the country of origin, the purpose of travel, eating style, and host factors.

According to retrospective studies of nearly 20,000 tourists, mostly from Switzerland and Germany, it has been possible to define three geographic risk zones for a traveler departing from the United States, Canada, or Europe (40). High-risk destinations, where the incidence of TD ranges from 20% to 50%, include most parts of Africa, Latin America, the Middle East, and Southern Asia. Intermediate-risk destinations, where the incidence of TD ranges from

10% to 20%, include Southern Europe, Israel, Northern Asia, South Africa, and certain Caribbean Islands. Low-risk destinations, where the incidence of TD is below 8%, include Northern Europe, the United States, Canada, Australia, and New Zealand.

In addition to the country of destination, the country of origin of the traveler is an important determinant of the risk of TD. Among political observers sent to Lebanon by the United Nations in 1958, 40% of those whose home country was in Europe developed TD compared to 10% of those from Asia or South America (41). Similar observations were made at international congresses in Teheran and Mexico City (17, 42, 43). Long residence in a tropical country leads to increased resistance to TD, but previous short-term travel to high-risk destinations has little influence on TD rates (43, 47). These data suggest that natural immunity does develop through exposure, but the immunity is not solid and long standing.

The purpose of travel and eating style of the traveler are also important determinants of the risk of TD (1, 40). The greatest frequency of TD occurs in people traveling as students or itinerant tourists, the lowest risk in those visiting relatives, and intermediate risk in business travelers. Traveler's diarrhea is acquired through ingestion of fecally contaminated food or beverages. High-level contamination with enteric bacteria is found in food from street vendors, school cafeterias, and restaurants (45). The safest place to eat is in a private home. High-risk foods and drinks include uncooked vegetables, meat, seafood, unpasteurized milk, and dairy products, sauces, and dressings in open containers on the table, unpeeled fruit, tap water, and ice. Low-risk foods and drinks include any item served steaming hot (>60°C), peeled fruit, bottled carbonated beverages (especially flavored beverages), wine, beer, hot coffee and tea, and water boiled or appropriately chlorinated. Bottled uncarbonated mineral water should not be considered risk-free for TD, since studies have shown that in some areas drinking of such water was associated with increased risk of waterborne infection (46, 47).

Host factors also play a role in determining the risk for development of TD. Young children (<4 years old) and travelers between 20 and 30 years old seem to have the highest rates of TD (40, 44). Lack of previous exposure to the causative agents of TD and immaturity of the immune system are the most likely reasons for the increased incidence of TD in young children. In young adults, it is not clear whether immunologic or epidemiologic factors—such as a more liberal or experimental eating style—are the causes for the increased incidence of TD. In addition to age, health-related and biologic host factors determine the susceptibility to TD. Gastric hypochlorhydria, immunodeficiency, and the presence of intestinal receptors required for the pathogenesis of certain TD pathogens may predispose the traveler to the illness (48).

V. PATHOGENESIS

Most work has focused on the pathogenesis of TD caused by enterotoxigenic *E. coli* (ETEC), the major pathogen in TD (49–52). This strain produces heat-labile toxin (LT), heat-stable toxin (ST), or both. Two types of genetic elements, usually plasmids, are required for pathogenicity of ETEC. The first genetic element encodes for fimbria or some other structure on the outer membrane that allows the bacterium to attach to the intestinal mucosa. The other genetic element encodes for production of toxin. The pathogenesis of heat-labile-toxin-producing ETEC and that of *V. cholerae* is similar, although not identical (53). Heat-labile toxin, like cholera toxin, attaches to the GM_1 ganglioside of the epithelial cell, followed by release of the A-subunit of the toxin hexamer. The A-subunit penetrates the epithelial cell and stimulates adenyl cyclase, which increases concentrations of cyclic adenosine monophosphate (cAMP). This alters the function of the sodium–potassium pump, with subsequent active excretion of sodium into the lumen, along with transfer of water, which leads to diarrhea.

Heat-stable toxin stimulates guanylate cyclase. The clinical picture caused by heat-labile and heat-stable toxins is similar, although heat-stable toxin may cause more vomiting and less diarrhea. The main site of activity in disease caused by heat-labile toxin is the small intestine, while disease caused by heat-stable toxin involves both the small intestine and colon. The clinical picture is not necessarily more severe when both heat-labile and heat-stable toxins are produced.

VI. CLINICAL FEATURES

Traveler's diarrhea does not begin immediately after arrival at the destination but generally 2–7 days later (1,54,55). Over 90% of the cases occur within two weeks after arrival. The abrupt onset of watery or loose bowel movements is the most common complaint, along with an array of associated or constitutional symptoms, such as nausea, vomiting, gas, cramps, fever, fecal urgency or tenesmus, abdominal pain, headache, fatigue, back pain, or arthralgias. Most patients have 3 to 5 loose stools a day, but about 20% pass 6 to 20 watery stools a day. The average duration of TD in untreated patients is 3 to 5 days (1,55,56). The illness lasts more than one week in 10% of TD sufferers, and 2% develop chronic diarrhea lasting a month or longer (6). Travelers with identifiable pathogens in their stools have a longer duration of diarrhea and more symptoms than those with culture-negative stools. Invasive enteric pathogens, especially *Shigella* or *Campylobacter*, are the usual causes of the most severe form of TD (50). Limited data suggest that young children are more prone to severe and long-lasting illness (44).

From a practical point of view, it is important to distinguish patients with potentially dangerous TD from those with the usual, milder form of the illness. Low-grade fever is not rare in TD and it seems to be more common in cases where a pathogen can be identified (54). However, high-grade fever and/or small volume mucoid and/or bloody bowel movements are most likely due to dysentery caused by *Shigella*, *Campylobacter*, or other invasive enteric pathogens. These cases should be recognized promptly and treated with antibiotics.

VII. PREVENTION

The various approaches to prevent TD can be classified into three general categories: 1. decreased risk of exposure to the causative pathogens of TD by education of the traveler, 2. various chemoprophylaxis methods against TD, and 3. immunoprophylaxis methods against TD.

Proper diet precautions are important not only to prevent TD but also other food-borne and water-borne infections, such as typhoid fever, hepatitis A, brucellosis, poliomyelitis, bovine tuberculosis, etc. The high-risk and low-risk foods and beverages for TD were reviewed above. The dietary rule “If you can’t cook it, peel it, or boil it—forget it” captures most of the relevant guidelines. The rate of TD was shown in one study to be reduced when travelers carefully followed guidelines for avoiding unsafe food and water (57). However, this was not a universal finding: in other studies dietary precautions did not lead to significant reduction of TD rates (58, 59). It seems that the main problem is not the inefficiency of dietary restrictions to prevent TD, but the traveler’s lack of strict adherence to guidelines. No more than 2% of Swiss and 5% of Finnish travelers were able to adhere strictly to the safe dietary guidelines (57,59). The adventurous travel style, including eating food from street vendors, has been associated with a higher risk of TD as well as increased incidence of multiple episodes of TD, which are rare in the regular course of the illness (40,44,60–63). On the other hand, more expensive hotels are not necessarily safer than low-priced hotels in terms of risk of TD (40,64–66). This may be partially explained by the fact that guests in a luxury hotel sometimes assume unwarranted protection from TD.

The value of improving the local hygiene level and the public health infrastructure of developing countries cannot be overemphasized in terms of decreasing the incidence of TD, other diarrheal diseases, and infectious diseases in general. In studies of British tourists to Spain, the installation of a high-quality water supply reduced the risk of TD (67).

Since the classic placebo-controlled trial by Kean and his collaborators in 1962 showed that antimicrobial drugs provide protection against TD, more than 20 placebo-controlled trials have been conducted (11,68–86). A number of orally administered antimicrobials, including doxycycline, trimethoprim-sulfamethoxazole, trimethoprim alone, mecillinam, erythromycin, norfloxacin, and ciprofloxacin, have been studied as prophylaxis for TD (Table 3) (68–83). In addition, orally administered but poorly absorbed antimicrobials, including neomycin, phthalylsulfathiazole, streptotriad, bicozamycin, and nifuroxazide, have been studied (Table 4) (11,68,84–86). Protection rates (defined as the relative reduction of TD rates in the drug group compared to placebo group) have varied from 32% to 100% in these studies. Lower protection rates were seen with the poorly absorbed neomycin, phthalysulfathiazole, and streptotriad, as well as with doxycycline in areas where implicated pathogens showed a high level of resistance to the drug. In studies employing trimethoprim-sulfamethoxazole or a fluoroquinolone (norfloxacin or ciprofloxacin), protection rates of 68% or above were accomplished.

The incidence of side effects of antimicrobial agents used for prevention of TD has varied considerably. Side effects are more common in prospective than in retrospective studies, most likely because of underreporting by travelers in the retrospective studies. About 2% of travelers report skin rash while taking norfloxacin and a higher number, 2%–14%, in travelers taking trimethoprim-sulfamethoxazole (72,74,79). Gastrointestinal complaints such as nausea, vomiting, or diarrhea are not uncommon with most antimicrobial agents. Antibiotic-associated colitis or *Candida* vaginitis may occur. Severe side effects such as blood disorders or Stevens-Johnson syndrome are rare.

An important concern with the use of antimicrobial drugs for prevention of TD is that their use by the millions of travelers can apply pressure to select for microorganisms resistant to antimicrobials. Although this issue has not been extensively studied in the field of TD, data from other studies on the problem of antimicrobial resistance support the position that the use of antimicrobial agents in general should be controlled and minimized to well-defined indications, with appropriate risk-benefit analyses and study of alternative strategies.

Besides antibiotics, other agents and compounds have been used for prevention of TD. Among them, bismuth subsalicylate has been used extensively and has been shown to have good results in placebo-controlled prevention trials (87–89). The bismuth moiety of bismuth subsalicylate has antibacterial activity in vitro at concentrations that can be achieved in the bowel (90). In addition, bismuth subsalicylate has salicylate-dependent antisecretory activity. The optimal dosage for adults is two 262-mg tablets or 30 mL of the liquid form of bismuth subsalicylate, four times a day, taken with meals and at bedtime. When taken conscientiously in this dosage, bismuth subsalicylate has a protection rate of about 65% against TD. With poor to moderate compliance, the protection drops to 30–35%. Short-term therapy for TD with bismuth subsalicylate is considered safe. The drug may cause transient tinnitus and harmless blacken-

Table 3 Available Trials with Oral Antimicrobials for Prophylaxis of Traveler's Diarrhea

Year	Ref.	Antimicrobial	Drug regimen	Patients studied	Destination	Protection rate (%)[a]
1978	[69]	Doxycycline	100 mg daily for 3 weeks	39	Kenya	90
1981	[70]	Erythromycin	1 g daily throughout the trip	48	Mexico	100
1981	[71]	Doxycycline	100 mg daily for 3 weeks	46	Kenya; Morocco	44
1982	[72]	TMP-SMX	160 mg TMP/day; 800 mg SMX/day for 3 weeks	147	Mexico	71
1983	[73]	Mecillinam	200 mg daily for 25 days	74	Egypt; Thailand; Japan; Philippines	75
1983	[74]	TMP-SMX	160 mg TMP/day; 800 mg SMX/day for 2 weeks	87	Mexico	94
1983	[74]	TMP	200 mg daily for 2 weeks	88	Mexico	58
1983	[75]	Doxycycline	200 mg on the first day then 100 mg daily until departure	145	Mexico	81
1984	[76]	Doxycycline	100 mg daily for 3 weeks	63	Thailand	59
1984	[77]	Doxycycline	100 mg daily for 3 weeks	44	Honduras	68
1985	[78]	Mecillinam	200 mg daily for 2 weeks	32	Mexico	66
1986	[79]	Norfloxacin	400 mg daily for 2 weeks	115	Mexico	89
1987	[80]	Norfloxacin	200 mg twice a day	115	Southern Europe; Africa; Asia; Latin America	68
1989	[81]	Ciprofloxacin	500 mg daily for 1 week	53	Tunisia	94
1990	[82]	Norfloxacin	400 mg daily for 1 week	222	Egypt	93
1994	[83]	Ciprofloxacin	250 mg daily for 4 weeks	21	Asia	100

Note: Number of patients refers only to the number of subjects fully evaluable for analysis.

$$\text{Protection rate} = 100 \times \frac{\text{\% of patients with diarrhea in placebo group} - \text{\% of patients with diarrhea in treatment group)}}{\text{\% of patients with diarrhea in placebo group}}$$

[a]Protection rate in comparison with placebo.

Source: Ref. 68.

Table 4 Available Trials with Poorly Absorbed Oral Antimicrobials for Prophylaxis of Traveler's Diarrhea

Year	Ref.	Antimicrobial	Drug regimen	Patients studied	Destination	Protection rate (%)[a]
1962	[11]	Neomycin sulfate	1 g daily	305	Mexico	32
1962	[11]	Phthalylsulfathiazole	2 g daily	336	Mexico	50
1967	[84]	Streptotriad	365 mg twice a day for 2 weeks; 365 mg daily in the third week	749	Africa; Middle East; north, south, central Europe; Asia; North and South America; Caribbean; Australia	—
1985	[85]	Bicozamycin	500 mg 4×/day for 3 weeks	30	Mexico	100
1986	[86]	Nifuroxazide	400 mg daily	266	Mexico; Egypt; Morocco	—

Note: Number of patients refers only to the number of subjects fully evaluable for analysis.

$$\text{Protection rate} = 100 \times \frac{\text{\% of patients with diarrhea in placebo group} - \text{\% of patients with diarrhear in treatment group)}}{\text{\% of patients with diarrhea in placebo group}}$$

[a]Protection rate in comparison with placebo.

Source: Ref. 68.

ing of the tongue and stools. Excessive doses of bismuth subsalicylate, especially in patients with underlying diseases, can cause myoclonic encephalopathy (91).

Another approach to prophylaxis against TD has been the use of various preparations of *Lactobacillus* and *Streptobacillus faecium* (SF 68). While the results of most trials using this approach to prevent TD have been disappointing, a preparation called *Lactobacillus GG* was shown to reduce TD by 40% in one of two studies in Turkey (92,93).

Halogenated hydroxyquinolines have been popular compounds in the prevention of TD, However, these drugs are not recommended because of their questionable efficacy and concerns for serious side effects including subacute myeloptic neuropathy (94,95). Also, the various popular starches, talc, chalk, and absorbent compounds, including kaolin and pectin, are not recommended as prophylactic measures against TD because of the lack of evidence for their efficacy.

Since the pathogens that cause TD are also frequent causes of acute diarrhea in children in developing countries, there is great interest in developing immunoprophylactic preventive approaches. An effective vaccine against ETEC would have a considerable impact on TD rates. An interesting approach has been the development of oral B-subunit/whole-cell cholera vaccine, which induces protection against ETEC (96). In addition, the possibility of passive immunity against TD has been explored, including the use of colostrum-derived antibodies against ETEC (97). Although several approaches utilizing active or passive immunity appear promising no vaccine or antibody preparation is currently recommended for prevention of TD.

A number of issues influence the recommendations regarding chemoprophylaxis for TD. To summarize, antimicrobial agents are not recommended for prevention of TD because of the risk of increasing antimicrobial resistance, the potential for causing side effects, and the false sense of security assumed by some travelers (68,98,99). In addition, there is rapid and effective treatment for the minority of travelers who will develop TD. All travelers should be advised to follow carefully the recommended dietary restrictions. Antimicrobial agents for prevention of TD could be considered for travelers with an underlying health problem that may increase the risk and/or severity of TD, such as gastric hypochlorhydria due to medications or disease, immunodeficiency state, inflammatory bowel disease, and insulin-dependent diabetes (68,99). When used, antimicrobial agents should begin the day of arrival at the high-risk destination and continue for 2 days after the return home. Chemoprophylaxis should not be used if the traveler spends more than 3–4 weeks in the high-risk destination.

VIII. TREATMENT

Recent recommendations for the management of TD emphasize the need for patient education and empiric self-treatment of the illness (99,100). This is justified by the fact that TD may occur when the traveler does not have access to medical care. In addition, most cases of TD are not severe, and they are easily controlled with appropriate therapy. There are three forms of therapy of TD: 1. fluid and electrolyte replacement, 2. nonspecific symptomatic therapy, and 3. antimicrobial agents. An algorithmic management of TD based on self-assessment and empiric self-treatment is shown in Figure 1. An important point in this algorithm is that treatment with antidiarrheal or antimicrobial drugs should not be started with the first or second passage of unformed stool. Indeed, in a study of U.S. adult travelers to Guadalajara, Mexico, 60% of untreated persons with mild diarrhea (defined as 1 or 2 loose stools per 24 hours and one symptom of enteric disease) did well by the second day (6). Another important point is that a physician should be consulted if symptoms of TD worsen or do not improve after 48 hours of appropriate treatment. A concern with this approach for the management of TD is that the determination of the severity of TD is done by the travelers themselves; thus careful traveler education is imperative.

A necessary component of the management of any form of diarrhea, including TD, is fluid and electrolyte replacement. Fortunately, fluid and electrolyte losses are mild or moderate in the majority of cases of TD, so they can be replaced with soft drinks, fruit juices, and soups and broths augmented with saltine crackers. However, more aggressive replacement of fluid and electrolyte losses is needed in infants, young children, and elderly travelers, particularly when diarrhea is severe (68,100).

Several antidiarrheal drugs have been used to treat TD, including antisecretory agents (bismuth subsalicylate), antimotility agents (loperamide, diphenoxylate, codeine, tincture of opiate, and paregoric), and water-absorbing agents (attapulgite). Among them, bismuth subsalicylate and loperamide combine good efficacy rates with relatively few side effects. Bismuth subsalicylate is particularly useful when vomiting is a major symptom. The optimal dosage of bismuth subsalicylate for the treatment of TD in adults is two 262-mg tablets or 30 mL of the liquid form every 30 minutes to 1 hour, as needed, up to 4 times within a 24-hour period. The same dosage can be repeated for one more day if needed. As discussed above, bismuth subsalicylate has antimicrobial activity besides its antisecretory properties. Other possible targets for pharmacologic intervention in enterotoxin-mediated diarrheal diseases, such as inhibition of calmodulin, have been explored (101). Zaldaride maleate, an intestinal calmodulin inhibitor, had promising results in the therapy of travelers' diarrhea (102).

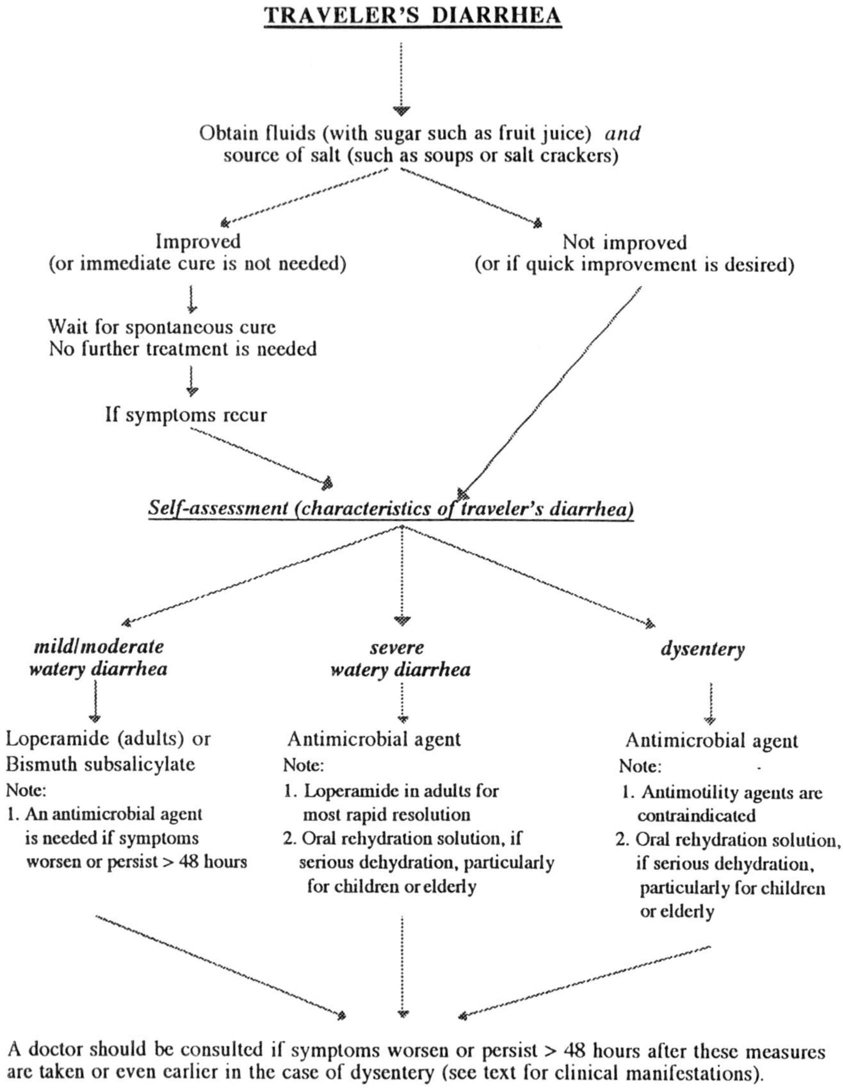

Figure 1 Self-assessment and empiric self-treatment of traveler's diarrhea: An algorithmic approach.

Among the antimotility agents, loperamide is usually recommended because it has fewer central side effects than the other synthetic or natural opiates from this class. The optimal dosage of loperamide for the treatment of TD in adults is 4 mg initially, followed by 2 mg after passage of each unformed stool, not

Table 5 Available Trials with Antimicrobial Drugs in the Treatment of Traveler's Diarrhea

Year	Ref.	Antimicrobial	Drug regimen	Patients studied	Destination	Improvement rate (%) drug	Improvement rate (%) placebo	p
1982	[103]	TMP-SMX	160 mg/800 mg *bid* for 5 days	110	Mexico	95	51	0.001
1982	[103]	TMP	200 mg *bid* for 5 days	110	Mexico	95	51	0.001
1984	[104]	Ampicillin	500 mg *qid* for 3 days	100	Mexico	49	NA	—
1986	[105]	TMP-SMX	160 mg/800 mg *bid* for 3 days	134	Mexico	100	88	<0.01
1986	[106]	Doxycycline	100 mg *bid* for 2 days	26	El Salvador, Columbia, Zaire, Brazil	85	33	0.02
1987	[107]	TMP-SMX	160 mg/800 mg *bid* for 5 days	181	Mexico	93	55	<0.0001
1987	[107]	Ciprofloxacin	500 mg *bid* for 5 days	181	Mexico	90	55	<0.0001
1988	[108]	Pivmecillinam	400 mg *tid* for 3 days	47	India	100	25	0.009
1989	[109]	Norfloxacin	400 mg *bid* for 3 days	447	Africa, Asia, Latin America	89	60	0.002
1991	[110]	Ciprofloxacin	500 mg *bid* for 3 days	104	Egypt	90	NA	—
1992	[111]	Ofloxacin	300 mg *bid* for 3 days	232	Mexico	95	71	<0.0001
1992	[111]	Ofloxacin	300 mg *bid* for 5 days	232	Mexico	89	71	<0.0001
1983	[112]	Bicozamycin	500 mg *qid* for 3 days	140	Mexico	98	57	0.0001
1984	[104]	Furazolidone	100 mg *qid* for 5 days	100	Mexico	74	NA	—

Note: Number of patients refers only to the number of subjects fully evaluable for analysis. The improvement rate (%) was calculated taking into account both patients cured and improved after each treatment. NA = Not available.
Source: Ref. 68.

to exceed 16 mg/day (the same dosage can be repeated for one more day if needed).

Several antimicrobial agents have been studied in trials of treatment of TD (Table 5) (68, 103–117). Among them, trimethoprim-sulfamethoxazole (TMP-SMX) and the quinolones have been used repeatedly with excellent results. The drug of choice is TMP-SMX in areas where most pathogens causing TD are susceptible to the drug. However, resistance to TMP-SMX and tetracycline has been increasing making the quinolones the preferred agents for the empiric treatment of TD in areas where susceptibility data are not available or where *Campylobacter jejuni* is a common cause of TD (118,119). The optimal duration of treatment of TD is not known. While a 5-day regimen is commonly recommended, several studies have shown that a 3-day regimen of TMP-SMX or a quinolone is adequate. Recent studies have shown that even a single dose of ciprofloxacin or fleroxacin is effective, although one study found that a 3-day regimen of ciprofloxacin was more effective than a single dose (113–115). There is interest in the use of orally administered, nonabsorbed antimicrobial agents for the treatment of TD, in view of their potential safety. Among these agents, aztreonam, and bicozamycin have shown good results in clinical studies (112,116).

Recent trials have compared the efficacy of the combination of an antidiarrheal drug and an antibiotic with each agent alone. In a study of travelers to Mexico, the combination of loperamide with TMP-SMX led to more rapid resolution of symptoms than treatment with either single agent (113). However, in two studies of U.S. military personnel in Egypt and Thailand, the addition of loperamide to ciprofloxacin for the treatment of TD offered only minimal additional benefits to therapy with ciprofloxacin alone (110,115). Although none of these studies showed any harm from the addition of loperamide to the antibiotic regimen, patients with dysentery should not be given antimotility agents, such as loperamide, because of the potential for facilitated intestinal invasion by bacteria due to increased time of contact between the pathogen and the mucosa (110,120).

REFERENCES

1. Steffen R, van der Linde F, Gyr K, Schar M. Epidemiology of diarrhea in travelers. JAMA 1983; 249:1176–1180.
2. Peltola H, Kyronseppä H, Hölsä P. Trips to the South—a health hazard. Morbidity of Finnish travellers. Scand J Infect Dis 1983; 15:375–381.
3. Gorbach SL. Travelers' Diarrhea. In: Gorbach SL, Bartlett JG, Blacklow NR, eds. Infectious Diseases. Philadelphia: W.B. Saunders, 1992:622–628.
4. Gorbach SL. Bacterial diarrhoea and its treatment. Lancet 1987; 2:1378–1382.
5. Thoren A. Enteric infections in the traveler: A socioeconomic perspective. Chemotherapy 1995; 41(Suppl 1):16–19.

6. Ericsson CD, Dupont HL. Travelers' diarrhea: approaches to prevention and treatment. Clin Infect Dis 1993; 16:616–624.
7. Hyams KC, Bourgeois AL, Merrell BR, et al. Diarrheal disease during Operation Desert Shield. N Engl J Med 1991; 325:1423–1428.
8. Bulmer E. A survey of tropical diseases as seen in the Middle East. Trans Roy SocTrop Med Hyg 1944; 37:225–242.
9. Kean BH, Waters SR. Incidence of diarrhea in travelers returning to the U.S. from Europe. AMA Arch Industr Hlth 1958; 18:148.
10. Kean BH, Smillie WG. Intestinal protozoa of American travelers returning to the United States from Mexico. AMA Arch Indust Health 1958; 18:148.
11. Kean BH, Schaffner W, Brennan RW, Waters SR. The diarrhea of travelers. V. Prophylaxis with phthalylsulfathiazole and neomycin sulfate. JAMA 1962; 180:367.
12. Kean BH. The diarrhea of travelers to Mexico: Summary of five-year study. Annals of Internal Medicine 1963; 59:605.
13. Kean BH, Waters SR. The diarrhea of travelers. Drug prophylaxis in Mexico. New England Journal of Medicine 1959; 216:71–74.
14. Gorbach SL, Kean BH, Evans DG, Evans DJ, Jr., Bessudo D. Travelers' diarrhea and toxigenic Escherichia coli. New England Journal of Medicine 1975; 292:933–936.
15. Rowe B, Taylor J, Bettelheim KA. An investigation of traveller's diarrhoea. Lancet 1970; 1:1–5.
16. Shore EG, Dean AG, Holik KJ, Davis BR. Enterotoxin-producing Escherichia coli and diarrheal disease in adult travelers: a prospective study. J Infect Dis 1974; 129:577–582.
17. Merson MH, Morris GK, Sack DA, et al. Travelers' diarrhea in Mexico. A prospective study of physicians and family members attending a congress. New England Journal of Medicine 1976; 294:1299–1305.
18. Levine MM. Escherichia coli that cause diarrhea: enterotoxigenic, enteropathogenic, enteroinvasive, enterohemorrhagic, and enteroadherent. J Infect Dis 1987; 155:377–389.
19. Black RE, Merson MH, Huq I, Alim AR, Yunus M. Incidence and severity of rotavirus and Escherichia coli diarrhoea in rural Bangladesh. Implications for vaccine development. Lancet 1981; 1:141–143.
20. Sack RB. Treatment and prevention of travelers' diarrhea. In: Holmgren J, Lindberg A, Mollby R, eds. Development of vaccines and drugs against diarrhea. Lund, Sweden: Studentlitteratur, 1986:289–301.
21. Black RE. Epidemiology of travelers' diarrhea and relative importance of various pathogens. Reviews of Infectious Diseases 1990; 12(suppl 1):S73–S79.
22. Petruccelli BP, Murphy GS, Sanchez JL, et al. Treatment of traveler's diarrhea with ciprofloxacin and loperamide. J Infect Dis 1992; 165:557–560.
23. Mattila L, Siitonen A, Kyronseppä H, et al. Seasonal variation in etiology of traveler's diarrhea. Finnish-Moroccan Study Group. J Infect Dis 1992; 165:385–388.
24. Mascola L, Tormey M, Ewert D, et al. Cholera associated with an international airline flight. Morb Mort Wkly Rep 1992; 41:134–135.

25. Vibrio vulnificus infections associated with raw oyster consumption—Florida, 1981-1992. Morb Mort Wkly Rep 1993; 42:405–407.
26. Parsonett J, Greene KD, Gerber AR, et al. *Shigella dysenteriae* type I infections in US travelers to Mexico (1988). Lancet 1989; 2:543.
27. Jokipii L, Jokipii AMM. Giardiasis in travelers: A prospective study. Journal of Infectious Diseases 1974; 130:295.
28. Jokipii L, Pohjola S, Jokipii AM. Cryptosporidiosis associated with traveling and giardiasis. Gastroenterology 1985; 89:838–842.
29. Gatti S, Cevini C, Bruno A, Bernuzzi AM, Scaglia M. Cryptosporidiosis in tourists returning from Egypt and the Island of Mauritius [letter]. Clin Infect Dis 1993; 16:344.
30. Bendall RP, Lucas S, Moody A, Tovey G, Chiodini PL. Diarrhoea associated with cyanobacterium-like bodies: a new coccidian enteritis of man. Lancet 1993; 341:590–592.
31. Hoge CW, Shlim DR, Rajah R, et al. Epidemiology of diarrhoeal illness associated with coccidian-like organism among travellers and foreign residents in Nepal. Lancet 1993; 341:1175–1179.
32. Ortega YR, Sterling CR, Gilman RH, et al. Cyclospora species—a new protozoan pathogen of humans (see comments). N Engl J Med 1993; 328:1308.
33. Vollett JJ, Ericsson CD, Gibson G, et al. Human rotavirus in an adult population with travelers' diarrhea and its relationship to the location of food consumption. Journal of Medical Virology 1979; 4:81–87.
34. Taylor DN, Echeverria P, Blaser MJ, et al. Polymicrobial aetiology of travellers' diarrhoea. Lancet 1985; 1:381–383.
35. Luscher D, Altwegg M. Detection of shigellae, enteroinvasive and enterotoxigenic Escherichia coli using the polymerase chain reaction (PCR) in patients returning from tropical countries. Mol Cell Probes 1994; 8:285.
36. Osterholm MT, MacDonald KL, White KE et al. An oubreak of a newly recognized chronic diarrhea syndrome associated with raw milk consumption. JAMA 1986; 256:484–490.
37. Parsonett J, Trock SC, Bopp CA, et al. Crhonic diarrhea associated with drinking untreated water. Ann Intern Med 1989; 110:985–991.
38. Afzalpukar RG, Schiller LR, Little KH, et al. The self-limited nature of chronic idiopathic diarrhea. N Engl J Med 1992; 327:1849–1852.
39. Castelli F, Carosi G. Epidemiology of traveler's diarrhea. Chemotherapy 1995; 41(suppl 1):20–32.
40. Steffen R. Epidemiologic studies of travelers' diarrhea, severe gastrointestinal infections, and cholera. Reviews of Infectious Diseases 1986; 8(suppl 2):S122–S130.
41. Haneveld D. Some epidemiological aspects of "travellers diarrhoea" in the Lebanon. Trop Geogr Med 1960; 12:339–344.
42. Kean BH. Turista in Teheran. Travellers' diarrhoea at the Eighth International Congresses of Tropical Medicine and Malaria. Lancet 1969; 2:583–584.
43. Loewenstein MS, Balows A, Gangarosa EJ. Turista at an international congress in Mexico. Lancet 1973; 1:529–531.

44. Pitzinger B, Steffen R, Tschopp A. Incidence and clinical features of traveler's diarrhea in infants and children. Pediatr Infect Dis J 1991; 10:719–723.
45. Wood LV, Ferguson LE, Hogan P, et al. Incidence of bacterial enterophathogens in foods in Mexico. Appl Environ Microbiol 1983; 46:328.
46. Blake PA, Rosenberg ML, Florencia J, et al. Cholera in Portugal, 1974. II. Transmission by bottled mineral water. Am J Epidemiol 1977; 105:344.
47. Harris, JR. Are bottled beverages safe for travelers? (editorial). Am J Public Health 1982; 72:787.
48. Wingate DL. Acid production and recurrent enteritis. Lancet 1990; 335:222.
49. DuPont HL. Pathogenesis of traveler's diarrhea. Chemotherapy 1995; 41(suppl 1):33–39.
50. Rowland HA. The pathogenesis of diarrhoea. Trans R Soc Trop Med Hyg 1978; 72:289–302.
51. Field M, Rao MC, Chang EB. Intestinal electrolyte transport and diarrheal disease. N Engl J Med 1989; 321:879–883.
52. Holmgren J, Svennerholm AM. Mechanisms of disease and immunity in cholera: a review. J Infect Dis 1977; 136(suppl):S105–S112.
53. Clements JD, Finkelstein RA. Demonstration of shared and unique immunological determinants in enterotoxins from Vibrio cholerae and Escherichia coli. Infect Immun 1978; 22:709–713.
54. Matilla L. Clinical features and duration of traveler's diarrhea in relation to its etiology. Clin Infect Dis 1994; 19:728.
55. Kateralaris PH, Farthing MJG. Traveler's diarrhea: Clinical presentation and prognosis. Chemotherapy 1995; 41(suppl 1):40–47.
56. Kollaritsch H. Traveller's diarrhea among Austrian tourists to warm climate countries: II. Clinical features. Eur J Epidemiol 1989; 5:355–362.
57. Kozicki M, Steffen R, Schar M. 'Boil it, cook it, peel it or forget it': does this rule prevent travellers' diarrhoea?. International Journal of Epidemiology 1985; 14:169–172.
58. Ryder RW, Oquist CA, Greenberg H, et al. Travelers' diarrhea in panamanian tourists in Mexico. Journal of Infectious Diseases 1981; 144:442–448.
59. Mattila L, Siitonen A, Kyronseppä H, Simula I, Peltola H. Risk behaviour for traveler's diarrhea among Finnish travelers. J Travel Med, In press.
60. Bryant HE, Csokonay WM, Love M, Love EJ. Self-reported illness and risk behaviours amongst Canadian travellers while abroad. Can J Public Health 1991; 82:316–319.
61. Tjoa WS, Dupont HL, Sullivan P, et al. Location of food consumption and travelers' diarrhea. American Journal of Epidemiology 1977; 106:61–66.
62. Blaser MJ. Environmental interventions for the prevention of travelers' diarrhea. Reviews of Infectious Diseases 1986; 8(suppl 2):S142–S150.
63. Kollaritsch H. Traveller's diarrhea among Austrian tourists n warm climate countries: I. Epidemiology. Eur J Epidemiol 1989; 5:74–81.
64. Reid D, Dewar RD, Fallon RJ, Cossar JH, Grist NR. Infection and travel: the experience of package tourists and other travellers. J Infect 1980; 2:365–370.

65. Cossar JH, Dewar RD, Redi D, Grist NR. Travel and health: illness associated with winter package holidays. J R Coll Gen Pract 1983; 33:642–645.
66. Cartwright RY. Epidemiology of travellers' diarrhoea in British package holiday tourists. PHLS Microbiol Dig 1992; 9:121–124.
67. Cartwright RY. Travellers' diarrhoea. Br Med Bull 1993; 49:348–362.
68. Scarpignato C, Rampal P. Prevention and treatment of traveler's diarrhea: A clinical pharmacological approach. Chemotherapy 1995; 41(suppl 1):48–81.
69. Sack DA, Kaminsky DC, Sack JN, Itotia RR, Arthur AZ, Kapikian F, Orskov F, Orskov I. Prophylactic doxycucline for travelers' diarrhea: results of a prospective double-blind study of Peach Corps volunteers in Kenya. N Engl J Med 1978; 298:758–763.
70. Andremont A, Tancrede C. Reduction of the aerobic gram negative bacterial flora of the gastrointestinal tract and prevention of travellers' diarrhoea using oral erythromycin. Ann Microbiol 1981; 132:419–427.
71. Santosham M, Sack RB, Froelich J, Greenberg H, Yolken R, Kapikain A, Javier C, Medina C, Orskov F, Orskov I. Biweekly prophylactic doxycycline for travelers' diarrhea. J Infect Dis 1981; 143:598–602.
72. DuPont HL, Evans DG, Rios N, Cabada FJ, Evans DJ, DuPont MW. Prevention of traveler's diarrhea with trimethoprim-sulfamethoxazole. Rev Infect Dis 1982; 4:533–539.
73. Black FT, Gaarslev K, Orskov F, Orskov I, Stenerup A, Stederup J, Christensen O. Mecillinam, a new prophylactic for travellers' diarrhoea: a prospective double-blind study in tourists travelling to Egypt and the Far East. Scand J Infect Dis 1983; 15:189–193.
74. DuPont HL, Galindo E, Evans DG, Cabada FJ, Sullivan P, Evans DJ. Prevention of travelers' diarrhea with trimethoprim-sulfamethoxazole and trimethoprim alone. Gastroenterology 1983; 84:75–80.
75. Freeman LD, Hooper DR, Lathen DF, Nelson DP, Harrison WO, Anderson DS. Brief prophylaxis with doxycycline for the prevention fo traveler's diarrhea. Gastroenterology 1983; 84:276–280.
76. Echeverria P, Sack RB, Blacklow NR, Bodhidatta P, Rowe B, McFarland A. Prophylactic doxycycline for traveler's diarrhea in Thailand: further supportive evidence of Aeromonas hydrophila as an enteric pathogen. Am J Epidemiol 1984; 120:912–921.
77. Sack RB, Santosham M, Froelich JL, Medina C, Orskov F, Orskov I. Doxycycline prophylaxis of travelers' diarrhea in Honduras, an area where resistance to doxycycline is common among enterotoxigenic *Escherichia coli*. Am J Trop Med Hyg 1984; 33:460–466.
78. Gaarslev K, Stenerup J. Changes during travel in the composition and antibiotic resistance pattern of the intestinal Enterobacteriaceae flora: results from a study of mecillinam prophylaxis against travellers' diarrhoea. Cur Med Res Opin 1985; 9:384–387.
79. Johnson PC, Ericsson CD, Morgan DR, DuPont HL, Cabada FJ. Lack of emergence of resistant fecal during successful prophylaxis of travellers' diarrhea with norfloxacin. Antimicrob Agents Chemother 1986; 30:671–674.

80. Wiström J, Norrby SR, Burman LG, Lundholm R, Jellheden B, Englund G. Norfloxacin versus placebo for prophylaxis against travellers' diarrhoea. J Antimicrob Chemother 1987; 20:563–574.
81. Rademaker CM, Hoepelman IM, Wolfhage MJ, Beumer H, Rozenberg-Arska M, Verhoef J. Results of a double-blind placebo-controlled study using ciprofloxacin for prevention of travelers' diarrhea. Eur J Clin Microbiol Infect Dis 1989; 8:690–694.
82. Scott DA, Harshbarger RL, Thornton SA, Hyam KC. Norfloxacin for the prophylaxis of traveler's diarrhea in US military personnel. Am J Trop Med Hyg 1990; 42:160–164.
83. Parry H, Howard AJ, Galpin OP, Hassan SP. The prophylaxis of travellers' diarrhoea: A double-blind placebo controlled trial of ciprofloxacin during a Himalayan expedition. J Infect 1994; 28:337–338.
84. Turner AC. Traveller's diarrhoea: a survey of symptoms, occurrence and possible prophylaxis. Br Med J 1967; 4:653–654.
85. Ericsson CD, DuPont HL, Galindo E, Mathewson JJ, Morgan DR, Wood LV, Mendiola J. Efficacy of bicozamycin in preventing traveler's diarrhea. Gastroenterology 1985; 88:473–477.
86. Bourée P, Kouchner G. Essai de chimioprophylaxie de la diarrhée du voyageur par le nifuroxazide. Pathol Biol 1986; 34:669–671.
87. DuPont HL, Sullivan P, Evans DG, et al. Prevention of traveler's diarrhea (emporiatric enteritis): Prophylactic administration of subsalicylate bismuth. JAMA 1980; 243:237–241.
88. Steffen R, DuPont HL, Heusser R, et al. Prevention of traveler's diarrhea by the tablet form of bismuth subsalicylate. Antimicrob Agents Chemother 1986; 29:625–627.
89. DuPont HL, Ericsson CD, Johnson PC, et al. Prevention of traveler's diarrhea by the tablet formulation of bismuth subsalicylate. JAMA 1987; 257:1347–1350.
90. Gorbach SL. Bismuth therapy in gastrointestinal diseases. Gastroenterology 1990; 99:863.
91. Mendelowitz PC, Hoffman RS, Weber S. Bismuth absorption and myoclonic encephalopathy during bismuth subsalicylate therapy. Ann Intern Med 1990; 112:140–141.
92. Black FT, Anderson PL, Orskow F, et al. Prophylactic efficacy of lactobacilli on traveler's diarrhea. Travel Med 1989; 8:333–335.
93. Oksanen P, Salminen S, Vapaatalo H, et al. Prevention of traveler's diarrhea by *Lactobacillus GG*. Ann Med 1990; 22:53–56.
94. Tsubaki T, Honma Y, Hoshi M. Neurologic syndrome associated with clioquinol. Lancet 1971; 1:696.
95. Baumgartner G, Gawel MJ, Kaeser HE, et al. Neurotoxicity of halogenated hydroxyquinolines: Clinical analysis of cases reported outside Japan. J Neurol Neurosurg Psychiatry 1979; 42:1073.
96. Peltola H, Siitonen A, Kyronseppä H, et al. Prevention of traveller's diarrhoea by oral B-subunit/whole-cell cholera vaccine. Lancet 1991; 338:1285–1289.

97. Tacket CO, Losonsky G, Link H, et al. Protection by milk immunoglobulin concetrate against oral challenge. N Engl J Med 1988; 318:1240.
98. Gorbach SL, Edelman R. Traveler's Diarrhea: National Institutes of Health Consensus Development Conference. Rev Infect Dis 1986; (suppl 2):S109.
99. DuPont HL, Ericsson CD. Prevention and treatment of traveler's diarrhea. N Engl J Med 1993; 328:1821–1827.
100. Farthing MJG, DuPont HL, Guadalini S, et al. Treatment and prevention of traveler's diarrhea. Gastroenterol Int 1992; 5:162–175.
101. Stoclet JC, Gerard D, Kilhoffer MC, et al. Calmodulin and its role in intracellural calcium regulation. Prog Neurobiol 1987; 29:321–364.
102. DuPont HL, Ericsson CD, Mathewson JJ, et al. Zaldaride maleate, an intestinal calmodulin inhibitor, in the therapy of travelers' diarrhea. Gastroenterology 1993; 104:709–715.
103. DuPont HL, Reves RR, Galindo E, Sullivan PS, Wood LV, Mendiola JG. Treatment of traveler's diarrhoea with trimethoprim/sulfamethoxazole and trimethoprim alone. N Engl J Med 1982; 307:841–844.
104. DuPont HL, Ericsson CD, Galindo E, Wood LV, Morgan D, Bistura JA, Mendiola JG, Furazolidone versus ampicillin in the treatment of travelers; diarrhea. Antimicrob Agents Chemother. 1984; 26:160–163.
105. Ericsson CD, Johnson PC, DuPont HL, Morgan DR. Role of a novel antidiarrheal agent, BW942C, alone or in combination with trimethoprim-sulfamethoxazole in the treatment of traveler's diarrhea. Antimicrob Agents Chemother 1986; 29:1040–1046.
106. Sack RB, Forehlich JL, Orskov F, Orskov I. Doxycycline is an effective treatment for travellers' diarrhoea. J Diarrhoeal Dis Res 1986; 4:144–148.
107. Ericsson CD, Johnson PC, DuPont HL, Morgan DR, Bitsura JA, De La Cabada FJ. Ciprofloxacin or trimethoprim-sulfamethoxazole as initial therapy for travelers' diarrhea: A placebo-controlled randomized trial. Ann Intern Med 1987; 106:216–220.
108. Christensen OE, Tuxen KK, Menday P. Treatment of travellers' diarrhoea with pivmecillinam. J Antimicrob Chemother 1988; 22:570–571.
109. Wiström J, Jertborn M, Hedstrom SA, Alestig K, Englund G, Jellheden B, Norrby SR. Short-term selftreatment of travellers' diarrhoea with norfloxacin: A placebo controlled study. J Antimicrob Chemother 1989; 23:905–913.
110. Taylor DN, Sanchez JL, Candler W, Thornton S, McQueen C, Echeverria P. Treatment of travelers' diarrhea: ciprofloxacin plus loperamide compared with ciprofloxacin alone. A placebo-controlled, randomized trial. Ann Intern Med 1991; 114:731–734.
111. DuPont HL, Ericsson CD, Mathewson JJ, DuPont MW. Five versus three days ofloxacin therapy of travelers' diarrhea: a placebo controlled study. Antimicrob Agents Chemother 1992; 36:87–91.
112. Ericsson CD, DuPont HL, Sullivan P, Gallindo E, Evans DG, Evans DJ. Bicozamycin, a poorly absorbable antibiotic effectively treats diarrhoea. Ann Intern Med 1983; 98:20–25.

113. Salem I, Katelaris P, Leigh-Smith S, et al. Randomised trial of single-dose ciprofloxacin for travellers' diarrhea (see comments). Lancet 1994; 165:557.
114. Steffen R, Jori R, Dupont HL, et al. Efficacy and toxicity of fleroxacin in the treatment of traveler's diarrhea. Am J Med 1993; 94:182S.
115. Petrucelli BP, Murphy GS, Sanchez JL, et al. Treatment of traveler's diarrhea with ciprofloxacin and loperamide. J Infect Dis 1992; 165:557–560.
116. DuPont HL, Ericcson CD, Mathewson JJ, et al. Oral aztreonam, a poorly absorbed yet effective therapy for bacterial diarrhea in US travelers to Mexico. JAMA 1992; 267:1932.
117. Ercsson CD, DuPont HL, Mathewson JJ, et al. Treatment of traveler's diarrhea with sulfamethoxazole and trimethopim and loperamide. JAMA 1990; 263:257–261.
118. Murray BE, Alvarado T, Kim KH, et al. Increasing resistance to trimethoprim-sulfamethoxazole among isolates of *Escerichia coli* in developing countries. J Infect Dis 1985; 152:1107–1113.
119. Villa J, Gascon J, Aballa S, et al. Antimicrobial resistance of Shigella isolates causing traveler's diarrhea. Antimicrob Agents Chemother 1994; 38:2668.
120. DuPont, H. L., Hornick, R. B. Adverse effect of lomotil therapy in shigellosis. JAMA 1990; 226:1525.

6

Intestinal Infections with *Salmonella* and *Yersinia* Species

DAVID W. K. ACHESON and GERALD T. KEUSCH
New England Medical Center, Boston, Massachusetts

I. INTRODUCTION

Salmonella and *Yersinia* are both invasive pathogens, usually entering the host across the gastrointestinal mucosa, and both cause intestinal and systemic disease. Interestingly, while the impact of diarrheal disease is, in general, most profound in the developing countries, salmonellosis and yersiniosis are more common problems of the industrialized world. This is the consequence of their individual ecological niches and the epidemiology surrounding transmission of these infections to humans. In addition, while the two genera share certain biological properties, such as invasion across mucosal surfaces, the disease spectrum they cause is often distinctive for each. This chapter will describe these organisms, the molecular mechanisms they employ during infection, and the resulting disease syndromes, while highlighting the basis for the differences between *Salmonella* and *Yersinia* where this is known.

II. SALMONELLOSIS

A. Introduction

It is a curious fact that the genus *Salmonella* is not named for its actual discoverer, Theobald Smith, who, working for the predecessor of the Department of Agriculture, believed he had identified the cause of hog cholera (1), but rather for his Bureau chief at the time, Daniel Salmon. While there is no genus named *Smithella*, Smith's seminal contribution to the definition of the prototypic *Salmonella*, the organism we now call *S. cholerasuis*, has been well recognized. Perhaps it would have been proper to name the genus after Gaffkey, who 10 years earlier had reported the isolation of *S. typhi* from the spleen of typhoid fever patients (2), but this would have led to an awkward genus name, *Gaffkeyella*. Over the century since the description of the typhoid bacillus and the first nontyphoidal *Salmonella*, over 2300 additional distinct members of the genus have been identified.

B. Microbiology

With but few exceptions (*S. typhi* and *paratyphi* C, which express a polysaccharide capsule called Vi) *Salmonella* are nonencapsulated gram-negative motile rods, possessing flagellae around the entire perimeter of the organism. They ferment glucose but not lactose, an important characteristic used in microbiological screening tests, and they generally produce H_2S, which can be recognized as a black reaction product in triple sugar–iron agar, a commonly used criterion for their presumptive identification. The more than 2300 *Salmonella* are differentiated from one another by the combination of somatic O (oligosaccharide) cell-wall antigens complexed to the core region of endotoxin and the expression of multiple protein flagellar H-antigens. Over the decades, it became common to name new isolates for the city in which they were first discovered, the person involved in their isolation, or the syndrome they cause, hence names like *S. dublin* or *newport, S. schottmuelleri* or *thompson*, or *S. cholerasuis* or *typhimurium* were coined. Over the past two decades, the classification has been increasingly based on genetic and biochemical properties, and the number of species has been whittled down to three, and most recently to just two, based on DNA relatedness. These are *S. bongori*, containing nonhuman organisms and *S. enterica*, consisting of six groups including human pathogenic strains, nearly all of which are in Group 1, *S. enterica* subspecies *enterica* (see Table 1).

The individual members of a subspecies are distinguished primarily by the serology of the carbohydrate O- and protein H-antigens. The major source of this variation comes from the ability of *Salmonella* to create mosaic flagellin genes by means of recombination and horizontal transfer, point mutations, and gene duplications. On this basis, such variants are properly considered to be serovars. Thus, the main cause of typhoid fever, typically called *S. typhi*, is properly classified as *S. typhi* subspecies *enterica* serovar Typhi, whereas the most common isolate in the United States, *S. enteritidis* should formally be called *S. enterica* subspecies enterica serovar Enteritidis. This is a bit awkward for clinicians and laboratory microbiologists both, and for the foreseeable fu-

Table 1 Taxonomy and Serogroup of Some Common Human Pathogenic *Salmonella*

Species	Subspecies	Serogroup	Common serovars
S. enterica	*enterica*	A	Paratyphi A
		B	Typhimurium
			Agona
			Derby
			Heidelberg
			Paratyphi B
		C	Cholerasuis
			Infantis
			Virchow
		D	Dublin
			Enteritidis
			Typhi
	salamae		
	arizonae		
	diarizonae		
	houtenae		
	indica		
S. bongori			

ture it is certain that these organisms will be known by their serovar name improperly raised to the level of a species. The serovar names will be exclusively used in this chapter.

In a clinical context, the initial data from the laboratory is usually the serogroup identification of a *Salmonella* isolate. This method uses the grouping of antisera to the major members of the 60 phase-1 somatic antigens and allows separation of *Salmonella* serogroups A, B, C, D etc. This remains useful to clinicians because it is now well known which important human *Salmonella* pathogens are included in Groups A–D. Armed with the serogroup and information about clinical presentation, an educated guess of etiology can be made and decisions reached about further diagnosis and therapy. Final identification may require sending the organism to a reference laboratory, and it may be weeks or months before the information is returned to the clinician.

C. Epidemiology

Salmonella are extraordinarily well adapted for survival. Some are highly host adapted to humans or certain animals, but most are not host adapted at all and can move between animals, the environment, and humans, creating an almost inexhaustible source of niches for the organism and opportunities for transmission to a susceptible human host. One reason *Salmonella* have become relatively more important in developed than developing countries is that they commonly find their way into processed or prepared foods and, in this manner, can be mass distributed. For example, industrial-scale preparation of powdered eggs or milk for inclusion in a variety of packaged foods will allow any contaminating *Salmonella* serovars to reach and infect large numbers of people over wide geographic areas, traveling along the routes of commercial distribution of foodstuffs rather than from host to host within a local area. In contrast, in Dhaka, Bangladesh, *Salmonella* serovars accounted for only 1.7% of the pathogens isolated in 1995, over half of which were serogroup B (Dr. M. J. Albert, personal communication), the majority of which were most likely *S. typhimurium*.

Over the past six decades, there has been a real increase in the incidence of *Salmonella* infections other than *S. typhi*, which are usually lumped together as nontyphoidal salmonellosis (Figure 1). One of the interesting epidemiological changes has been the recent rise in isolation of *S. enteritidis* (that is, S. *enterica* subspecies *enterica* serovar Enteritidis), which has become the most common isolate in the United States in the past five years, displacing the previous leading isolate, *S. typhimurium*, to second place. Similar changes in isolates rates for these two organisms have been observed in Europe as well (3). A major reason for this has been the increase in isolation of this organism from commercially produced grade A eggs (4). Originally thought to be a problem largely due to cracked eggs, it is now known that *Salmonella* can penetrate intact eggs lying in feces or bedding of naturally infected layer hens via mi-

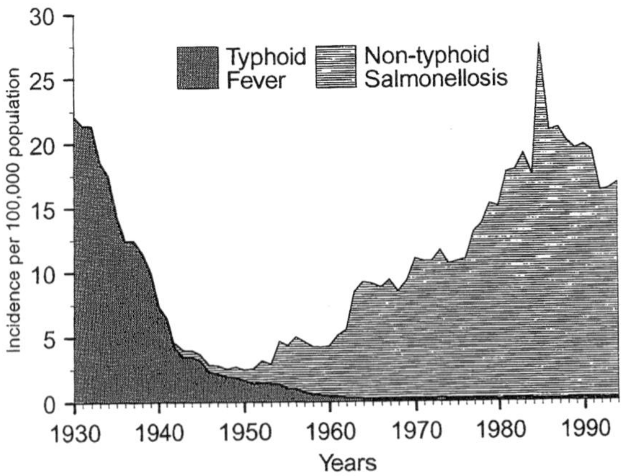

Figure 1 Annual incidence of typhoid fever and nontyphoidal salmonellosis in the United States, 1930–1994. Courtesy of R. V. Tauxe, Centers for Disease Control and Prevention.

croscopic pores in the shell—or even infect transovarially during egg development, before the shell is even formed. The initial contamination usually involves low numbers of organisms, but if cold temperature control is not continuously maintained after laying, the number of viable organisms can rise dramatically to a sufficient number to survive cooking and constitute an infectious inoculum to a susceptible host.

The majority of nontyphoidal salmonellosis is acquired from the ingestion of contaminated food. Common sources are poultry, eggs, milk, and foods containing raw or powdered eggs or milk, such as mayonnaise or hollandaise sauce (5–7). A handful of serovars account for the majority of infections. In fact, 10 of the over 2300 serovars accounted for over two-thirds of the human isolates in the United States in 1994 (see Table 2), and the top 20 isolates accounted for 30,318/38,336 (80%) of the total isolations reported to the Centers for Disease Control and Prevention (CDC) in 1994.

The isolation of certain serotypes may also provide a clue to the source. For example, *S. hadar* has been associated with contact with pet ducklings (8), *S. arizonae* is associated with ingestion of rattlesnake meat, often used as a special therapeutic agent in the southwestern United States (9,10), *S. dublin* commonly follows ingestion of raw milk or raw cow liver used as an alternative cancer therapy (11), *S. poona, chester,* or *javiania* often are transmitted by ingestion of raw fruits or vegetables, while *S. muenchen* has been related to the use of contaminated marijuana (12).

Table 2 The Ten Most Common *Salmonella* Isolates in the United States as Reported to the Centers for Disease Control and Prevention in 1994

Rank	Serovar	Isolations	Percent
1	Enteritidis	10009	26.1 (26.1)[a]
2	Typhimurium	8479	22.1 (48.2)
3	Heidelberg	1855	4.8 (53.0)
4	Newport	1698	4.4 (57.4)
5	Hadar	1033	2.7 (60.1)
6	Agona	766	2.0 (62.1)
7	Montevideo	639	1.7 (63.8)
8	Oranienburg	616	1.6 (65.4)
9	Muenchen	562	1.5 (66.9)
10	Thompson	560	1.5 (68.4)

Source: Centers for Disease Control and Prevention, Annual Surveillance Data, 1994.

[a]Cumulative percentage.

The most common causes of typhoid fever, *S. typhi*, and *S. paratyphi* A and B, are all highly human-host adapted serovars. While rare presentations of the syndrome can be due to the nonhost adapted serovar *S. typhimurium*, typhoid is typically traceable to another human, often an asymptomatic and unsuspecting carrier. Direct contact is, however, not the classic mode of transmission; rather the intervention of a food or water vehicle contaminated by a carrier is the more general rule. Given the changing prevalence of typhoid fever in the United States, the chronic carrier is now more likely to be a female over 50 years of age, often with chronic subacute cholecystitis and cholelithiasis. *S. typhi* can survive indefinitely deep within gallstones, protected from antibiotics excreted into bile. From this protected niche, the organism may be intermittently excreted in the stool thereafter. Indigenously acquired typhoid fever in the United States today can be characterized as a "grandmother connection," that is to say transmission from a chronic carrier grandmother to her grandchild. In addition to acquisition from known or newly diagnosed carriers, typhoid infection occurring in the United States also occurs in large common-source or small family, food-borne outbreaks, often related to kitchen or domestic workers or nannies who are recent immigrants from typhoid-endemic countries.

In fact, most typhoid in the United States is acquired abroad, targeting children, adolescents, and young adults (13). Approximately 500 cases per year of typhoid are currently reported to the CDC with Mexico the leading source overall. Regional differences exist, depending on travel patterns, and in New York City, for example, most cases are acquired in South and Southeast Asia. There are several known global hotspots where typhoid is highly endemic and travelers are common. These include Lima and elsewhere in Peru, Alexandria and elsewhere in Egypt, Jakarta and elsewhere in Indonesia, and all of India, Pakistan, and Nepal. Santiago, Chile, was previously one of these select typhoid hyperendemic sites; however, recent efforts to improve water quality and the infrastructure for sewage and waste disposal has resulted in a dramatic reduction in transmission.

D. Pathogenesis

Regardless of the vehicle of transmission, typhoid bacilli gain entry to the host by the oral route, and they must successfully pass the nonspecific gastric acid barrier in order to cause disease. Volunteer human experiments conducted with either *S. typhi* or nontyphoidal salmonellas, in which the inoculum is given in an isotonic salt solution, often with a large volume of bicarbonate to buffer gastric acid, has suggested that both nontyphoidal salmonellosis and typhoid fever are large inoculum infections, with doses of 10^5 organisms or more required. However, this is not a good representation of natural infection, usually transmitted in the context of a meal, which itself will buffer gastric acid. These studies suggest that the infectious inoculum is considerably less than 100,000 organisms (14). At least for *S. typhi*, there is no evidence that increasing inoculum results in more severe illness. A recent analysis of multiple studies of experimental typhoid infection with the Quailes strain, a reference laboratory strain, revealed an increase in the attack rate and a decrease in the mean incubation time with increasing inocula, but no change in any of the markers employed to describe disease severity (see Table 3) (15). Severity may be determined by specific host or pathogen properties, as discussed below.

It has previously been considered that gastric acid was a simple nonspecific host defense mechanism, disrupted by diseases or drugs that interfere with acid production. A more contemporary view suggests that gastric acid represents an environmental signal to the microorganisms that they are entering a potential host, and that it is time to turn on the synthesis of necessary virulence factors. Acid exposure may be one of these signals for Salmonella, since some 40 genes are now known to respond to low pH, typically by enhanced synthesis of the gene product. This so-called adaptive acid-tolerance response may be one of the keys to disease severity, as organisms surviving passage through the stomach may be made more virulent after upregulation of certain of these genes.

Subsequent events have been pieced together from in vitro data combined with limited in vivo data, primarily from *S. typhimurium* infections in mice, which result in the murine equivalent of typhoid fever. Sometimes the host range for *Salmonella* is sharp, as emphasized by the fact that *S. typhi* infection of mice is rapidly cleared from Peyer's patches and is not associated with clinical disease (16). The general events common to typhoid and nontyphoidal salmonellosis are translocation across the intestinal mucosa, which may occur by microbial transcytosis, preferentially across the M cells in Peyer's patches (17), or possibly across the enterocytes (18), leading in either case to transient bacteremia. In the case of typhoid, the organisms are rapidly taken up by mononuclear cells within local draining lymph nodes, liver, and spleen, where multiplication of the organism occurs, sequestered from humoral host defenses (19,20). *S. typhi* is covered by a polysaccharide capsular antigen, Vi, which

Table 3 Relationship of Inoculum Size, Attack Rate, and Incubation Period in Volunteers Experimentally Infected with *Salmonella typhi* Strains

Inoculum	Attack rate (percent)	Mean incubation (days)
10^3	0/13 (0)	—
10^5	77/200 (38.5)	9.3
10^7	13/27 (48.1)	7.4
10^{8-9}	24/25 (96.0)	4.7

Source: Ref. 15.

inhibits neutrophil phagocytosis and complement mediated bacteriolysis via the alternative pathway. When there are preexisting opsonizing antibodies to surface components, including Vi, the organism is rapidly taken up by neutrophils and killed, which explains some of the protection afforded by traditional killed parenteral typhoid vaccines or the parenteral Vi polysaccharide vaccine.

Both host and bacterial factors alter the survival of intracellular organisms within macrophages. The best-defined host genetic locus was first described on chromosome 1 in mice and named *ity* for its role in immun*ity* and susceptibil*ity* to *S. typhimurium* (21). Similar loci, described by other workers, mediated murine responses to leishmania (*lsh* locus) and Bcg, the tuberculosis vaccine mycobacterium strain (*bcg* locus). It was not very long, however, before it was realized that these were functional descriptions of the same genetic loci and the term Ity/Lsh/Bcg locus was coined (22). This has taken on additional significance with the discovery of the human *ity* homologue on human chromosome 2q35. These genes are now named Nramp, the natural resistance-associated macrophage protein, a family of a minimum of 3 genes encoding a macrophage-specific membrane transport protein (23), Nramp is involved in some manner in the early killing of intracellular pathogens by different mechanisms than those involved in cytocidal and cytostatic responses of activated macrophages (24). Nramp is linked to the IL-8 receptor gene cluster in humans, but the significance of this observation is unclear (25).

The cell invasive process appears similar to *S. typhi* and nontyphoidal salmonellas (26). When studied by vital cinemicroscopy of cultured mammalian cells, cell invasion by living *Salmonella* begins with a dramatic active ruffling of the host cell membrane, similar to that observed in cells exposed to growth factors (27). Ruffling is the visual consequence of extensive cytoskeletal rearrangements induced by the host–pathogen interaction, which ultimately leads to the entry of organisms in phagocytic vesicles comprised of host membrane. These vesicles contain lysosomal markers but exclude extracellular markers that would be taken up by nonspecific fluid phase endocytosis. This mechanism is analogous to the microbial-directed phagocytosis induced by *Shigella* spp. during invasion of host cells. A correlation has been observed between the ability to form and maintain spacious phagosomes in mouse macrophages and mouse virulence (28). *S. typhi* induced similar structures in human macrophages.

Whereas *Shigella* subsequently escape the vesicle to the cytoplasm and multiply intracellularly, *Salmonella* transmit to the basal membrane without multiplication, where they exit to the lamina propria. During this transit through the epithelial cell, initial alterations of the brush border are repaired and the gut cell is, apparently, unharmed. Virulent *Salmonella* are also endowed with the ability to resist the lethal effects of cryptins, antibacterial peptides produced by intestinal epithelial cells (20). The ability of *Salmonella* serovars to bind host plasminogen and convert this to enzymatically active plasmin (30) may assist the organism in degrading the extracellular matrix to cross the basement membrane and spread within the lamina propria. Plasmin bound to the surface of the organism potentiates the penetration of *Salmonella* through an artificial basement membrane preparation, Matrigel, when it is reconstituted on membrane filters (31).

In contrast to *S. typhi*, which are rapidly sequestered within host macrophages after initial entry into the blood stream, nontyphoidal *Salmonella* reach the circulation and, in the view of the authors, should be universally recoverable by blood cultures if obtained early enough in the course of the infection. With the exception of certain serovars (*S. typhimurium, S. enteritidis, S. dublin,* and *S. cholerasuis*), nontyphoidal *Salmonella* reaching the blood stream are generally rapidly cleared and killed by normal host defenses. Serovars with survival advantages in the host are better able to spread systemically and they more commonly cause focal and systemic infections rather than diarrhea alone. Whenever mononuclear phagocytes are defective, as occurs in patients with sickle cell anemia, in whom ingestion of heme products from chronic hemolysis leads to functional impairment and autosplenectomy, the risk of invasive *Salmonella* is increased tenfold over that of normal subjects. Increased incidence and severity of *Salmonella* infection also occurs in T-lymphocyte immunosuppressed patients, whether due to leukemia, lymphoma, or AIDS.

Molecular studies of *Salmonella* invasion mechanisms have been done with just a few serovars, but it is very likely that most, if not all, serovars use a similar array of genes (32). A critical chromosomal invasion locus, *inv*, best studied in *S. typhimurium*, includes at least 14 genes, a number of which have both sequence and functional homology to genes in other invasive organisms, including *Shigella* and *Yersinia* (33). The *inv* genes regulate the assembly of supramolecular structures on the bacterial cell surface. The earliest change is the appearance of appendages on the organism within 15 minutes of contact with the host cell, as determined by low-voltage scanning electron microscopy (34). By 30 minutes, ruffles form on the host cell and the bacterial appendages disappear (35). Pathogenic *Salmonella* need to assemble these structures and also be able to shed them. For example, avirulent *inv*A or E mutants assemble appendages but never lose them. The *inv*C or G mutants, which never assemble appendages, are avirulent as well.

The process of invasion is associated with the activation of a number of signaling pathways (36). The initial biochemical event detected is the activation of the mitogen-activated protein (MAP) kinase via a cell surface receptor. In turn, MAP kinase activates phospholipase A_2 (PLA_2), releasing arachidonic acid and initiating the subsequent production of prostaglandins and leukotrienes, in particular LTD_4, and there is an accompanying sharp increase in intracellular calcium concentration (37). It should be noted that some of these mediators are known to alter electrolyte and water transport across the gut and can cause diarrhea in other settings. It has been known for a number of years that both invasion and inflammation are necessary, but not sufficient, to cause *Salmonella* diarrhea in experimental animal models. More recent studies have revealed that disease causing but not avirulent *Salmonella* elicit transepithelial signals for the recruitment of neutrophils (38). Attachment of the organism to the cell surface stimulates this process while the cells remain intact and able to secrete the neutrophil chemoattractant chemokine, IL-8 (39). Any IL-8 secreted into the matrix underlying the epithelium is imprinted and resists the diluting effects of fluid movement. It is also directional, dependent on epithelial cell protein synthesis, and may be blocked by anti-IL-8 or by antibody to the IL-8 receptor on the neutrophil (40).

Highly invasive nontyphoidal serovars, such as *S. dublin*, possess a virulence plasmid, which shares a conserved 8-kb region of DNA in which a set of *spv* genes (for *Salmonella* plasmid virulence) are located, including both structural (*spvABCD*) and regulatory (*spvR*) genes (41). The spv genes are not generally expressed in vitro, but are rapidly turned on after entry into macrophages and nonphagocytic epithelial cells (42). The conditions for activation of these plasmid genes, required for systemic invasion, differs from those employed to induce invasion across the intestinal mucosa (43). The regulatory gene, *spvR*, is turned on by nutrient limitation when *Salmonella* enter eukaryotic cells (for example, low iron conditions) in concert with the chromosomal *rpoS* gene (44), which controls a stationary phase sigma factor (45). Expression of both *rpoS* and *spvR* is required to activate the *spv* structural genes. Another plasmid gene, *rck*, enhances virulence by encoding resistance to complement by blocking the assembly of the terminal attack complex on the cell surface. There are additional, as yet uncharacterized, virulence genes on the plasmid as well.

Similar to invasive nontyphoidal *Salmonella*'s need for mechanisms to invade and survive within the host, an essential characteristic of serovars causing typhoid fever is the ability to survive and multiply intracellularly within mononuclear phagocytes. As discussed above, this property is controlled by both microbial and host genes, and has been studied best in the mouse model of typhoid fever caused by *S. typhimurium* infection. *S. typhimurium* virulence is regulated by a two-component system, known as the PhoP locus, consisting of at least two genes, PhoP and PhoQ, although the majority of PhoP/Q-controlled genes are actually not involved in virulence (46). PhoP resembles a number of other bacterial regulator/signal receiving proteins while PhoQ is similar to the carboxy terminus of some microbial sensor/transmitter proteins (47). This system permits the organism to sense environmental signals and initiate adaptive responses by modifying gene expression. Recent data suggest that Mg^{2+} may be the principal signal regulating the PhoP/Q system (48). The periplasmic domain of PhoQ responds to Mg^{2+} concentration by conformational changes, indicating that this region is the Mg^{2+} sensor. The repertoire of twenty or more PhoP/Q regulated genes includes both PhoP/Q activated genes, collectively termed pags, and PhoP/Q-repressed genes, or prgs. In the examples studied thus far, regulation proceeds via transcriptional factors binding to enhancer DNA sequences that replace the usual -35 region upstream of the promoter region of the particular PhoP/Q regulated gene. Mutations in PhoP/Q have been described that decrease microbial survival in macrophages, increase sensitivity to acid pH and mammalian antimicrobial peptides, and attenuate virulence in vivo (49,50).

E. Clinical Manifestations, Diagnosis, and Therapy

Specific *Salmonella* serovars cause distinctive syndromes, including typhoid fever, gastroenteritis, septicemia, arteritis, various focal infections, and chronic carrier states. Although there are over 2300 different *Salmonella* serovars, it is possible to predict the most likely causes of each syndrome using a combination of clinical and epidemiological data.

1. Typhoid Fever

Although the portal of entry of the bacteria is the intestinal tract, and because not all cases are due to *S. typhi*, some have preferred to call this syndrome "enteric fever." However this name is no more precise since typhoid is in essence an acute systemic infection of the mononuclear phagocyte system and not an enteric infection. The term "paratyphoid fever" is used by some clinicians when the illness is due to *S. paratyphi* A, B, or C, however this leaves a rare nosologic gap when the syndrome is associated with *S. typhimurium* infection. Since these infections are, in essence, similar but milder forms of typhoid, they will not be separately discussed in this chapter. The characteristic feature of typhoid fever, whatever its microbial cause, is bacterial invasion of macrophages leading to sustained bacteremia but not septic shock, prolonged high fever, marked catabolism of lean body mass induced by cytokine activation, and inflammatory damage of the lower intestine, leading on occasion to enteric complications including bleeding, toxic megacolon, or perforation.

After a dose-regulated incubation period ranging from a few days to a few weeks, corresponding to the initial invasion of mononuclear phagocytes and intracellular multiplication, the classic typhoid fever case is characterized by a stepwise increase in temperature over several days to a sustained high fever, usually in the range of 40–41°C. In some instances, the prefebrile period is characterized by inflammatory diarrhea with leukocytes and increased protein in the stool, especially in the very young, or by a change from the normal bowel habits to constipation (51). Most often, however, the patient is asymptomatic until the febrile phase begins. With this, there may be a faint, evanescent salmon-colored macular-papular rash, primarily over the trunk, termed "rose spots." However rose spots are not often helpful in diagnosis, as the majority of patients do not exhibit this rash, it may be difficult to discern in dark-skinned patients, and rarely, rose spots may be seen in other infections, for example shigellosis. Initial manifestations are usually accompanied by nonspecific symptoms including chills, sweats, headache, muscle aches, and weakness, all characteristic of cytokine-mediated catabolism and altered regulation of body temperature. Some patients experience epistaxis and some complain of abdominal pain.

With the sustained high fever, typhoid patients look ill, usually glassy eyed, lethargic, and they may be confused and disoriented, a combination of features often characterized as "toxic" appearing. In a small number of patients, severe typhoid can present with psychiatric symptoms and be misdiagnosed as an acute psychotic illness; however, these manifestations clear with antibiotic therapy. Progression to an encephalopathic state may occur—with seizures, delirium or coma—and is an ominous finding associated with increased fatality rates (52).

Physical examination sometimes reveals a relative bradycardia in relation to the height of the fever, but not all patients exhibit this finding, believed to be an excellent clinical clue in typhoid. Approximately half of the patients have hepatosplenomegaly when first seen. Diffuse abdominal tenderness may be detected, and in the small proportion of typhoid patients with clinical hepatitis, cholecystitis, or pancreatitis, focal tenderness over these organs can be present. Otherwise, the physical examination is rather unrevealing and nonspecific. It is this lack of characteristic findings—and the relative infrequency with which the classic presentation with all the features of typhoid occurs—that makes this a difficult diagnosis.

Despite the continuous bacteremia, focal seeding of organisms is generally restricted to a few preferred sites, such as the gall bladder and the Peyer's patches of the intestine. The former is the source of the prolonged carrier state that may develop, especially in individuals with gall stones, and the latter induces an inflammatory response that can lead to bleeding, perforation, or toxic dilatation. These complications generally happen after the first week of illness and peak in the second–third weeks of fever. Interestingly, seeding of the heart valves or the meninges during the continuous bacteremia phase of typhoid is distinctly uncommon. Rarely, patients develop other complications, including hepatitis or cholecystitis, meningitis, nephritis, myocarditis, pneumonia, arthritis, osteomyelitis, pancreatitis, parotitis, or orchitis.

Untreated typhoid continues on for 6–8 weeks or more before the fever abates, with persistent high fever, anorexia and muscle wasting, and weight loss. The latter, evidence of the catabolic toll on host nutritional state and muscle wasting, will take months to reverse, even when the patient has access to a complete and nutritious diet. This prolonged debilitation may make the patient susceptible to other intercurrent infections and may be the reason for late fatalities. Initial morbidity and mortality is directly related to the rapidity of diagnosis and the prompt initiation of appropriate antibiotic therapy. In a few patients, the illness takes a fulminant course, progressing to disseminated intravascular coagulation, central nervous system involvement, and death. This is more typical of typhoid in young children than adults. Typhoid in infancy is more common than previously thought, and neonates may acquire severe infection via vertical transmission from an infected mother or from exogenous sources. Early and effective therapy has reduced the frequency of these complications. In fact, the only complication that has not been significantly impacted by early effective therapy is relapse, which may affect 10–20% of patients. Relapse is not due to selection of antimicrobial resistant organisms and is generally milder and may be treated by the same antibiotic used initially.

Diagnosis depends first on raising the possibility and then using the laboratory appropriately to confirm this. The most common trigger is sustained and unexplained high fever in a patient who has been potentially exposed via recent travel to a typhoid-endemic country of by contact with known carriers or recent immigrants from endemic countries. The diagnosis may be more likely in patients with hepatosplenomegaly or a typical rose spot rash, if there is relative bradycardia for the height of the fever, or if there is relative leukopenia in relation to the height of the fever, especially neutropenia, with a modest monocytosis. The patient is, however, able to respond appropriately to superimposed complications, and toxic dilatation or perforation, for example, are accompanied by brisk leukocytosis.

Definitive diagnosis is microbiological, and the most definitive finding is isolation of the organism, usually from blood culture. The diagnostic yield from cultures is very much dependent on what is cultured, when, and how. Blood yields the highest proportion of positives, over 90% in untreated patients, in the first week of illness, but this drops to only 50% positives in the third week, even in the absence of treatment. The number of positives is increased by culturing bone marrow as well, especially in those with false-negative cultures due to antimicrobial administration. The old trick of culturing ear lobe blood, where monocytes and, therefore, organisms, were thought to concentrate, does not seem to add very much. Culturing the buffy coat may reduce the time it takes for a culture to turn positive, but does not significantly increase the yield and is not commonly done. Stool cultures are typically negative in the first week, and then the count rises as the organism invades the Peyer's patch, and 75% of stool cultures in week three may be positive in untreated patients. By

8 weeks, no more than 10% are positive by stool culture, but the yield is increased if bile is sampled for culture, for example by the string test (53).

In individuals without recent immunization to typhoid, the Widal test, which measures agglutinating antibody titers to the O-antigen of the organism, is a simple and helpful test. In such persons, a titer of > 1:160 is suggestive, and > 1:640 is highly suggestive of acute typhoid (54). Because nontyphoidal *Salmonella* of groups A, B, and D can share the O-antigenic determinant measured in the Widal test, the serology cannot be definitive. Additional testing for flagellar H antigens is not of great help, because these are even more cross reactive among different *Salmonella* serovars. The traditional serological criterion of a fourfold rise in antibody holds for typhoid as well, but this does not help in the acute diagnosis and the titer ruse can be blunted by early and effective antibiotic therapy. Greater specificity can be obtained by testing for the presence of an antibody to Vi, and new, rapid latex or coagglutination tests have been developed with a sensitivity exceeding 95% (55). The test is not specific for *S. typhi*, since positive results may be obtained from other Vi-positive organisms, including *S. paratyphi* A, which can cause typhoid fever, or *C. freundii*, which does not. When studied in endemic regions, coagglutination may be more sensitive than culture, because many patients receive antibiotics before coming for medical attention (56). Unfortunately, this test is not likely to be available at this time in the clinical microbiology laboratory. New immunoassays to detect *Salmonella* outer membrane proteins and excellent and specific polymerase chain reaction (PCR) protocols have been developed, but are also not in general use.

The breakthrough in therapy of typhoid occurred nearly 50 years ago, when chloramphenicol was first used in this disease (57). To the present, no drug has ever been significantly better, and many have been considerably worse. For chloramphenicol-sensitive organisms, the clinical response begins soon after treatment begins, usually within 48 hours of the initial dose when divided doses of 3–4 g/day are given to adults or 50–75 mg/kg are given to children. Most patients are afebrile by day 5 and the dose can be reduced to 2 g/day or 30 mg/kg in adults and children, respectively, and continued for a total of two weeks. While chloramphenicol has been extensively used in the developing world, because it is both very effective and very inexpensive, the association of the drug with aplastic anemia has limited its use wherever other options are available (58). Thus, first-line oral regimens in the United States have included trimethoprim-sulfamethoxazole (320/1600 mg twice daily in adults, or 185 mg/m^2 of the trimethoprim component in children), amoxicillin (4–6 g/day or 100 mg/kg in adults and children, respectively, in 4 divided doses), or for individuals over 17, a fluoroquinolone such as ciprofloxacin (500 mg twice daily) (59) or comparable doses of related drugs, for example ofloxacin (60). There has been concern about the toxicity of quinolones in children, and these drugs are not recommended by the U.S. Food and Drug Administration for use in individuals under 17 years of age. In a review article from the manufacturer, reversible arthralgia was noted in 36 of 1113 (3%) patients under the age of 18 who received ciprofloxacin because of complications of cystic fibrosis; however, there was no radiologic evidence of cartilage damage (61). Recent attempts to objectively evaluate this concern have concluded that the benefit-to-risk ratio is high (62,63). Alternative, safe and effective oral regimens for either drug sensitive or resistant strains in children include furazolidone (7.5 mg/kg per day) (64,65) or cefixime (5 mg/kg every 12 h) for 3–7 days (66). Therapy for carriers will be discussed below.

Intravenous antibiotics are used for severe illness or for initial therapy of patients unable to take oral medication. A variety of proven effective choices are available, including chloramphenicol, trimethoprim-sulfamethoxazole, high-dose ampicillin, ciprofloxacin, and third-generation cephalosporins such as cefotaxime and cephoperazone (67). However, no parenteral drug is as effective and easy to administer as ceftriaxone, and short courses of 2–4 g once daily for 3 days in adults and 50–80 mg/kg once daily for 5 days in children have been shown to be equally effective as full 7-day courses (68). Multidrug-resistant strains of *S. typhi*, including strains with increased resistance to quinolones (69), have become quite common in the Indian subcontinent, including India (70) and Pakistan (71), in Southeast Asia (72,73), and in Africa (74). At the present time, either ciprofloxacin or ceftriaxone are recommended, and in fact these drugs should be the initial choice in suspected typhoid patients who may have acquired infection in regions where multidrug resistance is prevalent. There are exceptions, however, and in one study, 7 days of parenteral ceftriaxone (3 g/d for 7 days) resulted in clinical failure in 6/22 (27%) of patients compared to 0/20 patients receiving oral ciprofloxacin (500 mg *bid* for 7 days) (75). The 6 ceftriaxone failures were then switched to ciprofloxacin, which resulted in defervescence within 48 hours. Similar data were reported from Viet Nam, where there were 6 acute failures and 1 relapse among 25 patients treated with 3 g of ceftriaxone once daily, compared to complete cure in 22 patients receiving 200 mg q 12 h of ofloxacin (76). If a quinolone is to be used for infections acquired in India or Pakistan, it is now recommended to increase the dose to 10 mg/kg twice daily (77). As an alternative, a recent study from Pakistan suggests that oral cefixime, 10 mg/kg in 2 divided doses, is as effective in children with multidrug-resistant typhoid as a single dose of parenteral ceftriaxone, 65 mg/kg, but at a significantly reduced cost (66).

Prolonged carriage, that is greater than 1 year, occurs in around 5% of typhoid patients. The likelihood is increased in patients with chronic cholecystitis and gall stones. It has been an important problem, since such individuals may need to be monitored by public health workers, and they may not be allowed to work at occupations that pose an increased risk of transmission to others, for example food handlers. Prior regimens using prolonged intravenous drugs have given way to the use of 6–8 weeks of amoxycillin or trimethoprim-sulfamethoxazole, which are reported to be around 80% effective in eradicating carriage (78,79). The advent of the new quinolones has further revolutionized this aspect of the management of typhoid patients. Because of its activity against the organism, its ability to concentrate in the bile, and its ability to penetrate macrophages, for the first time an oral drug, ciprofloxacin or another fluoroquinolone, can reasonably be expected to eradicate the carrier state in nearly all patients (80).

In a placebo-controlled double-blind study in Indonesia of patients with severe typhoid fever and central nervous system manifestations ranging from delirium to coma, the use of high-dose intravenous dexamethasone (3 mg/kg as a loading dose over 30 minutes, followed by 1 mg/kg every 6 h for 24–48 h) in addition to chloramphenicol reduced the mortality rate from 56% to 10% (52). As a result of these data, it has been recommended that patients with severe typhoid manifesting delirium, obtundation, stupor, coma, or shock receive steroids. In spite of the high fever, it is not recommended to administer antipyretics, since the risk of bleeding may be increased. The frequency of ileal perforation in typhoid-endemic countries approximates 3%, with an overall reported mortality of 40% (81). Prompt surgical management of this severe complication significantly reduces typhoid mortality, which is usually due to peritonitis under these circumstances (82). Modern imaging methods, including angiography, isotopic scanning, and sometimes endoscopy may localize the site of perforation and facilitate operative repair. In developing countries, it has often been recommended that conservative measures be used. With improvements in management in many areas, simple closure of perforations in two layers without resection is now the treatment of choice (83). When accompanied by brisk fluid replacement and the use of an inexpensive broad antibiotic regiment for bowel flora, including chloramphenicol, metronidazole, and gentamicin, this regimen would be expected to reduce mortality rates from in excess of 30% to less than 10% (84).

2. *Gastroenteritis*

The most common manifestation of *Salmonella* infection is diarrhea, usually following ingestion of an inoculum in food or water. Nontyphoidal salmonellosis is the common cause of febrile "food-poisoning" occurring 24–48 hours after a suspect meal. The initial symptoms are nonspecific and include nausea, vomiting, and headache followed by chills, fever, abdominal cramps, and watery diarrhea. Fecal losses are usually moderate, but on occasion a prodigious cholera-like syndrome may occur. Uncommonly, salmonellosis presents with bloody diarrhea, or rarely, clinical dysentery can develop, with frequent small-volume bloody stools, abdominal cramps, and tenesmus. The typical watery diarrhea is self-limited and of short duration, and it is questionable if antibiotic therapy is required in most cases (see below).

Salmonella gastroenteritis can be particularly severe in neonates and in the elderly and, especially if due to a hyperinvasive serovar such as *S. dublin*, can lead to systemic sepsis and death. A recent study in Belgium demonstrated positive blood cultures in 71/1380 (5.1%) of patients with *S. typhimurium* infection and 32/280 (11%) of patients with *S. enteritidis*[3]. Although there are no data to substantiate our impression, the authors believe that transient bacteremia is the rule early in *Salmonella* gastroenteritis, based on the invasive mechanisms of pathogenic strains. Whether or not bacteremia is detected depends on the timing of cultures (most will be taken too late, when diarrheal symptoms have already developed and the transient bacteremia has been cleared), host factors that may influence the extent of invasion (for example age), and the efficacy of host defenses in clearing organisms from the blood stream (for example, patients with chronic hemolytic diseases or HIV). Interestingly, in the Belgium study, the rate of blood isolates increased after the first decade of life, and while some of the increase in young adults could be related to HIV infection, the rate continued to increase into the eighth decade of life.

Thus, the mere isolation of *Salmonella enterica* serovars from the blood stream is not necessarily a worrisome finding, indicative of systemic spread, sustained bacteremia, and focal infection, especially in healthy patients who are clinically improving. These complications are much more likely in at-risk hosts, for example patients at the extremes of life, immunosuppressed patients including those with lymphoma and leukemia, and those with prosthetic valves or vascular grafts. A recent retrospective chart review compared 51 non-HIV infected patients presenting clinically with primary nontyphoidal *Salmonella* bacteremia in the absence of intestinal symptoms, to 58 patients with diarrhea and nontyphoidal secondary *Salmonella* bacteremia (85). The former were older (51 vs 33% were over 60 years of age, $p < 0.05$)), were more commonly receiving steroids (41 vs 13%, $p < 0.01$), and were more frequently immunosuppressed (65 vs 14%, $p < 0.01$). The primary bacteremia patients were also more likely to have hematological malignancies, solid tumors, or connective tissue disease, and in 8 of the 51 subjects, primarily *Salmonella* bacteremia was the harbinger of the serious underlying disease. Patients with acute or chronic hemolysis such as malaria, bartonellosis, or sickle cell disease are also at risk (86). In these patients, ingestion of hemoglobin and erythrocyte ghosts by macrophages can interfere with their phagocytic and microbicidal capacity for the invading *Salmonella*, increasing the likelihood of focal infections developing. The isolation of *Salmonella* from the bloodstream should raise questions about the host and his/her risk factors, and clinical judgement is needed to decide which patients to treat.

The diagnosis of Salmonella gastroenteritis is laboratory based. The diagnosis may be suspected in individuals involved in food-borne outbreaks and in whom the presenting symptoms are febrile watery diarrhea. If the stool contains considerable numbers of leukocytes, the most likely diagnosis is either salmonellosis or shigellosis, and stool culture is necessary to distinguish between the two. In most cases, by the time an organism is identified, the patients are clinically improved. If the patient presents with fever and chills and appears ill, a blood culture may be obtained, especially in an at-risk host. Several days can elapse before an organism is isolated and identified, and the patient may also be clinically improved by that time, with or without specific therapy.

The issue of therapy was a simple one, since antibiotics did not alter the clinical course of the illness, might contribute to development of complications such as antibiotic-associated colitis, and often prolonged the period of convalescent excretion of the pathogen, constituting a public health risk of transmission to others (87–89). Therefore, the recommendation was clear: antibiotics play no role in the treatment of *Salmonella* gastroenteritis and should not be used. With the advent of the new quinolone class of drugs, initial studies suggested that, for the first time, there was a clinically effective drug available for the diarrhea (90). This has not been borne out, however, as subsequent studies have failed to confirm a beneficial effect of these agents (91), including a high relapse rate and delayed eradication of the organism from the stool (92–95). The current state of the art once again suggests that antibiotic therapy be withheld in *Salmonella* diarrhea unless there are specific reasons to treat, for example severe illness related to the extremes of age, patients with immunodeficiencies including AIDS, asplenia, and certain chronic diseases such as hemolytic anemias and chronic renal failure (96).

3. *Invasive Salmonellosis and Focal Infections*

Prolonged febrile illness, with multiple positive blood cultures, can be produced by highly invasive *Salmonella* including *S. dublin* (97) and *S. cholerasuis*. These are generally unaccompanied by diarrhea, and the diagnosis is made when a positive blood culture is obtained. Although there are some typhoid-like features to this acute febrile illness, none of the typical signs associated with typhoid fever, such as rose spots, relative bradycardia, or leukopenia are present, and the patients are often severely ill. Without prompt systemic treatment with ceftriaxone or a fluoroquinolone, the mortality is high. In one unconfirmed study, 47 neonates with documented intestinal or extraintestinal *S. typhimurium* infection were randomized to receive cefoperazone (group 1, 22 infants) or the same drug plus intravenous immunoglobulin, 500 mg/kg on days 1, 2, 3, and 8 (group 2, 25 infants) (98). Bacteremia was detected in 31% of group 1 and

8% in group 2 ($p < 0.05$), 41% of group-1 infants died compared to 12% in group 2 ($p < 0.05$), and among the survivors, duration of illness was reduced from 15 to 8 days in the IV globulin group ($p < 0.01$).

One consequence of *Salmonella* bacteremia is endovascular infection. *S. cholerasuis* has a predilection for causing mycotic aneurysm, generally in pre-existing infrarenal aortic aneurysms—due to arteriosclerotic disease in men over the age of 50—or in a prosthetic vascular graft. Mycotic aneurysms of the thoracic aorta or arch are exceedingly rare, and the outcomes are far worse than disease of the abdominal aorta (99). However, due to the low prevalence of this serovar, most endovascular infections are actually caused by *S. typhimurium*. Such infections should be suspected when an elderly patient with a known or palpable aneurysm or a known vascular graft presents with a febrile illness associated with back, abdominal, or chest pain. Imaging studies are helpful in establishing the diagnosis (100) and are also useful to direct surgical therapy, which is often necessary in addition to prolonged antibiotic treatment. Currently recommended first-line therapy is either ceftriaxone or a fluoroquinolone for a minimum duration of 6 weeks. In some instances where surgical intervention is precluded, indefinite suppressive therapy with a quinolone has been effective for prolonged periods (101). It is curious that, in spite of the continued bacteremia associated with these invasive vascular infections, *Salmonella* endocarditis remains an uncommon complication. It should also be appreciated that only 5 cases of *Salmonella* prosthetic valve endocarditis have been reported (102,103).

Recurrent clinically relevant bacteremia due to *Salmonella* spp, very often *S. typhimurium*, has been observed in AIDS patients. The incidence is estimated to be between 46 and 384 per 100,000, which is 100–1000 times greater than the calculated incidence in the general population of 0.3/100,000. In Africa, this has been one of the more common causes of fever of undetermined etiology in AIDS patients (104). An aggressive approach to treatment is warranted, with a 6–8 week course of antibiotics, including an initial several weeks of intravenous therapy followed by oral drugs depending on response and antibiotic susceptibility of the isolate. With the first relapse, it may be better to consider indefinite prophylaxis, once the illness is resolved (105). If the organism is susceptible, and the patient tolerates it, trimethoprim-sulfamethoxazole can serve for both *Salmonella* and *Pneumocystis carinii* prophylaxis. If the patient is on a regimen for mycobacterial infection that includes a fluoroquinolone, this will cover the *Salmonella* as well (106). As the AIDS population ages with better treatment and longer survival, it is to be expected that arteritis and mycotic aneurysm of the aorta will occur if the prevalence of Salmonella bacteremia continues to be high. Such patients have already been reported (107,108).

Focal infections include arthritis and osteomyelitis. The former is conditioned by corticosteroid immunosuppression, sickle cell disease, prosthetic joints, or known aseptic necrosis, presumably becoming infected during a transient *Salmonella* bacteremia. Septic arthritis due to *Salmonella* should not be confused with reactive arthritis in patients with *Salmonella* gastroenteritis. Among 113 Swedish physicians surveyed following an outbreak of *S. enteritidis* enteritis at a radiology congress, 17 (15%) developed reactive arthritis (109). The rate was the same among individuals who were treated with appropriate antibiotics (10/65, 15.4%) for a mean of 9.1 days and those who were not treated initially (7/48, 14.6%). Antibiotic treatment also had no impact on the persistence of symptoms at 6 months. Reactive arthritis is considered to be an immunologically mediated process, with a specific predilection for individuals expressing the HLA-B27 antigen, which is common among Scandinavians. It is not specific for salmonellosis and is also associated with other invasive diarrheal diseases, including, in particular, infections with *S. flexneri* and *Y. enterocolitica*. The specific antigenic constituents involved and the mechanism for activation of inflammatory processes within the synovia are not well understood. Salmonella osteomyelitis is well described in association wit sickle cell disease, sickle-thalassemia, and sickle-hemoglobin C disease. It is typically seen in children and young adults and generally occurs in long bones. The therapy for septic arthritis is always drainage and antibiotics; osteomyelitis often requires debridement of necrotic bone and appropriate drug therapy for a prolonged period, usually 6 or more weeks.

Salmonella can also cause cholecystitis, cholangitis, splenic abscess, meningitis (especially in neonates), pneumonia or empyema (in patients with preexisting pulmonary diseases or predisposing conditions such as diabetes or alcoholism), or urinary-tract infections (in patients with *Schistosoma hematobium* or renal tuberculosis causing obstructive uropathy). Therapy includes antibiotics and surgical drainage or debridement whenever appropriate.

F. Vaccines and Control

Considerable effort has gone into the development of *Salmonella* vaccines. There have been significant advances in new vaccines for *S. typhi* (110), but not much progress in vaccines for nontyphoidal infections. The original typhoid vaccine was a phenol extract of whole organisms, often combined with a similar preparation from *S. paratyphi* A and B, known as TAB vaccine. This is, essentially, a preparation of lipopolysaccharide (LPS), and it induces anti-O-antigen antibodies, at a cost of local reactogenicity, including pain, redness, and swelling at the site of the injection associated with mild fever. The effect of this vaccine is to induce circulating bactericidal antibodies that assist in the opsonization of organisms during the initial phagocytosis, which leads to rapid phagocytosis and killing by neutrophils. In the absence of these antibodies, organisms are taken up and survive within monocytes. Protective efficacy to

S. typhi has been estimated to be around 60% but this lasts just a few months, and immunity wanes beyond 6 months. Because there are no efficacy data for the antigens and because paratyphoid fever is generally a milder illness, LPS from *paratyphi* A and B has been removed from this form of typhoid vaccine produced in the United States.

Reactogenicity and limited efficacy of the killed vaccine has prompted the search for a better vaccine. The second generation of typhoid vaccine, now licensed and available, is a live, orally administered, attenuated *S. typhi* vaccine strain, defective in the galactose epimerase gene. This organism is able to invade cells but cannot metabolize galactose, and it is incapable of progressive replication in the host. Thus it induces immunity but causes no infection. Vaccine trials have suggested the mean efficacy of this vaccine to be in the same range as the old killed vaccine, but without the side effects. Three oral doses have been required for a primary immunization series. Protection lasts several years and it may be boosted.

The next vaccine to be field tested will be Vi polysaccharide (111). This induces immunity in a single injection and is much better tolerated than killed phenol-extracted vaccine. The efficacy appears to be similar to that of killed vaccine and protection lasts for several years, but the vaccine is not very effective in young children below 2 years of age who are unable to respond well to polysaccharide antigens. Attempts are being made to conjugate Vi to protein antigens in order to convert Vi from a T-independent to a T-dependent antigen to provide for memory responses (112); however, no conjugate typhoid vaccine product is ready for testing.

Other investigators are experimenting with auxotrophic mutant strains for attenuation. Mutations in the aromatic pathway appear to provide the needed attenuation without interfering with the generation of protective immune responses, but humoral and cell-mediated. This approach appears promising, since the auxotrophic mutants engage both the humoral and the cell-mediated pathways for immunization. A recent analysis of the cost–benefit relationship of typhoid vaccine in British travelers, regardless of the vaccine used, concluded that the cost of the vaccine greatly exceeded the cost of treating the low incidence of typhoid (estimated to be 0.2% of travelers), and therefore it was recommended that the National Health Service not support this program (113).

III. YERSINIOSIS

A. Introduction

Two of the three human pathogenic members of the genus *Yersinia*—*Y. enterocolitica* and *Y. pseudotuberculosis*—are enteric pathogens while *Y. pestis* is the infamous cause of plague and will not be discussed further. The others are principally environmental organisms and rarely cause human disease. *Y. enterocolitica* is the more common cause of intestinal disease, first described to cause human illness in the 1930s. It was originally named *Bacterium enterocolicum* (114), but was renamed *Y. enterocolitica* after the suggestion of Frederiksen that this organism be included in the family Enterobacteraceae (115). *Y. pseudotuberculosis* was probably described in 1883, when Mallasez and Vignal reported on a bacillus causing a granulomatous disease in guinea pigs which they named pseudotuberculosis (116). An interesting property of this organism was that it multiplied at 4°C, and grew better at 22°C than at 37°C. *Y. pseudotuberculosis* was first recovered from mesenteric lymph nodes in a patient presenting with clinical appendicitis by Masshoff in 1953 (117). Originally classified as a *Pasturella* spp., related to the plague organism then called *P. pestis*, the name was changed to *Y. pseudotuberculosis* when the genus was created 25 years ago.

B. Microbiology

Y. enterocolitica and *Y. pseudotuberculosis* are nonlactose fermenting gram-negative organisms but may be distinguished by biochemical and serological criteria (see Table 4). The former, a facultative anaerobic rod with peritrichous flagella, is divided into biogroups according to biochemical properties (see Table 5). Serotyping based on the more than 50 described O-antigens is used to designate strains although there may be some cross-reactivity between pathogenic and nonpathogenic types. The majority of human isolates are of serotypes O3, O8, or O9 and biotypes 2, 3, and 4 (118). Six serotypes of *Y. pseudotuberculosis* have been described with four subtypes, of which serotype O1 accounts for approximately 80% of human cases.

Table 4 Laboratory Features of *Y. enterocolitica* and *Y. pseudotuberculosis*

Characteristic	*Y. enterocolitica*	*Y. pseudotuberculosis*
Motility at 25°C	+	+
at 37°C	–	–
Oxidase	–	–
Urease	+	+
Indole	V	+
Nitrate reduction	+	+
Fermentation		
Glucose	+	+
Lactose	–	–
Sucrose	+	–

Source: Ref. 170.
Key: + = positive; – = negative; V = variable.

Table 5 Main Biochemical Features of Biogroups of *Y. enterocolitica*

	Biogroups						
Characteristic	1	American strains	2	3	3A[a],3B[b]	4	5
Lipase activity	+	+	–	–	–	–	–
Esculin hydrolysis	+/–	–	–	–	–/(+)	–	–
Indole production	+	+	(+)	–	–	–	–
Acid from xylose	+	+	+	+	–	–	v
Voges–Proskauer test	+	+	+	+	–	+	+/(+)
Ornithine decarboxylase	+	+	+	+	+	+	–
Pyrazinamidase activity	+	–	–	–	+	–	–

Source: Ref. 118.

+, positive; –, negative; parentheses, delayed reaction; v, 11–89% of strains positive.

[a]Positive for acid production from sorbose and inositol.

[b]Negative for acid production from sorbose and inositol.

C. Epidemiology

Yersinia enterocolitica can be isolated from patients around the world and is a significant cause of morbidity in developed countries. The epidemiological distribution correlates with temperate climates such as Northern Europe, Scandinavia, Canada, Japan,and the United States, suggesting that the distribution of the organism has more to do with climate than socioeconomic factors. The organism is rarely found in patients in tropical countries. At the International Center for Diarrheal Diseases Research in Dhaka, Bangladesh (ICDDR,B), a dedicated group of *Yersinia* microbiologists spent a year looking for the organism among the 100,000 patients evaluated microbiologically in the inpatient and outpatient settings and found just one isolate (personal communication, Dr. M. J. Albert, Director, Clinical Microbiology Laboratory, ICDDR,B). As a result, this organism is no longer sought at ICDDR,B. Epidemiologic studies in various countries have shown that *Y. enterocolitica* can be recovered from stool specimens in 6.7% of specimens in British Columbia, 5.9% in Belgium, 4.7% in Finland, 2.9% in the Netherlands, 1.4% in Italy, and 1% in the United States (119). The prevalence of this pathogen in these countries may rival that of *Campylobacter* or *Salmonella* spp, as a cause of bacterial diarrhea.

The reported incidence of *Y. enterocolitica* has increased over the last 20 years, probably largely due to increased awareness of the organism and improved diagnostic techniques. Not all serotypes of *Y. enterocolitica* are equally pathogenic to humans and their distribution varies in different parts of the world. Thus, most isolates from Scandinavia and Europe are serotypes O3 and O9, while in the United States the majority are O4, O8, O13, O18, O20, and O21 (120–123). Outbreaks of *Y. enterocolitica* are common in the United States (124,125), whereas sporadic illness is more typical in Europe. Although *Y. enterocolitica* is distributed widely in nature—and human pathogenic serotypes have been recovered from dogs, cats, cattle, and sheep—swine are the major reservoirs, especially serotypes O3 and O9 (126) and are a likely zoonotic source of human disease (127,128). Outbreaks have also been associated with milk and milk products, both pasteurized and nonpasteurized (129,130).

Yersinia pseudotuberculosis is isolated primarily from children undergoing surgery for presumed appendicitis who, instead, are found to have acute mesenteric lymphadenitis (131). The organism is distributed worldwide, and like *Y. enterocolitica*, with a higher reported frequency in Europe and Scandinavia. It has been recovered from both wild and domestic animals including cattle, horses, goats, sheep, rodents, cats, and dogs, as well as fowl. The disease predominates in children and most cases are sporadic, although small outbreaks may occur (132). Transmission to humans has been associated with ingestion of water or unpasteurized milk, but the source of most infections is not determined (119).

D. Pathogenesis

Different serotypes of *Y. enterocolitica* have a varying pattern of virulence factors and as a consequence are heterogeneous in their ability to cause disease. Infection is usually initiated following oral ingestion of a sufficient inoculum of bacterium, which find their way to the terminal ileum where they are able to bind to intestinal epithelial cells (133). They penetrate the intestinal mucosa through M cells and colonize local lymphoid follicles (Peyer's patches). From there, *Yersinia* can enter the lymphatics and disseminate.

The ability of *Y. enterocolitica* to survive in organs such as the liver and spleen is associated with the presence of a 70-kDa virulence plasmid (pYV). This appears to be essential for the virulence of *Yersinia* species (134), although strains cured of the pYV plasmid are still able to cross the intestinal epithelial cell barrier in animal models. The invasive characteristics of *Y. enterocolitica* correlate with their ability to cause disease. This property is associated with three invasion genes: *inv, ail*, and *yadA*, each of which promotes cell invasion (135–137). Both *inv* and *ail* are on the *Yersinia* chromosome, whereas *yadA* is plasmid encoded. Invasin, which is the principal invasion factor produced by both *Y. enterocolitica* and *Y. pseudotuberculosis* binds to a subset of β1-chain integrin receptors on the host cell, which potentiates the internalization of *Yersinia* (138). *Y. enterocolitica* invasin is a 92-kDa protein, which is highly homologous to the 103-kDa invasin of *Y. pseudotuberculosis*. It is maximally expressed at 28°C (139), suggesting that it may function early in infection when the organisms penetrate lymphoid follicles. Leong et al. determined that the C-terminal 192 amino acids of invasin contain the integrin-binding domains and are sufficient for the invasion phenotype (140). This domain is, when coated onto the outer surface of *Staphylococcus aureus*, able to mediate cell penetration (141).

The *ail* gene is also important for cellular invasion, but unlike invasin, *ail*-mediated invasion has cell-line specificity. An *ail* gene deletion results in some loss of invasive capacity, but not as much as an *inv* deletion mutantation. In *Y. enterocolitica, ail* is a 17-kDa protein with significant homology with *ail* from *Y. pseudotuberculosis*.

The *yadA* gene forms multimeric fibrillae on the surface of the pathogen. It mediates the binding of *Y. enterocolitica* to collagen, fibronectin, and mucus and is also responsible for other characteristics such as autoagglutination and hemagglutination (119). The *yadA* gene may also utilize β-1 chain integrin receptors for internalization (142).

Entry of *Y. enterocolitica* into mammalian cells is not a property of the organism alone, but rather is dependent on events within the host cells. Cell penetration by *Yersinia* is accompanied by marked cytoskeletal rearrangements, in contrast to the events during the entry of *Salmonella typhimurium* (143).

These rearrangements are related to tyrosine phosphorylation, since they are blocked by inhibitors of tyrosine protein kinase (144), which also prevent invasion of *Y. enterocolitica* but not *S. typhimurium*. After invading epithelial cells, *Y. enterocolitica*, like *Salmonella*, localize within lymphoid tissues in Peyer's patches.

Following this initial invasion, the bacteria can disseminate and multiply in different organs of the host. The ability of *Y. enterocolitica* to spread systemically is dependent on its capacity to avoid host defenses. This is largely due to a series of proteins encoded by the 70-kDa virulence plasmid, pYV (145,146). When animals are infected with either isogenic plasmid-bearing or cured strains, only the plasmid-positive strains proliferate and disseminate. Those lacking the plasmid are able to bind to intestinal epithelial cells, invade and colonize Peyer's patches, but are then cleared by the host defenses (147).

The pYV plasmid encodes proteins known as Yops (*Yersinia* outer membrane proteins) which endow the organism with the capacity to overcome host defenses and are highly conserved among *Yersinia* species. The genes for the 10 known Yops are distributed throughout the pYV plasmid in both monocistronic and polycistronic operons (146). Additional operons, *ysc*, encode regulatory proteins involved in Yop secretion. At 37°C the Yop and ysc operons are regulated by intracellular calcium levels and nucleotides such as ATP and GTP (148). The secretion of Yops is complex and appears to require multiple gene products from several operons, including the *ysc* locus, and the low calcium response (LCR) *lcrB* locus and the *lcrDR* locus (149). The V antigen is a 37–41-kDa protein that is subject to the same regulation as the Yops (150). It is considered to have a regulatory role in the low-calcium response as well as an "antihost" function and is known as LcrV: LcrV is a protective antigen in humans. The Yops fall into two general classes, including those like YopM and YopE with purely antihost functions, and those like YopN, YopD, and LcrG that have regulatory and/or Yop targeting functions, although LcrV and YopH appear to be bifunctional (146) (Table 6).

Clinical isolates of *Y. enterocolitica* have been shown to produce a 30 amino acid, heat-stable enterotoxin, Yst, similar to the heat-stable enterotoxins (ST) produced by *Escherichia coli*. Like E. coli ST, Yst is an activator of guanylate cyclase resulting in the net secretion of fluid in the intestine (151). Interestingly this toxin is not produced at temperatures above 30°C, and because of this, its clinical relevance has been questioned. *Y. enterocolitica* produce siderophores and a 65-kDa iron-repressible outer membrane protein, known as Irp65, has been identified in mouse-lethal strains of *Y. enterocolitica*. *Y. enterocolitica* O3 and O9 strains may also acquire iron by the use of nonbiological exogenous siderophores such as desferrioxamine, used for iron chelation in iron overload diseases. This is the explanation for the association of desferrioxamine therapy with severe systemic *Y. enterocolitica* infection in humans.

Table 6 Plasmid Encoded Virulence Factors

Virulence factor	Size (kDa)	Function
YopE	23	Cytotoxin, antiphagocytic effect
YopD	33	Required for entry of YopE into target cells
YopB	42	Similar to hemolysin and IpaB of *S. flexnerei* and the RTX family of hemolysins and toxins
YopH	51	Protein tyrosine phosphatase; involved in antiphagocytic properties of the organisms
YopM	42	Binds human α-thrombin, may sequester thrombin, inhibits platelet aggregation
YopJ	31	Unclear
YopO	82	Autophosphorylating enzyme
LcrV	37–41	Regulatory and antihost function
YadA	50	Bacterial binding, autoagglutination, and hemagglutination

Source: Ref. 119.

E. Clinical Manifestations, Diagnosis, and Therapy

Y. enterocolitica, like *Salmonella* spp, is able to cause diarrhea and a variety of other clinical syndromes, including mesenteric adenitis, terminal ileitis, erythema nodosum, and septicemia. The diarrhea due to *Y. enterocolitica* is usually watery but bloody diarrhea occurs in a quarter of the patients, with fever, abdominal pain, and vomiting in some. Stool examination reveals leukocytes and erythrocytes in about half of the patients. Marks et al. (152) studied 181 children with *Y. enterocolitica* infection and reported a stooling rate of 5–10 movements per day in the first week, with a mean total duration of diarrhea of 14 days (range 1–46 days). Twenty-six percent of the patients noted blood in their stool. Duration of fecal excretion of *Y. enterocolitica* varied between 14 and 97 days with a mean of 42 days. Although most infections are self-limited, a variety of complications can occur (discussed further below).

Yersinia enterocolitica has become famous as a cause of "pseudoappendicitis." Patients may present with fever, right lower quadrant abdominal pain, and tenderness and leukocytosis, with or without diarrhea. The clinical presentation is indistinguishable from appendicitis in up to 20% of patients subsequently shown to have *Y. enterocolitica* infection (153). At surgery, the appendix is found to be normal, but a marked terminal ileitis with inflammatory mesenteric lymph nodes is present and the surgeon closes the wound without resection. Ultrasonograph appears to be of some use in distinguishing true appendicitis from terminal ileitis and mesenteric adenitis due to *Y. enterocolitica* (154).

The nongastrointestinal manifestations of *Y. enterocolitica* are numerous and include cutaneous lesions, including erythema nodosum, erythema multiforme-like eruptions, and maculopapular rashes. The bacteria have been isolated from surgical wounds, pustulae, and skin ulcerations (153). Exudative pharangitis has been reported in association with *Y. enterocolitica* (155) and may be a cause of cervical adenopathy, with or without an enteric presentation. Reactive arthritis has been recognized as a complication of *Y. enterocolitica* infection since the late 1960s. Arthritis can develop during the acute gastrointestinal illness or may occur weeks to months after the initial presentation. The arthritic symptoms often persist for several months and they may become chronic, especially in individuals positive for the HLA-B27 antigen. A study of 85 patients with *Yersinia* arthritis over a 10 year period showed that 51.8% of patients continued to have some joint symptoms during the follow up period (156). Development of new reactive arthritis (4.7%) or chronic arthritis (2.4%) was uncommon; 14.1% of patients (all HLA-B27 positive) had acute iritis and 2.4% had conjunctivitis during the follow up period. Eighty percent of the patients in the study showed the presence of HLA-B27 were more likely to have lower back pain and sacroiliitis. While the synovial fluid is sterile, *Yersinia* antigens can be detected in the synovial fluid from the majority of patients with *Yersinia*-associated arthritis (157). *Y. enterocolitica* is known to express antigens with T-cell superantigen activity (158). This may be important in relation to the reported associations between *Y. enterocolitica* and an increased incidence of several inflammatory diseases including ankalosing spondylitis, Reiter's syndrome, myocarditis, glomerulonephritis, and thyroid disease (119). In a recent series of *Y. enterocolitica* infections among children, enteric disease occurred in 114 of 125 patients, including enteritis in 92, pseudoappendicitis in 20, and chronic ileitis in 2 (159). Seventeen of these 114 patients, and 11 others without enteric disease, had extramesenteric manifestations, especially in children above 6 years of age. Thirteen had arthritis, 11 had extensive lymphadenopathy, and 4 had erythema nodosum. In addition, one patient each had septicemia with pleurisy, vasculitis, and cholecystitis.

One of the most severe complications of *Y. enterocolitica* infection is septicemia. The case fatality rate varies in different studies but may be as high as 50% (160). Severe *Yersinia* sepsis is most often reported in immunocompromised patients, although 22% of cases in one series were previously healthy individuals (161). Conditions associated with iron-overload such as hemochromatosis, chronic hemolytic anemias, and, as previously noted, use of iron chelation therapy with desferrioxamine are predisposing factors to the development of *Y. enterocolitica* septicemia. In a recent series of 114 Italian thalassemic patients, mean age of 12.8 years, and 100 controls, mean age 12.1 years, symptomatic *Y. enterocolitica* infection occurred in 12 (10%) of the thalassemics and 2 (2%) of the controls. Of the former, 8 had enteritis, 1 had tonsillitis, and 5 (36%) had a septicemic presentation. Of the 2 infected controls, 1 had enteritis and the other tonsillitis (162).

Other associated predisposing factors include cirrhosis, immunosuppressive therapy, diabetes mellitus, alcoholism, and malnutrition (119). Bacteremia due to blood transfusion is also a documented problem, typically involving blood that has been stored for more than 25 days (163). This may be a consequence of the ability of *Yersinia enterocolitica* to survive and proliferate at 4°C during prolonged blood storage, analogous to cold enrichment for isolation. The circumstances of the initial contamination are unclear, but in some instances the donors have reported recent diarrheal illnesses (164).

The clinical features of *Y. pseudotuberculosis* infection are very similar to those of *Y. enterocolitica*. Intestinal symptoms such as diarrhea, abdominal pain, and fever are the most common signs. The presentation may be a pseudoappendicitis, and mesenteric lymphadenopathy is a common finding at laparotomy. Complications include sepsis, liver, abscess, erythema nodosum, and reactive arthritis. Severe systemic disease has been reported in Japanese children in association with *Y. pseudotuberculosis,* with high fever, a desquamative rash, lymphadenopathy, and conjunctivitis (165).

Diagnosis is microbiological. The organisms may be isolated from a variety of clinical specimens, including stool, peritoneal fluid, blood, lymph nodes, or pharyngeal exudate. *Y. enterocolitica* can be grown from stool on commonly used enteric media such as MacConkey agar, on which it appears as lactose-negative colonies after 48 h of growth at 25–28°C. Prior cold-enrichment growth may be required for isolation, but this can take up to 3 weeks. However, culturing *Yersinia* from stool is difficult, especially with serotypes other than O3 and O9. Potassium hydroxide treatment of stool samples has been suggested as a rapid and sensitive alternative to cold enrichment (166). Aside from the delays entailed, another problem with some of the enrichment procedures is that they are not selective for pathogenic *Yersinia*. Therefore simple and accessible tests for pathogenicity are desirable. Candidate tests include assessment of autoagglutination, Congo red absorption, crystal violet binding, pyrazinamidase activity, salicin fermentation, and esculin hydrolysis (119). The application of PCR to detect specific virulence genes would be a sensitive and specific way to identify pathogenic strains, but is not yet a routine clinical procedure.

Serological testing is of some use in diagnosis of *Yersinia* infection. The saline agglutination titer (SAT) is simple but not as sensitive as a Coomb's test or indirect immunofluorescence (167). Other available methods include enzyme immunoassay (ELISA) and radioimmunoassay. One of the problems with serological testing is the need to be able to detect the host response to the multiple pathogenic serotypes. Newer assays that utilize nonserotype specific antigens may eliminate this problem (168). Unfortunately, the utility of classical serological testing for *Yersinia* is diminished by false-positive reactions with other gram-negative bacteria. For this reason it is still preferable to try to isolate the bacteria whenever possible. In a recent series of 125 patients with proven *Y. enterocolitica* infection (159), the diagnosis was established by culture in 100 (80%) and by agglutination in 11/45 (24%) tested. However, circulating specific anti-IgA and anti-IgG to Yop proteins was present in 47/48 (98%), and antigen was detected in biopsy specimens in 28/33 (85%) of children tested.

Antibiotic therapy has not been shown to have a major impact on the outcome of *Y. enterocolitica* enteritis or mesenteric adenitis. Despite this, in part due to the invasive nature of the organism and its capacity to cause serious systemic illness, these infections are usually treated with antibiotics (Table 7), although the relatively mild nature of illness in young children suggests a strategy in which antibiotics are considered primarily in those over 6 or in those with a preexisting condition predisposing to severe, systemic, or complicated infection. The production of β-lactamases in certain serotypes and biotypes has made the use of older beta-lactam antibiotics unreliable and best avoided; thus penicillin, ampicillin, and first generation cephalosporins are ineffective. Nei-

Table 7 Antimicrobial Therapy for Systemic Infection with *Y. enterocolitica*

Effective agents	Drugs of choice for serious infections
Aminoglycosides	Fluoroquinolones
Trimethoprim-sulfamethoxazole	Ceftriaxone
Doxycycline	
Chloramphenicol	
Imipenem	
Aztreonam	

Source: Ref. 169.

ther the carboxy penicillins nor second generation cephalosporins are active against *Yersinia*, whereas aztreonam and imipenem/cilastatin are likely to be active. Third generation cephalosporins, especially ceftriaxone, are highly active in vitro and clinical data suggest they are efficacious, although there have been clinical failures (169). Some success is reported using amoxicillin/clavualate, however the other major choice at the present time would be a fluoroquinolone, although the FDA does not recommend the use of the drug in pediatric patients under 17 years because of the potential of bone and cartilage damage. As discussed in the section on the therapy for salmonellosis, recent studies have failed to substantiate a significant risk of these complications, and the risk of toxicity must be weighed against the risk of an untoward outcome in the seriously ill patient with *Yersinia* infection.

Antibiotics are without question appropriate in patients with disseminated *Yersinia* infection, using intravenous ceftriaxone or ciprofloxacin, or in pediatric patients allergic to ceftriaxone, trimethoprim-sulfamethoxazole. The duration of therapy in different studies has been between 2–6 weeks. To complete the course of treatment, initial intravenous antibiotic may be followed by an oral agent to which the isolate is sensitive.

Y. pseudotuberculosis enteritis or mesenteric adenitis does not routinely require therapy. Bacteremic patients have in the past been successfully treated with streptomycin (15mg/kg every 12 hours IM) or with tetracycline 20–30 mg/kg/day. Ampicillin remains an effective drug for *Y. pseudotuberculosis*. However, there is no reason to believe that ceftriaxone or a fluoroquinolone would not be highly efficacious, and these drugs would be the first choice until the organism was identified and antibiotic sensitivity data were available.

REFERENCES

1. Smith T. The hog-cholera group of bacteria. US Bur Anim Ind Bull 1894; 6:6–40.

2. Gaffkey G. Zur aeatiologie der abdominal typhus. Mitt Gesundheitsamte 1884; 2:372–342.
3. LeBacq F, Louwagie B, Verhaegen J. *Salmonella typhimurium* and *Salmonella enteritidis*: Changing epidemiology from 1973 until 1992. Eur J Epidemiol 1994; 10:367–371.
4. Mishu B, Koehler J, Lee JA, Rodrigue D, Brenner FH, Blake P, Tauxe RV. Outbreaks of *Salmonella enteritidis* infections in the United States, 1985–1991. J Infect Dis 1994; 169:547–552.
5. Chalker RB, Blaser MJ. A review of human salmonellosis: III. Magnitude of salmonella infection in the United States. Rev Infect Dis 1988; 10:111–124.
6. Mishu B, Griffin PM, Tauxe RV, Cameron DN, Hutcheson RH, Schaffner W. *Salmonella enteritidis* gastroenteritis transmitted by intact chicken eggs. Ann Intern Med 1991; 115:190–194.
7. Ryan CA, Nickels MK, Hargrett-Bean NT, et al. Massive outbreak of antimicrobial-resistant salmonellosis traced to pastueurized milk. JAMA 1987; 258:3269–3274.
8. Centers for Disease Control and Prevention. *Salmonella hadar* associated with pet ducklings -- Connecticut, Maryland and Pennsylvania. MMWR 1991; 41:182–187.
9. Waterman SH, Juraez G, Carr SJ, Kilman L. *Salmonella arizonae* infections in latinos associated with rattlesnake folk medicine. Am J Public Health 1990; 80:286–289.
10. Cortes E, Zuckerman MJ, Ho H. Recurrent *Salmonella arizona* infection after treatment for metastatic carcinoma. J Clin Gastroenterology 1992; 14:157–159.
11. Fang FC, Fierer J. Human infection with *Salmonella dublin*. Medicine 1991; 70:198–207.
12. Taylor DN, Wachsmuth IK, Shangkuan YH, et al. Salmonellosis associated with marijuana. N Eng J Med 1982; 306:1249–1253.
13. Mathieu JJ, Henning KJ, Bell E, Frieden TR. Typhoid fever in New York City, 1980 through 1990. Arch Int Med 1994; 154:1713–1718.
14. Blaser MJ, Neuman LS. A review of human salmonellosis. I Infective dose. Rev Infect Dis 1982; 4:1096–1106.
15. Glynn JR, Hornick RB, Levine MM, Bradley DJ. Infecting dose and severity of typhoid: analysis of volunteer data and examination of the influence of the definition of illness used. Epidemiol Infect 1995; 115:23–30.
16. Pascopella L, Raupach B, Ghori N, Monack D, Falkow S, Small PLC. Host restriction phenotypes of *Salmonella typhi* and *Salmonella gallinarum*. Infect Immun 1995; 63:4329–4335.
17. Clark MA, Jepson MA, Simmons NL, Hirst BH. Preferential interaction of *Salmonella typhimurium* with mouse Peyer's patch M cells. Res Microbiol 1994; 145:543–552.
18. Garcia-del Portillo F, Finlay BB. Invasion and intracellular proliferation of *Salmonella* within non-phagocytic cells. Microbiologia 1994; 10:229–238.
19. Foster JW, Spector MP. How *Salmonella* survive against the odds. Ann Rev Microbiol 1995; 49:145–174.

20. Dunlap NE, Benjamin WH Jr, McCall RD Jr, Tilden AB, Briles DE. A "safe-site" for *Salmonella typhimurium* is within splenic cells during the early phase of infection in mice. Microb Pathogen 1991; 10:297–310.
21. Zwilling BS, Hilburger ME. Macrophage resistance genes: Bcg/Ity/Lsh. Immunol Series 1994; 60:233–245.
22. Vidal S, Tremblay ML, Govoni G, Gauthier S, Sebastiani G, Malo D, Skamene E, Olivier M, Jothy S. Gros P. The Ity/Lsh/Bcg locus: natural resistance to infection with intracellular parasites is abrogated by disruption of the Nramp1 gene. J Exp Med 1995; 182:655–666.
23. Cellier M, Govoni G, Vidal S, Kwan T, Groulx N, Liu J, Sanchez F, Skamene E, Schurr E, Gros P. Human natural resistance-associated macrophage protein: cDNA cloning, chromosomal mapping, genomic organization, and tissue-specific expression. J Exp Med 1994; 180:1741–1752.
24. Blackwell JM, Barton CH, White JK, Roach TI, Shaw MA, Whitehead SH, Mock BA, Searle S, Williams H, Baker AM. Genetic regulation of leishmanial and mycobacterial infections: the Lsh/Ity/Bcg gene story continues. Immunol Lett 1994; 43:99–107.
25. White JK, Shaw MA, Barton CH, Cerretti DP, Williams H, Mock BA, Carter NP, Peacock CS, Blackwell JM. Genetic and physical mapping of 2q35 in the region of the NRAMP and IL8R genes: identification of a polymoprhic repeat in exon 2 of NRAMP. Genomics 1994; 24:295–302.
26. Mills SD, Finlay BB. Comparison of *Salmonella typhi* and *Salmonella typhimurium* invasion, intracellular growth and localization in cultured human epithelial cells. Microbial Pathogen 1994; 17:409–423.
27. Francis CL, Ryan TA, Jones BD, Smith SJ, Falkow S. Ruffles induced by *Salmonella* and other stimuli directed micropinocytosis of bacteria. Nature 1993; 364:639–642.
28. Alpuche-Aranda CM, Berthiaume EP, Mock B, Swanson JA, Miller SI. Spacious phagosome formation within mouse macrophages correlates with *Salmonella* serotype pathogenicity and host susceptibility. Infect Immun 1995; 63:4456–4462.
29. Miller SI, Pulkkinen WS, Selsted ME, Mekalanos JJ. Characterization of defensin resistance phenotypes associated with mutations in the *phoP* virulence regular of *Salmonella typhimurium*. Infect Immun 1990; 58:3706–3710.
30. Sjobring U, Pohl G, Olsen A. Plasminogen, absorbed by *Escherichia coli* expressing curli or by *Salmonella* expressing thin aggregative fimbriae, can be activated by simultaneously captured tissue-type plasminogen activator (t-PA). Molec Microbiol 1994; 14:443–452.
31. Lahteenmaki K, Virkola R, Pouttu R, Kuusela P, Kukkonen M, Korhonen TK. Bacterial plasminogen receptors: in vitro evidence for a role in degradation of the mammalian extracellular matrix. Infect Immun 1995; 63:3659–3664.
32. Finlay BB. Molecular and cellular mechanisms of *Salmonella* pathogenesis. Curr Top Microbiol Immunol 1994; 192:163–185.
33. Galan J, Ginocchio C. The molecular genetic basis of *Salmonella* entry into mammalian cells. Biochem Soc Trans 1994; 22:301–306.
34. Ginocchio CC, Olmstead SB, Wells CL, Galan JE. Contact with epithelial cells

induces the formation of surface appendages on *Salmonella typhimurium*. Cell 1994; 76:717–724.
35. Stein MA, Mills SD, Finlay BB. *Salmonella*: now you see it, now you don't. Bioessays 1994; 16:537–538.
36. Pace J, Hayman MJ, Galan JE. Signal transduction and invasion of epithelial cells by *Salmonella typhimurium*. Cell 1993; 72:505–514.
37. Pace J, Hayman MJ, Galan JE. Signal transduction and invasion of epithelial cells by *S. typhimurium*. Cell 1993; 72:505–514.
38. McCormick BA, Miller SI, Carnes D, Madara JL. Transepithelial signaling to neutrophils by salmonellae: a novel virulence mechanism for gastroenteritis. Infect Immun 1995; 63:2302–2309.
39. Eckmann L, Kagnoff M, Fierer J. Epithelial cells secrete the chemokine interleukin-8 in response to bacterial entry. Infect Immun 1993; 61:4569–4574.
40. Mcormick BA, Hofman PM, Kim J, Carnes DK, Miller SI, Madara JL. Surface attachment of *Salmonella typhimurium* to intestinal epithelia imprints the subeipthelial matrix with gradients chemotactic for neutrophils. J Cell Biol 1995; 131:1599–1680.
41. Guiney DG, Fang FC, Krause M, Libby S. Plasmid-mediated virulence genes in non–typhoid *Salmonella* seovars. FEMS Microbiol Lett 1994; 124:1–9.
42. Fierer J, Eckmann L, Fang F, Pfeifer C, Finlay BB, Guiney D. Expression of the *Salmonella* virulence plasmid gene *spvB* in cultured macrophages and nonphagocytic cell lines. Infect Immun 1993; 61:5231–5236.
43. Guiney DG, Libby S, Fang FC, Krause M, Fierer J. Growth-phase regulation of plasmid virulence genes in *Salmonella*. Trends in Microbiol 1995; 3:275–279.
44. Spink JM, Pullinger GD, Wood MW, Lax AJ. Regulation of *spvR*, the positive regulatory gene of *Salmonella* plasmid virulence genes. FEMS Microbiol Lett 1994; 116:113–121.
45. Chen CY, Buchmeier NA, Libby S, Fang FC, Krause M, Guiney DG. Central regulatory role in the RpoS sigma factor in expression of *Salmonella dublin* plasmid virulence genes. J Bacteriol 1996; 177:5303–5309.
46. Miller SI, Kukral AM, Mekalanos JJ. A two-component regulatory system (*phoP phoQ*) controls *Salmonella typhimurium* virulence. Proc Natl Acad Sci (USA) 1989; 86:5054–5058.
47. Garcia Vescovi E, Soncini FC, Groisman EA. The role of the PhoP/PhoQ regulon in *Salmonella* virulence. Res Microbiol 1994; 145:473–480.
48. Garcia Vescovi E, Soncini FC, Groisman EA. Mg^{2+} as an extracellular signal: environmental regulation of *Salmonella* virulence. Cell 1996; 84:165–174.
49. Miller SI, Mekalanos JJ. Constitutive expression of the *phoP* regulon attenuates *Salmonella* virulence and survival in macrophages. J Bacteriol 1990; 172:2485–2490.
50. Groisman EA, Parra CA, Salcedo M, Lipps CJ, Heffron F. Resistance to host antimicrobial peptides is necessary for *Salmonella* virulence. Proc Natl Acad Sci (USA) 1992; 89:11939–11943.
51. Butler T, Islam A, Kabir I, Jones PK. Patterns of morbidity and mortality in typhoid fever dependent on age and gender: review of 552 hospitalized patients with diarrhea. Rev Infec Dis 1991; 13:85–90.

52. Hoffman SL, Punjabi NH, Kumala S, Moechtar MA, Pulungish SP, Rivai AR, Rockhill RC, Woodward TE, Loedin AA. Reduction of mortality in chloramphenicol-treated severe typhoid fever by high-dose dexamethasone. New Eng J Med 1984; 310:82–88.
53. Antony TJ, Patwari AK, Anand VK, Pillai PK, Aneja S, Sharma D. Duodenal string test in typhoid fever. Ind Pediat 1993; 30:643–647.
54. Rasaily R, Dutta P, Saha MR, Mitra U, Bhattacharya SK, Manna B, Mukherjee A, Chakravorty S, Pal SC. Value of a single Widal test in the diagnosis of typhoid fever. Ind J Med Res 1993; 97:104–107.
55. Jesudason MV, Srigharan G, Mukundan S, John TJ. Vi-specific latex agglutination for early and rapid detection of *Salmonella* serotype typhi in blood cultures. Diagnost Microbiol Infect Dis 1994; 18:75–78.
56. Mukherjee C, Malik A, Khan HM, Malik A. Rapid diagnosis of typhoid fever by coagglutination in an Indian hospital. J Med Microbiol 1993; 39:74–77.
57. Woodward TE, Smadel JE, Ley HL, Green R, Mankikar DS. Preliminary report on the beneficial effect of chloromycetin in the treatment of typhoid fever. Ann Int Med 1948; 29:131–134.
58. Wallerstein RO, Condit PK, Kasper CK, Brown JW, Morrison FR. Statewide supply of chloramphenicol therapy and fatal aplastic anemia. JAMA 1969; 208:2045–2050.
59. DuPont HL. Quinolones in *Salmonella typhi* infections. Drugs 1993; 45 (Suppl 3):119–124.
60. Tran TH, Bethell DB, Nguyen TT, Wain J, To SD, Le TP, Bui MC, Nguyen MD, Pham TT, Walsh AL, et al. Short course ofloxacin for treatment of multidrug-resistant typhoid. Clin Infect Dis 1995; 20:917–923.
61. Kubin R. Safety and efficacy of ciprofloxacin in paediatric patients -- review. Infection 1993; 21:413–421.
62. Pradhan KM et al. Safety of ciprofloxacin therapy in children: magnetic resonance images, body fluid levels of fluoride and linear growth. Acta Paediatrica 1995; 84:555–560.
63. Schaad UB. Use of quinolones in paediatrics. Drugs 1993; 45 (Suppl 3):37–41.
64. Dutta P, Rasaily R, Saha MR, Mitra U, Mann B, Chakraborty S, Mukherjee A. Randomized clinical trial of furazolidone for typhoid fever in children. Scand J Gastroenterology 1993; 28:168–172.
65. Sethuraman S, Mahamood M, Kareem S. Furazolidone in multi-resistant childhood typhoid fever. Ann Trop Paediat 1994; 14:321–324.
66. Bhutta ZA, Kahn IA, Molla AM. Therapy of multidrug-resistant typhoid fever with oral cefixime vs. intravenous ceftriaxone. Pediat Infect Dis J 1994; 13:990–994.
67. Soe GB, Overturf GD. Treatment of typhoid fever and other systemic salmoneloses with cefotaxime, cefoperazone, and other newer cephalosporins. Rev Inect Dis 1987; 9:719–736.
68. Acharya G, Butler T, Ho M, Sharma PR, Tiwari M, Adhikari RK, Khagda JB, Pokhrel B, Pathak UN. Treatment of typhoid fever: randomized trial of a three-day course of ceftriaxone versus a fourteen day course of chloramphenicol. Am J Trop Med Hyg 1995; 52:162–165.

69. Lewin CS, Nandivada LS, Amyes SG. Multiresistant *Salmonella* and fluoroquinolones. J Antimicrob Chemother 1991; 27:47–49.
70. Threlfall EJ, Ward LR, Rowe B, Raghupathi S, Chandrasekaran V, Vandepitte J, Lemmens P. Widespread occurrence of multiple drug-resistant *Salmonella typhi* in India. Eur J Clin Microbiol Infect Dis 1992; 11:990–993.
71. Bhutta ZA, Naqvi SH, Razzaq RA, Farooqui BJ. Multidrug resistant typhoid in children: presentation and clinical features. Rev Infect Dis 1991; 13:832–836.
72. Oh HM, Chew SK, Monteiro EH. Multidrug resistant typhoid fever in Singapore. Singapore Med J 1994; 35:599–601.
73. Tran TH, Bethell DB, Nguyen TT, Wain J, To SD, Le TP, Bui MC, Nguyen MD, Pham TT, Walsh AL, White NJ. Short course of ofloxacin for treatment of multidrug-resistant typhoid. Clin Infect Dis 1995; 20:917–923.
74. Coovadia YM, Gathiram V, Bhamjee A, Garratt RM, Mlisana K, Pillay N, Madlalose T, Short M. An outbreak of multiresistant *Salmonella typhi* in South Africa. Quart J Med 1992; 82:91–100.
75. Wallace MR, Yousif AA, Mahroos GA, Mapes T, Threlfall EJ, Rowe B, Hyams KC. Ciprofloxacin versus ceftriaxone in the treatment of multiresistant typhoid fever. Eur J Clin Microbiol Infect Dis 1993; 12:907–910.
76. Smith MD, Duong NM, Hoa NT, Wain J, Ha HD, Diep TS, Day NP, Hien TT, White NJ. Comparison of ofloxacin and ceftriaxone for shor-course treatment of enteric fever. Antimicrob Agents Chemother 1994; 38:1716–1720.
77. Lewin CS. Treatment of multiresistant *Salmonella* infection. Lancet 1991; 337:41.
78. Nolan CM, White PCJ. Treatment of chronic typhoid carrier with amoxicillin. JAMA 1978; 239:2352–2354.
79. Brodie J, MacQueen IA. Effect of trimethoprim-sulfamethoxazole on typhoid and *Salmonella* carriers. Br Med J 1970; 3:318–319.
80. Ferrecio C, Morris GJ, Valivieso C. Efficacy of ciprofloxacin in the treatment of chronic typhoid carriers. J Infect Dis 1988; 157:1235–1239.
81. van Basten JP, Stockenbrugger R. Typhoid perforation: A review of the literature since 1960. Trop Geograph Med 2994; 46:336–339.
82. Bitar R, Tarpley J. Intestinal perforation in typhoid fever: a historical and state-of-the-art review. Rev Infect Dis 1985; 7:257–271.
83. Butler T, Knight J, Nath SK, Speelman P, Roy SK, Azad MD. Typhoid fever complicated by intestinal perforation: a persisting fatal disease requiring surgical management. Rev Infect Dis 1985; 7:244–256.
84. Mock C, Visser L, Denno D, Maier R. Aggressive fluid resuscitation and broad spectrum antibiotics decrease mortality from typhoid ileal perforation. Trop Doctor 1995; 25:115–117.
85. Ramos JN, Garcia-Corbeira P, Aguado JM, Arjona R, Ales JM, Soriano F. Clinical significance of primary vs. secondary bacteremia due to nontyphoid *Salmonella* in patients without AIDS. Clin Infect Dis 1994; 19:777–780.
86. Gopinath R, Keystone JS, Kain KC. Concurrent falciparum malaria and salmonella bacteremia in travelers: report of two cases. Clin Infect Dis 1995; 20:706–708.
87. Aserkoff B, Bennett JV. Effect of antibiotic therapy in acute salmonellosis on the fecal excretion of salmonellae. New Eng J Med 1969; 281:636–640.

88. Kazemi M, Gumbert TG, Marks MI. A controlled trial comparing sulfamethoxazole-trimethoprim, ampicillin, and no therapy in the treatment of salmonella gastroenteritis. J Pediat 1973; 83:646–650.
89. Ashkenazi S, Cleary TG. Antibiotic treatment of bacterial gastroenteritis. Pediat Infect Dis J 1991; 10:140–148.
90. Pichler HET, Diridl G, Stickler K, Wolf D. Clinical efficacy of ciprofloxacin compared with placebo in bacterial diarrhea. Am J Med 1987; 82(Suppl 4A):329–332.
91. Sanchez C, Garcia-Restoy E, Garau J, Bella F, Freixas N, Simo M, Lite J, Sanchez P, Espejo E. Cobo E, et al. Ciprofloxacin and trimethoprim-sulfamethoxazole versus placebo in acute uncomplicated *Salmonella* enteritis: a double-bline trial. J Infect Dis 168:1304–1307.
92. Carlstedt G, Dahl P, Niklasson PM, Gullberg K, Banck G. Norfloxacin treatment of salmonellosis does not shorten the carrier state. Scand J Infect Dis 1990; 2:553–556.
93. Neill MA, Opal SM, Heelan J, Giusti R, Cassidy JE. Failure of ciprofloxacin to eradicate convalescent fecal excretion after acute salmonellosis: experience during an outbreak in health care workers. Ann Int Med 1991; 114:195–199.
94. Wistrom J, Jertborn M, Ekwall E, Norlin K, Soderquist B, Stromberg A, Lundholm R, Hogevik H, Lagergren L, Englund G. Empiric treatment of acute diarrheal disease with norfloxacin. A randomized, placebo-controlled study. Ann Int Med 1992; 117:202–208.
95. Funke G, Nemes P, Luthy-Hottenstein J, Altwegg M. Effect of ciprofloxacin therapy in duration of bacterial excretion in acute *Salmonella* gastroenteritis. Schweiz Med Wochenschr 1993; 123:1935–1940.
96. Akalin HE. Quinolones in the treatment of acute bacterial diarrhoeal diseases. Drugs 1993; 45(Suppl 3):114–118.
97. Fang FC, Fierer J. Human infection with *Salmonella dublin*. Medicine 1991; 70:198–207.
98. Gokalp AS, Toksoy HB, Turkay S, Bakici MZ, Kaya R. Intravenous immunoglobulin in the treatment of *Salmonella typhimurium* infections in preterm neonates. Clin Pediat 1994; 33:349–352.
99. Meerkin D, Yinnon AM, Munter RG, Shemesh O, Hiller N, Abraham AS. *Salmonella* mycotic aneurysm of the aortic arch: case report and review. Clin Infect Dis 1995; 21:523–528.
100. Chan P, Tsai CW, Huang JJ, Chuang YC, Hung JS. Salmonellosis and mycotic aneurysm of the aorta. A report of 100 cases. J Infect 1995; 30:129–133.
101. Donabedian H. Long-term suppression of *Salmonella* aortitis with an oral antibiotic. Arch Intern Med 1989; 149:1452–1453.
102. Choo PW, Gantz NM, Anderson C, Maguire JH. *Salmonella* prosthetic valve endocarditis. Diag Microbiol Infect Dis 1992; 15:273–276.
103. Lee YH, Lai LP, Shyu KG, Kuan P, Lien WP. *Salmonella* prosthetic valve endocarditis. Angiol 1994; 45:245–247.
104. Gilks CF, Brindle RJ, Otieno LS, Simani PM, Newnham RS, Bhatt SM, Lule GN, Okelo GB, Watkins WM, Waiyaki PG. Life threatening bacteraemia in HIV-

1 seropositive adults admitted to hospital in Nairobi, Kenya. Lancet 1990; 336:545–549.

105. Nelson MR, Shanson DC, Hawkins DA, Gazzard BG. *Salmonella, Campylobacter* and *Shigella* in HIV-seropositive patients. AIDS 1992; 6:1495–1598.

106. Jacobson MA, Hahn SM, Gerberding JL, Lee B, Sande MA. Ciprofloxacin for salmonella bacteremia in the acquired immunodeficiency syndrome (AIDS). Ann Intern Med 1989; 110:1027–1029.

107. Gouny P, Valverde A, Vincent D, Fadel E, Lenot B, Tricot JF, Rozenbaum W, Nussaume O. Human immunodeficiency virus and infected aneurysm of the abdominal aorta: report of three cases. Ann Vasc Surg 1992; 6:239–243.

108. Buff DD, Patel AD, Neches RB. *Salmonella cholerasuis* bacteremia and endocarditis in a patient with acquired immunodeficiency syndrome. NY State J Med 1993; 93:147–149.

109. Locht H, Kihlstrom E, Lindstrom FD. Reactive arthritis after *Salmonella* among medical doctors - study of an outbreak. J Rheumatol 1993; 20:845–848.

110. Ivanoff B, Levine MM, Lambert PH. Vaccination against typhoid fever: present status. Bull WHO 1994; 72:957–971.

111. Plotkin SA, Bouveret-LeCam N. A new typhoid vaccine composed of the VI capsular polysaccharide. Arch Int Med 1995; 155:2293–2299.

112. Szu SC, Taylor DN, Trofa AC, Clements JD, Shiloach J, Sadoff JC, Bryla DA, Robbins JB. Laboratory and preliminary clinical characterization of Vi capsular polysaccharide-protein conjugate vaccines. Infect Immun 1994; 62:4440–4444.

113. Behrens RH, Roberts JA. Is travel prophylaxis worth while? Economic appraisal of prophylactic measures against malaria, hepatitis A, and typhoid in travelers. Brit Med J 1994; 309:9180–922.

114. Schleifstein J, Coleman MB. An unidentified microorganism resembling *B. ligneri* and *Past. pseudotuberculosis* and pathogenic for man. NY State J Med 1939; 39:1749–1753.

115. Frederiksen W. In: Proceedings of the XIV Scandinavian Congress of Pathology and Microbiology. Universitests Trykningssentral, Oslo, 1964:103–104.

116. Mallasez L, Vignal W. Tuberculox zoologique (forme ou aspect on tuberculose sans bacillus). Arch Physiol Norm Pathol 1883; 53:2.

117. Masshoff W. Eine neuartige form der mesenterialen lymphadenitis. Deutsche Med Wchnschr 1953; 78:532–535.

118. Cornelis G, Laroche Y, Balligand G, Sory MP, Wauters G. Yersinia enterocolitica, a primary model for bacterial invasiveness. Rev Infect Dis 1987; 9:64–87.

119. Cover TL. *Yersinia enterocolitica* and *Yersinia pseudotuberculosis*. In: Blaser MJ, Smith PD, Ravdin JI, Greenberg HB, Guerrant RL. Infections of the Gastrointestinal Tract. New York: Raven Press, 1995:811–823.

120. Hoogkamp-Korstanje JAAA, de Koning J, Samsom JP. Incidence of human infection with *Yersinia enterocolitica* serotypes O3, O8 and O9 and the use of indirect immunofluorescence in diagnosis. J Infect Dis 1986; 153:138–141.

121. Shayegani M, DeForge I, McGlynn DM, Root T. Characteristics of *Yersinia*

enterocolitica and related species isolated from human, animal, and environmental sources. J Clin Microbiol 1981; 14:304–312.
122. Bissett ML. *Yersinia enterocolitica* isolates from humans in California, 1968–1975. J Clin Micro 1976; 4:137–144.
123. Kay BA, Wachsmuth K, Gemski P, Feeley JC, Quan TJ, Brenner DJ. Virulence and phenotypic characterization of *Yersinia enterocolitica* isolated from humans in the United States. J Clin Microbiol 1983; 17:128–138.
124. Tacket CO, Narain JP, Sattin R et al. A multistate outbreak of infections cause by *Yersinia enterocolitica* transmitted by pasteurized milk. JAMA 1984; 251:483–486.
125. Nolan C, Harris N, Ballard J, Allard J, Kobayashi J. Outbreak of *Yersinia enterocolitica* - Washington State. Morbid Mortal Wkly Rept 1982; 41:562–564.
126. Toma S, Deidrick VR. Isolation of *Yersinia enterocolitica* from swine. J Clin Microbiol 1975; 2:478–481.
127. Tauxe RV, Vandepitte J, Wauters G, et al. *Yersinia enterocolitica* infections and pork: the missing link. Lancet 1987; 1:1129–1132.
128. Lee LA, Gerber AR, Lonsway DR, et al. *Yersinia enterocolitica* O:3 infections in infants and children, associated with the household preparation of chitterlings. N Engl J Med 1990; 322:984–987.
129. Greenwood MH, Hooper WL. Excretion of *Yersinia* species associated with consumption of pastuerized milk. Epidemiol Infect 1990; 104:345–350.
130. Hughes D. Repeated isolation of *Yersinia enterocolitica* from pasteurized milk in a holding vat at a dairy factory. J Appl Bacteriol 1980; 48:383–385.
131. Knapp W. Mesenteric adenitis due to *Pasteurella pseudotuberculosis* in young people. N Engl J Med 1958; 259:776–778.
132. Randall KJ, Mair NS. Family outbreak of *Pasteurella pseudotuberculosis* infection. Lancet 1962; 1:1042–1043.
133. Grutzkay A, Hanski C, Hahn H, Riecken EO. Involvement of M cells in the bacterial invasion of Peyer's patches: a common mechanism shared by *Yersinia enterocolitica* and other enteroinvasive bacteria. Gut 1990; 31:1011–1015.
134. Hanski C, Naumann M, Hahn H, Riecken EO. Determinants of invasion and survival of *Yersinia enterocolitica* in intestinal tissue. Med Microbiol Immunol 1989; 178:289–296.
135. Isberg RR, Falkow. A single genetic locus encoded by *Yersinia pseudotuberculosis* permits invasion of cultured animal cells by *Escherichia coli* K-12. Nature (London) 1985; 317:262–264.
136. Miller VL, Falkow S. Evidence for two genetic loci in *Yersinia enterocolitica* that can promote invasion of epithelial cells. Infect Immun 1988; 56:1242–1248.
137. Yang Y, Isberg RR. Cellular internalization in the absence of invasin expression is promoted by the *Yersinia pseudotuberculosis yad A* product. Infect Immun 1993; 61:3907–3931.
138. Isberg RR, Leong JM. Multiple β-1 chain integrins are receptors for invasin, a protein that promotes bacterial penetration into mammalian cells. Cell 1990; 60:861–871.
139. Isberg RR, Swain A, Falkow S. Analysis of expression and thermoregulation of

the *Yersinia pseudotuberculosis inv* gene with hybrid proteins. Infect Immun 1988; 56:2133–2138.

140. Leong JM, Fournier R, Isberg RR. Identification of the integrin binding domain of *Yersinia pseudotuberculosis* invasin protein. EMBO J 1990; 9:1979–1989.
141. Rankin S, Isberg RR, Leong JM. The integrin-binding domain of invasin is sufficient to allow bacterial entry into mammalian cells. Infect Immun 1992; 60:3909–3912.
142. Bliska JB, Compass MC, Falkow S. The *Yersinia pseudotuberculosis* adhesin YadA mediates intimate bacterial attachment to and entry into Hep-2 cells. Infect Immun 1993; 61:3914–3921.
143. Young VB, Falkow S, Schoolnik GK. The invasin protein of *Yersinia enterocolitica*: internalization of invasin-bearing bacteria by eukaryotic cells is associated with reorganization of the cytoskeleton. J Cell Biol 1992; 116:197–207.
144. Rosenshine I, Duronio V, Finlay BB. Tyrosine protein kinase inhibitors block invasin-promoted bacterial uptake by epithelial cells. Infect Immun 1992; 60:2211–2217.
145. Brubaker RR. Factors promoting acute and chronic diseases caused by *Yersiniae*. Clin Microbiol Rev 1991; 4:309–324.
146. Straley SC, Skrzypek E, Plano GV, Bliska JB. Yops of *Yersinia* spp. pathogenic for humans. Infect Immun 1993; 61:3105–3110.
147. Hanski C, Naumann M, Hahn H, Riecken EO. Determinants of invasion and survival of *Yersinia enterocolitica* in intestinal tissue: an in vivo study. Med Microbiol Immuol 1989; 178:289–296.
148. Straley SC, Perry RD. Environmental modulation of gene expression and pathogenesis in *Yersinia*. Trends in Microbiol 1995; 3:310–317.
149. Straley SC, Plano GV, Skrzypek E, Haddix PL, Fields KA. Regulation by Ca^{2+} in the *Yersinia* low Ca^{2+} response. Molec Microbiol 1993; 8:1005–1010.
150. Brubaker RR. The V antigen of yersiniae: an overview. Contrib Microbiol Immunol 1991; 12:127–133.
151. Robins-Browne RM, Still CS, Miliotis MD, Koornhof HJ. Mechanism of action of *Yersinia enterocolitica* enterotoxin. Infect Immun 1979; 25:680–684.
152. Marks MI, Pai CH, Lafleur L, Lackman L, Hammerberg O. *Yersinia enterocolitica* gastroenteritis: a prospective study of clinical, bacteriologic, and epidemiologic features. J Pediat 1980; 96:26–31.
153. Vantrappen G, Geboes K, Ponette E. *Yersinia* enteritis. Med Clin N Am 1982; 66:639–653.
154. Puylaert JBCM, Vermeijden RJ, van der Werf SDJ, Doornbos L, Koumans RKJ. Incidence and sonographic diagnosis of bacterial ileocaecitis masquerading as appendicitis. Lancet 1989; 2:84–86.
155. Rose FB, Camp CJ, Antes EJ. Family outbreak of fatal *Yersinia enterocolotica* pharangitis. Am J Med 1987; 82:636–637.
156. Leirisalo-Repo M, Suoranta H. Ten-year follow-up study of patients with *Yersinia* arthritis. Arthritis Rheum 1988; 31:533–537.
157. Granfors K, Jalkanen S, von Essen R, et al. *Yersinia* antigens in synovial-fluid cells from patients with reactive arthritis. N Engl J Med 1989; 320:216–221.

158. Stuart PM, Woodward JG. *Yersinia enterocolitica* produces superantigenic activity. J Immunol 1992; 148:225–233.
159. Hoogkamp-Korstanje AJ, Stolk-Engelaar VM. *Yersinia enterocolitica* infection in children. Pediatr Infect Dis J 1995; 14:771–775.
160. Gayraud M, Scavizzi MR, Mollaret HH, Guillevin L, Hornstein MJ. Antibiotic treatment of *Yersinia enterocolitica* septicemia: a retrospective review of 43 cases. Clin Infect Dis 1993; 17:405–410.
161. Bouza E, Dominguez A, Meseguer M et al. *Yersinia enterocolitica* septicemia. Am J clin Pathol 1980; 74:404–409.
162. Cherchi GB, Pacifico L, Cossellu S, Gallisai D, Zanetti S, Fadda G, Chiesa C. Prospective study of *Yersinia enterocolitica* infection in thalassemic patients. Pediatr Infect Dis J 1995; 14:579–584.
163. Ardunio MJ, Bland LA, Tipple MA, Aguero SM, Favero MS, Jarvis WR. Growth and endotoxin production of *Yersinia enterocolitica* and *Enterobacter agglomerans* in packed erythrocytes. J Clin Micro 1989; 27:1483–1485.
164. Jensenius M, Hoel T, Heier HE. *Yersinia enterocolitica* septicemia after blood transfusion. Tidsskrift for Den Norske Leageforening 1995; 115:9540–9542.
165. Sato K, Ouchi K, Taki M. *Yersinia pseudotuberculosis* infection in children, resembling Izumi fever and Kawasaki syndrome. Pediatr Infect Dis 1983; 2:123–126.
166. Weissfeld AS, Sonnenwirth AC. Rapid isolation of *Yersinia* spp. from feces. J Clin Microbiol 1982; 15:508–510.
167. Cafferkey MT, Buckley TF. Comparison of saline agglutination, antibody to human gammaglobulin, and immunofluorescence tests. I the routine serological diagnosis of yersiniosis. J Infect Dis 1987; 156:845–848.
168. Maki-Ikola O Heesemann J, Lahesmaa R, Toivanen A Granfors K. Combined use of released protein and lipoplysaccharide in enzyme-linked immunosorbent assay for serologic screening of *Yersinia enterocolitica* infections. J Infect Dis 1991; 163:409–412.
169. Johnson RH. Yersinia. In: Schlossberg D, ed. Current Therapy of Infectious Disease. St. Louis: Mosby, 1996:480–481.
170. Boyce JM. *Yersinia* species. In: Mandell GL, Douglas RG, Bennett JE, eds. Principles and Practice of Infectious Diseases. Chichester: Wiley Medical, 1986:1296–1301.

7

Small and Large Bowel Infections in AIDS

MICHAEL S. KARASIK and NEZAM H. AFDHAL
Boston University School of Medicine, Boston, Massachusetts

I. INTRODUCTION

Human immunodeficiency virus (HIV) infects a wide variety of organ systems and cell types (1). Mononuclear cells of the immune system appear to be the primary target (2–5). Immunosuppression resulting from their destruction and dysfunction is ultimately responsible for the majority of the morbidity and mortality of AIDS. Persons with AIDS characteristically demonstrate reduced numbers of T helper and T suppressor cells. However, T-helper cells (CD4+) appear to be the most affected (6–8), resulting in a reversal of the normal T-helper/T-suppressor cell ratio (9,10). Peripheral blood CD4 counts correlate well with the development of various opportunistic infections and have served as reliable markers to gauge the degree of immune suppression (10–13). Other mononuclear cell abnormalities demonstrated in patients with AIDS include abnormal B-cell activation and regulation (3), altered Langerhan cell activity (4), and impaired cytokine production (5). Although immunosuppression in AIDS results in the development of opportunistic infections in all organ systems, the gastrointestinal tract appears to be particularly susceptible. Altered intestinal mucosal immunity, impaired gastric acid secretion, intestinal dysmotility, and nutritional deficiencies are likely to be responsible for this particular predilection.

As the interface between environmental pathogens and potential human hosts, the gastrointestinal tract has developed a number of protective mechanisms that are often lost in persons with advanced HIV infection. Of these, intestinal mucosal immunity is the most important. Patients with AIDS have greatly reduced cell-mediated and humoral immune processes. Alterations of T-helper and T-suppresser cell counts within the lamina propria are similar to those occurring in peripheral blood (14–16). Decreased numbers of secretory IgA-producing plasma cells in the lamina propria and reduced secretion of soluble IgA also occur (17). Nutritional deficiencies, even less well understood, are extremely common in AIDS patients with diarrhea and have been associated with inhibition of mucosal defenses (18,19). Nonimmune intestinal clearance mechanisms are also impaired in persons with AIDS. Gastric acid, which inhibits bacterial colonization (20–23), is commonly reduced in persons with AIDS (24–26). Achlorhydria in AIDS has correlated highly with the development of opportunistic infections, independent of CD4 cell count (26). This appears to be particularly true for *Mycobacterium-avium* complex infections. AIDS autonomic neuropathy (27) and intestinal dysmotility may also enhance access to intestinal pathogens that would normally be cleared in the fecal stream.

Epidemiologic statistics corroborate the predilection and significance of intestinal infections in AIDS. It is estimated that 20 million people have been infected by HIV and that at least 4.5 million cases of AIDS have occurred worldwide (28). Clinically significant gastrointestinal disease occurs in 50–90% of infected patients (29) and presents as diarrhea in 60–90% of persons with AIDS (30–33). The immunosuppression associated with HIV predisposes to both common and opportunistic intestinal pathogens. The risk of each, however, may vary with individual risk factors, i.e., degree of immunosuppression, geographic location, and sexual practices, as well as the extent of investigation. Further, up to 30% of patients with AIDS and diarrhea will have multiple concomitant pathogens (34–36).

This chapter is not intended to review all of the potential small- and large bowel infections that may occur in persons with HIV infection. Rather, it will highlight those enteric infections that are particularly important either because they are unique to persons with AIDS, or because their epidemiology or clinical course is significantly altered by HIV immunosuppression. The management of AIDS-related chronic diarrhea will also be discussed in detail with emphasis on cost-benefit consideration. An individualized algorithmic approach, based upon the clinical features of each person's illness, is provided.

II. BACTERIAL INFECTIONS OF THE SMALL AND LARGE BOWEL

Persons with HIV infection are susceptible to the same range of enteric bacterial pathogens as HIV-seronegative individuals. The clinical course of several of these pathogens, namely *Salmonella, Shigella, Campylobacter*, and *C. difficile*, however, is altered in HIV-seropositive hosts.

A. *Salmonella* sp.

The incidence of Salmonellosis appears to be approximately 20 times increased in persons with AIDS and bacteremia is up to 5 times more common in this population (37). Bacteremia may appear without diarrhea in up to 20% of cases (38) and stool cultures may be negative despite diarrhea (39–41). Fever is common with bacteremia, enteritis, or colitis. Approximately 50% of *Salmonella* species are resistant to ampicillin (42). Following treatment, recurrence rates as high as 50% have been reported, particularly in persons with AIDS (43) and in persons initially presenting with septicemia (38). The risk of recurrence appears to be reduced by use of TMP-SMX, ciprofloxacin, or AZT (44,45).

B. *Shigella* sp.

Shigellosis does not appear to be more common in patients with HIV; however, the incidence of bacteremia does appear to be increased in seropositive individuals (43). Persistent infection and antibiotic insensitivity may also be seen in patients with AIDS (46), as compared to the typical self-limited and antibiotic-sensitive infections usually occurring in HIV-seronegative individuals. The typical presentation of acute colitis and fever is seen in approximately 50% of the cases.

C. *Campylobacter jejuni*

In Los Angeles county, the incidence of *Campylobacter* infection was reported to be up to 39 times increased in persons with AIDS (47). Although uncommon, bacteremia is also more frequently seen in persons with AIDS. Normally a self-limited illness in immunocompetent patients, *Campylobacter* infection may result in chronic diarrhea in patients with AIDS (48,49). Persistence has been associated with the development of antibiotic resistance. Affected individuals may present with colitis or ileitis. Mucosal biopsy cultures may detect cases of *Campylobacter* not found in routine stool cultures (50).

D. *Clostridium difficile*

Although HIV infection does not appear to be an independent risk factor for *Clostridium difficile* infection, persons with advanced HIV infection are clearly predisposed by frequent antibiotic usage and greater numbers of hospitalizations (51,52). Although we have not noticed any significant difference in the character of *C. difficile* infections in our HIV-seropositive patients, Bartlett has suggested that the severity may be increased and the response to treatment reduced in this group (52).

III. MYCOBACTERIAL INFECTIONS OF THE SMALL AND LARGE BOWEL

A. Overview

Although the incidence of active tuberculosis has risen exponentially with the AIDS epidemic, gastrointestinal disease is still extremely uncommon. The opposite is true for atypical mycobacterial infections, however. Prior to AIDS, *Mycobacterium-avium* complex (MAC) infections were rare and primarily responsible for pulmonary disease. Neither gastrointestinal nor disseminated infections were described. In the past decade MAC has become the most common mycobacterial infection and one of the most common opportunistic infections overall in persons with AIDS. In contrast to infection by M. tuberculosis, which is often latent, MAC infections are usually acute (53), presenting as disseminated disease in patients with significant HIV-associated immunosuppression. The CD4 counts are generally less than 50 cells/mm^3. In addition to constitutional symptoms of fever, night sweats, anorexia, and malaise, most of the manifestations of MAC infection are gastrointestinal in nature. Diarrhea, hepatosplenomegaly, cholestatic hepatitis, abdominal pain (often secondary to mediastinal lymphadenopathy), and wasting are common. Although multidrug antituberculosis regimens are often successful for the treatment of tuberculosis in persons with HIV, they have had only limited success for the treatment of MAC. Clarithromycin, however, is a new agent that is demonstrating considerable in vivo activity as a single agent for MAC. The determination of optimal dosage for this agent, particularly in combination with other active agents, offers an opportunity to improve survival and quality of life in infected patients. Prophylaxis against MAC is also becoming feasable.

B. *Mycobacterium-avium* Complex

1. Epidemiology

Mycobacterium avium and *Mycobacterium intracellulare*, two species of pathogenic atypical mycobacterium found throughout the environment, cannot be differentiated biochemically or morphologically and have been referred to, collectively, as *Mycobacterium-avium–intracellulare* (MAI) or *Mycobacterium-avium* complex (MAC). The mycobacterium MAC is ubiquitous. Cultured from soil (54), dust (55), and fresh water (56), it is estimated to contaminate 30–40% of drinking water reservoirs in the United States (57). Recently, however, an epidemiologic study of MAC infection in San Francisco suggested that the soil may be a more important reservoir of infection (58). Although MAC is also responsible for infections in poultry and swine, animal–human and human–human transmissions do not occur. The gastrointestinal and respiratory tracts are presumed to be the primary routes of acquisition from the environment.

The epidemiology of MAC infection has changed considerably since the beginning of the AIDS epidemic. Prior to AIDS, MAC infection was uncommon, usually occurring in patients with chronic obstructive pulmonary disease who were residing in the rural southeast United States (59). *M. intracellulare* accounted for almost half of these infections and disseminated disease was exceedingly rare. In contrast, *M. avium* accounts for over 95% of MAC infections occurring in persons with AIDS (60) and no geographic variations have been noted. Localized disease is now uncommon; dissemination and gastrointestinal involvement have become the rule. The GI tract is both a major route of acquisition of MAC, following ingestion of contaminated water or foodstuffs (61,62), and is likely also a main site of origin prior to dissemination (63).

Mycobacterium-avium complex infection invariably occurs late in the course of HIV disease (64). Most patients with disseminated MAC have already had an opportunistic infection and have CD4 cell counts less than 50/mm^3. In a prospective study of 1006 HIV-seropositive patients from Parkland Memorial Hospital, Dallas, the annual incidence of disseminated MAC was 39% in persons with CD4 cell counts of less than 10/mm^3 as compared to 15% in those with counts of 40–59/mm^3, and 3% in those with counts of 100–199/m^3. Overall, 20% of the patients developed disseminated MAC infection annually. Autopsy studies, by contrast, now demonstrate disseminated MAC in as many as 30–50% of AIDS patients at the time of death (65,66). It is expected that the incidence of MAC will continue to rise as the duration of survival of patients with advanced HIV-immunosuppression continues to improve (67,68).

2. *Clinical Presentation*

Mycobacterium-avium complex usually presents as disseminated disease in persons with AIDS and any organ can be involved (59,69). The diagnosis is often made post-mortem. The most characteristic signs and symptoms are nonspecific and include fever (87%), night sweats (78%), diarrhea (47%), weight loss greater than 20 pounds (38%), and abdominal pain (35%), and nausea/vomiting (26%) (70). The diarrhea associated with MAC is variable in volume and frequency depending upon the site and extent of GI tract involvement. Intra-abdominal lymphadenopathy is seen in approximately 40% and may be associated with severe abdominal pain. Hepatosplenomegaly is present in approximately 25%. Eighty-five percent of patients are severely anemic (hematocrit < 25%) and hepatic cholestasis is seen in over 50% (71). In our experience, persistent high levels of alkaline phosphatase and gamma-glutamyl transpeptidase (10–20 times elevated) are highly suggestive of liver involvement by

MAC. Other causes in persons with AIDS include HIV cholangiopathy and extra-hepatic biliary obstruction, as from choledocholithiasis or neoplasia.

3. *Diagnosis*

The diagnosis of disseminated MAC is made by its identification in one or more tissue sites, the most common being blood, but biopsy of bone marrow, liver or lymph nodes may be required. Blood cultures are the most sensitive test (72) and once positive, over 97% of subsequent blood cultures remain positive in untreated patients.

The value of stool studies for MAC-related disease is less clear. Prospective studies comparing screening blood cultures, stool cultures, and smears have demonstrated negative stool studies in 60–80% of patients who develop bacteremia (73,74). And although intestinal involvement by disseminated MAC is usually associated with bacteremia, bowel colonization without dissemination probably occurs as well. High numbers of MAC have been seen in the GI tract of AIDS patients with negative blood cultures up to 8 months prior to evidence of dissemination (73,74). Further, MAC has been identified in the stools of up to 10–22% of HIV seronegative individuals and 1.3–12% of HIV infected non-AIDS patients (75,76). Therefore, the finding of MAC by stool culture or smear should not be used to diagnose disseminated MAC. It should be noted, in addition, that stool smears appear to be inferior to fecal cultures for the detection of MAC. In one large multicenter study, 393 of 2176 stool specimens were positive for MAC by stool culture. The use of AFB smears alone identified only 16 additional cases and failed to identify 50% of those positive by stool culture (77,78). The sensitivity of AFB smears in this study was 34% and its specificity 99%. Unfortunately this study did not concomitantly evaluate patients for bacteremia.

Mycobacterium-avium complex may be identified in either the small or large intestine endoscopically, although there is no specific appearance. A "frosted" duodenal mucosa with diffuse 1–3 mm white plaques (Figure 1a) has been most commonly associated with MAC (79), however, the duodenum may appear granular or normal. Biopsy specimens reveal sheets of mycobacteria with foamy macrophages (Figure 1b) and may demonstrate poorly formed granulomas. Similar histology may be seen in the colon although we are unaware of any characteristic colonoscopic findings.

4. *Therapy*

Mycobacterium-avium complex has significant resistance to antimicrobial therapy. Experience, however, has demonstrated clinical responses (reduced fever and night sweats) in association with reduced levels of bacteremia. Although these factors, rather than alterations in mortality rates, have generally been used as markers of successful treatment, it is expected that clearance of bacteremia

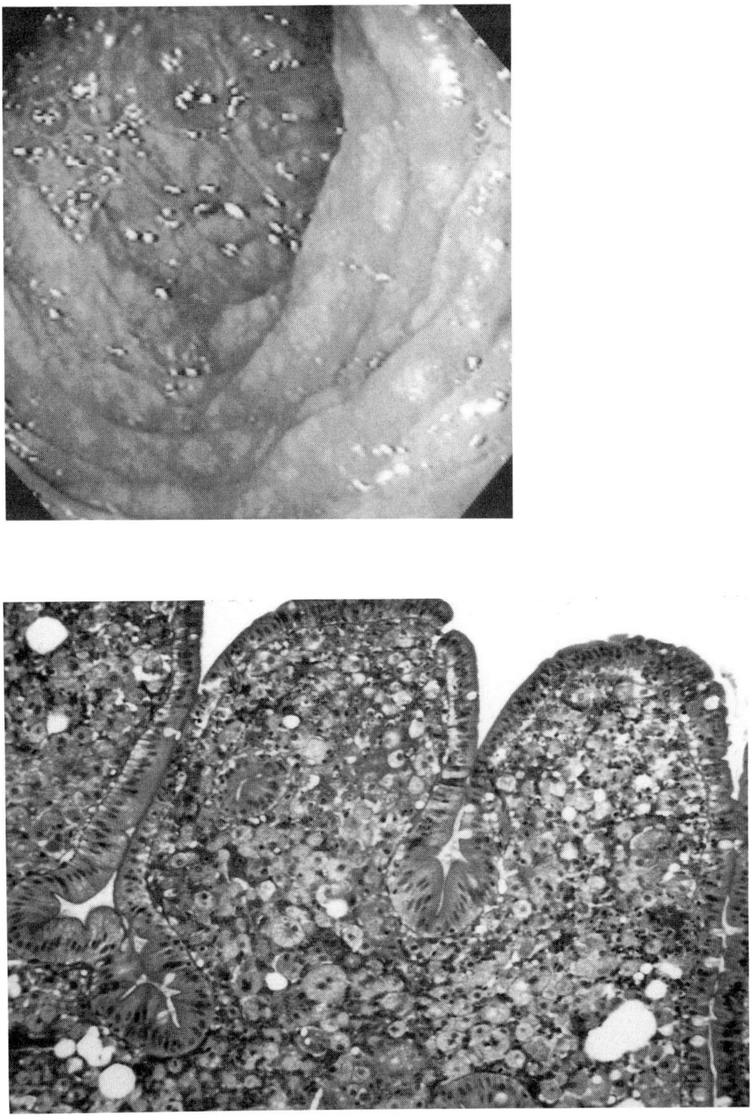

(A)

(B)

Figure 1 A "frosted" duodenal mucosa, although nonspecific, should raise suspicion for MAC infection (A). These small white/yellow duodenal plaques represent dense infiltrates of foamy macrophages (arrow, B). PAS and AFB staining usually reveals numerous rod-like bacilli within cytoplasm and stroma. (Courtesy of Dr. Sigfus Nikulasson, Mallory Institute of Pathology, Boston University School of Medicine.)

would result in improved survival just as disseminated disease has been associated with reduced survival (69,80–82). Although placebo-controlled trials are lacking to test this hypothesis, a prospective observational study (83) and retrospective analyses (70,83) have demonstrated improved survival with treatment. The development of antibiotic resistance, bacteremia recurrences, and drug-related toxicities (primarily gastrointestinal) remain as significant problems.

Several factors are presumed to contribute to *Mycobacterium-avium* complex resistance in patients with AIDS. The organisms is shielded from high levels of antibiotic by both its intracellular growth and an outer polysaccharide wall (85). Of MAC species, *M. avium* is more common than *M. intracellulare* in persons with AIDS and is the more resistant of the two species (60). Additionally, MAC infections may be polyclonal, composed of multiple, genetically diverse strains with differing sensitivities (86,87). Further, as compared to patients with *M. tuberculosis* infections and AIDS, the immunosuppression associated with disseminated MAC is generally far more advanced (64,88). These factors, in addition to providing antimicrobial resistance, also greatly increase the risk of developing resistant mycobacterial strains following treatment and support the use of multiagent therapy, as is recommended for *M. tuberculosis* (89).

Initial therapeutic offers, based upon in vitro data, were primarily centered on available antituberculous agents. As compared to *M. tuberculosis*, however, MAC is 10 to 100 times less sensitive to first-line antituberculosis agents (59). Of these, only ethambutol has demonstrated significant in vitro activity (90). Rifabutin is more effective than the related, less-lipophilic rifampin (91–93). Second-line antituberculous regimens may be slightly better but are significantly more toxic. Clofazamine, a leprosy drug, has also demonstrated modest activity against MAC but may require up to several months to achieve inhibitory serum and tissue concentrations (94).

Fluoroquinolone, macrolide, and aminoglycoside antibiotics have also been evaluated for treatment of MAC. Although ciprofloxacin has activity against many atypical mycobacterium, less than 50% of MAC isolates appear to be susceptible at doses commonly used in vivo (90). The macrolide antibiotics clarithromycin and azithromycin, in contrast, have demonstrated excellent activity against MAC, possibly because of improved intracellular penetration (95). Unfortunately, animal models have demonstrated the development of MAC resistance when so treated. In one in vitro system, however, the coadministration of amikacin was able to prevent the development of resistance to clarithromycin (96).

In clinical trials, regimens composed of ethambutol/rifampin/ciprofloxacin with or without amikacin or clofazamine (97–99) have generally demonstrated significant reductions in bacterial colony counts (blood) and improved or resolved MAC symptomatology for at least the duration of therapy in patients with AIDS and disseminated MAC. Bacterial clearance has been less common. Further, drug toxicities (primarily gastrointestinal) have resulted in withdrawal of approximately 40% of the patients in these studies (100). In another trial, the addition of clarithromycin to ciprofloxacin, with reduced dosing of amikacin, was associated with enhanced efficacy against MAC and a reduction in the incidence and severity of related toxicities (101). Unfortunately, the multiagent design of these studies have complicated assessment of either the importance or toxicity of any of the individual agents.

Single-agent studies have primarily focused on the use of clarithromycin. In a study by Dantzenberg et al., clarithromycin treatment (500–2000 mg/d) was associated with dose-dependent clearance of MAC bacteremia in 60–98% of patients by 6–12 weeks and significantly reduced colony counts, fever, and night sweats in the majority of patients remaining bacteremic (102). A similar dose-dependent benefit was also seen by Gupta et al. (103) and by Chaisson and the ACTG Protocol 157 study team (104). In this latter study, dosing of 2 gm *bid* was associated with a more rapid reduction in blood colony counts than doses of 500 mg *bid* or 1 gm *bid*; however, no difference in the percent of MAC-free blood cultures was seen between the 3 doses of clarithromycin at 12 weeks. Survival was best in those patients receiving 500 mg *bid* and was not associated with the initial level of bacteremia, time from first positive blood culture to enrollment, or CD4 cell count.

Despite these dramatic effects, recurrences following discontinuation of clarithromycin therapy have been reported in approximately 25% of patients and have been associated with the development of clarithromycin resistance (102). This has been more likely in patients who had had an interruption of drug administration for 7 or more days, usually as a result of drug toxicity. The development of clarithromycin resistance has also been associated with higher initial colony counts but not to drug dosing (100). Patients receiving the highest doses in that study, however, were more likely to discontinue therapy than patients receiving either lower dose. The most common toxicities were gastrointestinal in nature and were dose limiting in up to 20%.

Clinical experience with other agents in monotherapy has been limited. Azithromycin, another macrolide antibiotic, has demonstrated significant reductions in bacterial burden, albeit less impressively than with clarithromycin (104). Another study evaluated independent therapy with ethambutol (15 mg/kg/d), clofazimine (200 mg/d), and rifampin (600 mg/d). Of these, only ethambutol resulted in a significant reduction in mycobacteremia (105).

Although responses to clarithromycin as part of multiagent therapy have thus far not been superior to clarithromycin monotherapy, multidrug regimens would seem to be necessary, at least to prevent the development of resistance by

MAC. However, the most efficacious regimen with the least toxicity has yet to be defined. With the notable exception of clarithromycin, and probably azithromycin, the in vitro activity of anti-MAC agents has not translated into clinical efficacy. Additional studies should determine the optimum dosing of clarithromycin, particularly when used in conjunction with other agents, as well as the required duration of therapy and duration of effect. The most recent recommendations from The Task Force on Prophylaxis and Therapy for *Mycobacterium-avium* Complex (1993) are to use at least two agents and one should be either clarithromycin or azithromycin (89). Ethambutol is usually included as a second agent (70). Third and fourth agents are usually chosen from among clofazimine, rifabutin, rifampin, ciprofloxacin, and amikacin (Table 1). Further, the task force also recommended life-long therapy for patients responding to therapy, as established by clearance of blood or by clinical parameters.

5. *MAC Prophylaxis*

Two trials have established rifabutin for prophylaxis against MAC in patients with AIDS. In each, rifabutin administration (300 mg/day) resulted in a 50% reduction in the incidence of MAC bacteremia as compared to placebo (106). No survival advantage was seen, however. Prophylaxis with clarithromycin (500 mg *bid*), in contrast was associated with a 60% reduction in the incidence of bacteremia and a small but significant reduction in mortality, as compared to

Table 1 Antibiotic Therapy for AIDS Diarrhea

Bacteria	
Salmonella sp.	Ceftriaxone, azithromycin, amoxicillin, TMP-SMX
Campylobacter jejuni	Ciprofloxacin, erythromycin
Shigella sp.	Ciprofloxacin, TMP-SMX, ampicillin
Clostridium difficile	Metronidazole, vancomycin
Aeromonas sp.	Ciprofloxacin, TMP-SMX
Plesiomonas shigelloides	Ciprofloxacin, TMP-SMX
Mycobacteria	
M. avium complex (MAC)	Clarithromycin and ethambutol +/- rifabutin, amikacin, clofazamine
Protozoa	
Cyclospora	TMP-SMX
Entameba histolytica	Metronidazole, tinidazole, iodoquinol
Giardia lamblia	Metronidazole
Isospora belli	TMP-SMX, pyrimethamine and folinic acid
Viruses	
Cytomegalovirus	Gancyclovir, foscarnet
Herpes simplex virus	Acyclovir, foscarnet

placebo (107). Results from a prophylaxis trial using combination therapy (ACTG 196) are pending. It is unclear if the effects of each will be additive, however, as the use of rifabutin has been associated with enhanced hepatic metabolism of clarithromycin.

Given the poor prognosis associated with MAC infection and the growing at-risk population, prophylaxis is clearly desirable. In addition to efficacy, however, a number of other potential problems must be overcome. Drug interactions can complicate therapy with rifabutin. The concomitant use of fluconazole has been associated with enhanced levels of rifabutin and is likely responsible for the high incidence (38%) of uveitis seen in patients with disseminated MAC treated with > 300 mg/day of rifabutin in the Canadian HIV Trials Network Study (108,109). As evidence against the use of clarithromycin, a retrospective review of prophylaxis in practice found 22% of breakthrough isolates to be resistant to clarithromycin as compared to 0% with rifabutin (110).

At the present time, recommendations from the U.S. Public Health Service and the Infectious Disease Society of America are for consideration of prophylaxis with rifabutin 300 mg/day for persons with AIDS and CD4 counts less than 75 cells/mm^3 (111). Clarithromycin 500 mg *bid* and azithromycin 500 mg *tiw* are recommended as alternatives.

IV. PROTOZOAN INFECTIONS OF THE SMALL AND LARGE BOWEL

Giardia lamblia, Entameba histolytica, and *Blastocytis hominis* do not appear to behave differently in patients with HIV infection (112) and will not be discussed here.

A. *Cyclospora* sp.

1. *Epidemiology*

Cyclospora species have only recently been recognized as enteric pathogens in humans. Endemic in developing countries, infection has primarily been documented in immunocompetent travelers to Nepal, Morocco, Pakistan, India, Mexico, and Peru (113–118). Additionally, although not identified directly by name, an organism of very similar appearance has been described in the feces of persons with chronic diarrhea in other areas of North, Central, and South America; Southeast Asia; Eastern Europe; and Carribean islands. Although rare within the United States, an outbreak has recently been reported in house-staff physicians at a Chicago medical center (114,119). This and other reports suggest that the infection is spread by ingestion of contaminated water (119,120). Although it would seem that the risk of *Cyclospora* infection is primarily a result of geographical location, there is evidence of substantially increased risk to persons immunocompromised by HIV (117,121,122). In one large cohort study of persons with chronic diarrhea in Haiti, the prevalence of *Cyclospora* was 11% in association with HIV infection and diarrhea, as compared to 0% in HIV seronegative patients with diarrhea, and 2% in patients without HIV infection and without diarrhea (122). Behaving as an opportunistic pathogen, over 90% of HIV seropositive patients infected by *Cyclospora* either had AIDS or developed AIDS within the ensuing several months. Despite this, however, it should be noted that *Cyclospora* infection is an extremely rare cause of illness in the patients seen at our AIDS center, even in those recently immigrated from Haiti and other developing countries. While a relatively uncontaminated environment and potential underreporting by less familiar investigators may contribute to this relative obscurity, the frequent administration of trimethoprim-sulfamethoxazole as prophylaxis against *Pneumocystis carinii* may also be an important factor.

2. *Clinical Syndrome*

Cyclospora infections are believed to be symptomatic in 11–28% of immunocompetent persons (118). The most common symptoms are those of diarrhea and abdominal cramping (117–119,123,124). The diarrhea may be severe, intermittent, and explosive, and periods of remission and relapse characteristically occur. A flu-like syndrome is also common. Muscle aches, anorexia, fever, nausea, and weight loss occur in approximately 50%. Chills, headache, vomiting, and constipation (during remissions) are described in 20–40%. Although *Cyclospora* infection results in a prolonged but self-limited illness of 1–6 weeks duration in immunocompetent individuals (116,119), chronic diarrhea and abdominal cramps of at least 4 months duration have been described in patients with AIDS (121,122).

3. *Diagnosis*

Cyclospora infection may be underreported due to difficulties in identifying this pathogen. The most sensitive assay appears to be kinyoun-modified acid-fast staining; however, fecal cyst staining is variable (117,125). As compared to this technique, however, wet mount preparations are only 75% sensitive and auramine/rhodamine or safranin staining is only 25–30% sensitive (122).

Cyclospora species have previously been referred to as cyanobacteria, or blue-green algae-like bodies, largely because of the characteristic ultraviolet fluorescence of its fecal cysts (117,119). They have been confused with cryptosporidia because of similarities in oocyte appearance and of the syndromes associated with their infection (118). *Cyclospora* oocytes, however, are approximately 8–9 μm in diameter, significantly larger than those of *Cryptosporidium parvum* and smaller than those of *Isospora belli*. Developmental observations have placed them within the coccidian genus *Cyclospora* (118) and the name *Cyclospora cayetanensis* has been proposed (126).

4. *Treatment*

Cyclospora is highly responsive to treatment with cral trimethoprim 160 mg–sulfamethoxazole 800 mg (TMP-SMX) in patients with or without AIDS (122,127). Of 43 AIDS patients with symptomatic infection who were treated with a 10-day course of TMP-SMX, four times daily, 100% had resolution of diarrhea and abdominal pain within 5 days (mean, 2.5 days) with clearance of the protozoan from the stool. Unfortunately, almost half (44%) of these developed a recurrence of their symptoms and *Cyclospora* in their stool within the following 3 days. Retreatment with trimethoprim-sulfamethoxazole, however, resulted in resolution of symptoms within 2 days. Following the second successful course of therapy, 12 patients were then followed for 7 months while taking a three-times-weekly prophylactic course of TMP-SMX. A second recurrence was seen in only 1 of these patients.

B. Cryptosporidia

Cryptosporidium is a eucoccidian protozoan that has recently been described as an enteric pathogen in both immunocompetent and immunocompromised individuals (128). Initially this organism was thought to cause disease only in animals but since 1980 has been associated with disease in humans (Table 2). The major difference between *Cryptosporidium* infection in normal hosts and the immunocompromised is that the disease is self-limited in the former whereas it is persistent and extremely debilitating in the latter.

1. *Epidemiology and Microbiology*

At least 17 species of *Cryptosporidium* have been described but only *parvum* and *muris* appear pathogenic in humans (129). *Cryptosporidium* is the commonest protozoan pathogen described in AIDS diarrhea and is seen in 16% of homosexual men, with and without AIDS (130–132). In the United States the prevalence in patients with AIDS is between 10 and 20% whereas it is much

Table 2 High-Risk Categories for *Cryptosporidium* Infection

Immunocompetent	Immunocompromised
Sporadic cases	Congenital immunodeficiency
Animal handlers	Immunosuppressive therapy
Homosexual men	AIDS
Traveler's diarrhea	
Hospital personnel	
Children in daycare	
Household contacts	
Water-borne epidemics	

higher and approaches 55% in developing countries (133–136). Although rarely a direct cause of death in AIDS patients, severe wasting, malnutrition, and general debilitation from this infection make it an important cause of severe morbidity. The cryptosporidial oocyst contains four naked sporozoites, is very small (2–5 μm in diameter) and resistant to most laboratory disinfectants, cold, and heat (137,138). This resistance of the oocysts makes it highly infectious when present in stool and increases risk of transmission to laboratory workers. The oocysts sporulate and excyst to release 4 thin, flat sporozoites, which are the infective form of the organism (139). *Cryptosporidium* has a monoxenous life cycle and is able to complete this cycle within a single host. The clinical importance of these unique developmental characteristics is that the organism has a tremendous potential for reinfecting the host. In AIDS patients this is reflected by chronic infection and persistent shedding of oocysts in the stool.

Worldwide, *Cryptosporidium* is a common cause of diarrhea, infecting as many as 10% of children in developing nations (140–142). *Cryptosporidium* is spread in a variety of different modes (143–145). Animal-to-human (zoonoses), human-to-human, and water-borne outbreaks have all been well documented. Epidemic transmission among schoolchildren and nosocomial spread in hospitals have been reported as well as several large water-borne outbreaks in San Antonio and Milwaukee (146–148). Therefore, *Cryptosporidium* should be considered a highly infectious and easily spread organism even in immunocompetent hosts.

2. *Pathology and Pathophysiology*

In AIDS patients *Cryptosporidium* has been found from the pharynx to the rectum as well as in the liver and biliary tract (149–156). The relationship of *Cryptosporidium* to the intestinal epithelium of the infected host has unique pathological features (1,157,158). *Cryptosporidium* does not invade the epithelial cell but is located adherent to the enterocyte surface, often enclosed in a membrane which may be derived from the cell. The enterocytes themselves appear intact but there can be associated villous blunting with crypt elongation and hyperplasia (Figure 2). An inflammatory cellular infiltrate is usually absent although increased numbers of intraepithelial cell lymphocytes have been described. The exact mechanism by which *Cryptosporidium* causes diarrhea is unknown. Clinically the diarrhea may present as malabsorption and these patients often have the above histological findings on small bowel biopsy. Many patients however have little epithelial cell injury but profound diarrhea that more closely resembles that seen with secretory diarrheas. An unidentified enterotoxin has been proposed as an explanation for the secretory nature of the diarrhea. *Cryptosporidium* has been identified adjacent and within M cells and can present antigens for processing to the gut-associated lymphoid tissue (158). Antibody responses with both IgM and IgG antibodies to *Cryptosporidium* have been

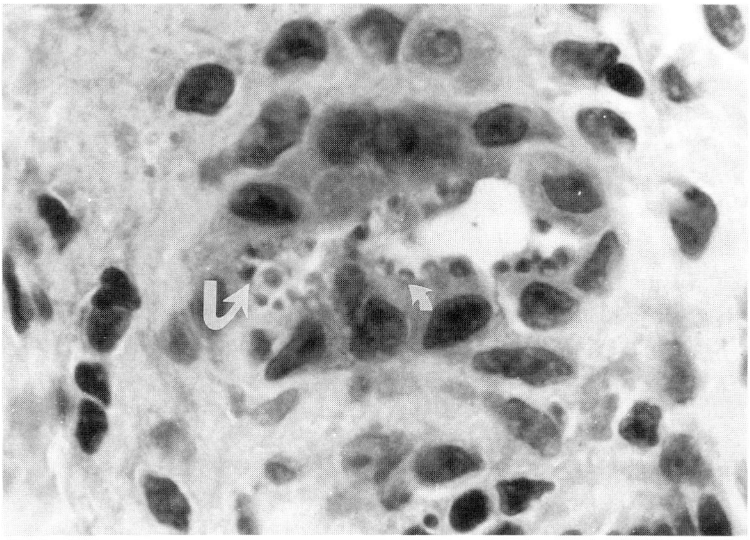

(A)

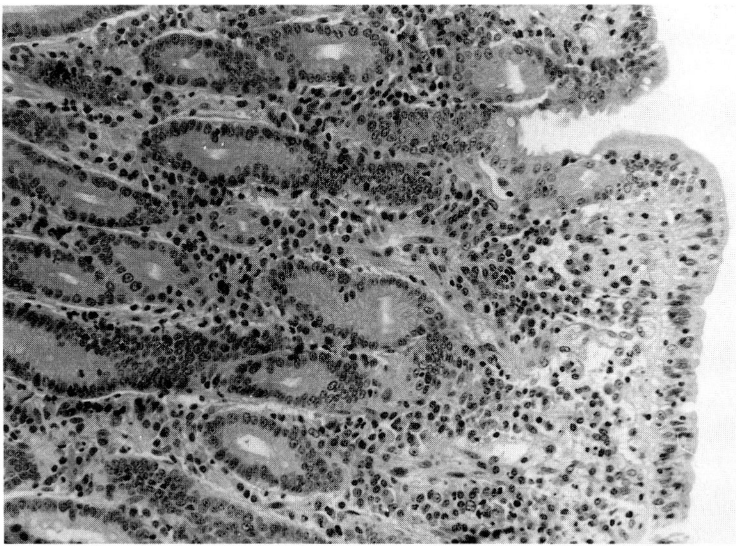

(B)

Figure 2 (A) Cryptosporidia visualized within a small intestinal crypt. (B) Same patient demonstrating nonspecific villous shortening, crypt hyperplasia, and lymphocytic infiltration within the epithelium. (Courtesy of Dr. Sigfus Nikulasson, Mallory Institute of Pathology, Boston University School of Medicine.)

identified serologically in immunocompetent and immunocompromised patients (159–161). These antibodies do not appear to be protective, particularly in the immunocompromised, but are useful for seroepidemiological study of this infection. Since chronic *Cryptosporidium* infection is also seen in patients with humoral immune deficiency, T-cell function is probably important for the eradication of infection and may explain why the disease is chronic in HIV-infected patients.

3. *Clinical Manifestations*

In humans the severity of cryptosporidial infection appears to be related to immune status. In the immunocompetent host, the disease is characterized by a 2–14 day incubation period followed by abdominal cramps, diarrhea, anorexia, nausea, and weight loss. Symptoms last for up to 14 days but oocysts can be shed in the stool for a further 2–3 weeks, and even without therapy the illness is self-limited. In AIDS patients, a severe diarrheal illness is usual and characterized by frequent (5–25), voluminous (1–25 liters) watery bowel movements. There is associated crampy abdominal pain, steatorrhea, and weight loss. Severe abdominal pain, fever, and bleeding are not seen and suggest other etiologies. We have observed protracted nausea and vomiting in some patients, which is often associated with colonization of the stomach by *Cryptosporidium*. Dehydration is common and requires intensive intravenous fluid replacement. *Cryptosporidium* can readily colonize both the gallbladder and the biliary tree where it can cause both cholecystitis or cholangitis (see Hepatic Infections). More commonly the gallbladder appears to act as a reservoir for the parasite from which recurrent infections can occur. In our opinion, once a patient has been diagnosed with *Cryptosporidium* infection, loss of the organism is rare even though the clinical symptoms may be temporarily controlled. Even though *Cryptosporidium* is rarely the immediate cause of death at our hospital, the median life expectancy after the diagnosis of infection is approximately 6 months.

4. *Diagnosis*

Cryptosporidium should be suspected in all AIDS patients with severe small-bowel type diarrhea, particularly those from developing nations and gay men. Diagnosis is confirmed by finding oocytes in fresh stool samples. Three separate stool specimens are recommended and special stains for *Cryptosporidium* should be requested. These stains include acid-fats stains such as both hot and cold Kinyoun, modified Ziehl–Nielsen, fluorescent auramine-rhodamine, PAS, and the carbofuschin-negative stains (162–168). All the stains appear to have similar sensitivity in detecting *Cryptosporidium* oocysts and in the hands of experienced observers identification of the oocysts is straightforward. We recommend either the acid-fast stain or Kinyoun since they are both reliable and inexpensive. Several techniques have been described to increase sensitivity including a sucrose flotation method (169) and the formalin-ether method of Ritchie (170). Concentration of stool is rarely necessary in acute cases but is useful in follow-up after therapy to confirm eradication of oocysts. We have rarely found it necessary to use duodenal aspiration or endoscopic biopsy to confirm the diagnosis since the oocysts are almost continuously shed in stool in active infection. If laboratory expertise in identifying oocysts is poor then a small-bowel biopsy examined by standard H and E light microscopy should be adequate. Electron microscopy is seldom necessary and very expensive. Newer techniques including a stool ELISA are currently under clinical evaluation.

5. *Treatment*

Unfortunately no specific anticryptosporidial therapy has been proven effective to date in eradicating *Cryptosporidium*, which is obviously the primary goal of therapy. However just as important to the patient are the secondary goals of reducing the frequency of bowel movements and improving general quality of life and nutritional status. Therefore, initial therapy should be supportive and focused on maintaining patient comfort, hydration, and restoring nutritional balance (see Section VII). When the volume of diarrhea permits, oral rehydration is possible and can be stimulated by addition of glucose polyelectrolyte solutions and a high refined-carbohydrate diet. Patients must drink up to 5 liters of fluids per day to replace losses of 1–2 liters in stool. Greater stool volumes or associated vomiting nearly always require IV rehydration, which can be achieved by nocturnal replacement of saline using a central venous access port or intermittent peripheral therapy. We favor the latter since it interferes less with the patient's daily activities. Nonspecific antidiarrheals should be used liberally and in large doses to attempt to control both the diarrhea and the cramps. Although not proven in randomized trials, sandostatin, an analog of somatostatin, can be useful in individual patients and can be combined with pancreatic supplements to counteract malabsorbtion (171,172).

Nutritional support is critical when weight loss and malabsorption are present. Oral intake should be low fat, high carbohydrate with avoidance of milk products. Supplements including medium-chain triglyceride preparations can be useful. However, approximately 50% of patients will require intravenous nutritional therapy for supplemental nutrition. Hypoalbuminemia and persistent negative nitrogen balance are associated with increased early mortality in AIDS patients.

Multiple therapies have been targeted against *Cryptosporidium* and deserve discussion despite apparent lack of efficacy. Initial enthusiasm for macrolide antibiotics including erythromycin, spiramycin, and azithromycin has faded since none of these agents have proven efficacious in eradicating *Cryptosporidium* (173,174). We do not routinely use any of these agents at the present time.

Recent open trials have suggested that paromomycin, an aminoglycoside, can reduce stool volume and decrease oocyst shedding in patients with *Cryptosporidium* but controlled trials are awaited (175,176).

Initial case reports suggest that bovine hyperimmune colostrum containing high titers of anticryptosporidial antibodies could eradicate infection (177). A powdered milk shake containing grams of anticryptosporidial antibody was administered until recently in stool volume or loss of oocysts in the feces were seen. More recently, in a small controlled study, this therapy was not proven efficacious compared to nonspecific immunoglobulin, but a type II error cannot be excluded. We believe this treatment modality needs further evaluation and have used hyperimmune globulin successfully in several patients and have found it particularly useful in neonates and infants with AIDS and *Cryptosporidium* infection. Eradication is unusual but we have seen marked reductions in stool output, intermittent loss of oocysts, and restoration of nutrition and growth in infants.

C. *Isospora belli*

Isospora, a coccidian protozoan that is endemic to tropical and subtropical climates, has been described in 15–20% of patients with AIDS from Haiti but in less than 2% of patients from the United States with AIDS and diarrhea (178,179). The clinical syndrome is indistinguishable from the diarrhea seen with *Cryptosporidium* except that peripheral eosinophilia is often seen with *Isospora* infection. Stool examination shows large 20–30 μm oocysts with 2 sporoblasts using modified Kinyoun acid-fast staining. Oocysts are shed intermittently in stool and analysis of 3 stools for ova and parasites are mandatory to rule out *Isospora*. Charcot–Leyden crystals have also been described in the stool secondary to intestinal eosinophilia.

Isospora infection responds promptly to therapy with oral trimethoprim and sulfamethoxazole given 4 times daily for ten days and then twice daily for three weeks (179,180). Diarrhea stops in nearly all patients within 2 weeks but 50% of patients relapse after cessation of therapy. Retreatment is effective and maintenance therapy may be necessary. Pyrimethamine plus folinic acid is an excellent alternative primary and maintenance therapy (180).

D. Microsporidia

Prior to the AIDS pandemic, Microsporidia rarely caused human infection, even in immunosuppressed patients. Since AIDS, however, several different genera have emerged as potentially important intestinal pathogens. Determination of the true incidence of microsporidiosis is made difficult because diagnosis depends upon the experience of the investigator, the specimen being evaluated and technique used, the protozoal burden, and erratic bowel shedding. Further complicating our understanding of the importance of intestinal microsporidial infection is the fact that some infected HIV patients are asymptomatic. Nevertheless, most studies have demonstrated an association between microsporidial infection and chronic diarrhea in AIDS.

1. *Epidemiology*

At least five species of Microsporidia have been associated with infection in humans (181). With the exception of scattered case reports in HIV-seronegative individuals, Microsporidia infects only patients with advanced HIV immunosuppression (CD4 cells < 100/mm^3). Within the intestinal and biliary tracts *Entercytozoon bieneusi* accounts for approximately 70–80% of microsporidial infections and *Septata intestinalis* most likely accounts for the remainder (182,183). Although one series reported *Encephalitozoon cuniculi*, another microsporidian, to be present in 31% of patients with intestinal microsporidial infection (182), in retrospect it seems more likely that the microsporidian species involved in these cases was the very similar-appearing *S. intestinalis*. In contrast to *E. bieneusi* and *S. intestinalis, Encephalitozoon* species are primarily associated with non-GI infections except for one case of peritonitis (184) and another of fulminant hepatocellular necrosis (185).

Microsporidia have only rarely been described in AIDS patients with CD4 counts > 100 cell/mm^3 (183,186). Most individuals with AIDS and microsporidiosis have already had an AIDS-defining diagnosis prior to the diagnosis of microsporidiosis. In contrast to HIV-seronegative individuals, in whom this pathogen has been associated with self-limited diarrhea (181,187,188), patients with advanced immunosuppression (CD4 cells < 100/mm^3) typically have more chronic symptoms (183,186,189,191). Further, of persons with AIDS and chronic diarrhea, lower CD4 counts and Karnofsky scores are seen in those with microsporidial infection as compared to those without (190). Microsporidial infection has been reported in 7–50% (182,189,190,192,193) of persons with AIDS and unexplained diarrhea.

2. *Clinical Manifestations*

Although small-bowel microsporidial infections are generally presumed to be responsible for diarrhea in patients with AIDS, this point is still somewhat controversial. A pathogenic role has been suggested by studies from Weber et al. who have identified the protozoan in 10–22% of HIV-seropositive persons with chronic diarrhea but not in individuals without chronic diarrhea (194,195) and by Molina et al. who demonstrated Microsporidia in 9 of 18 patients with AIDS and chronic diarrhea (190). Microsporidia were the only pathogens identified in 8 of these 9 cases. Some HIV-infected individuals, with and without AIDS, appear to have asymptomatic microsporidial carriage (186,196). However, Rabeneck et al. demonstrated no difference in the incidence of intestinal Microsporidia between AIDS patients with and without diarrhea and found no correlation between the presence/absence of diarrhea, CD4 count, or the intensity of microsporidial infection (196). Moreover, a number of studies have shown patients with Microsporidia and diarrhea to continue to excrete microsporidial spores despite resolution of diarrhea following administration of agents postulated to have antimicrosporidial activity (183,186,190,197). Interpretation of these contradictory findings is further complicated by difficulties in the identification of this protozoa. Additionally, villous atrophy, malabsorption of fat and D-xylose have only been seen in some patients with diarrhea and intestinal microsporidiosis (183,186,190,191). Although malabsorption may result from protozoal damage (191), alternative explanations include progressive immunodeficiency, altered immunoregulation (198,199), small-bowel bacterial overgrowth (183,200), malnutrition (183,201,202), other pathogens (183), or HIV enteropathy.

Diarrhea in persons with AIDS and Microsporidia ranges in frequency from 1–10 times/day (183,186,190,191), is often intermittent, may be loose or watery and is nonbloody. Diarrhea may be exacerbated by eating. Abdominal cramps and bloating are common; however, fevers, rigors, tenesmus, and fecal leukocytes are not seen. Significant weight loss, dehydration, malnutrition, and electrolyte abnormalities can occur in more severe cases. Microsporidiosis of the small bowel has been implicated as a cause for “Slim Disease,” the AIDS-associated wasting syndrome first described in Africa (203,204). Retrospective studies in the United States have demonstrated microsporidiosis in up to 25% of persons with wasting syndrome as the initial AIDS-defining diagnosis (183).

Enterocytozoon infections have also been associated with right upper quadrant pain, elevated serum alkaline phosphatase, gamma glutamyl-transpeptidase, and dilated bile ducts in persons with AIDS. Such cases most likely represent ongoing HIV cholangiopathy and both *E. bieneusi* and *S. intestinalis*, amongst other infectious agents, have been implicated in its pathogenesis (205).

3. Diagnosis

The diagnosis of intestinal microsporidiosis is often delayed, partly owing to the intermittent nature and the nonspecificity of associated symptoms. Intestinal microsporidiosis may be identified in the supranuclear region of infected small-intestinal enterocytes by either light or electron microscopy (EM) examination of mucosal biopsies or cytology specimens. Parasites may also be identified by light microscopic examination of stools and have uncommonly been associated with colonic infection (196). Differences in investigator experience, variable protozoal burdens, and erratic fecal shedding (190,206) contribute to questions regarding the predictive value of a negative test (191) and uncertainty regarding the true incidence of infection.

Until recently EM was considered the best study for identification of Microsporidia, but ultrastructural examination is not a practical screening technique (207). Light microscopy, in contrast, is widely available and relatively inexpensive but is less sensitive, particularly using routine hematoxylin and eosin staining. Special stains, including tissue Gram's stain (Brown and Hopps or Brown and Brenn methods), Geimsa stain, and Warthin–Starry stain, have demonstrated variable success, largely dependent upon the experience of the pathologist evaluating the specimen. Two relatively new staining techniques include modified trichrome staining (195), and chemofluorescence staining (182). Although neither is as yet widely available, both appear to offer significantly enhanced sensitivity for identification of Microsporidia. Additional advantages of the latter method include its ease of use, rapidity and reliability. In one large study (182), this technique identified Microsporidia in 186 of 186 fecal smears from 19 patients with known *E. bieneusi*. Despite erratic shedding of this organism, Uvitex-2B chemofluorescence identified *E. bieneusi* in 40 consecutive daily stool specimens in one patient and identified cessation of *Encephalocitozoon* spore shedding in another patient who simultaneously had a clinical response with albendazole.

Serologic testing does not appear to have clinical utility at the present time (208,209). In the future, immunofluorescent techniques may allow microsporidial detection and species differentiation. The development of such techniques, however, is dependent upon the development of long-term culture systems, as yet unsuccessful for *E. bieneusi*.

4. *Treatment*

No specific therapy has clearly demonstrated benefit in patients with microspordial diarrhea and AIDS. Published studies have been either retrospective or nonblinded and uncontrolled (183,186,189,197,210). These series have primarily evaluated two agents, metronidazole and albendazole. Determination of response to these agents has been complicated by the intermittent nature of microsporidial diarrhea and the inability to demonstrate eradication of Microsporidia in patients in whom the diarrhea has improved.

Reports on metronidazole have demonstrated variable success. Schattenkirk et al. treated 13 AIDS patients with presumptive microsporidial diarrhea and noted either resolution or improvement within several days in 10 out of the 13 (186). However, symptomatic responses were not associated with Microsporidia eradication. This group also tried primaquine without any response in symptoms. In contrast, a minimal and transient response to a two-week course of metronidazole has been described by Molina et al. (190) and Asmuth et al. (183). Albendazole has also been tried with only temporary improvement and without protozoal clearance. Of 10 patients treated with albendazole by Asmuth et al., 3 demonstrated a significant and rapid response, 3 a partial response, and 4 no response. Interestingly, 2 of the 3 responders to metronidazole and 2 of the 3 rapid responders to albendazole were infected by *S. intestinalis*, suggesting a possible susceptibility in this species. In contrast to these responses, however, it should also be noted that 8 of another 9 patients with microsporidiosis in this study had significant improvement without antibiotics when placed on a low fat, low residue diet. The best responses to albendazole thus far have been reported by Dieterich et al. (197). These investigators demonstrated a good response to albendazole 400 mg *bid* in 13 of 23 patients and a partial response in 9 others. Only 4 of 23 patients had a poor response. All patients demonstrated a reduction in stool frequency. Regardless of the improvement in symptoms, however, all 23 patients demonstrated persistence of Microsporidia.

V. VIRAL INFECTIONS OF THE SMALL AND LARGE BOWEL

Viral infections of the large and small bowel are common in patients with advanced HIV infection. Cytomegalovirus (CMV) and Herpes Simplex Virus (HSV) commonly infect the large intestine; CMV may also infect the small bowel. Although these infections are generally responsive to therapy, posttreatment recurrences are common. Additionally, human immunodeficiency virus also appears to directly infect intestinal tissues. Intestinal HIV infection has been implicated as a potential cause of otherwise unexplained diarrhea and/or weight loss in some HIV-seropositive persons.

A. Cytomegalovirus

Cytomegalovirus (CMV) is the commonest cause of life-threatening viral infection in AIDS patients (211), and CMV can cause primary (212), latent (213) and persistent (214) infections in patients with AIDS. Antibodies to CMV are found in 90% of homosexuals and female prostitutes and the virus can be transmitted sexually, through IV drug use, and by vertical transmission from mother to child (215–217). Due to this high prevalence of antibodies, serological tests are virtually useless for making the diagnosis of active CMV infection. Although evidence of CMV infection is also seen in 90% of AIDS patients at autopsy (218) and viremia may be present in up to 50% of patients prior to death, clinical CMV disease appears to occur in only about 7% of patients, with the GI tract being involved in 2.5% of patients (211). Gastro intestinal involvement is predominantly seen as acute esophagitis, gastritis, and colitis. In this chapter we will focus on the manifestations of CMV colitis (Figure 3).

1. *Pathophysiology*

After primary infection, which is often asymptomatic, CMV may be shed in semen and urine for years and remain clinically dormant. As immunosuppression progresses and the CD4 count falls below 100/mm^3, reactivation of CMV can result in clinical infection. Colitis caused by CMV has the pathologic features of a small-vessel vasculitis. The colonic mucosa is grossly ulcerated with scattered focal 0.5–1 cm ulcers. Occasionally both a large-mass lesion (CMVoma) or a large transmural ulcer may be seen (219). Histologically there is often a diffuse active inflammatory infiltrate and intranuclear inclusions are pathognomic for CMV (220). Inclusion bodies are often best seen in the granulation or connective tissue associated with the ulceration or else within the endothelial cells. Occasionally neutrophilic infiltration of endothelial cells confirms the presence of a small-vessel endarteritis. Viral cultures of the inflamed tissue are usually positive for CMV.

2. *Clinical Manifestations*

Cytomegalovirus presents as an acute colitis with abdominal pain and diarrhea (221–224). The diarrhea is watery, occasionally bloody, small volume, and

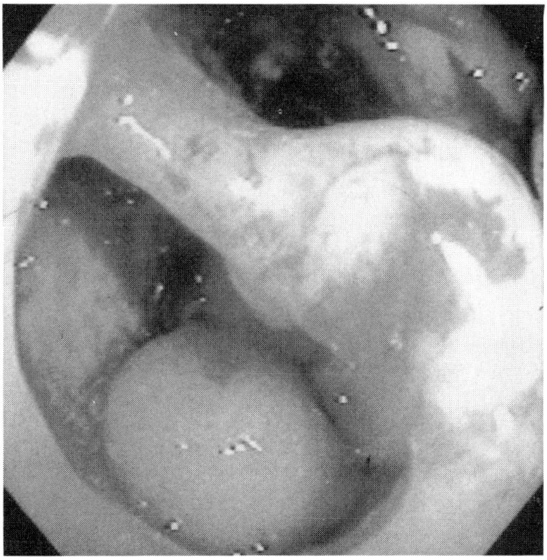

(A)

Figure 3 Cytomegalovirus infection of the colon may have a number of different endoscopic appearances. The CMVoma (A) may look most like a colonic neoplasm, especially when viewed by barium radiograph. Seen here is deep undermining by a large cecal ulcer with secondary mucosal bridging and bulging of adjacent mucosa. Another appearance is that of shallow, irregularly shaped ulcerations (B). These may be isolated or diffuse. Pseudomembranes may also be associated with CMV colitis. Biopsies generally confirm the diagnosis (C). Characteristically, intranuclear (large arrow) and intracytoplasmic (small arrow) inclusion bodies are seen. There is a predilection for endothelial involvement. (Courtesy of Dr. Sigfus Nikulasson, Mallory Institute of Pathology, Boston University School of Medicine.)

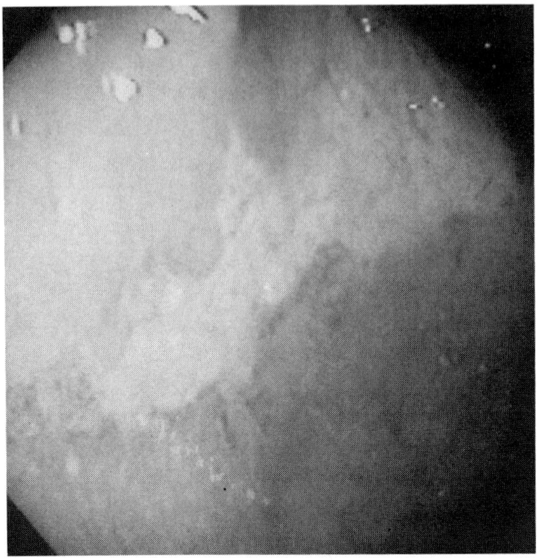

(B)

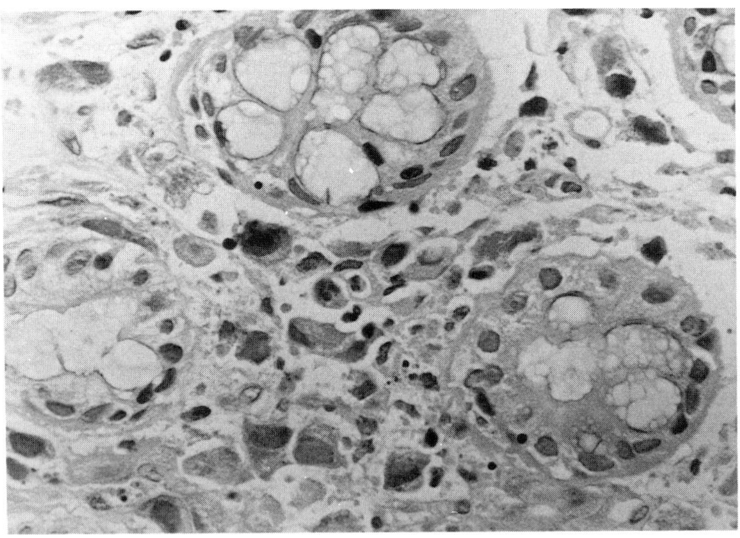

(C)

Figure 3 Continued

frequent (up to 20 times/day). Fever is seen in over half the patients with active colitis. The pain may be crampy but in our experience it is more often severe, continuous, and often localized to the left or right iliac fossa. The differential diagnosis includes bacterial colitis, diverticulitis, clostridium difficile colitis, and mesenteric ischemia. The majority of patients present with chronic symptoms for several weeks but an acute presentation of massive lower gastrointestinal bleeding or perforation has been reported. The disease is often focal and segmental and presentation with an abdominal mass mimicking carcinoma or abscess has been described (219). In view of the high risk of perforation, we investigate patients with colonic symptoms and negative stool bacterial cultures promptly for CMV colitis. If rectal symptoms such as tenesmus are present, a left-sided colonoscopy or flexible sigmoidoscopy should be performed. Symptoms of right-sided pain, focal tenderness, or an abdominal mass require a full colonoscopy. Findings on colonoscopy vary from a diffuse nonspecific colitis to focal small and large ulcers. Biopsy and viral culture are mandatory to confirm the diagnosis. In patients with abdominal pain, a CT scan may show focal thickening of the bowel, particularly in right-sided colitis. Stool cultures and positive biopsies with CMV inclusion bodies from areas of normal mucosa are not useful for the diagnosis of active infection. Once the diagnosis is suspected and biopsies have been taken, we prefer to start empiric therapy for CMV, especially in patients with severe colitis or large focal ulcers.

3. *Treatment*

Gastrointestinal CMV is one of the readily treatable causes of colitis in AIDS patients (221–224). Gancyclovir, an analog of thymidine, is active against all herpesviruses after intracellular conversion to gancyclovir triphosphate, a potent DNA polymerase inhibitor (225). Cells infected with CMV convert gancyclovir more rapidly to the monophosphate than normal cells and then cellular kinases convert the monophosphate to the active triphosphate. Gancyclovir is ten times more active than acyclovir against CMV and appears very specific in its antiviral activity with little effect on growth and metabolism of normal mammalian cells. Gancyclovir is not metabolized in humans and is excreted unchanged in the urine. Gancyclovir is given intravenously, preferably via a central vein. In patients with normal renal function, the induction dose is 2.5 mg/kg every 8 hours, followed by a maintenance dose of 5 mg/kg every 24 hours. A new oral form of gancyclovir has recently become available for clinical trials and we have used this for maintenance therapy successfully in two patients with CMV colitis. Gancyclovir was recently used in large study of 31 patients with CMV colitis with good clinical response in 70% and virological response with negative urine cultures in a similar percentage (223). After cessation of therapy 33–50% of patients have a relapse of CMV when no antiviral therapy is given. Thus standard practice is to continue maintenance IV therapy with hope that the new oral therapy will prove efficacious in the near future. The major toxicity of gancyclovir is hematological and the CBC should be monitored on therapy. Neutropenia is the most serious adverse effect and may require cessation of drug therapy, which usually results in restoration of the neutrophil content.

Foscarnet (trisodium phosphonoformate), an alternative therapy for CMV, is a potent inhibitor of herpesvirus DNA polymerase and also retroviral reverse transcriptase (224,226). Foscarnet does not require phosphorylation to an active form and can therefore be used in gancyclovir resistant patients. Foscarnet has a 60% efficacy both clinically and virologically in CMV colitis and about 20% of patients will relapse within 6 months of stopping therapy. Foscarnet is usually given via a central line as a continuous intravenous infusion of 200 mg/kg per day. Side effects include hypomagnesemia, hypocalcemia, hypophosphatemia, renal insufficiency, and bone marrow suppression. This side-effect profile makes gancyclovir the drug of first choice in clinical management of CMV.

B. Herpes Simplex Virus

Herpes simplex virus infection will be discussed only briefly here, primarily as it pertains to specific clinical differences between patients with and without HIV coinfection. A more detailed discussion of HSV proctitis can be found in Chapter 16 which deals with the gay bowel syndrome.

Herpes simplex infection in HIV-seronegative persons differs in a number of respects from that in persons with AIDS. Although both these groups may develop proctitis and/or perianal disease, chronic infection is more likely in HIV-seropositive individuals (227–233). Also, whereas most cases of symptomatic HSV proctitis in HIV-seronegative persons are felt to represent primary infection, they are more likely to result from reactivation of latent infection in persons with AIDS (234,235). Reactivation is particularly common when CD4 counts drop below 50 cells/mm^3.

The primary presentation of HSV proctitis is tenesmus. Urinary retention can result from sacral nerve involvement. Although patients may complain of diarrhea, they actually have frequent passage of mucus or pus rather than stool; constipation is typical (34). Extrarectal intestinal infections by HSV are exceedingly rare, even in patients with AIDS. Rarely HSV enterocolitis can lead to perforation (236). Chronic acyclovir use may be associated with the development of resistant mutant strains (237), however, these infections generally respond to foscarnet (238). This mutant strain appears to be killed by foscarnet, however, because subsequent reactivations demonstrate acyclovir sensitivity again.

C. Human Immunodeficiency Virus and HIV-Enteropathy

Despite intensive investigations, no pathogen can be identified in at least 15% of AIDS patients with diarrhea (34) who also have small intestinal villus atrophy, malabsorption, and weight loss. Although the presence of unrecognized pathogens cannot be excluded, accumulating evidence suggests that so-called "HIV enteropathy" may result from intestinal epithelial infection by HIV itself (239).

Detected in intestinal epithelium (239–245), HIV has been shown to replicate in tissue-culture cell lines derived from gastrointestinal mucosa (246–249). In vitro, infection and intraepithelial replication by HIV has resulted in structural abnormalities, including shortening and disorganization of microvilli similar to that seen in vivo in HIV-seropositive patients with "HIV enteropathy." (248) These abnormalities are also similar to those in children with microvillus inclusion disease (250), another condition associated with malabsorption, enhanced secretion, and chronic diarrhea. Further, direct GI infection by HIV has been associated in vivo with small-bowel atrophy, defective enterocyte maturation (251), and altered epithelial function (252,253).

Immunologic evidence also supports a direct relationship between HIV infection and diarrhea. In a group of 48 HIV seropositive persons with diarrhea, only 31% of whom had an identifiable pathogen, Mathewson et al. demonstrated anti-p24 secretory IgA in 67% of those with diarrhea, as compared to 10% in those without diarrhea, and 0 out of 23 HIV seronegative persons with diarrhea (254). It is unclear, however, if this implies that HIV-induced intestinal damage is occurring through virus-mediated cytotoxicity or the immune response it triggers. Allergic mechanisms have also been implicated. In one small series HIV antigen was shown to induce histamine release via a type 1 IgE-mediated reaction in 9 out of 12 AIDS patients but 0 out of 10 healthy controls (255).

Symptoms of diarrhea have, in many cases, correlated with the presence of HIV (251,254). Fifty-five percent of infants and children with HIV infection and persistent diarrhea had stools containing HIV nucleic acids, compared to 10% of HIV patients without diarrhea, and none of 21 HIV seronegative patients with diarrhea (256). To our knowledge no formal studies have evaluated antiretroviral therapy or antihistamine therapy for diarrhea in HIV-seropositive persons with chronic diarrhea. The use of AZT, however, has been associated with weight gain in some seropositive persons (257).

VI. MANAGEMENT STRATEGIES IN HIV-SEROPOSITIVE PERSONS WITH CHRONIC DIARRHEA

A. Overview

A variety of approaches have been proposed for the management of persistent diarrhea in persons with HIV infection (258–261), each with its own merits and weaknesses. While the most common focus has been on pathogen identification, a role for empiric therapies has also been emphasized. Rather than using a standardized diagnostic protocol, we believe that a more individualized approach, based upon each patient's clinical features, may provide a more cost-effective management strategy for patients with AIDS and diarrhea.

When AIDS was new and our experience with associated opportunistic enteric pathogens was limited, it seemed logical to thoroughly evaluate all persons with severe or chronic diarrhea. Rigorous evaluations including stool studies, blood cultures, upper (EGD) and lower endoscopy, duodenal fluid collection, malabsorptive and ultrastructural (EM) studies have been demonstrated to identify at least one potential pathogen in up to 85% of patients with AIDS and diarrhea (34,259). However, while this strategy maximizes diagnostic yield, it is not very cost effective. Experience has proven that we are unable to eradicate many AIDS-related pathogens, and even if we do, relapses are common. These factors, taken together with the intermittent nature of diarrhea and variable responses to nonspecific antidiarrheal agents, have made the value of a rigorous diagnostic evaluation less clear.

The issue of cost-effectiveness was initially addressed by Johanson and Sonnenberg using a decision-analysis model (258). In 1000 hypothetical patients with nonbloody chronic diarrhea and AIDS, they compared potential patient outcomes associated with "minimal," "limited," and "full" diagnostic evaluations. A minimal evaluation consisted of a single stool culture for enteric bacterial pathogens. A limited exam included an additional three stool ova and parasite studies, a stool stain for protozoa, and two blood cultures. A full exam included endoscopy and colonoscopy, each with biopsies. When a pathogen was identified, a patient was assumed, depending on available therapy, to have either a successful or unsuccessful response. Average prevalence, treatment response, and recurrence rates were estimated from previously reported clinical investigations. Based upon the available data, the authors determined that each of the three diagnostic strategies was equally efficacious for relieving diarrhea. Further, a stepwise progression from minimal to limited or full evaluation, for those patients failing a less extensive workup, did not alter the conclusion that the minimal evaluation was most cost-effective.

Johanson and Sonnenberg's study strongly supports the use of limited investigations into the etiology of diarrhea in persons with AIDS and diarrhea and suggests a potential role for empiric antidiarrheal therapy. The generalizability of these conclusions is, however, questionable. An inherent problem of this and other decision analyses is that the conclusions derived can only be as correct as the appropriateness of the data-based assumptions used to derive them. In our experience, the epidemiology of gastrointestinal infections is clearly not the same in all persons with AIDS. In addition to bloody diarrhea, an exclusion criteria in the above mentioned study, we have found that a number of clinical factors may aid in the determination of subgroups in which offending pathogens may more easily be identified or treated (Table 3). For example, while Johanson and Sonnenberg's conclusions argue against endoscopic examination, a diagnosis of viral colitis cannot be made without it. This is extremely important because viral colitis can be effectively treated which specific therapy. Further, CMV colitis, when left untreated, may become complicated by bleeding, bowel perforation, or bowel ischemia.

An NIH Consensus Conference in 1992 supported the use of empiric antidiarrheal agents in AIDS patients with stool studies negative for treatable pathogens (259). Their recommended stool studies included three samples each for enteric pathogen cultures and for ova and parasite staining. Stools would be examined with saline, iodine, trichrome, and acid-fast preparations and assayed for *C. difficile* toxin. Failing this initial more cost-effective strategy, however, they urged rigorous endoscopic investigation of all affected individuals not responding to nonspecific antidiarrheal agents.

Although we, too, agree with a step-up approach we have difficulty supporting the widespread use of comprehensive studies in every person who has failed less extensive evaluation. Some patients are as likely to benefit from limited endoscopy as from panendoscopy. Subgroups of patients—for example, those with anorectal symptoms—are likely to have treatable pathogens identified by flexible sigmoidoscopy alone (262). Additionally, neither electron microscopy for microsporidia and adenovirus, or colonic cultures for adenovirus are cost-effective until specific, effective agents are available to eradicate these infec-

Table 3 Predictive Factors for Treatable Causes of Diarrhea in Persons with HIV

1. CD4 cell count > 200/mm^3 and no previous opportunistic infections
2. Geographic risk factors:
   a. Persons recently residing in Haiti, Central or South America, suspect *Isospora*
   b. Persons in these regions and in Nepal or Morocco, suspect *Cyclospora*
3. Symptoms, signs, and basic laboratory findings:
   a. Severe, refractory, chronic abdominal pain, suspect CMV, MAI
   b. Bloody diarrhea, suspect colitis from CMV, *C. difficile*, HSV
   c. Tenesmus, suspect proctitis secondary to CMV, HSV, *C. difficile*
      If gay and sexually active then also suspect *N. gonnorrhea* and *Chlamydia sp.*
   d. Eosinophilia (peripheral smear), suspect *Isospora, Strongylloides*, lymphoma
   e. Markedly thickened colon or colonic segment, suspect CMV, *C. difficile*, lymphoma

Note: No signs or symptoms are specific for any one pathogen and several pathogens may be identified in any one patient. These factors highlight a subgroup of persons with AIDS and persistent diarrhea who are more likely to be infected by a pathogen for which specific antimicrobial therapy is effective.

tions. Submitting mucosal specimens for mycobacterial cultures is also not necessary as blood cultures are cheaper and as effective (263).

Additional support for empiric therapy has recently come from Dupont and Marshall (260) who proposed that persons with AIDS, diarrhea, and negative stool studies be given an empiric course of quinolone antibiotics. If there is no response and if patients are afebrile and their stools without gross blood then they recommend symptomatic treatment with nonspecific antidiarrhea agents, as proposed by Johanson and Sonnenberg (258). A more thorough investigation for bowel pathogens is reserved only for patients with persistent diarrhea. Although we are unaware of any controlled trials to evaluate the use of empiric antibiotic therapy, there is good rationale for such an approach. Accumulating evidence suggests a reduced sensitivity of stool cultures for identifying enteric bacterial pathogens in many persons with AIDS and diarrhea (264–267). Cultures of blood and other tissues may identify a pathogen in some of these cases. In one large series, bacterial pathogens including *Campylobacter jejuni*, multiple *Salmonella* sp., and *Shigella sonnei* were identified in 24 out of 290 cases by culturing colonic mucosal biopsies (mostly from the rectosigmoid), up to a third of which were not identified by cultures of stool (52). Interestingly, 11 out of 14 (79%) of positive *Campylobacter jejuni* cultures were obtained from patients with normal-appearing colonic mucosa. Enteroadherent bacteria are another cause of culture negative, chronic diarrhea in persons with AIDS (268). Virulence in these pathogens results from a plasmid-associated adherence factor (269,270). While the incidence of this type of infection is unknown, the use of ciprofloxacin has been associated with resolution of associated diarrhea (268). Further, quinolone antibiotics may be helpful in those patients with diarrhea secondary to bacterial overgrowth. Reduced gastric acid and autonomic neuropathy, presumptive risk factors for bacterial overgrowth in HIV-seronegative persons, appear to be more common in patients with AIDS (271,272). Although the potential role and timing of empiric antibiotics for culture-negative diarrhea awaits formal clinical investigation, we suggest that some patients, particularly those with fever and CD4 counts > 200 cells/mm^3, are good candidates for empiric therapy.

Mayer and Wanke have recently suggested that individualized management (261) should be based on each patient's clinical presentation. These investigators attempt to determine the most likely pathogens and sites of intestinal infection based upon the patient's history, physical examination, and basic laboratory studies. Historical information thought to be most important include diarrhea characteristics and duration, amount of associated weight loss, most recent CD4 cell count, and history of potential exposures. They also recommend multiple stool and blood cultures, particularly for febrile patients, to exclude *Salmonella* sp. and other enteric bacterial pathogens. Patients with persistent diarrhea and small-bowel symptomatology (i.e., high-volume or malabsorptive type diarrhea) should undergo EGD with luminal fluid collection and mucosal biopsies, including EM. Colonoscopy is reserved for persons with large bowel symptomatology (i.e., frequent, small-volume diarrhea, with/without tenesmus, mucus, or hematochezia).

In our practice we also support an individualized management approach based upon a patient's particular clinical features, rather than systemic exclusion of all potential etiologic agents. Until pathogen-specific effective therapy is available for adenovirus, Cryptosporidia, and Microsporidia, we agree with Johanson and Sonnenberg (258) that a specific diagnosis is not always necessary. Due to the multiplicity of infections and the severity of diarrhea in some AIDS patients, the differential diagnosis may be quite lengthy. Rather than stratifying patients solely for diagnostic purposes, we sometimes find it helpful to stratify patients according to predicted response. Although we recognize that clinical features are nonspecific, certain features may suggest a diagnosis for which specific and effective therapy is available (Table 3). These patients may be better candidates for an empiric trial of antibiotics than with nonspecific antidiarrhea agents. Additionally, we believe some clinical features can identify patients in whom it would seem more cost-effective to alter the order of performed studies. For example, patients with anorectal symptoms may be best served by sigmoidoscopic evaluation as the initial investigation.

The extent of immunosuppression strongly influences the course of diarrhea, the likelihood of pathogen identification, the spectrum of potential pathogens, and patient survival. When CD4 counts drop below 150 $/mm^3$, opportunistic protozoan and viral pathogens become prevalent and diarrhea becomes persistent. In contrast, nonopportunistic enteric pathogens occur in HIV-seropositive persons with CD4 counts $> 200\ /mm^3$, as in HIV-seronegative individuals (261). Effective specific therapy is available in most cases, even for opportunistic pathogens like cryptosporidia (273). Thus, we believe that HIV-seropositive patients with persistent diarrhea but without AIDS defining criteria (CD4 counts $< 200\ /mm^3$ or who have not previously had an opportunistic infection or the wasting syndrome (274)) should be evaluated in the same fashion as HIV-seronegative patients. The importance of CD4 cell count for determining the extent of diarrhea investigations is less clear in persons with AIDS. Although a potential diarrhea-producing pathogen is more often identified in persons with AIDS and CD4 count of $< 100\ /mm^3$ than in those with AIDS and a CD4 count $> 100\ /mm^3$ (275), a significantly better survival has been seen in those individuals in whom a diagnosis could not be made (275–277).

Independent of CD4 cell count, the presence of anorectal symptoms (i.e., tenesmus) greater than 5–10 small bowel movements/day with or without blood or mucus, fecal leukocytes, and anorectal pains, signals a high likelihood of proctocolitis in persons with HIV infection. Common bacterial causes of colitis include *Salmonella* sp., *Shigella* sp., *Campylobacter* sp., and *C. difficile*.

In at-risk individuals, gay-bowel pathogens, particularly *N. gonorrhea* and *C. trachomatis*, must also be considered (131). Viral proctocolitis is more common in the severely immunosuppressed. This appears to be particularly true for CMV and, in our own experience, appears to be independent of sexual orientation.

Extremely severe and persistent abdominal pain, usually nonradiating and often episodic is suggestive, in our experience, of colonic ulceration in persons with persistent diarrhea and CD4 counts < 100 /mm^3. Cecal CMV lesions may present with pain localized to the right lower quadrant, while transverse colon and rectosigmoid involvement is often associated with mid-abdominal and left lower quadrant pain, respectively. A CAT scan, usually performed for abdominal pain rather than diarrhea, can also be suggestive of infectious colitis. In addition to CMV colitis, markedly thickened segments of colon on CAT scan should raise suspicion for *Clostridium difficile* colitis (Figure 4) or lymphoma in persons with AIDS. As with proctitis, endoscopic visualization of the colon

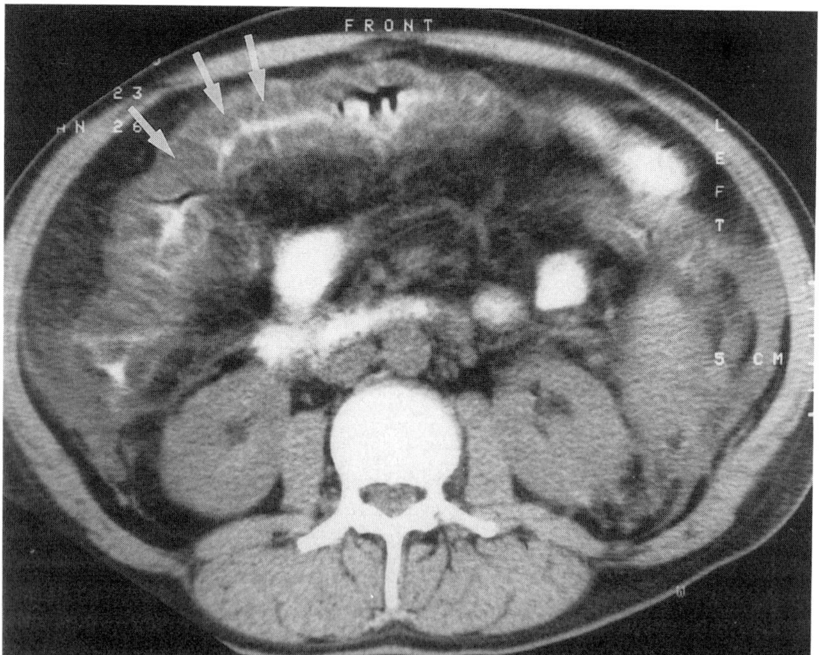

Figure 4 A CT scan of the abdominal cavity may demonstrate marked colonic thickening involving either a segment of colon or the entire large bowel. The most common etiologies include CMV colitis (seen here) and *C. difficile* colitis.

is recommended when viral colitis is suspected. Bloody diarrhea generally indicates colitis and warrants gentle colonoscopic examination.

Fever in patients with AIDS-associated diarrhea usually is associated with bacterial or viral infections. Thus, diarrhea with fever should raise suspicion of *Salmonella, Shigella*, and *Campylobacter* and blood cultures should be obtained. The addition of night sweats, hepatosplenomegaly, and cholestatic LFTs in persons with persistent diarrhea, negative stool cultures, and CD4 counts $<$ 100 /mm^3 is suggestive of mycobacterial infection and prompts duodenal, liver, and/or bone marrow biopsy when blood cultures are negative.

Geographic background can also be an important determinant of patterns of infection and should be taken into account in the management of unexplained diarrhea in patients with AIDS. Enteric infections in AIDS are far more common and serious in developing regions of the world, where diarrhea is the initial presentation of AIDS in up to 90% of cases, 2–3 times more often than in persons in North America or Europe (30–33). While protozoans are the most commonly identified pathogens, effective specific therapy is only available for *Isospora belli, Cyclospora, Giardia lamblia*, and *Entameba* spp.

Eosinophilia on peripheral blood smear, although nonspecific, may also signal the presence of pathogens for which effective treatment is available. Eosinophilia has been associated with *Isospora belli* and/or *strongyloides stercoralis* infection and with intestinal lymphoma.

VII. AN ALGORITHM FOR THE INDIVIDUALIZED MANAGEMENT OF AIDS DIARRHEA

Based upon the available data and extensive personal experience we suggest the following approach to persistent diarrhea in persons with AIDS. An algorithm outlining this strategy is seen in Figure 5.

At least one standard bacterial stool culture and *Clostridium difficile* cytotoxin assay should be performed in all persons with AIDS and persistent diarrhea. Although we recommend that most patients submit three stool samples for bacterial culture and three for oocyte and parasite staining, the presence of anorectal symptoms mandates flexible sigmoidoscopy with biopsy and culture as an initial test (Figure 6). Although an empiric trial of acyclovir can be administered, postponing a sigmoidoscopic examination pending a response to acyclovir can prolong symptoms of severe pain and diarrhea that may necessitate hospitalization. If clinical suspicion is high for HSV we recommend an empiric trial of acyclovir be initiated after cultures and histopathology have been sent. While empiric use of gancyclovir or foscarnet for presumed viral proctocolitis may allow coverage of both CMV and HSV infections, in our opinion they are usually too toxic for an empiric trial of more than a few days.

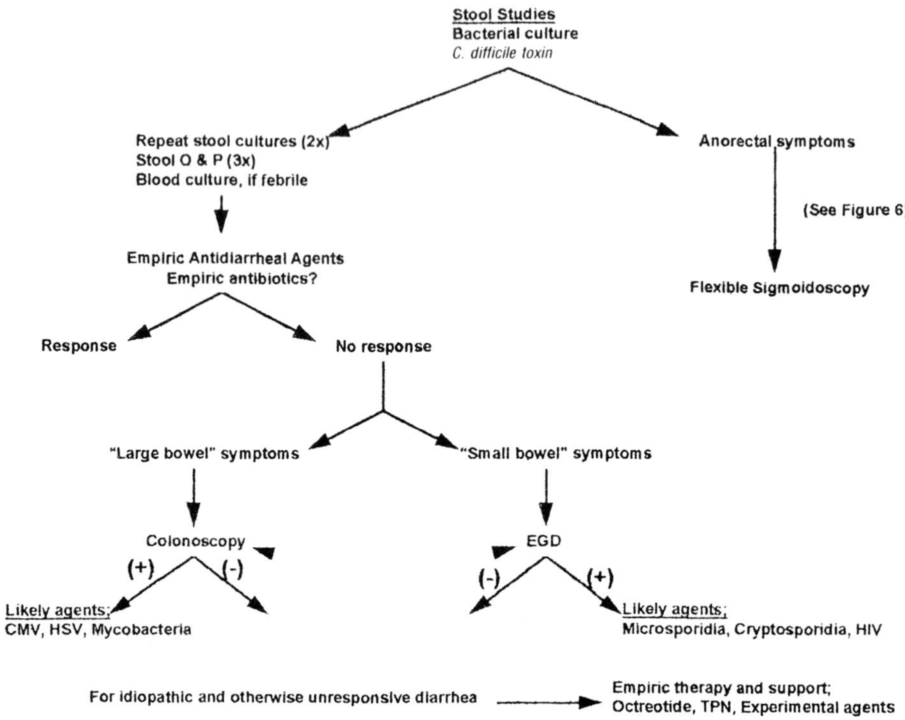

Figure 5 An algorithm for management of AIDS diarrhea.

Many AIDS patients with diarrhea will have intermittent symptoms that are at least partially responsive to antidiarrheal agents (278). We have had good success with loperamide but often use dehydrogenated tincture of opium (DTO), which can be tapered to suit the severity of diarrhea and is well tolerated. We do not generally recommend the use of narcotics like oxycodone, fentanyl (patch), or morphine sulfate. Nevertheless, some patients do respond best to these agents.

Some AIDS patients with diarrhea should receive an initial course of antibiotics rather than empiric nonspecific antidiarrheal agents. For example, ciprofloxacin may be useful in patients with chronic diarrhea, particularly those who are febrile, have symptoms of colitis, and have negative blood cultures and stool studies. Although no clinical trials have yet evaluated such a course of action, we feel it is reasonable when there is strong suspicion of a bacterial pathogen. Nonresponders to empiric therapy will require more invasive investigations, especially if diarrhea is complicated by dehydration. The use of TMP-SMX can be considered if there is suspicion for *Isospora belli*, i.e., chronic diarrhea with

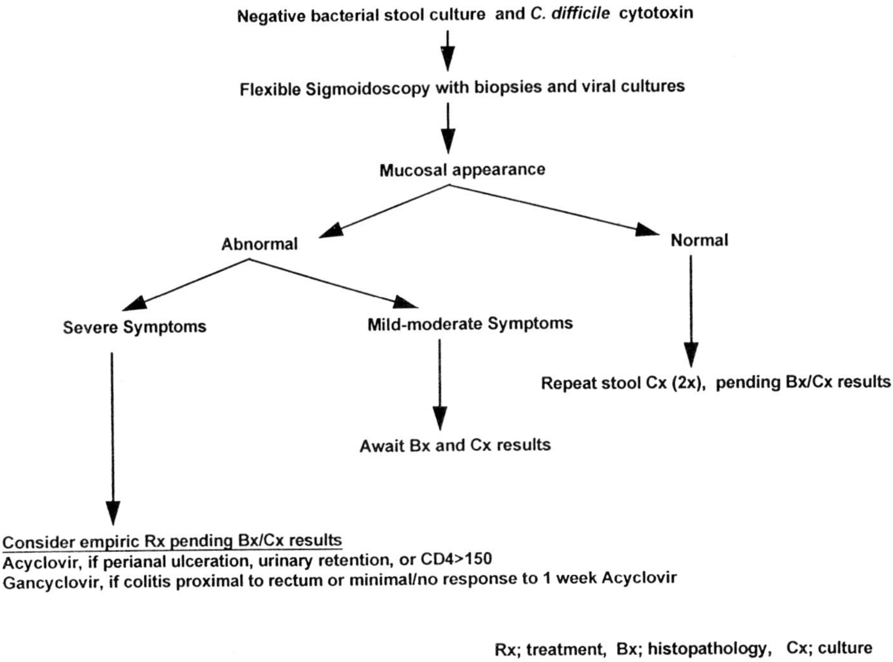

Figure 6 Management of diarrhea with anorectal symptoms (tenesmus, LLQ pain, hematochezia, or fecal WBCs).

peripheral eosinopilia in a person from Haiti or from other developing nations where it is endemic. Patients with AIDS and negative stool studies, who are from or have recently visited the Caribean, Central or South America, or regions near Nepal where *Cyclospora* is endemic should also be considered for a trial of TMP-SMX.

Although we attempt to group patients into those with large- vs. small-bowel symptoms, based on stool characteristics, these are often intermediate or ill defined in nature. For those patients with typical symptoms of large-bowel infection we proceed next to colonoscopy. Right-sided abdominal pain, particularly when located in the right lower quadrant, is suspicious of proximal colonic or terminal ileal inflammation. Both sites can usually be reached and biopsied during colonoscopy. In patients with symptoms consistant with more proximal small-bowel involvement, endoscopy is recommended. In our experience we have found upper endoscopy to be extremely insensitive in identifying responsible pathogens, treatable or otherwise, but occasionally *Giardia lamblia* or *Strongyloides stercoralis* may be found in duodenal fluid, or MAC may be identified in duodenal mucosal biopsies. Until specific effective therapy is available we do not believe there is a role for electron microscopic investigations for microsporidia, adenovirus, or other, as yet, untreatable pathogens. When either initial endoscopy or colonoscopy fails to identify a treatable pathogen, the other is then performed.

Empiric management is recommended for persistent diarrhea that is associated with nontreatable pathogens or is idiopathic. Many of these patients have diarrhea that is intermittent and does not result in dehydration. Usually some response to antimotility agents can be expected. Patients with persistent or voluminous diarrhea may become dehydrated and are less likely to respond to loperamide or diphenoxylate. When this occurs we suggest a trial of dehydrated tincture of opium (DTO).

Persons reaching this point in the management algorithm have either "idiopathic" diarrhea or are infected by pathogens for which effective specific therapy is not available. Some of these patients may respond to octreotide, a synthetic analog of somatostatin, with reduction in stool frequency, volume, and reversal of weight loss (171). Response to octreotide is significantly better in those individuals in which no pathogen can be identified, although this is controversial (172). In our own experience octreotide has been helpful in some patients with chronic refractory diarrhea. We initially prescribe 100 micrograms of octreotide sq *tid* and titrate upwards by 100 micrograms *tid* every three days to a maximal dose of 500 micrograms *tid*. The latter dose has been associated with pancreatic exocrine insufficiency and may exacerbate diarrhea in some instances. Oral pancreatic enzyme replacement may be helpful in some cases and some patients may require DTO while trying octreotide.

Some patients refractory to octreotide who have severe malabsoptive-type diarrhea have benefited from a course of total parenteral nutrition (TPN) with bowel rest. Surprisingly, after 2–3 weeks of TPN, some patients are able to start eating again without diarrhea, though unfortunately the diarrhea often recurs. Patients with refractory diarrhea and recurrent dehydration occasionally need chronic TPN. These patients are given a long-term in-dwelling catheter, as for chemotherapy. We prefer to give these patients night time infusions to avoid interfering with their daily activities as much as possible.

REFERENCES

1. Donaldson YK, Bell JE, Ironside JW, Brettle RP, Robertson JR, Busuttil A, Simmonds P. Redistribution of HIV outside the lymphoid system with onset of AIDS. Lancet 1994; 343:382–5.
2. Ho DD, Rota TR, Hirsch MS. Infection of monocyte/macrophages by human T lymphotropic virus type III. J Clin Invest 1986; 77:1712–5.
3. Lane HC, Masur H, Edgar LC, Whalen GB, Rook AH, Fauci AS. Abnormalities of B-cell activation and immunoregulation in patients with the acquired immunodeficiency syndrome. N Engl J Med 1983; 309:453–8.

4. Belsito DV, Sanchez MR, Baer RL, Valentine F, Thorbecke GJ. Reduced Langerhans' cell Ia antigen and ATPase activity in patients with the acquired immunodeficiency syndrome. N Engl J Med 1984; 310:1279–82.
5. Murray HW, Rubin BY, Masur H, Roberts RB. Impaired production of lymphokines and immune (gamma) interferon in the acquired immunodeficiency syndrome. N Engl J Med 1984; 310:883–9.
6. Schnittman SM, Psallidopoulos MC, Lane HC, Thompson L, Baseler M, Massari F, Fox CH, Salzman NP, Fauci AS. The reservoir for HIV-1 in human peripheral blood is a T cell that maintains expression of CD4. Science 1989; 245:305–8.
7. Embretson J, Zupancic M, Ribas JL, Burke A, Racz P, Tenner-Racz K, Haase AT. Massive covert infection of helper T lymphocytes and macrophages by HIV during the incubation period of AIDS. Naure 1993; 362:359–62.
8. Pantaleo GB, Graziosi C, Butini L, Pizzo PA, Schnittman SM, Kotler DP, Fauci AS. Lymphoid organs function as major reservoirs for human immunodeficiency virus. Proc Natl Acad Sci USA 1991; 88:9838–42.
9. Fahey JL, Prince H, Weaver M, Groopman J, Visscher B, Schwartz K, Detels R. Quantitative changes in T helper or T supressor/cytotoxic lymphocyte subsets that distinguish aquired immune deficiency syndrome from other immune subset disorders. AM J Med 1984; 76:95–100.
10. Lane HC, Masur H, Gelmann EP, Longo DL, Steis RG, Chused T, Whalen GB, Edger LC, Fauci AS. Correlation between immunologic function and clinical subpopulations of patients with the acquired immune deficiency syndrome. Am J Med 1985; 78:417–22.
11. Flanigan T, Whalen C, Turner J, Soave R, Toerner J, Havlir D, Kotler D. Cryptosporidium infection and CD4 counts. Ann Intern Med 1992; 116:840–2.
12. Jacobson MA, Hopewell PC, Yajko DM, Hadley WK, Lazarus E, Mohanty PK, Modin GW, Feigal DW, Cusick PS, Sande MA. Natural history of disseminated *Mycobacterium avium* complex infection in AIDS. J Infect Dis 1991; 164:994–8.
13. Polk BF, Fox R, Bookmeyer R, Kanchanaraksa S, Kaslow R, Visscher B, Rinaldo C, Phair J. Predictors of acquired immunodeficiency syndrome developing in a cohort of seropositive homosexual men. N Engl J Med 1987; 316:61–6.
14. Rodgers VD, Fassett R, Kagnoff MF. Abnormalities in intestinal mucosal T cells in homosexual populations including those with the lymphadenopathy syndrome and acquired immunodeficiency sydyndrome. Gastroenterology 1986; 90:552–8.
15. Ellakany S, Whiteside Tl, Schade RR, van Thiel DH. Analysis of intestinal lymphocyte subpopulations in patients with Acquired Immunodeficiency Syndrome (AIDS) and AIDS-related complex. AM J Clin Pathol 1987; 87:356–64.
16. Budhraja M, Levendoglu H, Kocka F, Mangkornkanok M, Sherer R. Duodenal mucosal T cell subpopulation and bacterial cultures in acquired immune deficiency syndrome. Am J Gastroenterol 1987; 82:427–31.
17. Kotler DP, Scholes JV, Tierney AR. Intestinal plasma cell alterations in acquired immunodeficiency syndrome. Dig Dis Sci 1987; 32:129–38.
18. Heise C, Dandekar SI, Kumar P, Duplantier R, Donovan RM, Halsted CH.

Human immunodeficiency virus infection of enterocytes and mononuclear cells in human jejunal mucosa. Gastroneterology 1991; 100:1521-7.

19. Chandra RK. Nutrition, immunity, and infection: Present knowledge and future directions. Lancet 1983; ii:688–91.
20. Bennett RG, Greenough WB. Approach to acute diarrhea in the elderly. Gastroenterol Clin North Am 1993; 22:517–33.
21. Roberts SH, James O, Jarvis EH. Bacterial overgrowth syndrome without "blind" loop": A cause for malnutrition in the elderly. Lancet 1977; ii:1193–5.
22. Ruddell WS, Losowsky MS. Severe diarhoea due to small intestinal colonisation during cimitidine treatment. Br Med J 1980; 281:273.
23. Draser BS, Shiner M, McLeod GM. Studies on the intestinal flora. 1. The bacterial flora of the gastrointestinal tract in healthy and achlorhydric persons. Gastrenterology 1969; 56:71-9.
24. Lake-Bakaar GB, Quadros E, Beidas SI, Elisakr M, Tom W, Wilson DE, Dincsoy HP, Cohen P, Straus EW. Gastric secretory failure in patients with acquired immunodeficiency syndrome (AIDS). Ann Intern Med 1988; 109:502–4.
25. Belitsos PC, Greenson JK, Sisler J, Yardley JH, Bartlett JG. Association of chronic wasting diarrhea with gastric hypoacidity and opportunistic enteric infections in patients with acquired immunodeficiency syndrome (AIDS). J Infect Dis 1992; 166:277–84.
26. Scott MK, Cello JP, Koch J. Achlorhydria in patients with HIV/AIDS: Correlation with opportunistic infections and malnutrition. AM J Gastroenterol 1995; A155.
27. Griffin GE, Miller A, Batman P, Forster SM, Pinching AJ, Harris JRW, Mathan MM. Damage to jejunal intrinsic autonomic nerves in HIV infection. AIDS 1988; 2:379–82.
28. World Health Organization. The current global situation of the HIV/AIDS pandemic. World Health Organization, Geneva, Switzerland, 1995.
29. Karasik MS, Afdhal NH. Clinical Syndromes: Gastrointestinal Manifestations. In: Libman H, Witzburg R, eds. HIV Infection: A Primary Care Manual. 3rd ed. Boston: Little, Brown, and Co., 1996:165–180.
30. Janoff EN, Smith PD. Perspectives on gstrointestinal infectrions in AIDS. Gastroenterol Clin North Am 1988; 17:451–63.
31. Dworkin B, Wormser GP, Rosenthal WS, Heier SK, Braunstein M, Weiss L, et al. Gastrointestinal manifestations of the acquired immunodeficiency syndrome: a review of 22 cases. AM J Gastroenterol 1985; 80:774–8.
32. Colebunders R, Francis H, Mann JM, Bila KM, Izaley L, Kimputu L, et al. Persistent diarrhea, strongly associated with HIV infection in Kinshasa, Zaire. Am J Gastroenterol 1987; 82:859–64.
33. Malebranche R, Arnoux E, Guerin JM, Pierre GD, Larouche AC, Pean-Guichard C, et al. Acquired immunodeficiency syndrome with severe gastrointestinal manifestations in Haiti. Lancet 1983; 2:873–8.
34. Smith PD, Lane HC, Gill VJ, Manischewitz JF, Quinnan GV, Fauci AS, Masur H. Intestinal infections in patients with the acquired immunodeficiency syndrome (AIDS). Etiology and response to therapy. Ann Intern Med 1988; 108:328–33.

35. Antony MA, Brandt LJ, Klein RS, Bernstein LH. Infectious diarrhea in patients with AIDS. Dig Dis Sci 1988; 33:1141–6.
36. Rene E, Marche C, Regnier B, Saimot AG, Vilde JL, Perrone C, Michon C, Wolf M, Chevalier T, Vallot T, et al. Intestinal infections in patients with acquired immunodeficiency syndrome. A prospectice study in 132 patients. Dig Dis Sci 1989; 34:773–80.
37. Celum CL, Chaisson RE, Rutherford GW, Barnhart JL, Echenberg DF. Incidence of salmonellosis in patients with AIDS. J Infect Dis 1987; 156:998–1002.
38. Nelson MR, Shanson DC, Hawkins DA, Gazzard BG. Salmonella, Campylobacter, and Shigella in HIV-seropositive patients. AIDS 1992; 6:1495–8.
39. Jacobs JL, Gold JWM, Murray HW, Roberts RB, Armstrong D. *Salmonella* infections in patients with the Acquired Immunodeficiency Syndrome. Ann Intern Med 1985; 102:186–8.
40. Glaser JB, Morton-Kute L, Berger SR, Weber J, Siegal FP, Lopez C, Robbins W, Landesman SH. Recurrent *Salmonella typhimurium* bacteremia associated with the acquired immunodeficiency syndrome. Ann Intern Med 1985; 102:189–93.
41. Profeta SI, Forrester C, Eng RHK, Liu R, Johnason E, Palinkas R, Smith SM. *Salmonella* infections in patients with acquired immunodeficiency syndrome. Arch Intern Med 1985; 145:670–2.
42. Rolston KV, Rodriguez SI, Mansell PW. Antimicrobial therapy for *Salmonella* infections in the acquire immunodeficiency syndrome. (Letter) Ann Intern Med 1988; 108:309.
43. Nelson MR, Shanson DC, Hawkins DA, Gazzard BG. *Salmonella, Campylobacter* and *Shigella* in HIV-seropositie patients. AIDS 1992; 6:1495–8.
44. Salmon D, Detruchis P, Leport C, Bouvet E, Karam D, Mehoyas MC, Couland JP, Vilde JC. Efficacy of zidovudine in preventing relapses of *Salmonella* bacteremia in AIDS. J Infect Dis 1991;163:415–1632.
45. Elwell LP, Ferone R, Freeman A, Fyfe JA, Hill JA, Ray PH, Richards CA, Singer SC, Knick VB, Rideout JL, et al. Antibacterial acitvity and mechanism of faction of 3′-azido-3′-deoxythymidine. Antimicrob Agents Chemother 1987; 31:274–80.
46. Blaser MJ, Recurrent *Shigellosis* complicating Human Immunodeficiency Virus infection failure of pre-existing antibodies to confer protection. Am J Med 1989; 86:105–7.
47. Sorvillo FJ, Lieb LE, Waterman SH. Incidence of campylobacteriosis among patients with AIDS in Los Angeles County. J Acquired Immune Defic Syndr 1991; 4:598–602.
48. Dworkin B, Wormser GP, Abdoo RA, Cabello F, Aguero ME, Sivak SL. Persistence of multiply antibiotic-resistant *Campylobacter jejuni* in patient with the acquired immune deficiency syndrome. Am J Med 1986; 80:965–70.
49. Perlman DM, Ampel NM, Schifman RB, Cohn DL, Patton CM, Aguirre ML, Wang WL, Blaser MJ. Persistent *Campylobacter jejuni* infections in patients infected with human immunodeficiency virus (HIV). Ann Intern Med 1988; 108:540–6.

50. Beaugerie L, Salauze B, Bure A, Deluol AM, Carbonnel F, Ngo Y, Cosnes J, Rozenbaum W, Nicolas JC, Gendre JP. Yield of culture for bacteria and fungi from colonic biopsy specimens in HIV-infected patients with diarrhea (290 patients). Gastroenterology 1995; 108:A779.
51. Hutin Y, Molina JM, Casin I, Daix V, Sednaoui P, Welker Y, Lagrange P, Deazes JM, Modai J. Risk factore for *Clostridium difficile*-associated diarrhea in HIV infected patients. AIDS 1993; 7:1441–7.
52. Bartlett JG. *Clostridium difficile*-associated diarrhea and colitis in patients with HIV infection. AIDS Clinical Care 1994; 6:99–102.
53. Horsburgh CR, Selik RM. The epidemiology of disseminated nontuberculous mycobacterial infection in the acquired immunodeficiency syndrome (AIDS). Am Rev Respir Dis 1989; 139:4–7.
54. Wolinsky E, Rynearson TK. Mycobacteria in soil and their relation to disease-associated strains. Am Rev Respir Dis 1968; 97:1032–7.
55. Reznikov M, Leggo JH, Dawson DJ. Investigation by seroagglutination of strains of *Mycobacterium-intracellulare-Mycobacterium scrofulaceum* group from house dusts and sputum in southeastern Queensland. Am Rev Respir Dis 1971; 104:951–3.
56. Goslee S, Wolinsky E. Water as a source of potentially pathogenic mycobacteria. Am Rev Respir Dis 1976; 113:287–92.
57. Kirshner RA, Parker BC, Falkinham JO. Epidemiology of infection by non tuberculosis mycobacteria. Am Rev Resp Dis 1992; 145:271–5.
58. Yajko DM, Chin DP, Gonzalez PC, Nassos PS, Hopewell PC, Reingold AL, Horsburgh CR Jr., Yakrus MA, Ostroff SM, Hadley WK. Mycobacterium avium complex in water, food, and soil samples collected from the environment of HIV-infected individuals. J Acquir Immune Defic Syndr Hum Retrovirol 1995: 9;176–82.
59. Wallace RJ Jr., O'Brien R, Glassroth J, Raleigh J, Dutt A. Diagnosis and treatment of disease caused by non tuberculous mycobacteria. Official Statement of the American Thoracic Society and the American Lung Association. Am Rev Respir Dis 1990; 142:940–53.
60. Guthertz LS, Damsker B, Bottone EJ, Ford EG, Midure TF, Janda JM. *Mycobacterium-avium* and *Mycobacterium-intracellulare* infectious in patients with and without AIDS. J Infect Dis 1989; 160:1037–41.
61. Hellyer TJ, Brown IN, Taylor MB, Allen BW, Easmon CSF. Gastro intestinal involvment in *Mycobacterium avium-intracellulare* infection of patients with HIV. Journal of Infection 1993; 26:55–66.
62. Horsburgh CR, Metchock BG, McGowan JE, Thompson SE. Clinical implications of recovery of *Mycobacterium avium* complex from the stool or respiratory tract of HIV-infected individuals. AIDS 1992; 6:512–4.
63. Damsker B, Bottone EJ. *Mycobacterium avium-mycobacterium intracellulare* from the intestinal tracts of patients with the acquired immunodeficiency syndrome: Concepts regarding acquisition and pathogenesis. J Infect Dis 1985; 151:179–81.
64. Nightingale SB, Byrd LT, Southern PM, Jockusch JD, Cal SX, Wynne BA.

Incidence of *Mycbacterium-avium-intracellulare* complex bacteremia in human immunodeficiency virus-positive patients. J Infect Dis 1992; 165:1082–5.

65. Hawkins CC, Gold JWM, Whimbey E, Kiehn TE, Brannon P, Cammarata R, Brown AE, Armstrong D. *Mycobacterium-avium* complex infections in patients with acquired immunodeficiency syndrome. Ann Intern Med 1986; 105:184–8.
66. Wallace JM, Hannah JB. *Mycobacterium avium* complex infection in patients with the acquired immunodeficiency syndrome; A Clinicopathologic Study. Chest 1988; 93:926–32.
67. Hoover DR, Saah AJ, Bacellar H, Phair J, Detels R, Anderson R, Kaslow RA. Clinical manifestations of AIDS in the era of *Pneumocystis carinii* prophylaxis. Multicenter AIDS Cohort Study. N Engl J Med 1993; 329:1922–6.
68. Havlik JA Jr, Horsburgh CR Jr, Metchock BG, Williams PP, Fann SA, Thompson SE III. Disseminated *Mycobacterium avium* complex infection: clinical identification and epidemiologic trends. J Infect Dis 1992; 165:577–80.
69. Chaisson R, Moore RD, Richman DD, Keruly J, Creagh T, the Zidovudine Epidemiology Study Group. Incidence and natural history of *Mycobacterium avium* complex infections in patients with advanced human immunodeficiency virus disease treated with zidovudine. Am Rev Respir Dis 1992; 146:2285–9.
70. Benson CA, Ellner JJ. *Mycobacterium avium* complex infection and AIDS: Advances in theory and practice. Clin Infect Dis 1993; 17:7–20.
71. Benson CA. Disease due to the *Mycobacterium avium* complex in patients with AIDS: epidemiology and clinical syndrome. Clinical Infectious Diseases 1994; 18 (suppl 3):S218–22.
72. Kiehn TE, Edwards FF, Brannon P, Tsang AY, Maio M, Gold JWM, Whimbey E, Wong B, McClatchy JK, Armstrong D. Infections caused by *Mycobacterium avium* complex in immunocompromised patients: Diagnosis by blood culture and fecal examination, antimicrobial susceptibility tests, and morphological and seroagglutination characteristics. J Clin Microbiol 1985; 21:168–173.
73. Chin DP, Hopewell PC, Yajko DM, et al. *Mycobacterium avium* complex (MAC) in respiratory or gastrointestinal tract preceds MAC bacteremia. In: Avium M, The Modern Epidemic, Cook JL, ed. Frontiers in Mycobacteriology. Denver: National Jewish Center for Immunology and Respiratory Medicine, 1992:15.
74. Havlik JA Jr, Metchock B, Thompson SE III, Barrett K, Rimland D, Horsburgh CR Jr. A prospective evaluation of *Mycobacterium avium* comples colonization of the respiratory and gastrointestinal tracts of persons with human immunodeficiency virus infection. J Infect Dis 1993; 168:1045–8.
75. Hellyer TJ, Brown IN, Taylor MB, Allen BW, Easmon CSF. Gastrointestinal involvement in *Mycobacterium avium-intracellulare* infection of patients with HIV, J Infect 1993; 26:55–66.
76. Colebunders R, Nembunzu M, Portaels F, Lusakumunu K, Kapita B, Piot P. Isolation of mycobacteria from stools and intestinal biopsies from HIV seropositive and HIV seronegative patients with and without diarrhea in Kinshasa, Zaire: preliminary results. Ann Soc Belge Med Trop 1990; 70:303–309.
77. Kiehn TE, Cammarata R. Laboratory diagnosis of mycobacterial infections in

patient with Acquired Immunodeficiency Syndrome. J Clin Microbiol 1986; 24:708–11.
78. Morris A, Reller LB, Salfinger M, Jackson K, Sievers A, Dwyer B. Mycobacteria in stool specimens: the nonvalue of smears for predicting culture results. J Clin Microbiol 1993; 31:1385–7.
79. Trujillo A, Cello JP, Scott MK, Herndier BG, Alonso J, Koch J. Correlation of endoscopic and histopathologic abnormalities of the duodenum in patients with HIV/AIDS. Am J Gastroenterol 1995; 90:A316.
80. Horsburgh CR Jr, Selik RM. The epidemiology of disseminated nontuberculous mycobacterial infection in acquired immunodeficiency syndrome (AIDS). Am Rev Respir Dis 1989; 139:4–7.
81. Bachetti P, Osmond D, Chaisson RE, et al. Survival patterns of the first 500 AIDS cases in San Francisco. J Infect Dis 1988; 157:1044–7.
82. Rothenberg R, Woelfel M, Stoneburner R, Milberg J, Parker R, Truman B. Survival with the acquried immunodeficiency syndrome: experience with 5833 cases in Ne York City. N Engl J Med 1987; 317:1297–302.
83. Chin DP, Reingold AL, Stone EN, Vittinghoff E, Horsburgh RC Jr., Simon EM, Yajko DM, Hadley WK, Ostroff SM, Hopewell PC. The impact of *Mycobacterium avium*-complex bacteremia and its treatment on survival of AIDS patients—A prospective study. J Inf Dis 1004; 170:578–84.
84. Ives DV, Davis RB, Currier JS. Impact of clarithromycin and azithromycin on patterns of treatment and survival among AIDS patients with disseminated *Mycobacterium avium* complex. AIDS 1995; 9:261–6.
85. Rastogi N, Frehel C, Ryter A, Ohayon H, Lesourd M, David HL. Multiple drug resistance in *Mycobacterium avium*: Is the wall architecture responsible for the exclusion of antimicrobial agents? Antimicrob Agents and Chemother 1981; 20:666–677.
86. Arbeit RD, Slutsky, Barber TW, Maslow JN, Niemczyk, Falkinham JO III, O'Connor GT, Fordham von Reyn C. Genetic diversity among strains of *Mycobacterium avium* causing monoclonal and polyclonal bacteremia in patients with AIDS. J Infect Dis 1993; 167:1384–90.
87. von Reyn CF, Jacobs NJ, Arbeit RD, Maslow JN, Niemczyk SI. Polyconal *Mycobacterium avium* infections in patients with AIDS: variations in antimicrobial susceptibilities of different strains of *M. avium* isolated from the same patient. J Clin Microbiol 1995; 33:1008–10.
88. Small PM, Schecter GF, Goodman PC, Sande MA, Chaisson RE, Hopewll PC. Treatment of tuberculosis in patients with adanced human immunodeficiency virus infection. N Engl J Med 1991; 324:289–94.
89. Masur H, the U.S. Public Health Service Task Force. Special Report: Recommendations on prophylaxis and therapy for disseminated *Mycobacterium avium* complex disease in patients infected with the human immunodeficiency virus. N Engl J Med 1993; 329:898–904.
90. Gay JD, DeYoung DR, Roberts GD. In vitro activities of Norfloxacin and Ciprofloxacin against *Mycobacterium tuberculosis, M. avium* Complex, *M. chelonei, M. fortuitum,* and *M. kansasii.* Antimicrob Agents Chemother 1984; 26:94–6.

91. Heifets LB, Iseman MD. Determination of in vitro susceptibility of mycobacteria to ansamycin. Am Rev Respir Dis 1985; 132:710–1.
92. Perronne C, Gikas A, Truffot-Pernot C, Grosset J, Pocidalo J-J, Vilde J-L. Activities of clarithromycin, sulfisoxazole, and rifabutin against *Mycobacterium avium* complex multiplication within human macrophages. Antimicrob Agents Chemother 1990; 34:1508–11.
93. Woodley CL, Kilburn JO. In vitro susceptibility of *Mycobacterium avium* complex and *Mycobacterium tuberculosis* strains to a spiro-piperidyl rifamycin. Am Rev Respir Dis 1982; 126:586–7.
94. Clofazimine for leprosy and *Mycobacterium avium* complex infections. Med Lett Drugs Ther 1987; 29:77–8.
95. Rapp RP, McCraney SA, Goodman NL, Shaddick DJ. New macrolide antibiotics: Usefulness in infections caused by mycobacteria other than *Mycobacterium tuberculosis*. Ann Pharmacother 1994; 28:1255–63.
96. Lounis N, Ji B, Truffot-Pernot C, Grosset J. Selection of clarithromycinresistant *Mycobacterium avium* complex during combined therapy using the beige: mouse model. Antimicrob Agents Chemother 1995; 39:608–12.
97. Chiu J, Nussbaum J, Bozzette SI, Tilles JG, Young LS, Leedom J, Hesletine PN, McCutchen JA. Treatment of *Mycobacterium avium* complex infection in AIDS with amikacin, ethambutol, rifampin, and ciprofloxacin. Ann Intern Med 1990; 113;358–61.
98. Kemper CA, Meng TC, Nussbaum J, Chiu J, Feigal DF, Bartok AE, Leedom JM, Tilles JG, Deresinski SC, McCutchen JA. Treatment of *Mycobacterium avium* complex bacteremia in AIDS with a four-drug oral regimen: rifampin, ethambutol, clofazimine, and ciprofloxacin. Ann Intern Med 1992; 166:466–72.
99. Benson CA. Treatment of dissemianted disease due to the *Mycobacterium avium* complex in patients with AIDS. Clin Inf Dis 1994; 18(suppl 3):S1237–42.
100. Chaisson RE, Benson CA, Dube MP, Heifets LB, Korvick JA, Elkin SI, Smith T, Craft JC, Sattler FR, the AIDS Clinical Trials Group Protocol 157 Study Team. Clarithromycin therapy for bacteremic *Mycobacterium avium* complex disease. A randomized, double-blind, dose-ranging study in patients with AIDS. Ann Intern Med 1994; 121:905–11.
101. de Lalla F, Maserati R, Scarpellini P, Marone P, Nicolin R, Caccamo R, Rigoli R. Clarithromycin-ciprofloxacin-amikacin for therapy of *Mycobacterium avium–Mycobacterium intracellulare* bacteremia in patients with AIDS. Antimicrob Agents Chemother 1992; 36:1567–9.
102. Dautzenberg B, Marc SI, Meyohas MC, Eliaszewitch M, Haniez F, Rogues AM, De Wit SI, Cotte L, Chausin JP, Grosset J. Clarithromycin and other antimicrobial agents in the treatment of disseminated *Mycobacterium avium* infections in patient with acquired immunodeficiency syndrome. Arch Intern Med 1993; 153:368–72.
103. Gupta SI, Blahunka K, Dellerson M, Craft JC, Smith T. Interim results of safety and efficacy of clarithromycin (C) in the treatment of disseminated *Mycobacterium avium* complex (MAC) infection in patients (Pts) with AIDS (abstract no. 892). In: Program and abstracts of the 32nd Interscience Conference on Antimi-

crobial Agents and Chemotherapy. Washington, DC: American Society for Microbiology, 1992:260.
104. Young LS, Wiviott L, Wu M, Kolonoski P, Boland R, Inderlied CB. Azithromycin for treatment of *Mycobacterium avium-intracellulare* complex infection in patients with AIDS. Lancet 1991; 338:1107–9.
105. Kemper CA, Havlir D, Haghighat D, Dube M, Bartok AE, Sison JP, Yao Y, Yangco B, Leedom JM, Tilles JG, et al. The individual microbiologic effect of three antimycobacterial agents, clofazimine, ethambutol, and rifampin, on *Mycobacerium avium* complex bacteremia in patients wtih AIDS. J Infect Dis 1994; 170:157–64.
106. Nightingale SB, Cameron DW, Gordin FM, Sullam PM, Cohn DL, Chaisson RE, Eron LJ, Sparts PD, Bihari B, Daufman DL, et al. Two controlled trials of rifabutin prophylaxis is against *Micobacterium avium* complex infection in in AIDS. N Engl J Med 1993; 329:828–33.
107. Pierce M, Lamarca A, Jablonowski H, Jemsek J, Faekenheuer G, Youle M, et al. a placebo-controlled trial of clarithromycin prophylaxis against MAC infection in AIDS patients (Abstract). In: Programs and Abstracts- 34th Interscience Conference on Antimicrobial Agnets and Chemotherapy, Orlando, October 1994. Washington, DC: American Society for Microbiology, 1994, A/2.
108. Gordin F, Wynne B, Schoenfelder J, Bailey B, Foard K, Sullam P. Uveitis Not Reported Following Dose Reduction of Rifabutin in Ongoing Study for the Treatment of *Mycobacterium avium* Complex (MAC), 087250: Rifabutin (RBT) or Placebo (PLA) Plus Clarithromycin (CLA) and Ethambutol (Eth). In: Program and Abstracts of the 35th Interscience Conference on Antimicrobial Agents and Chemotherapy. San Francisco, CA: American Society for Microbiology, 1995, Abstract I208.
109. Shafran SD, Singer J, the MAC Study Group. Uveitis in AIDS Patients with MAC Decreases Markedly at Lower Rifabutin Doses in Combination with Ethambutol and Clarithromycin. In: Program and Abstracts of the 35th Interscience Conference on Antimicrobial Agents and Chemotherapy San Francisco, CA: American Society for Microbiology, 1995, Abstract I209.
110. Asmuth D, Slim J. Evaluation of Resistance Patterns of Rifabutin (RBU) and Macrolides (MCL) as Prophylaxis for Disseminated Mycobacterium avium Complex (dMAC) Disease. In: Program and Abstracts of the 35th Interscience Conference on Antimicrobial Agents and Chemotherapy. San Francisco, CA: American Society for Microbiology, 1995, Abstract E1.
111. USPHS/IDSA Guidelines for the prevention of opportunistic infections in persons infected with the human immunodeficiency virus. MMWR 1995; 40:RR–8.
112. Guerrant RL, Bobak DA. Medical Progress: Bacterial and protozoal gastroenteritis. N Engl J Med 1991; 325:327–340.
113. Taylor DN, Houston R, Shlim DR, Bhaibulaya M, Ungar BLP, Echevarria P. Etiology of diarrhea among travelers and foreign resident in Nepal. JAMA 1988; 260:1245–8.
114. Outbreaks of diarrheal illness associated with cyanobacteria (blue-green algae-like bodies) Chicago and Nepal, 1989 and 1990. MMWR Morb Mortal Wkly Rep 1991; 40:325–7.

115. Hoge CW, Shlim DR, Rajah R, Triplett J, Shear M, Rabold JG, Echeverria P. Epidemiology of diarrhoel illness associated with coccidian-like organism among travelers and foreign resident in Nepal. Lancet 1993; 341:1175–9.
116. Shlim DR, Cohen MT, Eaton M, Rajah R, Long EG, Ungar BL. An alga-like organism associated with an outbreak of prolonged diarrhea among foreigners in Nepal. Am J Trop Med Hyg 1991; 45:383–9.
117. Long EG, Ebrahimzadeh A, white EH, Swisher B, Callaway CS. Alga associated with diarrhea in patients with acquired immunodeficiency syndrome and in travelers. J Clin Microbiol 1990; 28:1101–4.
118. Ortega YR, Sterling CR, Gilman RH, Cama VA, Diaz F. Cyclospora species—a new protozoan pathogen of humans. N Engl J Med 1993; 328:1308–12.
119. Huang P, Weber JT, Sosin DM, Griffin PM, Long EG, Murphy JJ, Kocka F, Peters C, Kallick C. The first reported outbreak of diarrheal illness associated with cyclospora in the United States. Ann Intern Med 195; 123:409–14.
120. Rabold JG, Hoge CW, Shlim DR, Kefford C, Rajah R, Echeverria P. Cyclospora outbreak associated with chlorinated drinking water (Letter). Lancet 1994; 344:1360–1.
121. Hart AS, Ridinger MT, Soundarajan R, Peters CS, Swiatlo AL, Kocka FE. Novel organisms associated with chronic diarrhoea in AIDS. Lancet 1990; 335:169–70.
122. Pape JW, Verdier R-I, Boncy M, Boncy J, and Johnson WD Jr. Cyclospora infection in adults infected with HIV. Clinical manifestations, treatment, and prophylaxis. Ann intern Med 1994; 121:654–7.
123. Wurtz RMk, Kocka FE, Peters CS, Weldon-Linne CM, Kuritza A, Yungbluth P. Clinical characteristics of seven cases of diarrhea associated with a novel acid-fast organism in the stool. Clin Infec Dis 1993; 16:136–8.
124. Bendall RP, Lucas S, Moody A, Tovey G, Ghiodini PL. Diarrhoea associated with cyanobacterium-like bodies: a new coccidian enteritis of man. Lancet 1993; 341:590–2.
125. Long EG, White EH, Carmichael WW, Quinlisk PM, Raja R, Swisher BL, Daugharty H, Cohen MT. Morphologic and staining characteristics of a cyanobacterium-like organism associated with diarrhea. J Infect Dis 1991; 164:199–202.
126. Ortega YR, Gilman RH, Sterling CR. A new coccidian parasite (Apicomplexa: Eimeridae) from humans. J Parasitol 1994; 80:625–9.
127. Madico G, Gilman RH, Miranda E, Cabrera L, Sterling CR. Treatment of cyclospora infections with co-trimoxazole. Lancet 1993; 342:122–3.
128. Soave R, Armstrong D. *Cryptosporidium* and cryptosporidiosis. Rev of Infec Dis 1986; 8(No.6), November-December.
129. Upton SJ, Current WL. The species of *Cryptospordium* (Apicomplexa: Cryptosprodiidae) infecting mammals. J Parasitol 1985; 71:625–9.
130. Smith PD, Lane Hc, Gill VJ, Manischewitz JF, Quinnan GV, Fauci AS, Masur H. Intestinal infections in patients with acquired immunodeficiency syndrome (AIDS). Etiology and response to therapy. Ann Intern Med 1988; 108:328–33.
131. Laughon BE, Druckman DA, Vernon A, Quinn TC, Polk BF, Modlin JF, Yolkin RH, Bartlett JG. Prevalence of enteric pathogens in homosexual men with and

without acquired immunodeficiency syndrome. Gastroenterology 1988; 94:984–93.

132. Janoff EN, Reller LB. *Cryptosporidium* and cryptosporiodiosis. Rev Infect Dis 1986; 8:1012–23.
133. Navin TR. Cryptosporidiosis in humans: review of recent epidemiologic studies. Eur J Epidemiol 1985; 1:77–83.
134. Jokipii L, Pohjola S, Jokipii AMM. Cryptosporidum: a frequent finding in patients with gastrointestinal symptoms. Lancet 1983; 2:358–61.
135. Holten-Anderson W. Gerstoft J, Henricksen SA, Pedersen NS. Prevalence of *Cryptpsporidium* among patients with acute enteric infection. J Infect 1984; 9:277–82.
136. Boagaerts J, Lepage P, Rouvroy D, Vandepitte J. *Cryptosporidium* species: a frequent cause of diarrhea in center Africa. J Clin Microbiol 1984; 20:874–6.
137. Tzipori S. Cryptosporidiosis in animals and humans. Microbiol Rev 1983; 47:84–96.
138. Anderson BC. Moist heat inactivation of *Cryptosprodium* sp. Am J Public Health 1985; 75:1433–4.
139. Phlenz J, Bemrick WJ, Moon HW, Cheville NF. Bovine crytpsporiodosis: a transmission and scanning electron microscopic study of some stages in the life cycle and of the host-parasite relationship. Vet Pathol 1978; 15:417–27.
140. Mata L, Bolanos H, Pizarro D, Vives M. Crytpsporidiosis in children from some highland Costa Rican rural and urban areas. Am J Trop Med Hyg 1984; 33:24–9.
141. Casemore DP, Jackson B. Sporadic crytpsporidosis in children. Lancet 1983; 2:258–61.
142. Hart CA, Baxby D, Blundell N. Gastroenteritis due to *Cryptosporidium* a prospective survey in a children's hospital. J Infect 1984; 9:264–70.
143. Wolfson JS, Richter JM, Waldron MA, Weber JD, McCarthy DM, Hopkins CC. Cryptosporidiosis in immunocompetent patients. N Engl J Med 1985; 312:1278–82.
144. Jokipii L, Pohjola S, Valle SL, Jokipii AM. Cryptosporidiosis associated with traveling and giardiasis. Gastroenterology 1985; 4:838–42.
145. Issacs D, Hunt GH, Phillips AD, Price EH, Raafat F, Walker-Smith JA. Crytpsporiodosis in immunocompetent children. J Clin Pathol 1985; 38:76–81.
146. Sloper KS, Dourmashkin RR, Bird RB, Slavin G, Webster ADB. Chronic malabsorption due to crytpsporidiosis in a child with immunoglobulin deficiency. Gut 1982; 23:80–2.
147. D'Antonio RG, Winn RE, Taylor JP, Gustafson TL, Current WL, Rhodes MM, Gary GW Jr, Zajac RA. A water-borne outbreak of cryptosporidiosis in normal hosts. Ann Intern Med 85; 103:886–8.
148. MacKenzie WR, Hoxie NJ, Proctor ME, Grodus MS, Blair KA, Peterson DE, Kazmierczak JJ, Addiss DG, Fox KR, Rose JB, et al. A massive outbreak in Milwaukee of cryptosporidiosis infected transmitted through the public water supply. New Engl J Med 1994; 331:161–7.
149. Guarda LA, Stein SA, Cleary KA, Ordonez NG. Human cryptosporidiosis in the

Acquired Immunodeficiency Syndrome. Arch Pathol Lab Med 1983; 107:562–6.
150. Weisburger WR, Hutcheon DF, Yardley JH, Roche JC, Hillis WD, Charache P. Cryptospridiosis in an immunosuppressed renal-transplant recipient with IgA deficiency. Am J Clin Pathol 1979; 72:473–8.
151. Meisel JL, Perera DR, Meligro C, Rubin CE. Overwhelming watery diarrhea associated with a *Cryptosporidium* in an immunosuppressed patient. Gastroenterology 1976; 70:1156–60.
152. Lasser KH, Lewin KJ, Ryning FW. Cryptosporidial enteritis in patient with congenital hypogammaglobulinemia. Hum Pathol 1979; 10:234–40.
153. Stemmermann GN, Hayashi T, Glober GA, Oishi N, Frankel RI. Crytpsporidiosis: report of a fatal case complicated by disseminated toxoplasmosis. Am J Med 1980; 69:637–42.
154. Pitlik SD, Fainstein V, Garza D, Guarda L, Bolivar R, Rios A, Hopfer RL. Human cryptosporidosis: spectrum of disease. Report of six cases and review of the literature. Arch Intern Med 1983; 143:2269–76.
155. Ferrucci MJ. Cytomegalovirus-and cryptosporidium-associated acalculous gangrenous cholecystitis. Am J Med 1984; 76:118.
156. Margulis SJ, Honig CL, Soave R, Govoni A, Jacobson IM. Biliary tract obstruction in the acquired immunodeficiency syndrome. Ann Intern Med 1986; 105:207–10.
157. Navin TR, Juranek DD. Crytpsporidiosis: clinical, epidemiologic, and parasitologic review. Rev Infect Dis 1984; 6:313–27.
158. Marcial MA, Madara JL. Cryptosporidum: cellular localization, structural analysis of absorptive cell-parasite membrane-membrane interactions in guinea pigs and suggestion of protozoan transport by M cells. Gastroenterology 1986; 90:582–94.
159. Campbell PM, Current WL. Demonstration of serum antibodies to *Cryptosporidium* sp. in normal and immunodeficient humans with confirmed infections. J Clin Microbiol 1983; 18:165–9.
160. Tzipori S, Campbell I. Prevalence of *Cryptospodidium* antibodies in 10 animals species. J Clin Microbiol 1981; 14:455–6.
161. Ungar BL, Soave R, Fayer R, Nash TE. Enzyme immunoassay detection of immunoglobulin M and G antibodies to *Cryptosporidium* in immunocompetent and immunocompromised patients. J Infect Dis 1986; 153:570–8.
162. Ma P, Soave R. Three-step stool examination for cryptosporidiosis in 10 homosexual men with protracted watery diarrhea. J Infect Dis 1983; 147:824–8.
163. Henricksen SA, Pohlenz JFL. Staining of crytpsporidia by a modified Ziehl–Neelsen technique. Acta Vet Scand 1981; 22:594–6.
164. Garcia LS, Bruckner DA, Brewer TC, Shimizu RY. Techniques for the recovery and identification of *Crytptosporidium* oocysts from stool specimens. J Clin Microbil 1983; 18:185–90.
165. Baxby D, Blundell N. Sensitive, rapid, simple methods for detecting *Cryptosporidium* in faeces (letter). Lancet 1983; 2:1149.

166. Horen WP. Detection of *Cryptosporidium* in human fecal specimens. J Parasitol 1983; 69:622–4.
167. Bronsdon MA. Rapid dimethyl sulfoxide-modified acid-fast stain of *Cryptosporidium* oocysts in stool specimens. J Clin Microbiol 1984; 19:952–3.
168. Casemore DP, Sands RL, Curry A. *Cryptosporidium* species a "new" human pathogen. J Clin Pathol 1985; 38:1321–36.
169. Sheather AL. The detection of intestinal protozoa and mange parasites by flotation technique. J Comp Pathol 1953; 36:268–75.
170. Ritchie LS, Pan C, Hunter GW. A comparison of the zincsulfate and the MGL (formalin-ether) techniques. J Parasitol 1952; 38:16.
171. Cello JP, Grendell JH, Basuk P, Simon D, weiss L, Wittner M, Rood RP, Wilcox CM, Forsmark CE, Read AE, et al. Effect of octreotide on refractory AIDS-associated diarrhea. Ann Intern Med 1991; 115:705–10.
172. Simon DM, Cello JP, Valenzuela J, Levy R, Dickerson GB, Goodgame R, Brown M, Lyche K, Fessel WJ, Grendell J, Wilcox CM, Afdhal N, Fogel R, Reeves-Darby V, Stern J, Smith O, Graziano F, Pleakow D, Flanigan T, Schubert T, Loveless M, Eron L, Basuk P, Bonacini M, Orenstein J. Multicenter trial of octreotide in patients with refractory acquired immunodeficiency syndrome-associated diarrhea. Gastroenterology 1995; 108:1753–60.
173. Portnoy D, Whiteside ME, Buckley E III, MacLeod CL. Treatment of intestinal cryptosporidiosis with spiramycin. Ann Intern Med 1984; 101:202–4.
174. Connolly GM, Dryden MS, Shanson DC, Gazzard BG. Cryptosporidial diarrhoea in AIDS and its treatment. Gut 1988; 29:593–597.
175. White AC Jr, Chappell CC, Hayat CS, Kimball KT, Flanigan TP, Goodgame RW. Paromomycin for cryptosporidiosis in AIDS: A prospective, double-blind trial. J Infect Dis 1994; 170:419–24.
176. Fichtenbaum CJ, Ritchie DJ, Powderly WG. Use of paramomycin for treatment of cryptosporidiosis in patients with AIDS. Clin Infect Dis 1993; 16:298–300.
177. Ungar BLP, Ward DJ, Fayer R, Quinn CA. Cessation of *Cryptosporidium*-associated diarrhea in an acquired immunodeficiency syndrome patient after treatment with hyperimmune bovine colostrum. Gastroenterology 1990; 98:486–89.
178. Soave R, Johnson WD Jr. *Cryptosporidium* and *Isospora belli* infections. J Infect Dis 1988; 157:225–29.
179. DeHovitz JA, Pape JW, Boncy M, Johnson WD Jr. Clinical manifestations and therapy of *Isopora belli* infection in patients with the acquired immunodeficiency syndrome. N Engl J Med 1986; 315:87–90.
180. Pape JW, Verdier RI, Johnson WD Jr. Treatment and prophylaxis of *Isopora belli* infection in patients with the acquired immunodeficiency syndrome. New Engl J Med 1989; 320:1044–7.
181. Weber R, Bryan RT, Schwartz DA, and Owen RL. Human microsporidial infections. Clin Microbiol Rev, Oct. 1994:426–61.
182. van Gool T, Sniijders F, Reiss P. Eeftinck Schattenkerk JKM, van den Bergh Weerman MA, Bartelsman JFWM, Bruins JJM, Canning EU, Dankert J. Diagnosis of intestinal and disseminated microsporidial infections in patients with HIV by a new rapid fluorescence technique. J Clin Pathol 1993; 46:694–699.

183. Asmuth DM, DeGirolami PC, Federman M, Ezratty CR, Pleskow DK, Desai Gautam, Wanke CA. Clinical features of microsporidiosis in patients with AIDS. J Infect Dis 1994; 18:819–25.
184. Zender HO, Arrigoni E, Eckert J, Kapanci Y. A case of *Encephalitozoon cuniculi* peritonitis in a patient with AIDS. Am J Clin Pathol 1989; 92:352–6.
185. Terada S, Reddy KR, Jeffers LJ. Cali A, Schiff ER. Microsporidian hepatitis in the acquired immunodeficiency syndrome. Ann Intern Med 1987; 107:61–2.
186. Eeftinck Schattenkerk JKM, van Gool T, van Ketel RJ, Bartelsman JFWM, Kuiken CL, Terpstra WJ, Reiss P. Clinical significance of small-intestinal microsporidiosis in HIV-1-infected individuals. Lancet 1991; 337:895–8.
187. Sandfort J, Hannemann A, Stark D, Owen RL, Ruf B. Enterocytozoon bieneusi infection in an immunocompetent HIV-negative patient with acute diarrhea. Clin Infect Dis 1994; 19:514–6.
188. Bretagne S, Foulet F, Alkassoum W, Fleury J, Develoux M. Prevalence of microsporidia spores in stools from children in Niamey, Niger. Workshop on Intestinal Microsporidia in HIV Infection, Paris, 1992 (Abstract).
189. Orenstein JM, Chiang J, Steinberg W, Smith PD, Rotterdam H, Kotler DP. Intestinal microsporidiosis as a cause of diarrhoea in human immunodeficiency virus-infected patients: a report of 20 cases. Hum Pathol 1990; 21:475–81.
190. Molina JM, Sarfati C, Beauvais B, Lemann M, Lesourd A, Ferchal F, Casin I, Lagrange P, Modigliani R, Derouin F, Modai J. Intestinal microsporidiosis in human immunodeficiency virus-infected patients with chronic unexplained diarrhea: prevalence and clinical and biologic features. J Infect Dis 1993; 167:217–21.
191. Kotler DP, Francisco A, Clayton F, Scholes JV, Orenstein JM. Small intestinal injury and parasitic diseases in AIDS. Ann Intern Med 1990; 113:444–449.
192. Field AS, Hing MC, Marriott DJ. Microsporidia in the small intestine of HIV infected patients: a new diagnostic technique and a new species. Med J Aust 1993; 158:390–4.
193. Lucas SB, Papadaki L, Conlon C, Sewankambo N, Goodgame R, Serwadda D. Diagnosis of intestinal microsporidiosis in patients with AIDS. J Clin Pathol 1989; 42:885–90.
194. Weber R, Sauer B, Ammann R, Briner J, Altwegg M, Pfyffer, Luthy R. Epidemiology of microsporidiosis in Switzerland—preliminary results of a prospective study. Workshop on Microsporidiosis and Cryptosporidiosis in Immunodeficient Patients, Ceske Budejovice. (Abstract.)
195. Weber R, Bryant RT, Owen L, Wilcox M, Gorelkin L, Visvesvara GS. Improved light-microscopical detection of microsporidia spores in stool and duodenal aspirates. N Engl J Med 1992; 326:161–6.
196. Rabeneck L, Gyorkey F, Genta RM, Gyorkey P, Foote LW, Risser MH. The role of microsporidia in the pathogenesis of HIV-related chronic diarrhea. Ann Intern Med 1993; 119:895–9.
197. Dieterich DT, Lew EA, Kotler DP, Poles MA, Orenstein JM. Treatment with albendazole for intestinal disease due to enterocytozoon bieueusi in patients with AIDS. J Infect Dis 1994; 169:178–83.

198. Elson CO, Reilly RW, Rosenberg IH. Small intestinal injury in the graft versus host reaction: an innocent bystander phenomenon. Gastroenterology 1977; 72:886–9.
199. Kloster BE, Tomar RH, Spira TJ. Lymphocytotoxic antibodies in the acquired immune deficiency syndrome (AIDS). Clin Immunol Immunopathol 1984; 30:330–5.
200. King CE, Toskes PP. Small intestinal bacterial overgrowth. Gstroenterology 1979; 76:1035–55.
201. Odeh M. The role of zinc in acquired immunodeficiency syndrome. J Int Med 1992; 231:463–9.
202. Beach RS, Mantero-Atienza R, Shor-Posner GB, et al. Specific nutrient abnormalities in asymptomatic HIV-1 infection. AIDS 1992; 6:701–8.
203. Serwadda D, Mugerwa RD, Sewankambo NK, et al. Slim disease: a new disease in Uganda and its association with HTLV-III infection. Lancet 1985; 2:849–52.
204. Lucas SB, Papadaki L, Conlon C, Sewankambo N, Goodgame R, Serwadda D. Diagnosis of intestinal microsporidiosis in patients with AIDS (Letter). J Clin Pathol 1989; 42:885–7.
205. Pol SI, Romana CA, Richard SI, Amouyal P, Desportes-Livage I, Carnot F, Pays JF, Berthelot P. Microsporidia infection in patients with the human immunodeficiency virus and unexplained cholangitis. N Engl J Med 1993; 328:95–9.
206. Weber R, Bryant RT, Vugia DJ, Kaiser L, Sauer B, Luthy R. Clinical manifestations and course of intestinal Enterocytozoon bieneusi microsporidiosis, 1993; abstracts book vol. 1, p. 5a7, abstract WS-B14-5. 9th Int Conf AIDS.
207. Schwartz DA, Bryant RT, Weber R, Visvesvara GS. Microsporidiosis in HIV positive patients: current methods for diagnosis using biospy, cytologic, ultrastructural, immunological, and tissue culture techniques. Folia parasitol 1994; 41:101–109.
208. Hollister WS, Canning EU. An enzyme-linked immunosorbent assay (ELISA) for detection of antibodies to *E. cuniculi* and its use in determination of infections in man. Parasitology 1987; 94:209–19.
209. Bryant RT. Microsporidia. In: Mandell GL, Bennett JE, Dolan R, eds. Principles and Practice of Infectious Diseases. 4th ed. New York: Churchill Livingstone, 1995:2513–2524.
210. Blanshard C, Ellis DS, Tovey DG, Dowell S, Gazzard BG. Treatment of intestinal microsporidiosis with albendazole in patients with AIDS. AIDS 1992; 6;311–3.
211. Jacobson MA, Mills J. Serious cytomegalovirus disease in the acquired immunodeficiency syndrome (AIDS). Ann of Intern Med 1988; 108:585–94.
212. Ho M. Epidemiology of cytomegalovirus infections. Rev Infect Dis 1990; 12:S701–10.
213. Jordan MC. Latent infection and the elusive cytomegalovirus. Rev Infect Dis 1983; 5:205–15.
214. Goodgame RW. Gastrointestinal cytomegalovirus disease. Ann Intern Med 1993; 119:924–35.
215. Mintz L, Drew WL, Miner RC, Braff EH. Cytomegalovirus infections in homosexual men: an epidemiologic study. Ann Intern Med 1983; 98:326–9.

216. Drew WL, Mintz L, Miner RC, Sands M, Ketterer B. Prevalence of cytomegalovirus in homosexual men. J Infect Dis 1981; 143:188–92.
217. Quinnan GV Jr, Masur H, Rook AH, Armstrong G, Frederick WR, Epstein J, Manischewitz JF, Macher AM, Jackson L, Ames J, et al. Herpesvirus infections in the acquired immune deficiency syndrome. JAMA 1984; 252:72–7.
218. Reichert CM, O'Leary TJ, Levens DL, Simerll CR, Macher AM. Autopsy pathology in the acquired immune deficiency syndrome. Am J Pathol 1983; 12:357–82.
219. Rich JD, Crawford JM, Kazanjiian SN, Kazanikian PH. Discrete gastrointestinal mass lesions caused by cytomegalovirus in patients with AIDS: Report of three cases and review. Clin Infect Dis 1992; 15:609–14.
220. Wu DG, Shintaku PI, Chien K, Geller SA. A comparison of routine light microscopy, immunohistochemistry, and in situ hybridization for the detection of cytomegalovirus in gastrointestinal biopsies. Am J Gastro 1989; 84:1517–20.
221. Dieterich DT, Rahmin M. Cytomegalovirus colitis in AIDS: Presentation in 44 patients and a review of the literature. J Acquired Immune Def Syndrome 1991; :S29–S35.
222. Francis, Boylston AW, Roberts AHG, Parkin JM, Pinching AJ. Cytomegalovirus infection in gastrointestinal tracts of patients infected with HIV-1 or AIDS. J Clin Pathol 1989; 42:1055–1064.
223. Chachoua A, Dieterich D, Krasinksi K, et al. 9-(1,3-dihydroxy-2-propoxymethyl) guanine (Ganciclovir) in the treatment of cytomegalovirus gastrointestinal disease with the acquired immunodeficiency syndrome. Ann of Intern Med 1987; 107:133–37.
224. Nelson MR, Connolly GM, Hawkins DA, Gazzard BG. Foscarnet in the treatment of cytomegalovirus infection of the esophagus and colon in patients with the acquired immune deficiency syndrome. Am J of Gastro 1991; 86:876–81.
225. Friedman LS, Dienstag JL, Watkins E, Hinkle CA. Evaluation of blood donors with elevated serum alanine aminotransferase levels. Ann Intern Med 1987; 107:137–44.
226. Blanshard C, Benhamou Y, Dohin, Lernesfedt JO, Gaazzard BG, Katlama C. Treatment of AIDS-associated gastrointestinal cytomegalovirus infection with foscarnet and ganciclovir: a randomized comparison. J Infect Dis 1995; 172:622–28.
227. Quinn TC, Stamm WE, Goodell SE, Mkrtichian E, Benedetti J, Grey L, Schuffler MD, Holmes KK. The polymicrobial origin of intestinal infections in homosexual men. N Engl J Med 1983; 309:576–82.
228. Lopez AP, Gorbach SL. Diarrhea in AIDS. Infect Dis Clin North Am 1988; 2:705–18.
229. Smith PD, Janoff EN. Infectious diarrhea in human immunodeficiency virus infection. Gastroenterol Clin North Am 1988; 17:587–98.
230. Laughon BE, Druckman DA, Vernon A, Quinn TC, Polk BF, Modilin JF, Yolken RH, Bartlett JG. Prevalence of enteric pathogens in homosexual men with and without the acquired immunodeficiency syndrome. Gastroenterology 1988; 94:984–93.

231. Siegal FP, Lopez C, Hammer GS, Brown AE, Kornfeld SJ, Gold J, Hassett J, Hirschman SZ, Cunningham-Rundles, Adelsberg BR, et al. Severe acquired immunodeficiency in male homosexuals manifested by chronic perianal ulcerative herpes simplex lesions. N Engl J Med 1981; 305:1439–44.
232. Law C. Sexually transmitted disease and enteric infection in the male homosexual population. Seminars in Dermatology 1990; 9:178–84.
233. Goodell SE, Quinn TC, Mkrtichian E, Schuffler MD, Holmes KK, Corey L. Herpes simplex proctitis in homosexual men. Clinical, sigmoidoscopic, and histopathological features. N Engl J Med 1983; 308:868–71.
234. Wasselle JA, Sedgwick JH, Dawson PJ, Fabri PJ. Intestinal herpes simplex infection presenting with intestinal perforation. Am J Gastroenterol 1992; 87:1475–7.
235. Bagdades EK, Pillay D, Squire B, O'Neil C, Johnson MA, Griffiths PD. Relationship between herpes simplex virus ulceration and CD4 cell counts in patient with HIV infection. AIDS 1992; 6:1317–20.
236. Mobley K, Rotterdam HZ, Lerner CW, Tapper ML. Autopsy findings in AIDS. Pathol Annu 1985; 20:45–65.
237. Erlich KS, Mills J, Chatis P, Martz GJ, Busch DF, Follensbee SE, Grant RM, Crumpacker CS. Acyclovir-resistant herpes simplex virus infections in patient with acquired immunodeficiency syndrome. N Engl J Med 1989; 320:293–6.
238. Chatis PA, Miller CH, Schrager LE, Crumpacker CS. Successful treatment with foscarnet in acyclovir-resistant mucocutaneous infection with herpes simplex virus in a patient with acquired immunodeficiency syndrome. N Engl J Med 1989; 320:293–6.
239. Ullrich R, Zeitz M, Heise W, L'age M, Hoffken G, Riecken E. Small intestinal structure and function in patients infected with human immunodeficiency virus (HIV): evidence for HIV-induced enteropathy. Ann Intern Med 1989; 111:15–21.
240. Mathijs JM, Hing M, Grierson J Dwyer DE, Goldschmidt C, Cooper DA, Cunningham AL. HIV infection of rectal mucosa. Lancet 1988; i:1111.
241. Nelson JA, Wiley CA, Reynolds-Kohler C, Reese CE, Mergaratten W, Levy JA. Human immunodeficiency virus detected in bowel epithelium from patients with gastrointestinal symptoms. Lancet 1988;i:259–62.
242. Heise C, Dandekar SI, Kumar P, Duplantier R, Donovan RM, Halsted CH. Human immunodeficiency virus infection of enterocytes and mononuclear cells in human jejunal mucosa. Gastroenterology 1991; 100:1521–7.
243. Fox CH, Kotler D, Tiernay A, Wilson CS, Faver AJ. Detection of HIV-1 rna in the lamina propria of patients with AIDS and gastrointestinal disease. J Infect Dis 1989; 159:467–71.
244. Kotler DP, Reka S, Borcich A, Cronin WJ. Detection, localization, and quantitation of HIV-associated antigens in intestinal biopsies from patients with HIV. Am J Pathol 1991; 139:823–30.
245. Bartlett JG, Belitsos PC, Sears CL. AIDS enteropathy. Clin Infect Dis 1992; 15:726–35.

246. Adachi A, Loenig S, Gendelman H, et al. Productive, persistent infection of human colorectal cell lines with human immunodeficiency virus. J Virol 1987; 61:209–13.
247. Moyer MP, Huot RI, Ramirez A, Joe S, Meltzer MS, Gendelman HE. Infection of human gastrointestinal cells by HIV-1. AIDS Res Hum Retroviruses 1990; 6:1409–15.
248. Fantini J, Yahi N, Baghdiguian S, Chermann JC. Human colon epithelial cells productively infected with human immunodeficiency virus show impaired differentiation and altered secretion. J Virol 1992; 66:580–5.
249. Fleming SC, Kaoembwa MS, MacDonald TT, Griffin GE. Direct in vitro infection of human intestine with HIV-1. AIDS 1992; 6:1099–1104.
250. Cutz E, Rhoads JM, Drumm B, Sherman PM, Durie PR, Forstner GG. Microvillus inclusion disease: an inherited defect of brush border assembly and differentiation. N Engl J Med 1989; 230:646–51.
251. Ullrich R, Zeitz M, Heise W, L'age M, Hoffken G, Riecken EO. Small intestinal structure and function in patients infected with human immunodeficiency virus (HIV): evidence for HIV-induced enteropathy. Ann Intern Med 1989; 111:15–21.
252. Kapembwa MS, Fleming SC, Sewankambo N, Serwadda D, Luccas S, Moody A, Griffin GE. Altered small intestinal permeability associated with diarrhoea in human immunodeficiency virus-infected Caucasian and African subjects. Clin Sci 1991; 81:327–34.
253. Sutherland LR, Church DL, Gill MJ, Kelly JK, Hwang WS. Gastrointestinal function and structure in HIV-positive patients. Can Med Assoc J 1990; 143:641–6.
254. Mathewson JJ, Jiang ZD, DuPont HL, Chintu C, Luo N, Zumla A. Intestinal secretory IgA immune response against human immunodeficiency virus among infected patients wtih acute and chronic diarrhea. J Inf Dis 1994; 169:614–7.
255. Pedersen M, Nielsen CM, Permin H, Norn S. HIV antigen stimulates basophil leukocytes from AIDS patients to release histamine due to type I allergy. Agents Actions 1989; 27:55–7.
256. Yolken RH, Shuojia L, Perman J, Viscidi R. Persistent diarrhea and fecal shedding of retroviral nucleic acids in children infected with human immunodeficiency virus. J Inf Dis 1991; 164:61–6.
257. Ullrich R, Heise W, Bergs C, Lage M, Riecken EO, Zeitz M. Effects of zidovudine treatment on the small intestinal mucosa in patients infected with the human immunodeficiency virus. Gastroenterology 1992; 102:1483–92.
258. Johanson JF, Sonnenberg A. Efficient management of diarrhea in the acquired immunodeficiency syndrome (AIDS): a medical decision analysis. Ann Intern Med 1990; 112:942–8.
259. Smith PD, Quinn TC, Strober W, Janoff EN, Masur H. Gastrointestinal infections in AIDS. Ann Intern Med 1992; 116:63–77.
260. DuPont HL, Marshall GD. HIV-associated diarrhoea and wasting. Lancet 1995; 346:352–6.

261. Mayer HB, Wanke CA. Diagnostic strategies in HIV-infected patients with diarrhea. AIDS 1994; 8:1639–48.
262. Wilcox CM, Schwartz DA, Cotsonis GB, Thompson SE. Evaluation of chronic unexplained diarrhea in human immunodeficiency virus (HIV) infection: final results of a prospective study. Am J Gastroent 1995; 90:1668, A453.
263. Trujillo A, Cello JP, Scott MK, Herndier BG, Alonso J, Koch J. Correlation of endoscopic and histopathologic abnormalities of the duodenum in patients with HIV/AIDS. Am J Gastroent 1995; 90:1633, A316.
264. Jacobs JL, Gold JWM, Murray HW, Roberts RB, Armstrong D. *Salmonella* infections in patients with the acquired immunodeficiency syndrome. Ann Intern Med 1985; 102:186–8.
265. Blaser MJ. Recurrent *Shigellosis* complicating human immunodeficiency virus infection: failure of preexisting antibodies to confer protection. Am J Med 1989; 86:105–7.
266. Baskin DH, Lax JD, Barenberg D. *Shigella* bacteremia in patients with the acquired immune deficiency syndrome. Am J Gastroent 1987; 82:338–41.
267. Perlman DM, Ampel NM, Schifman RB, Cohn DL, Patton CM, Aquirre ML, Wang W-N L, Blaser MJ. Persistent *Campylobacter jejuni* infections in patients infected with human immunodeficiency virus (HIV). Ann Intern Med 1988; 108:540–6.
268. Kotler DP, Orenstein JM. chronic diarrhea and malabsorption associated with enteropathogenic bacterial infection in a patient with AIDS. Ann Intern Med 1993; 119:127–8.
269. Rothbaum R, McAdams AJ, Gianella R, Partin JC. A clinicopathologic study of enterocyte-adherent Escherichia coli: a cause of protracted diarrhea in infants. Gastroenterology 1982; 83:441–54.
270. Dougan GB. Molecular characterization of bacterial virulence factors and the consequences for vaccine design. J Gen Microbiol 1989; 135:1397–406.
271. Batman PA, Miller ARO, Sedgwick PM, Griffin GB. Autonomic denervation in jejunal mucosa of homosexual men infected with HIV. AIDS 1991; 5:1247–52.
272. Bartlett JG, Belitsos PC, Sears CL. AIDS Enteropathy. Clin Infect Dis 1992; 15726–35.
273. Flanigan T, Whalen C, Turner J, et al. Crlyptosporidium infection and CD_4 counts. Ann Intern Med 1992; 116:840–2.
274. Centers for Disease Control and Prevention. 1993 Revised classification system for HIV infection and expanded surveillance case definitions for AIDS among adolescents and adults. Morb Mortal Wkly Rpt 1992; 41:1–11.
275. Wilcox CM, Schwartz DA, Cotsonis GB, Thompson SE, III. Chronic unexplained diarrhea in Human Immunodeficiency Virus infection: determination of the best diagnostic approach. Gastroenterology 1996; 110:30–37.
276. Blanshard C, Gazzard BG. Natural history and prognosis of diarrhea of unknown cause in patients with acquired immunodeficiency syndrome. Gut 1995; 36:283–286.

277. Connolly GM, Forbes A, Gazzard BG. Investigation of seemingly pathogen-negative diarrhoea in patients infected with HIV1. Gut 1990; 31:886–89.
278. Sorvillo Lieb L, Iwakoshi K, Waterman SD. Isospora belli and the acquired immunodeficiency syndrome (letter). N Engl J Med 1990; 322:131.

8

Campylobacter Infections

J. THOMAS LAMONT
Beth Israel Hospital and Harvard Medical School, Boston, Massachusetts

I. INTRODUCTION

Campylobacter enteritis is now recognized as one of the most commonly diagnosed forms of enterocolitis in developing countries and in Western industrial societies. The annual incidence of infection in developed countries, based on laboratory cultures, is approximately 50 to 100 cases per 100,000 population (1,2), while the incidence in tropical and developing countries may be 5 to 10 times greater, especially during the first 5 years of life. *Campylobacter* infections of sheep were first described early in the twentieth century (3), but human infection was not documented until 1957 (4). The first human isolates were thought to be related to *Vibrios*, but in 1963 these organisms were assigned to a new genus, *Campylobacter* (5). This genus includes *Helicobacter* species that produce gastric infections in animals and man (see Chapter) and *Arcobacter* species, which have recently been identified as a cause of human and primate dysentery (6). The widespread use of selective media has led to the recognition that *Campylobacter* species have virtually worldwide distribution. In addition to typical bacterial dysentery, *Campylobacter* may cause a wide spectrum of extraintestinal manifestations involving virtually every organ system including the central nervous system.

II. BACTERIOLOGY

Two *Campylobacter* species, *C. jejuni* and *C. coli*, account for more than 98% of isolates from patients with diarrhea, and *C. jejuni* alone accounts for at least 90% of clinical isolates in most series (Table 1). *Campylobacters* are curved, gram-negative rods that are classified as microaerophilic bacteria; that is, they tolerate only low concentrations of oxygen, approximately 5 to 10%. At higher oxygen concentrations, as found in room air, growth is inhibited. Laboratory diagnosis of *Campylobacter* requires careful handling of clinical specimens and meticulous culture techniques (7). Rectal swabs and stool cultures should be plated as soon as possible after collection (preferably within a few hours) to avoid drying and exposure to oxygen. Refrigeration or transport in special transport medium may improve culture yield. *Campylobacter* grow best on enriched culture media that contain antimicrobials to inhibit the growth of normal stool flora. Most clinical laboratories use a selective media called Campy-BAP that contains Brucella agar supplemented with 5% sheep blood and antibiotics. Optimum growth occurs at 42°C in sealed containers with 5% oxygen and 7.5% carbon dioxide. Recently, some laboratories have employed filtration of liquid stool samples to select for *Campylobacters,* as these organisms are capable of passing through 0.45 or 0.65 micron filters that retard other bacteria. Filtration techniques are particularly useful for isolation of *C. coli*, a species that accounts for less than 5% of isolates in North America or Western Europe, but up to 30% in certain developing countries. Certain other *Campylobacter* species cannot be isolated using these techniques. Rarely, *C. cinaedi, C. fenneliae, C. upsaliensis, C. hyointestinalis*, and *C. butzleri*, can be isolated from patients with diarrhea and other intra-abdominal infections using special culture and identification techniques (8) (Table 1).

Specific identification of *C. jejuni* on stool culture plates is generally not difficult. *C. jejuni* grows as shaggy grey nonhemolytic colonies. The organism has a characteristic curved appearance by gram stain and exhibits darting motility by phase microscopy. *C. jejuni* is oxidase and catalase positive and is usually hippurate positive. Further typing of *C. jejuni* and other *Campylobacters* has been performed using molecular and serologic techniques, but these are not used in routine clinical practice.

III. PATHOGENESIS

C. jejuni can be transmitted in humans experimentally by ingestion of only 80 organisms, compared to inocula of 10^5 or higher for *Salmonella* (9). The number of bacteria required to cause infection in nonimmune hosts may be influenced by gastric pH, quantity and quality of intestinal mucus secretions, and nonspecific host defenses such as lysozyme. The endogenous host microflora

Table 1 Disease-Causing *Campylobacters* and Related Species

Species	Approximate frequency of isolation	Comments
Typical forms		
C. jejuni	80–90%	Causes typical dysentery
C. coli	5–10%	Similar to *C. jejuni*
Atypical forms		
C. fetus	Rare	Associated with extraintestinal manifestations and chronic infections in gay men or immunocomprimised hosts
C. upsaliensis	1–2%	Diarrhea or bacteremia in patients with co-morbid conditions
C. hyointestinalis	Rare	Diarrhea and bacteremia in humans, enteritis in pigs
C. concisus	Unknown	Periodontal disease
C. sputorum	Unknown	Abscesses
Helicobacter cinaedi and fennelliae	Rare	Proctitis, diarrhea and bacteremia in gay males
Arcobacter butzleri	Rare	Bloody diarrhea, appendicitis, abdominal pain

probably provides a barrier to colonization by *Campylobacter* species and other pathogenic bacteria.

A. Virulence Factors

Three bacterial virulence factors for *Campylobacter* infections have been identified: invasiveness, enterotoxin production, and cytotoxin production (Table 2). Blood stools, abdominal pain, fever, and leukocytosis in patients with *C. jejuni* enteritis suggest that mucosal invasion is common, but entry into the blood stream or spread of infection to extraintestinal sites is uncommon compared to *Salmonella*. While several bacterial proteins have been linked to invasiveness of *C. jejuni* (10,11), none have been fully characterized and no strains of *C. jejuni* have been isolated that are consistently more invasive than other strains. Klipstein (12) reported that all strains isolated from patients with bloody diarrhea were strongly positive for a bacterial antigen detected by ELISA, while strains isolated from patients with nonbloody diarrhea, or from asymptomatic patients, lacked this antigen. However in a human inoculation study, a putative invasive strain of *C. jejuni* produced less severe diarrhea than a noninvasive strain (9).

C. jejuni produces an enterotoxin and a cytotoxin, although not all strains produce both toxins. Most strains isolated from patients with watery diarrhea produce a heat-labile enterotoxin that causes morphologic changes in Chinese hamster ovary (CHO) cells, increased capillary permeability following intradermal injection in rabbits, and fluid secretion in ligated ileal loops of rodents (12). *C. jejuni* enterotoxin is neutralized with antisera against *E. coli* heat-labile enterotoxin (LT), as well as antisera to cholera toxin (CT), suggesting structural homology among these toxins (13). The enterotoxin of *C. jejuni* has not yet been purified, nor has its precise mechanism of action on a cellular level been elucidated.

Cytotoxicity in *C. jejuni* culture supernatants can be demonstrated by rounding of Vero or HeLa cells in culture (14,15). *C. jejuni* cytotoxic activity is not neutralized by antibody to LT, suggesting that the enterotoxin and cytotoxin are immunologically distinct. Enterotoxin production was observed in 62% of Costa Rican children with watery diarrhea, but none of these strains produced cytotoxin (16). Moreover, only 10% of strains isolated from children with bloody diarrhea and 17% from chickens with diarrhea produced cytotoxin in vitro. These observations suggest that *C. jejuni* cytotoxin is probably not required for pathogenesis.

B. Experimental *Campylobacter* Enteritis

Chickens developed enteritis after oral inoculation of a *C. jejuni* strain isolated from a patient with severe diarrhea (17). An inoculum of only 90 bacteria was

Table 2 Virulence Factors of *Campylobacter jejuni*

Factor	Structure	Receptor	Effects on Cell Tissues
Enterotoxin	Heat-labile protein	GM_1 ganglioside	Fluid secretion from ileum Elongation of cultured cells
Cytotoxin	Unknown	Unknown	Rounding of Vero or HeLa cells
Invasion-related antigens	Glycoprotein	Unknown	Mediates adherence to and penetration of host epithelial cells

also capable of producing diarrhea in 90% of test animals. Lethal enteritis occurred in 32% of chickens between 4 and 7 days after infection, and all of these had positive blood cultures. Mucosal damage and inflammation occurred in the terminal ileum and proximal large bowel where penetration of enterocytes by *Campylobacters* was observed. Similar results were reported in rabbits inoculated orally with 1000 *C. jejuni* organisms (18). As in chickens, acute inflammatory lesions occurred in the ileum and colon with goblet cell depletion, superficial mucosal erosions, and an acute inflammatory exudate. Interestingly, rabbit enterocolitis can only be induced in animals whose intestinal motility is reduced by a temporary ligature around the terminal ileum, which is released 4 hours after inoculation.

Human volunteers developed diarrheal illness after oral inocula of 80 to 2×10^9 *C. jejuni* (9). In contrast, *Vibrios, Salmonella*, and *Aeromonas* require ingestion of at least 10^5 viable organisms. The volume of diarrhea in these experiments was also strain specific with one strain causing an average of 5 stools with a total volume of 500 mL/day while a more virulent strain produced 15 stools with a total volume of 1500 mL/day. Onset of symptoms occurred approximately 72 hours post-exposure, but only 50% of patients with positive stool cultures developed any symptoms. Asymptomatic fecal excretors (carriers) of *C. jejuni* have also been observed during community-acquired enteritis in developing countries (19). Twenty-four hours following ingestion of live organisms colonization of the duodenum was documented, followed by positive stool cultures at 48 to 72 hours. All volunteers with diarrhea had fecal leukocytes, approximately half had fever, but none had positive blood cultures.

IV. IMMUNITY

Immunity to *Campylobacter* infections has not been extensively studied, and vaccination procedures are not established. Natural and experimental infection in humans (9) and primates (20) appears to afford protection against subsequent exposure to *C. jejuni*. The titer of antibodies to *C. jejuni* is higher in patients with diarrhea than in asymptomatic carriers (9). For example, human volunteers who developed acute diarrhea after oral ingestion of *C. jejuni* did not develop diarrhea when rechallenged with the same strain one month later. However, all rechallenged patients became colonized with *C. jejuni* and excreted the organism in stool (9), suggesting that antibodies to the pathogen protect against symptomatic infection but not against colonization. Children infected with enterotoxigenic strains of *C. jejuni* developed serum IgG antibody to the enterotoxin in 1-month convalescent serum (21). Persistent, severe *C. jejuni* infections have been reported in HIV patients in whom the humoral IgG, IgA, and IgM responses to bacterial antigens were impaired, compared to normal human volunteers (22). Intestinal IgA antibody directed against *C. jejuni* outer membrane antigens appear in the feces of patients within 10 to 11 days of naturally acquired infections (23).

Secretory IgA directed against *C. jejuni* are present in colostrum and breast milk. Longitudinal studies in Mexico indicate that breast milk with high titers of *C. jejuni* antibodies prevented diarrhea in children between birth and six months of age (24). The protective antibody in breast milk was directed against flagellar proteins of the protein. Recently a group of basic *Campylobacter* proteins have been identified that are recognized by antisera from recently infected patients (25). Antisera to one of these basic proteins recognizes all *C. jejuni* and *C. coli* isolates tested, suggesting that this protein could be a potential vaccine candidate.

V. EPIDEMIOLOGY

Incidence

In developing countries *Campylobacter jejuni* is now recognized as one of the commonest causes of acute diarrheal infections, accounting for more cases of acute infections and diarrheas than *Shigella, Salmonella*, and *Yersinia* combined. *Campylobacter* diarrhea is a warm-weather illness in temperate climates with peak incidence from May through August (26). Children below age 10 and adults age 20–29 are most likely to be infected, with equal sex distrubtion.

Campylobacter species are distributed worldwide, even in sparsely populated areas, where the organism can be cultured from groundwater. In developing countries of Central and South America and Africa, *Campylobacter* diarrhea is extremely common, particularly in young children between the age of weaning (6–18 months) and 5 years. In developing countries, frequent infections during the first 5 years of life probably confers lasting immunity, as the rate of infection in older adults is much less than in childhood. In Scandinavia, approximately 40–70% of *Campylobacter* infections are acquired by adult travelers to the Mediterranean and Asia, with the remainder acquired domestically (27).

Most cases of *C. jejuni* infections diagnosed in doctor's offices are sporadic, without evidence of point-source infection. Infection occurs either through contact with an infected patient or animal or by ingestion of contaminated food, particularly poultry. The organism lives in the intestinal tract of domestic and wild birds, and droppings of the latter may account for contaminated groundwater in remote rural areas. Chicks are not colonized with *C. jejuni* at birth, but acquire infection two or three weeks after hatching (28). Infection of poultry is generally asymptomatic and spreads rapidly through the block because of intense crowding. At the slaughterhouse, nearly all chicken carcasses become fecally contaminated during handling and dipping into scald tanks to remove feathers. During meal preparation, *C. jejuni* is spread from the contaminated meat to cutting boards, counters, knives, and dishes. Up to 75% of raw chicken and turkey on sale in the United States is contaminated with *C. jejuni*, while pork and beef contamination is usually below 5% (29). Undercooked poultry, particularly grilled, barbecued, or fried broiler chicken has been implicated in several outbreaks, as well as in sporadic infection (30). Exposure to puppies and kittens with diarrhea has also been associated with human infection (31,32). A five-year longitudinal survey of commercially reared beagles revealed that approximately one-third of asymptomatic dogs were carriers of *C. jejuni*, while 80% of dogs with diarrhea were infected (33).

Other potential sources of human infection are asymptomatic postconvalescent adult and pediatric carriers. Patients may shed *C. jejuni* for several weeks after recovery from fever or diarrhea, although chronic carriage is rare (34). In developing countries where *C. jejuni* is endemic, asymptomatic infection is common in children (35).

VI. CLINICAL FEATURES AND DIAGNOSIS

Symptoms of *C. jejuni* usually occur within 48 to 72 hours of inoculation from an infected contact or ingestion of contaminated food or water. The onset of illness may be heralded by prodromal symptoms of headache, myalagias, and fever to 39°C (36,37). In the majority of patients diarrhea is the first symptom and is usually accompanied by crampy or colicky lower abdominal pain (Table 3). A small percentage of patients may experience such severe abdominal pain that a surgical emergency may be suspected. Indeed, some patients with acute *C. jejuni* enteritis have undergone laparotomy for suspected acute appendicitis (pseudoappendicitis). Approximately 50% of patients with *C. jejuni* infections will complain of vomiting, nausea, and anorexia. Rectal bleeding and tenesmus occur in up to 50% of patients, but this is usually flecks of blood or bloody mucus rather than frank hematochezia. A biphasic illness is occasionally seen in which patients appear to recover spontaneously after 4 to 5 days of illness, only to relapse several days later with similar or worse diarrhea. Physical examination in acute enteritis reveals lower abdominal tenderness with hyperactive bowel sounds in a febrile, acute ill-appearing patient. The presence of mucoid bloody stool is highly predictive of an enteric infection with *Campylobacter, Shigella, Salmonella*, or enterohemorrhagic *E. coli.*

Routine laboratory tests other than stool cultures are seldom required in the diagnosis of *Campylobacter* dysentery. Approximately one third of hospitalized patients have leukocytosis with immature forms of peripheral smear. Electrolyte abnormalities, azotemia, or dehydration are distinctly unusual in *C. jejuni* infection except in debilitated or immunosuppressed patients, or infants with severe diarrhea.

Table 3 Typical Clinical Features of *Campylobacter* Enteritis

Symptom	% of patients
Diarrhea	98–100
Diarrhea > 10 times daily	30
Malaise	90–95
Abdominal pain	90–95
Fever	60–90
Fever > 39°C	20–40
Nausea	60–70
Vomiting	30–50
Arthralagias	20–30
Visible blood in stool	30–50
Microscopic blood in stool	40–50
Leukocytes in stool	75
Peripheral blood leukocytes	60–75
Bacteremia	1–2

The demonstration of *C. jejuni* or other *Campylobacter* species by stool culture is the single most important diagnostic test. Accurate laboratory diagnosis of *Campylobacter* infection requires that a fresh stool specimen be delivered promptly to the laboratory, where it should be plated on selective medium and cultured under ideal conditions for *Campylobacter* growth. Fresh stool should also be examined for the presence of fecal leukocytes, present in approximately 75% of patients with acute infection.

Radiologic and endoscopic tests are seldom required to diagnose *Campylobacter* enteritis except in severe illness or to rule out surgical conditions, idiopathic inflammatory bowel disease (38), or intestinal ischemia. Barium enema or computerized tonography of the abdomen may demonstrate edema, thickening, and ulceration of the colon or ileum (39). The sigmoidoscopic findings of edema, friability, and small ulcerations are nonspecific and may be seen in any acute infectious colitis and also in some patients with acute flares or ulcerative colitis or Crohn's colitis.

A. Pathology

The pathologic features of patients infected with *C. jejuni* are similar to those described in *Shigella* or *Salmonella* dysentery (40–42). During the first week of illness the colonic mucosa is infiltrated with neutrophils, with microulceration of the surface epithelium. Mucin depletion of colonic goblet cells is prominent, and small crypt abscesses may be present, but crypt architecture is well preserved. During recovery (7–14 days from onset) epithelial regeneration occurs with healing of ulcers and erosions and disappearance of edema and inflammatory infiltrate. Healing is usually complete by two weeks except in complicated cases. Pathologic examination of rectal biopsies can be especially valuable in helping to differentiate acute bacterial colitis from acute ulcerative colitis, especially when stool culture results are not available or are confusing (43). The major diagnostic features of acute ulcerative colitis are diffuse abnormalities of crypt architecture with distortion or branching of crypts, atrophy of crypts, or villiform projections from the surface epithelium.

B. Complications

Complications of *Campylobacter* infection include gastrointestinal and intra-abdominal conditions, as well as extraintestinal or systemic manifestations (Table 4). In several large series, complications of various sorts, most of them mild, were recorded in 10–20% of patients (44,45). Abdominal complications include acute inflammation of the gallbladder, pancreas, liver, and peritoneum. Children or young adults with acute *C. jejuni* infection in whom fever, leukocytosis, and right lower quadrant abdominal pain are prominent may be misdiagnosed as having acute appendicitis. The presence of persistent or frequent diarrhea is rare in patients with acute appendicitis and, if present, should allow correct diagnosis. A form of peritonitis resulting from *Campylobacter* infection occurs in chronic peritoneal dialysis patients. These patients may develop an indolent or relapsing peritonitis that is resistant to antibiotic therapy (46).

Hemolytic-uremic syndrome is rare complication of bacterial dysenteries including *Campylobacter* (47,48), *Shigella*, and enterohemorrhagic *E. coli* (0157:H7). Typical manifestations are acute renal failure, thrombocytopenia, and hemolytic anemia occurring during or shortly after a bout of acute enteritis. This syndrome is being recognized with increasing frequency in children

Table 4 Complications of *C. jejuni* Infection

Abdominal	Extraintestinal
Cholecystitis	Guillain–Barre syndrome
Pancreatitis	Hemolytic-uremic syndrome
Pseudoappendicitis	Bacteremia
Peritonitis in chronic peritoneal dialysis patients	Reactive arthritis (Reiter's Syndrome)
Superimposed on ulcerative colitis or Crohn's disease	

and is accompanied by bleeding disorders, disseminated intravascular coagulation, neurologic sequellae including stroke, and acute renal failure.

Reiter's syndrome or reactive arthritis occurs one to three weeks after the onset of bacterial dysentery from *Campylobacter* or other pathogens. In a outbreak of *C. jejuni* enteritis affecting 35 guests at a party, 7 developed arthritis during or after the diarrheal illness (49). Patients who developed arthritis had higher serum IgM antibody titers than patients without arthritis, supporting the theory that this complication is immune mediated. The migratory arthritis affects the hands, wrist, knees, and ankles, and complete recovery without deformity usually occurs within a month of onset, although a more chronic evolution is occasionally seen. Reiter's syndrome occurs more frequently in patients with HLA B27 histocompatibility antigen.

Guillain–Barré syndrome has recently been identified as a late sequellae of *Campylobacter* enteritis (50,51). This postinfective polyneuropathy is characterized by muscle weakness, sensory abnormalities, and autonomic dysfunction. A causal relationship between acute bacterial or viral infection and subsequent Guillain–Barré syndrome has been suspected for many years because of the repeated observation that acute infectious diarrhea precedes the neurologic symptoms by 1 to 3 weeks in 10 to 30% of patients. Approximately one-third of Guillain-Barré patients have evidence of *Campylobacter* infection including positive stool cultures or elevated antibodies to *Campylobacter jejuni* antigens. Serum antibodies to *C. jejuni* lipopolysaccharide share antigenic determinants with brain gangliosides, suggesting that cross-reacting antibodies might contribute to the development of nerve damage following *Campylobacter* enteritis (52).

VII. TREATMENT

Therapy for acute *Campylobacter* infections should be based on severity of disease. Mild symptoms in previously healthy adults can be treated at home, while severe infections in infants, elderly patients, or immunosuppressed patients may require aggressive inpatient therapy (Table 5). All patients with *Campylobacter* enteritis require adequate rehydration and electrolyte replacement. Since most patients do not require hospitalization, hydration can usually be accomplished at home with oral fluid replacement in the form of clear liquids (broth, water, soda, tea) or by the use of commercial oral rehydration solutions containing electrolytes and glucose. The use of antidiarrheal agents in infectious diarrheas carries the potential risk of delaying the clearance of pathogens and their toxins from the colon. However, diphenoxylate or codeine in low doses are probably safe in patients with mild *Campylobacter* infection and may provide relief from abdominal cramping and tenesmus. Hospitalization is indicated for dehydrated patients especially infants or adults with vomiting who are unable to take adequate fluids by mouth. Patients with compli-

Table 5 Therapy of *Campylobacter jejuni* Infection

Severity of illness	Therapy
1. Mild watery diarrhea without fever or abdominal pain	Oral rehydration Full fluid diet Bismuth subsalicaylate or diphenoxylate
2. Eight or more stools stools per day with blood, fever > 100°F or abdominal pain	Oral rehydration Clear liquid diet Erythromycin 500 mg po *bid* × 5d or Norflaxacin 400 mg po *bid* × 5d
3. As in 2, with significant-co-morbidity, age> 60, fever>102°F, vomiting, rigors or significant dehydration, or any extraintestinal manifestation	Hospitalize for intravenous rehydration Bowel rest Antibiotics as in 2

cations of peritonitis, suspected bacteremia, or serious coexistent medical conditions may also require brief hospitalization.

The advisability of antibiotic therapy for *Campylobacter* enteritis is still somewhat controversial. Several controlled therapeutic trials suggest that antibiotics may shorten the duration of diarrhea by 1 or 2 days and reduce the duration of fecal excretion of organisms (53–55). However, some investigators report little or no benefit of antibiotic therapy in acute *C. jejuni* infections (56,57). Many patients with mild to moderate acute diarrhea are already recovering by the time they visit their physician and are often better by the time the results of stool cultures become available (58). Accordingly, antibiotic therapy should be reserved for patients with moderate to severe dysentery at the time of presentation, for patients with significant co-morbidity (AIDS, diabetes, cirrhosis, peritoneal dialysis), for patients with suspected bacteremia (fever, rigors, leukocytosis), and infants or infirm elderly patients. Early treatment with antibiotics will be based on a presumptive diagnosis of bacterial dysentery (*Campylobacter, Shigella, Salmonella*) prior to the availability of stool culture results.

The two most frequently used antibiotics for *Campylobacter* infection are erythromycin and ciprofloxacin. Despite decades of widespread use, erythromycin resistance among *Campylobacter* isolates has remained less than 5% in most developed countries and less than 20% in developing countries (59,60). Erythromycin reduces the duration of diarrhea, but only when given early in the course of illness. A typical dosage schedule is erythromycin stearate 500 mg *bid* for 5 days.

Norfloxacin has been tested recently in acute diarrhea caused by *Campylobacter, Salmonella*, and *Shigella* (54). Norfloxacin 400 mg *bid* for 5 days reduced the number of loose stools and hastened elimination of Campylobacter from stools (Figure 1). A growing concern with quinolone antibiotics is the emergence of resistant strains in humans following treatment. In the study quoted above, norfloxacin-resistant strains developed in two-thirds of patients

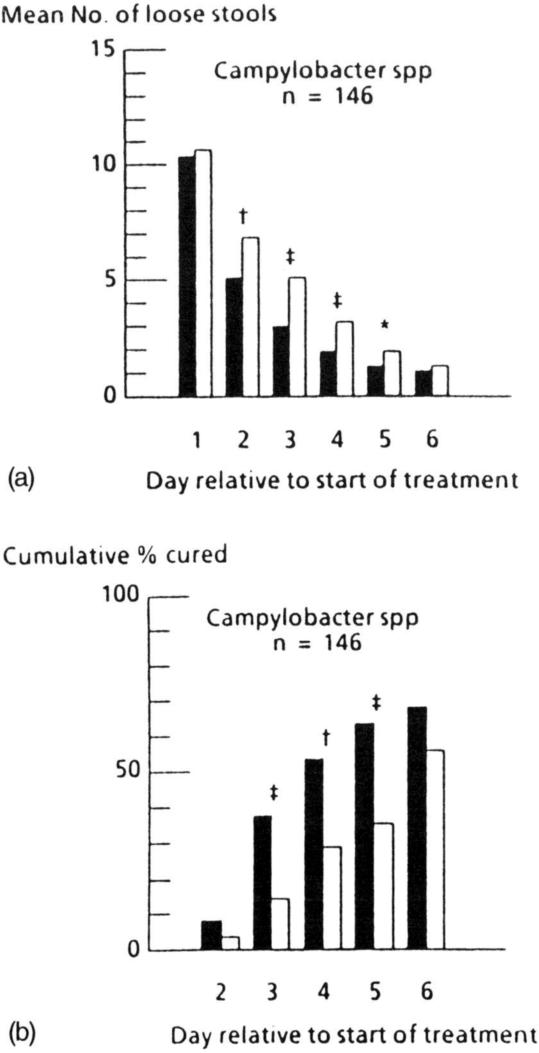

Figure 1 Effects of empiric treatment of campylobacter enteritis with norfloxacin 400 mg *bid* for 5 days or placebo. (a) Effects on diarrhea. (b) Effects on clinical recovery. $^{*}p < 0.05$; $^{+}p > 0.01$; $^{\ddagger}p < 0.001$. (From Ref. 55.)

tested. This suggests that treatment with quinolones should be reserved for seriously ill patients who are unable to take erythromycin.

VIII. SUMMARY

Intestinal infection with *Campylobacter* species is one of the commonest causes of acute infectious diarrhea in our society. This organism invades the mucosa to produce diarrhea that is sometimes bloody, and is usually accompanied by abdominal cramps and fever. Children less than age 5 and young adults between age 20 and 30 are most commonly infected. *Campylobacters* are widespread in domestic and wild animals, and milk and poultry products often are contaminated with this organism. Infection is spread by the fecal-oral route during contact with an infected person, or by ingestion of contaminated food or water. While *C. jejuni* infection is usually self-limited, very young, elderly, or immunosuppressed patients may develop severe or prolonged illness requiring hospitalization for intravenous rehydration and electrolyte replacement. Hemolytic-uremic syndrome, reactive arthritis, and Guillain-Barré syndrome are recognized sequelae of *C. jejuni* infection. Antibiotic therapy with erythromycin or ciprofloxacin may reduce the severity of diarrhea and other symptoms, especially when given early in the course of infection.

REFERENCES

1. Skirrow MB. A demographic survey of *Campylobacter, Salmonella*, and *Shigella* infections in England. Epidemiol Infect 1987; 99:647–57.
2. Popovic-Uroic T. *Campylobacter jejuni* and *Campylobacter coli* diarrhea in rural and urban populations in Yugoslavia. Epidemiol Infect 1989; 102:59–67.
3. McFadyean J, Stockman S. Report of the Departmental Committee Appointed by the Board of Agriculture and Fisheries to inquire into Epizootic Abortion. London: His Majesty's Stationary Office, 1913.
4. King EO. Human infections with *Vibrio fetus* and a closely related *Vibrio*. J Infect Dis 1957; 101:119–128.
5. Cebald M, Veron M. Teneur en bases de l'Adn et classification des vibrions. Ann Inst Pasteur 1963; 105:897–910.
6. Van Damme P, Pugina P, Benzi G, Van Etterijck R, Vlaes L, Kersters K, Butzler JP, Lior H, Lauwers S. Outbreak of recurrent abdominal cramps associated with *Arcobacter butzleri* in an Italian school. J Clin Microbiol 1992; 30:2335–2337.
7. Blaser MJ. *Campylobacter* enteritis. In: Ellner PD, ed. Infectious Diarrheal Diseases. New York:Marcel Dekker, 1984:1–12.
8. Kiehlbauch JA, Brenner DJ, Nicholson MA, Baker CN, Patton CM, Steigerwalt AG, Wachsmuth IK. *Campylobacter butzleri* sp. nov. isolated from humans and animals with diarrheal illness. J Clin Microbiol 1991; 29:376–385.
9. Black RE, Levine MM, Clements ML, Hughes TP, Blaser MJ. Experimental *Campylobacter jejuni* infection in humans. J Infect Dis 1988; 157:472–479.

10. Konkel ME, Joens LA. Adhesion to and invasion of Hep-2 cells by *Campylobacter* spp. Infect Immun 1989; 57:2984–2990.
11. Konkel ME, Babakhani F, Joens LA. Invasion-related antigens of *Campylobacter jejuni*. J Infect Dis 1990; 162:888–895.
12. Klipstein FA, Engert RF. Properties of crude *Campylobacter jejuni* heat-labile enterotoxin. Infect Immun 1984; 45:314–319.
13. Klipstein FA, Engert RF. Immunologic relationship of the B subunits of *Campylobacter jejuni* and *Escherichia coli* heat-labile enterotoxins. Infect Immun 1985; 48:629-633.
14. Yeen WD, Puthucheary SD, Pang T. Demonstration of a cytotoxin from *Campylobacter jejuni*. J Clin Pathol 1983; 36:1237–1240.
15. Klipstein FA, Engert RF, Short H, Schenk EA. Pathogenic properties of *Campylobacter jejuni*: assay and correlation with clinical manifestations. Infect Immun 1985; 50:43–49.
16. Florin I, Antillon F. Production of enterotoxin and cytotoxin in *Campylobacter jejuni* strains isolated in Costa Rica. J Med Microbiol 1992; 37:22–29.
17. Ruiz-Palacios GM, Escamilla E, Torres N. Experimental *Campylobacter* diarrhea in chickens. Infect Immun 1981; 34:250–255.
18. Caldwell MB, Walker RI, Stewart SD, Rogers JE. Simple adult rabbit model for *Campylobacter jejuni* enteritis. Infect Immun 1983; 42:1176–1182.
19. Rajan DP, Mathan VI. Prevalence of *Campylobacter fetus* sub sp. *jejuni* in healthy populations in Southern India. J Clin Microbiol 1982; 15:749–751.
20. Russell RG, Blaser MJ, Sarmiento JI, Fox J. Experimental *Campylobacter jejuni* infection in *Macaca nemestrina*. Infect Immun 1989; 57:1438–1444.
21. Ruiz-Palacios GM, Lopez-Vidal Y, Torres J, Torres N. Serum antibodies to heat-labile enterotoxin of *Campylobacter jejuni*. J Infect Dis 1985; 152:413–416.
22. Perlman DM, Ampel NM, Schifman RB, Cohn DL, Patton CM, Aguirre ML, Wang WL, Blaser MJ. Persistant *Campylobacter jejuni* infections in patients infected with human immunodeficiency virus (HIV). Ann Int Med 1988; 108:540–546.
23. Winsor DK, Mathewson JJ, Dupont HL. Western blot analysis of intestinal secretory immunoglobulin A response to *Campylobacter jejuni* antigens in patients with naturally acquired *Campylobacter* enteritis. Gastro 1986; 90:1217–1222.
24. Ruiz-Palacios GM, Calva JJ, Pickering LK, Lopez-Vidal Y, Volkow P, Pezzarossi H, West MS. Protection of breast-fed infants against *Campylobacter* diarrhea by antibodies in human milk. J Pediatr 1990; 116:707–713.
25. Pei ZH, Ellison RT, Blaser MJ. Identification, purification and characterization of major antigenic proteins of *Campylobacter jejuni*. J Biol Chem 1991; 266:16363–16369.
26. Skirrow MB. Food-born illnesses: *Campylobacter*. Lancet 1990; 336:921–923.
27. Svedhem A, Kaijser V. *Campylobacter fetus* sub sp. *jejuni*: a common cause of diarrhea in Sweden. J Infect Dis 1980; 142:353–359.
28. Humphrey TL. Human *Campylobacter* infections: epidemiology and control. Science Progress 1995; 78:135–146.
29. Harris NV, Weiss NS, Nolan CM. The role of poultry and meats in the etiology of *Campylobacter jejuni/coli* enteritis. Am J Public Health 1986; 76:407–411.

30. Kapper UDG, Skjerve E, Bean NH, Ostroff SM, Lassen J. Risk factors of sporadic *Campylobacter* infections: results of a case-controlled study in Southeastern Norway. J Clin Microbiol 1992; 30:3117–3121.
31. Blaser MJ, LaForce FM, Wilson NA, Wang WL. Reservoirs for human Campylobacteriosis. J Infect Dis 1980; 141:665–669.
32. Saeed AM, Harris NV, DiGiacomo RF. The role of exposure to animals in the etiology of *Campylobacter jejuni/coli* enteritis. Am J Epiemiol 1993; 137:108–114.
33. Fox JG, Claps MC, Taylor NS, Maxwell KO, Ackerman JI, Hoffman SB. *Campylobacter jejuni/coli* in commercially reared beagles: prevalence and serotypes. Lab Anim Sci 1988; 38:262–265.
34. Albert MJ, Leach A, Asche V, Hennessy J, Penner JL. Serotype distribution of *Campylobacter jejuni* and *Campylobacter coli* isolated from hospitalized patients with diarrhea in Central Australia. J Clin Microbiol 1992; 30:207–210.
35. Haq JA, Rahman KM. *Campylobacter jejuni* as a cause of acute diarrhoea in children: a study at a urban hospital in Bangladesh. J Trop Med Hyg 1991; 94:50–54.
36. Blaser MJ, Berkowitz ID, LaForce FM, Cravens J, Reller LB, Wang WL. *Campylobacter* enteritis: clinical and epidemiologic features. Ann Int Med 1979; 91:179–185.
37. Drake AD, Gilchrist MJ, Huizenga KA, Van Scoy RE. Diarrhea due to *Campylobacter fetus* sub sp *jejuni*. Mayo Clin Proc 1981; 56:414–423.
38. Blaser MJ, Hoverson D, Ely IG, Dunkin DJ, Wang WL, Brown WR. Studies of *Campylobacter jejuni* in patients with inflammatory bowel disease. Gastro 1984; 86:33–38.
39. Brodey PA, Fertig S, Aron JM. *Campylobacter* enterocolitis: radiographic features. Amer J Radiol 1982; 139:1199–1201.
40. Lambert ME, Shofield PF, Ironside AG, Mandel BK. *Campylobacter* colitis. Br Med J 1979; 1:857–859.
41. Price AB, Jewkes J, Sanderson PJ. Acute diarrhoea: *Campylobacter* colitis and the role of rectal biopsy. J Clin Path 1979; 32:990–997.
42. Colgan T, Lambert JR, Newman A, Luk SC. *Campylobacter jejuni* enterocolitis. Arch Path Lab Med 1980; 104:571–574.
43. Surawicz SM, Haggitt RC, Husseman M, McFarland LV. Mucosal biopsy diagnosis of colitis: acute self-limited colitis in idiopathic inflammatory bowel disease. Gastro 1994; 107:755–763.
44. Schmidt U, Chmel H, Kaminski Z, Sen P. The clinical spectrum of *Campylobacter fetus* infections: report of five cases and review of the literature. Quarterly J Med 1980; 49:431–442.
45. Pitkanen T, Ponka A, Pettersson T, Kosunen TU. *Campylobacter* enteritis in 188 hospitalized patients. Arch Int Med 1983; 143:215–219.
46. Wood CJ, Flemming V, Turnidge J, Thompson N, Atkins RC. *Campylobacter* peritonitis in continous peritoneal dialysis: a report of eight cases and a review of the literature. Am J Kidney Dis 1992; 19:257–263.
47. Delans RJ, Biuso JD, Saba SR, Ramierz G. Hemolytic uremic syndrome after *Campylobacter*-induced diarrhea in an adult. Arch Int Med 1984; 144:1074–1076.

48. Haq JA, Raham KM, Akbar MS. Haemolytic-uraemic syndrome and *Campylobacter*. Med J Aust 1985; 142:662-663.
49. Bremell T, Bjelle A, Fvedhem A. Rheumatic symptoms following an outbreak of *Campylobacter* enteritis: a five-year follow-up. Ann Rheum Dis 1991; 50:934–938.
50. Mishu B, Blaser MJ. Role of infection due to *Campylobacter jejuni* in the initiation of the Guillain-Barre syndrome. Clin Infect Dis 1993; 17:104–108.
51. Mishu B, Ilyas AA, Koski CL, Vriesendorp F, Cooke SD, Mithen FA, Blaser MJ. Serologic evidence of previous *Campylobacter jejuni* infection in patients with the Guillain-Barre syndrome. Ann Int Med 1993; 118:947–953.
52. Yuki N, Taki T, Inagaki F, Kasama T, Takahashi M, Saito K, Handa S, Miyatake T. A bacterium lipopolysaccharide that elicits Guillain-barre syndrome has a GM_1 ganglioside-like structure. J Exp Med 1993; 178:1771–1775.
53. Pichler H, Diridl G, Stickler K, Wolf D. Clinical efficacy of ciprofloxacin compared with placebo in bacterial diarrhea. Amer J Med 1987; 82(suppl 4A):329–332.
54. Goodman LJ, Trenholme GM, Kaplan RL, Segreti J, Hines D, Petrak R, Nelson JA, Mayer KW, Landau W, Parkhurst GW, Levin S. Empiric antimicrobial therapy of domestically acquired acute diarrhea in urban adults. Arch Int Med 1990; 150:541-546.
55. Winstrom J, Jertvorn M, Ekwall E, Norlin K, Soderquist V, Stromberg A, Lundholm R, Hogevik H, Lagergren L, Englund G, Norrby R. Empiric treatment of acute diarrheal disease with norfloxacin. Ann Int Med 1992; 117:202–208.
56. Williams MD, Schorling JB, Barrett L, Dudley SM, Orgel I, Koch WC, Shields DS, Thorson SM, Lohr JA, Guerrant RL. Early treatment of *Campylobacter jejuni* enteritis. Antimicrob Agents Chemother 1989; 33:248–250.
57. Petruccelli VP, Murphy GS, Sanchez JL, Waltz S, DeFraites R, Gelnett J, Haberberger RL, Echeverria P, Taylor DN. Treatment of traveller's diarrhea with ciprofloxacin and lopermaide. J Infect Dis 1992; 165:557–560.
58. Tabibian N, Clarridge JE, Smith JL, Alpert E, Shaw I, Graham DY. Clinical impact of stool cultures for *Campylobacter* in adults with acute or chronic diarrhea. Southern Med J 1987; 80:709–711.
59. Reina Borrell N, Serra A. Emergence of resistance to erythromycin and fluoroquinolones in thermo-tolerant *Campylobacter* strains isolated from feces 1987–1991. Eur J Clin Microbiol Infect Dis 1992; 11:1163–1166.
60. Taylor DE. Antimicrobial resistance of *Campylobacter jejuni* and *Campylobacter coli* to tetracycline, chloramphenicol and erythromycin. In: Nachamkin I, Blaser MJ, Thompkins LS, eds. *Campylobacter jejuni*: current status and future trends. Washington DC: Am Soc Microbiol 1992; 74–86.

9

Shigella Infections

KAREN L. KOTLOFF and MYRON M. LEVINE
University of Maryland School of Medicine, Baltimore, Maryland

I. INTRODUCTION

Shigella infections persist as a major cause of diarrheal morbidity and mortality throughout much of the world. Direct fecal-oral spread is fostered in situations where hygiene and sanitation are compromised, making control of transmission difficult. Antimicrobial therapy is often indicated for suspected shigellosis, thus raising complex issues associated with widespread use of antibiotics such as cost, availability, and emergence of resistant strains.

II. NOMENCLATURE AND CLASSIFICATION

Shigellae, gram-negative, nonlactose-fermenting, nonmotile bacilli of the family Enterobacteriaceae, are classified into four species: *S. dysenteriae, S. flexneri, S. boydii,* and *S. sonnei,* also designated Groups A, B, C, and D, respectively. Groups A, B, and C contain multiple serotypes (13, 6 [13 including subtypes] and 18, respectively), whereas Group D contains only a single serotype.

III. EPIDEMIOLOGY

A. Transmission

The predominant mode of transmission is by fecal-oral contact, and a low infectious inoculum renders Shigellae highly contagious for humans, the only natural host for *Shigella*. An example of the potential for *Shigella* to disseminate widely and rapidly comes from an outbreak that occurred at a mass outdoor gathering and involved an unusual antibiotic-resistant strain of *S. sonnei,* which made tracking possible (1). The gathering was held at a natural forest campsite with rudimentary sanitation facilities. Over a several week period, it was estimated that more than 50% of the 12,700 attendees became ill. Dispersal of the group resulted in nationwide dissemination of the organism during the two months after participants returned home.

Persons symptomatic with diarrhea are primarily responsible for transmission. This was exemplified by successful control of a daycare center outbreak of shigellosis that was resistant to all antibiotics routinely used to treat shigellosis in children. The outbreak was terminated by instituting appropriate interventions (hand washing, education, and excluding food preparers from child care) even though untreated convalescent children were permitted to return and untreated asymptomatic children were not excluded (2). Segregation of ill persons is a critical factor for interrupting transmission during institutional outbreaks (3).

Outbreaks related to contaminated food and water occur occasionally. The most common vehicle for food-borne transmission is salad; contamination is generally related to a breech in hygienic practices by an infected food handler (4). Although spread by fomites is possible, the organism generally survives poorly in the environment. In certain settings where disposal of human feces is inadequate, houseflies can serve as a mechanical vector for transmission. The impact of fly-borne transmission was demonstrated in a cross-over trial conducted in two Israeli military camps (5). As new recruits arrived, baited fly traps were introduced at one of the camps, while the other served as a control. After 11 weeks a second cohort of recruits arrived, and the fly traps were discontinued at the intervention camp and introduced to the control camp. During the intervention phases, there was a 64% decline in fly density associated with an 85% reduction in clinic visits for shigellosis and a 76% decrease in seroconversion to *Shigella* antibodies.

B. Incidence and Risk Factors

1. Industrialized Countries

Dramatic declines in the incidence of shigellosis in the United States followed improvements in hygiene and socioeconomic conditions. Currently endemic foci persist primarily among indigent persons living in inner cities and in some Native American communities (6). An elevated risk of shigellosis is also present in settings where hygiene is difficult to maintain, such as daycare centers (2), custodial institutions (3), travel to less-developed countries (7), and soldiers in field conditions (8). Venues supporting transmission of *Shigella* tend to suffer also from high rates of hepatitis A, a disease that shares many of the same risk factors as shigellosis (6).

The incidence of shigellosis in the United States has been estimated based on national laboratory surveillance data collected by the Centers for Disease Control and Prevention (CDC) (6). Isolation rates are calculated using the number of culture-confirmed cases reported weekly to the CDC by the state health departments, in concert with census estimates of the population. These figures most certainly represent an underestimation, because only about 5% of all symptomatic cases are reported. Since the 1960s, isolation rates of *Shigella* in the United States have followed periodic peaks and troughs ranging from 5.4 to 10.1 isolations per 100,000 population. The highest rates are reported from the western states (with most isolates coming from California), followed by the south, north central, and northeastern regions. Seasonal peaks occur in the late summer and fall.

Worldwide, the incidence of shigellosis is highest among children one to four years old, a trend also reflected in the CDC's surveillance data, which show the highest rates of culture-proven cases among children in this age group (6). Nonetheless, compared to other enteropathogens, *Shigella* infection is uncommon in the United States and accounts for fewer than 5% of episodes of diarrhea among children younger than five years (9).

Two notable demographic trends were reported in recent years from the United States. Between 1967 and 1988, marked increases occurred in the rate of infection among women of childbearing age (6). Presumed to reflect transmission from infected children to their mothers [in households with small children, transmission rates can exceed 50% (10)], this trend could be accounted for by the steady increase in the use of daycare facilities whose role in disseminating shigellosis to persons in the community is recognized (11). An increase in isolation of *S. flexneri* from adult men has been linked to oral-anal transmission among homosexuals (12).

2. *Developing Countries*

S. dysenteriae type 1, also known as Shiga bacillus, has been recognized as the major cause of epidemic dysentery for nearly 100 years. During the past 30 years, pandemics of Shiga dysentery have spread across Central America, Bangladesh, South Asia, and Central and East Africa (13–15). The pandemic that began in Central Africa in 1979 progressed to East Africa and has since become particularly problematic among refugee populations (15). The pandemic strains afflict up to 10% of the population, exhibit multiple antibiotic resistances and induce severe illness with high case fatality in all age groups (16,17). In general, both the incidence and the fatality rates are highest among the very young and the elderly.

Although epidemic Shiga dysentery is the most dramatic manifestation of *Shigella* infection in developing countries, the majority of *Shigella* infections are due to endemic shigellosis. Endemic *Shigella* is responsible for approximately 10% of all diarrheal episodes among children younger than five years living in developing countries (18). In Bangladesh alone, *Shigella* dysentery causes 75,000 deaths among children in this age group annually during peak epidemic years and an estimated 35,000 deaths in nonepidemic years (16). The Institute of Medicine estimates that each year *Shigella* causes 250 million cases of diarrhea and 650,000 deaths worldwide (19).

C. Epidemiologic Patterns According to Serogroup

The predominant serogroup of *Shigella* circulating in a community appears to be related to the level of development. *S. sonnei* is the main type found in industrialized countries while *S. flexneri*, followed by *S. dysenteriae*, predominates in less-developed countries. Endemic transmission of *S. dysenteriae* no longer occurs in the United States; this species is seen exclusively among traveler's returning from less-developed countries. There is a tendency for *S. sonnei* to replace *S. flexneri* as the predominant *Shigella* species as socioeconomic conditions improve (20). It has been postulated that widespread immunization against *S. sonnei* occurs in less-developed countries because surface water is often contaminated with bacterial species such as *Plesiomonas shigelloides* that may possess antigens that cross-react with *S. sonnei* (21). Observations in Israel lend credence to an alternate hypothesis. Increasing antimicrobial resistance was found among clinical strains of *S. sonnei* to a far greater extent than has been found among isolates of *S. flexneri*, suggesting that antibiotic pressures are responsible for the emergence of *S. sonnei* in more-developed countries (22).

IV. PATHOGENESIS

A. Inoculation

The low oral infective dose of *Shigella* when administered without buffer or food is unique among other bacterial enteropathogens. In adult volunteers, as few as 10 organisms, administered without buffer, were sufficient to cause dysentery (23). In contrast, the infective dose without buffer of *Vibrio cholerae* is 10^8 cfu (24) and for enterotoxigenic *Escherichia coli* 10^{10} cfu (25). The relative acid resistance of *Shigella* compared to other enteropathogens may enable the organism to survive the gastric acid barrier (26).

B. Plasmid Encoded Virulence Factors and Inflammatory Response

After oral inoculation, Shigellae pass to the terminal ileum and colon where they invade and proliferate within enterocytes, produce cell death, incite an inflammatory reaction, and induce intestinal fluid secretion. This multistep process involves many highly regulated virulence properties encoded by both chromosomal and plasmid genes (Table 1).

A cardinal pathogenic feature is invasion of intestinal epithelial cells. This process involves a bacteria–host cell interaction in which Shigellae penetrate host cells by a mechanism that resembles phagocytosis in that it requires actin polymerization and myosin accumulation at the site of entry (27). The specialized antigen-processing cells of the intestine called M cells, located over mucosal lymphoid follicles, appear to be the major initial target of cell entry (28). Invasion of epithelial cells occurs at a later time and requires bacterial contact with the basolateral cell surface that is not exposed to the intestinal lumen (29). Invasion requires the expression of a series of genes located on a 31 kb region of the 140 MDA virulence plasmid (30). These include the *ipa*B–D, which encode invasion polypeptides, and the *mxi-spa*-encoded Ipa secretory apparatus (31).

Table 1 Critical Steps in the Pathogenesis of *Shigella*-Associated Invasive Diarrhea

Oral inoculation
Invasion of specialized antigen-processing "M cells" overlying lymphoid follicles in the terminal ileum and colon
Translocation to intraepithelial and subepithelial spaces
Early inflammatory response with destruction of follicular architecture
Proinflammatory cytokine production
Polymorphonuclear leukocyte (PMN) chemotaxis
PMN migration from lamina propria to lumen, disrupting intercellular spaces
Mucosal ulceration
Formation of microabscesses
Invasion of epithelial cells at basolateral surface via endocytosis
Lysis of endocytotic vacuole with entry into cytoplasm
Intracytoplasmic proliferation
Intracellular movement via manipulation of host cell cytoskeleton
Formation of cellular protrusions that are endocytosed by adjacent epithelial cells, repeating the cycle
Eventual epithelial cell apoptosis

After entry into M cells, Shigellae are translocated to the intraepithelial and subepithelial areas, often remaining extracellular (28). This process evokes an intense inflammatory response characterized by edema and infiltration of the lamina propria with polymorphonuclear (PMN) leukocytes and mononuclear cells, and formation of mucosal microabscesses and ulcerations. The PMN migrate through the intercellular space to reach luminal organisms. Migration by PMN may actually facilitate bacterial invasion of epithelial cells by disrupting the intercellular space and opening a pathway for invasive organisms to access the basolateral surface of enterocytes (32).

Within epithelial cells, Shigellae express IpaB, which lyses the phagocytic vacuole and allows organisms to gain access to the cytosol where they multiply rapidly and are free to scavenge nutrients (33). To navigate intracellularly and to spread from cell-to-cell, Shigellae move in a polar fashion again by reorganizing the host cell cytoskeleton, a process that is mediated by the protein encoded by *ics*A (also designated *vir*G) (34). Ultimately some bacteria are propelled toward the cell surface, which leads to the development of protrusions that penetrate the basolateral membrane of adjacent epithelial cells. Finally, the Shigellae lyse their two surrounding membranes via expression of the plasmid-encoded *ics*B and reach the cytoplasm of the adjacent cell (35). Intracellular bacteria eventually kill host epithelial cells by a mechanism that involves blocking respiration (36). As contiguous cells die, additional areas of mucosal ulceration and hemorrhage are formed.

A well-established animal model of *Shigella* pathogenicity is the Sereny test. The Sereny test evaluates the ability of Shigellae to elicit purulent keratoconjunctivitis in guinea pigs following inoculation into the conjunctival sac and demonstrates the ability of the organism to invade epithelial cells and evoke an inflammatory reaction (37).

C. Chromosomal Virulence Factors

The *Shigella* chromosome contains numerous genes involved in regulating plasmid-encoded virulence properties such as invasion, intercellular spread, and host-cell death. Some regulatory loci on the chromosome are sensitive to environmental signals such as temperature and osmolarity (38). Teleologically, these feedback systems allow bacterial metabolic expenditure to be conserved until the milieu of the human intestine is encountered.

The *Shigella* chromosome also contains virulence genes. Expression of the lipopolysaccharide (LPS) molecule (smooth phenotype) is chromosomally encoded (39), with the exception of *S. sonnei*, which carries the genes for expression of the O antigen on the 120 MDa virulence plasmid (40), and *S. dysenteriae* 1, which contains 6 MDa plasmid that encodes O-antigen expression in conjunction with chromosomal genes (41). In experimental models, the

Lipid A, or endotoxin component of LPS, induces a range of pathophysiologic reactions, including fever, hypotension, and disseminated intravascular coagulation (42). Accordingly, this molecule has been incriminated as a cause of the severe systemic illness associated with shigellosis, and LPS also plays a role in bacterial resistance to host defenses such as opsonization, phagocytosis, and intracellular killing (42).

Other chromosomal genes allow *Shigella* to scavenge nutrients essential for survival. These include *iucA-iut* (which encodes the siderophore aerobactin) (43) and multiple *aro* genes of the paraaminobenzoic acid (PABA) biosynthesis pathway (44).

D. Toxins

Until recently, the pathogenesis of the watery diarrhea that typically precedes dysentery (45) and that is often the sole clinical manifestation of mild infection (46) remained enigmatic. Several observations in animals have strongly predicted the existence of enterotoxins in *S. flexneri* (47). Two novel *Shigella* enterotoxins have been incriminated as the likely mediators of the watery diarrhea often seen with shigellosis. These enterotoxins, designated *ShET*1 and *ShET*2, are excreted by Shigellae grown in Fe^{++}-depleted medium. The *ShET*1 gene has been cloned from the *S. flexneri* 2a chromosome and the *ShET*2 gene is located on the *Shigella* virulence plasmid (48,49). The enterotoxic activity of *ShET*1 has been demonstrated in the rabbit ileal loop (where it elicits fluid accumulation) and in the Ussing chamber model (where it increases short circuit current). Sera from volunteers recovering from infection with wild type *S. flexneri* 2a contain antibodies that neutralize the Ussing chamber activity of *ShET*1 and that recognize *ShET*2 proteins on western blot.

Although all *Shigella* species produce varying quantities of exotoxins, only *S. dysenteriae* 1 produces the highly potent cytotoxin called Shiga toxin. Shiga toxin is a chromosomally encoded 70 kDa heterodimeric protein that comprises an enzymatically active A subunit and five smaller B subunits, similar in structure to cholera toxin and the heat-labile toxin of *E. coli*. The B subunit is responsible for binding of the holotoxin molecule to host-cell glycosphingolipid globotriosylceramide (Gb3) receptors. The toxin enters the cell by receptor-mediated endocytosis whereupon the A subunit irreversibly inhibits protein synthesis by ribosomes (50,51).

The precise role played by Shiga toxin in the pathogenesis of dysentery is still not entirely clear. Mutants of *S. dysenteriae* 1 that are invasive but do not express Shiga toxin, nevertheless, have caused typical Shiga diarrhea and dysentery when fed to monkeys and volunteers, although less endothelial damage to intestinal microvasculature is evident (52). One hypothesis is that Shiga toxin increases the severity of disease by destroying the endothelium in the local capillary loops and causing ischemia in the intestinal tissue. Enterohemorrhagic *E. coli* (EHEC) produces a biologically similar toxin and, like *S. dysenteriae*, induces an illness with bloody diarrhea that is associated with the hemolytic-uremic syndrome, further supporting a role for toxin in the pathogenesis of these events. The thrombotic microangipathy that characterizes hemolytic-uremic syndrome is thought to result from the action of systemically absorbed toxin on endothelial cells.

V. CLINICAL FINDINGS

A. Gastroenteritis

Shigellosis typically evolves through several phases. The incubation period is one to four days, but may be as long as eight days with *S. dysenteriae* (52). First there is fever and other constitutional symptoms such as headache, malaise, anorexia, and occasional vomiting, followed in several hours by watery diarrhea (Table 2). However, progression within a few hours or days to frank dysentery may occur with frequent small stools containing blood and mucus, accompanied by lower abdominal cramps and rectal tenesmus. Patients with severe infection may pass more than 20 dysenteric stools in one day (53). With repeated infections by the same serotype, illness is absent or attenuated and excretion is diminished (18,54,55). Most cases of shigellosis in the United States are due to *S. sonnei* (6), which more commonly results in mild disease (18,46,56).

B. Extraintestinal Manifestations

A variety of unusual but important extraintestinal manifestations may occur. Seizures are reported in 12–45% of hospitalized children and are the most common extraintestinal manifestation (57,58). Seizures frequently occur in the presence of fever and may precede the onset of diarrhea. Encephalopathy is encountered rarely; symptoms include headache, lethargy, confusion, and hal-

Table 2 Clinical Manifestations of Shigellosis

Fever
Headache
Malaise
Anorexia
Diarrhea
Dysentery
Abdominal cramps
Rectal tenesmus

lucinations (58). Microangiopathic hemolytic anemia can complicate infection with Shiga toxin-producing organisms, manifesting as the hemolytic-uremic syndrome in children and as thrombotic thrombocytopenia purpura in adults (59). Another hematologic complication encountered with *S. dysenteriae* 1 infection is a leukemoid reaction with polymorphonuclear counts exceeding 50,000–100,000/mm^3 (60). Reports of focal infections such as *Shigella* meningitis (56), arthritis (61), splenic abscess (62), and osteomyelitis (63) have been rare.

C. Acute Complications

Most episodes of shigellosis in otherwise healthy individuals are self-limited and resolve within 5–7 days without sequelae. Acute, life-threatening complications occur most frequently among infants and young children living in developing countries, particularly when there is concomitant malnutrition (Table 3) (64). Although epidemics of *S. dysenteriae* 1 are associated with dramatic increases in mortality, in highly endemic areas any species of *Shigella* may cause severe illness or death. Dehydration, hyponatremia, and hypoglycemia are the most common metabolic derangements associated with a poor outcome (16,65,66). Intestinal complications include toxic megacolon, rectal prolapse from tenesmus, and intestinal perforation (64). *Shigella* sepsis is rare. It occurs most often in young malnourished children and rarely in other hosts and can be fatal (67). In the United States, *Shigella* bacteremia has occasionally been reported among HIV-infected and other immunocompromised patients (68).

D. Long-Term Complications

Persistent diarrhea and malnutrition are long-term complications of shigellosis seen primarily among children from developing countries (Table 3). The du-

Table 3 Complications of Shigellosis

Acute	Subacute	Late
Seizures	Hemolytic-uremic syndrome	Reactive arthritis
Encephalopathy	Thrombotic thrombocytopenia purpura	Reiter's syndrome
Leukemoid reaction	Persistent diarrhea	Malnutrition
Focal infection	Hypoproteinemia	
Dehydration		
Hypoglycemia		
Hyponatremia		
Toxic megacolon		
Rectal prolapse		
Intestinal perforation		
Sepsis		

ration of illness due to *Shigella* exceeds 14 days in 15–20% of children from these areas (69). Persistent diarrhea can have a profound negative impact on nutritional status (70). This can be compounded by the common occurrence of intestinal protein loss in shigellosis. Extensive damage to the intestinal mucosa of young children can cause marked exudation of proteins, eventually leading to hypoproteinemia and kwashiorkor (71).

An uncommon late sequela of *Shigella* infection seen primarily in adults is reactive inflammatory arthritis, alone (72) or as part of a constellation of arthritis, conjunctivitis, and urethritis known as Reiter's syndrome (Table 3) (73). Arthritis has an acute onset usually two to four weeks after the intestinal illness and most often follows infection with *S. flexneri* serotypes. Joint symptoms can range from mild arthralgia to severe polyarthritis, which may become chronic in about 10% of cases. Individuals with the HLA-B27 histocompatibility antigen are predisposed, accounting for approximately one-half of the cases (74). To explain the pathogenesis of arthritis, the phenomena of molecular mimicry has been invoked, in which the host immune response to a preceding *Shigella* infection cross-reacts with self antigens (75). It has been suggested that there are "arthritogenic" strains that carry a small plasmid encoding a cross-reactive peptide (76). Another possible mechanism is pathogen-induced immunomodulation with activation of autoreactive T cells at synovial sites (77).

VI. IMMUNITY

A. Infection-Derived Immunity

Wild type *Shigella* infection confers serotype-specific immunity. The incidence of disease declines with the duration of stay in high-risk settings such as military camps (78). In endemic areas, the incidence of shigellosis peaks during the first 5 years of life and declines thereafter, suggesting that immunity develops after repeated exposures during childhood (46). Compelling evidence of natural immunity comes from a longitudinal study of a cohort of Chilean children in whom primary *Shigella* infection conferred 76% protective efficacy against reinfection with the same serotype (18). Finally, adult volunteers who were experimentally infected with either *S. sonnei* or *S. flexneri* were significantly protected against illness following rechallenge with the homologous strain (64–74% protective efficacy) (54,55).

B. Protective Immune Responses

The specific immune responses that confer protection against shigellosis have not been clearly elucidated. Several lines of evidence suggest that anti-LPS antibodies are protective. Most notably, naturally acquired immunity appears to be serotype specific (18,54,55,79). Furthermore, Israeli soldiers who lacked anti-LPS antibody were significantly more likely than seropositives to develop illness following exposure to the homologous *S. sonnei* or *S. flexneri* strain during military camp outbreaks (80). Similarly, volunteers who received bivalent *Salmonella typhi* Ty21a-*S. sonnei* vaccine but lacked anti-LPS antibody were 3–7 times more likely to develop shigellosis following wild type *S. sonnei* challenge, compared with seropositive vaccine recipients (81).

Immune responses to *Shigella* plasmid-encoded outer membrane proteins (*ipa*A, B, C, and D and virG) are also encountered (82). In contrast to the O antigen, these peptides are shared among the four serogroups; however, their clinical significance is uncertain.

Although systemic humeral immune responses have been correlated with resistance to shigellosis, the first line of defense must occur at the mucosal level. The importance of mucosal immunity is illustrated by the efficacy of passively transferred oral immunoglobulin in preventing shigellosis (83) and the possible role of secretory antibody in limiting the duration of illness (84). Breast milk sampled from mothers living in highly endemic areas contains *Shigella* antibodies (85). This may explain the protective effects of breast feeding on the severity of shigellosis among infants from developing countries (86). Although a specific immunoprotective response at the level of the intestinal mucosa has not been identified, volunteer studies have suggested that the number of O-specific IgA antibody-secreting mononuclear cells circulating in the peripheral blood seven days after vaccination is a measure of intestinal priming that correlates with vaccine efficacy (87).

VII. DIAGNOSIS

A. Stool Microscopy

If shigellosis is suspected, an examination for fecal leukocytes should be performed as follows. A drop of fresh stool (preferably mucus) is mixed with 0.1 ml of methylene blue stain on a glass slide with a cover slip and immediately examined by light microscopy. Large numbers of fecal leukocytes in a patient with acute diarrheal illness suggests that a bacterial pathogen has invaded the colonic mucosa and produced inflammation (88). Stool microscopy is also useful for distinguishing enteroinvasive bacterial infection from amebic dysentery (89). However, this test is nonspecific because other bacterial pathogens, such as nontyphoidal *Salmonella, Campylobacter jejuni, Yersinia enterocolitica,* and enteroinvasive *E. coli*, can cause dysentery accompanied by fecal leukocytes.

B. Culture

There is no commercially available serologic assay to aid in the diagnosis of shigellosis. Definitive diagnosis of *Shigella* infection is made by culturing the organism from a stool specimen. Areas of fecal mucus are optimal for sampling. If whole stool is not available, comparable culture results can be obtained by gently swabbing the rectal mucosa with a cottontip applicator inserted into the anus (90). Shigellae are extremely fastidious and survive poorly in stool samples that are left in ambient temperature; therefore, the sample should be fresh. If it cannot be plated quickly onto solid media, the specimen should be inoculated into transport media and refrigerated. Buffered glycerol saline is preferable to Cary Blair as a transport media (91). Culture of two or more stool specimens before initiation of antibiotic therapy increases the likelihood of isolating *Shigella*.

Media appropriate for culturing *Shigella* include mildly selective media, such as MacConkey, deoxycholate citrate, and eosin-methylene blue, and more highly selective media such as xylose-deoxycholate (XLD), Hektoen, and *Salmonella-Shigella* (SS) agar. Most laboratories use a combination of the two. If *S. dysenteriae* is suspected, Tergitol-7 agar is particularly useful, but XLD can also isolate this serogroup. Yield of culture can be enhanced by the addition of enrichment media such as gram-negative (GN) broth. Susceptibility testing should be performed. Most commercial laboratories serogroup but serotyping is usually delegated to reference laboratories.

It should be kept in mind that stool culture for enteric pathogens is one of the most costly microbiologic tests. To be cost effective, patient characteristics have been sought that are associated with a low likelihood of identifying a bacterial enteropathogen. It is recommended that a stool smear be evaluated for leukocytes in patients who have symptoms suggestive of enteroinvasive bacterial enteritis, namely abrupt onset of diarrhea, frequent stools (more than four per day), and no vomiting before the onset of diarrhea. If more than five leukocytes are detected per high-power field, a stool culture should be performed. This algorithm detects 70% of those with positive cultures and results in unnecessary cultures on 5% of negatives (92). On the other hand, published results indicate that bacterial enteropathogens are identified in fewer than 1% of adults and children with diarrhea who have been hospitalized for more than three days. It is recommended that stool cultures from these patients be restricted unless suggestive clinical or epidemiologic features are present (93).

VIIII. TREATMENT

A. Supportive Therapy and Oral Rehydration

Careful attention to the patient's fluid and electrolyte balance with correction of deficits and replacement of ongoing losses is a central feature of management. Oral rehydration therapy is effective in treating dehydration due to *Shigella* diarrhea (94). The clinician should be alerted to other possible complications of shigellosis that may require specific therapy, such as seizures and intestinal perforation.

B. Nonspecific Antidiarrheal Therapy

No evidence suggests that common antidiarrheal preparations, such as kaolin-pectin formulas, lactobacilli, or bismuth-salicylate, have a significant beneficial effect, nor does evidence suggest that these agents are deleterious and therefore contraindicated. Agents that suppress intestinal motility, such as diphenoxylate, loperamide, and tincture of opium, are not generally recommended in known or suspected shigellosis because of safety concerns. Animals with shigellosis had higher mortality when given opium (95). Diphenoxylate appeared to prolong the clinical and bacteriologic course of experimental shigellosis in volunteers (96). In children with watery diarrhea, shock and enterocolitis were reported after treatment with loperamide (97,98).

Nonetheless, a double-blind, placebo-controlled, randomized trial recently demonstrated that adults with dysentery due to *Shigella* (predominantly *S. flexneri*) or the closely related enteroinvasive *E. coli* who were treated with loperamide plus ciprofloxacin had significantly fewer diarrheal stools (median 2.0 stools) compared with subjects treated with ciprofloxacin alone (median 6.5 stools), and a significantly shorter duration of diarrhea (19 hours versus 42 hours, respectively) (99). Adverse effects from loperamide were not detected.

These findings suggest that loperamide may offer additional benefit to ciprofloxacin in adults with *Shigella* dysentery. However, loperamide should not be given to children, debilitated, or immunocompromised patients, to patients who may be infected with ciprofloxacin-resistant strains, or to those infected with *S. dysenteriae*.

C. Antibiotic Therapy

1. General Approach

Many controlled clinical trials have demonstrated that appropriate antibiotics significantly decrease the duration of fever, diarrhea, intestinal protein loss, and excretion of the pathogen in shigellosis. Most patients in these studies were infected with either *S. flexneri* or *S. dysenteriae* (71,100). The advantages of treating *S. sonnei*, which is usually self-limited, are less clear. For these patients, benefit is likely to be greatest when therapy is initiated early in the course of illness. Nonetheless, this cumulative experience, in conjunction with the fact that treatment may interrupt person-to-person transmission, provides the rationale for treating patients with shigellosis with antibiotics. This must be reconciled with the reality that only a few antibiotics have proven to be clinically efficacious (although many show activity in vitro), and resistant *Shigella* strains may eventually emerge from widespread use of these antibiotics.

Several principles can be used to guide the choice of antimicrobials to treat shigellosis. The drug should achieve concentrations in serum well above the minimal inhibitory concentration (MIC) of the infecting strain of *Shigella*. Experience with nonabsorbable antibiotics with in vitro activity against *Shigella*, such as furazolidone (101), provide evidence that stool concentrations of the drug in the absence of serum levels are not sufficient to ensure a satisfactory clinical outcome. In contrast, ampicillin and trimethoprim-sulfamethoxazole (TMP-SMX), administered intravenously, are effective therapeutic agents, even when appreciable fecal levels were not achieved (102,103).

Not all antibiotics that exceed the minimal inhibitory serum concentrations are effective. In one small study, the therapeutic and bacteriologic cure rates of oral amoxicillin were inferior (though not significantly) to the less well-absorbed (i.e. higher fecal concentrations) analogue ampicillin despite higher serum concentrations of the former (104). Oral cephalosporins such as cefixime (105) and the parenterally administered cephalosporin cephamandole (106) are not consistently effective in treating shigellosis despite in vitro susceptibility and appreciable serum concentrations. Failure of cephalosporins has been attributed to their lack of intracellular activity. An exception is the reported efficacy of parenteral ceftriaxone, but this may be related to excretion of its active form in bile (107).

2. *Treatment Options (Table 4)*

Susceptible strains can be treated with ampicillin (but not amoxicillin) or TMP-SMX. These drugs are inexpensive, available in oral form, and safe for children. However, since the mid 1980s, strains of *S. dysenteriae, S. flexneri,* and *S. sonnei* that are resistant to one or both drugs have been identified with increasing frequency in Asia, Africa, and North America (108). For infections acquired in the United States for which susceptibility is unknown, TMP-SMX is given for 5 days, unless resistance is suspected or proven. Fewer than 5% of domestically acquired isolates are resistant to TMP-SMX while about 10% are resistant to ampicillin (108). However, if there is a history of recent foreign travel in the patient or a household member with diarrhea, approximately 20% of isolates may be resistant to TMP-SMX and 60% may be resistant to ampicillin (108). In this instance, the quinolones (nalidixic acid, ciprofloxacin, norfloxacin) and third generation cephalosporins (ceftriaxone) are good choices.

In developing countries, most strains are now resistant to tetracyclines, chloramphenicol, and sulfonamides. Nalidixic acid has been used most often to treat *Shigella* in areas where these multiresistant strains prevail. In contrast to other quinolones, nalidixic acid is inexpensive. However, introduction into communities has been followed by rapid emergence of chromosomally mediated resistance among *Shigella* and other *Enterobacteriaceae* (109).

Table 4 Antimicrobial Therapy of Shigellosis

Clinical venue	Antibiotic	Route	Adult Dose	Pediatric Dose
Empiric therapy				
Endemic infection	TMP/SMX	PO,IV	160 mg TMP/800 mg SMX *bid* × 5d	5 mg/kg TMP/25 mg/kg SMX *bid* × 5d
Travel-related	Ciprofloxacin	PO,IV	500 mg *bid* × 1–5 d	Not recommended
	Norfloxacin	PO	400 mg *bid* × 1-5d	Not recommended
	Nalidixic acid	PO	Not commonly used	55 mg/kg/day divided into 4 doses × 5d
	Ceftriaxone	IV, IM	1–4 g divided into 1–2 doses × 5 d	50 mg/kg/day divided into 1–2 doses × 5d
Susceptible strains	Ampicillin	PO, IV	500 mg *qid* × 5 d	25 mg/kg/day divided into 4 doses × 5d

TMP/SMX = trimethoprim/sulfamethoxazole; *bid* = twice daily; *qid* = four times daily; d = days.

Most *Shigella* strains that are resistant to ampicillin, TMP-SMX, and nalidixic acid remain susceptible to the newer quinolones. In controlled trials, ciprofloxacin is more effective than ampicillin for treatment of adults with shigellosis (110), and in smaller studies norfloxacin and enoxacin are comparable to nalidixic acid or TMP-SMX and superior to placebo (111-113). In developing countries where costs of therapy are a great concern, short one-to-three day courses of oral quinolones are effective for milder illness caused by serotypes other than *S. dysenteriae* 1; however, a five-day course of therapy should be administered for severe illness or for suspected Shiga dysentery (114). With the exception of severely ill patients, therapy can be administered orally.

Two concerns have been raised regarding the use of quinolones. The safety of these agents in children has been questioned because of the observation that they cause arthropathy when given in high doses to immature animals that belong to several different species. This has not been a major problem to date in humans (115). However, these concerns have stopped the Food and Drug Administration from granting approval of the newer quinolones for use in children. Nalidixic acid is approved for use in children older than two months because the review predated the observations of arthropathy in animals.

A second concern is that the high cost of the newer quinolones render them unaffordable within the constraints of the health-care budgets of many developing countries. Options for inexpensive oral therapy are thus limited in these settings. Pivmecillinam has been shown to be more effective than nalidixic acid and equivalent to TMP-SMX in controlled trials of acute shigellosis in children (116,117). It may provide a useful alternative, but it is expensive, and resistance has already been reported. Injectable cephalosporins, such as ceftriaxone, are effective but impractical in developing countries. There is a pressing need for more effective control measures, such as vaccination and improved hygiene and sanitation.

IX. CONTROL AND PREVENTION

A. Sanitation and Hygiene

Prevention of shigellosis could be achieved with provision of a safe water supply and sanitary disposal of fecally contaminated materials; however, the cost of these measures is beyond the resources of many developing countries. Interruption of transmission by individual hygienic behavior such as hand washing is also effective in controlling endemic transmission and in interrupting outbreaks (2,118), but these measures are difficult to implement on a large scale in developing countries. Segregation of ill persons is an important factor in interrupting transmission in settings where hygienic practices are difficult to enforce, such as outbreaks occurring in institutions for the mentally handicapped (3). Antibiotics should not be used to prevent transmission.

B. Vaccine Development

1. Noninvasive Live Oral Attenuated Vaccines

As cited above, observations in field settings and in experimental models indicate that natural infection induces protection against illness following homologous reinfection. These findings suggest that if a safe vaccine could be developed that mimics natural infection, protective immunity could be induced. When parenteral killed whole-cell vaccines failed to elicit immunity in volunteers despite stimulating high levels of anti-LPS antibody (119), efforts were shifted toward developing oral vaccines to target the mucosal immune system and simulate natural immunity.

During the 1960s, two prototypic live, oral attenuated *Shigella* vaccines were developed that were highly efficacious in field trials. It is now appreciated that the noninvasiveness is a result of spontaneous deletions of the plasmid genes encoding invasion antigens and intercellular spread of *Shigella* (120). In field trials in China, the T32-ISTRATI strain of *S. flexneri* 2a appeared to provide protection against infection with heterologous *S. flexneri* serotypes (121). It should be noted that heterologous protection has not been observed elsewhere in either humans or animals (79,122). The second live, oral vaccine was composed of various combinations of streptomycin-dependent *Shigella* strains (79). However, drawbacks were recognized that precluded continued use of these vaccines, such as the need for multiple doses and the large number of vaccine organisms required per dose (which affected cost), occasional genetic reversions (123), and the need for annual booster doses to maintain protection (124). Thus while these sentinel trials demonstrated that prevention of shigellosis through vaccination is an attainable goal, it was recognized that more immunogenic and genetically stable vaccines would be needed for effective public health tools.

2. Invasive Oral Attenuated Hybrids and Deletion Mutant Vaccines

Molecular technology is currently being used to develop live, attenuated oral vaccine candidates. Many modern vaccines have been designed to invade the intestinal epithelium to increase stimulation of the mucosal immune system, while lacking full virulence to ensure clinical safety. There are two areas of active research. One approach is to construct hybrid vaccines in which critical *Shigella* genes (such as the chromosomal genes responsible for expression of the putatively immunoprotective O antigen and the invasiveness plasmid) are introduced into a commensal *E. coli* (125) or other carrier strains (81). The second strategy involves making defined deletions in virulence genes of wild type Shigellae or genes that affect the ability to survive or proliferate in vivo, for example *vir*G, *aro, gua*B-A, and *iuc*A-*iut* (126–129). Several of these constructs have entered clinical trial (126–128).

3. *Parenteral Conjugate Vaccines*

Robinson and Schneerson have pursued parenteral vaccines consisting of detoxified O-specific polysaccharides of *S. dysenteriae* 1, *S. flexneri* 2a, and *S. sonnei* conjugated to a protein to create T-cell-independent antigens (130). They hypothesize that serum anti-LPS IgG antibodies will confer immunity because these antibodies are detectable in the intestinal fluid and may extravasate into the submucosa to provide protection at the sites of invasion. Preliminary data from a field trial in Israel demonstrates that the *S. sonnei* construct can confer short-term protective immunity (131).

REFERENCES

1. Wharton M, Speigel RA, Horan JM, Tauxe RV, Wells JG, Barg N, Herndon J, Meriwether RA, MacCormack JN, Levine RH. A large outbreak of antibiotic-resistant shigellosis at a mass gathering. J Infect Dis 1990; 162:1324–1328.
2. Centers for Disease Control and Prevention. Multiply resistant shigellosis in a day-care center - Texas. MMWR 1986; 35:753–755.
3. Mahoney FJ, Farley TA, Burbank DF, Leslie NH, McFarland LM. Evaluation of an intervention program for the control of an outbreak of shigellosis among institutionalized persons. J Infect Dis 1993; 168:1177–1180.
4. Black RE, Craun GF, Blake PA. Epidemiology of common-source outbreaks of shigellosis in the Unites States, 1961–1975. Am J Epidemiol 1978; 108:47-52.
5. Cohen D, Green M, Block C, Slepon R, Ambar R, Wasserman SS, Levine MM. Reduction of transmission of shigellosis by control of houseflies (*Musca domestica*). Lancet 1991; 337:993–997.
6. Lee LA, Shapiro CN, Hargrett-Bean N, Tauxe RV. Hyperendemic shigellosis in the United States: A review of surveillance data for 1967–1988. J Infect Dis 1991; 164:894–900.
7. Parsonnet J, Green KD, Gerber AR, Tauxe RV, Vellej Aguilar OJ, Blake PA. *Shigella dysenteriae* type 1 infections in US travellers to Mexico, 1988. Lancet 1989; 2:543–545.
8. Sharp TW, Thornton SA, Wallace MR, Defraites RF, Sanchez JL, Batchelor RA, Rozmajzl RJ, Hanson K, Echeverria P, Kapikian AZ, Xiang XJ, Estes MK, Burans JP. Diarrheal disease among military personnel during Operation Restore Hope, Somalia. Am J Trop Med Hyg 1995; 52:188–193.
9. Kotloff KL, Wasserman SS, Steciak JY, Tall BD, Losonsky GA, Nair P, Morris JG., Jr., Levine MM. Acute diarrhea in Baltimore children attending an outpatient clinic. Pediatr Infect Dis J 1988; 7:753–759.
10. Wilson R, Feldman RA, Davis J, LaVenture M. Family illness associated with *Shigella* infection: The interrelationship of age of the index patient and the age of household members in acquisition of illness. J Infect Dis 1981; 143:130–132.

11. Centers for Disease Control and Prevention. Shigellosis in child day care centers - Lexington-Fayette County, Kentucky, 1991. MMWR 1992; 41:440–442.
12. Tauxe RV, McDonald RC, Hargrett-Bean N, Blake PA. The persistence of *Shigella flexneri* in the United States: Increasing role of adult males. Am J Public Health 1988; 78:1432–1435.
13. Mata L, Gangarosa E, Caceres A, Perera D, Mejicanos M. Epidemic *Shiga bacillus* dysentery in Central America. I. Etiologic investigations in Guatemala, 1969. J Infect Dis 1970; 122:170–180.
14. Rahaman MM, Khan MM, Aziz KM, Islam MS, Kibriya AK. An outbreak of dysentery caused by *S. dysenteriae* type 1 on a Coral Island in the Bay of Bengal. J Infect Dis 1975; 132:15–19.
15. Centers for Disease Control and Prevention. Health status of displaced persons following civil war-Burundi, December 1993-January 1994. MMWR 1994; 43:701–703.
16. Bennish ML, Wojtyniak BJ. Mortality due to shigellosis: Community and hospital data. Rev Infect Dis 1991; 13[Suppl 4]:S245–S251.
17. Tuttle J, Ries AA, Chimba RM, Perera CU, Bean NH, Griffin PM. Antimicrobial-resistant epidemic *Shigella dysenteriae* type 1 in Zambia: Modes of transmission. J Infect Dis 1995; 171:371–375.
18. Ferreccio C, Prado V, Ojeda A, Cayyazo M, Abrego P, Guers L, Levine MM. Epidemiologic patterns of acute diarrhea and endemic *Shigella* infections in children in a poor periurban setting in Santiago, Chile. Am J Epidemiol 1991; 134:614–627.
19. Institute of Medicine. The prospects for immunizing against *Shigella spp*. In: New Vaccine Development: Establishing Priorities: Vol. 2. Diseases of Importance in Developing Countries. Washington, D.C.: National Academy Press, 1986:329–337.
20. Kostrzewki J, Stypulkowska-Misiurewicz H. Changes in the epidemiology of dysentery in Poland and the situation in Europe. Arch Immunol Ther Exp 1968; 16:429–451.
21. Sack DA, Hoque ATMS, Hug A, Etheridge M. Is protection against shigellosis induced by natural infection with *Plesiomanas shigelloides*? Lancet 1994; 343:1413–1415.
22. Ashkenazi S, May-Zahav M, Dinari G, Gabbay U, Zilberberg R, Samra Z. Recent trends in the epidemiology of *Shigella* species in Israel. Clin Infect Dis 1993; 17:897–899.
23. DuPont HL, Levine MM, Hornick RB, Formal SB. Inoculum size in shigellosis and implications for expected mode of transmission. J Infect Dis 1989; 159:1126–1128.
24. Cash RA, Music SI, Libonati JP, Snyder MJ, Wenzel RP, Hornick RB. Response in man to infection with *Vibrio cholerae*. I. Clinical, serologic, and bacteriologic responses to a known inoculum. J Infect Dis 1974; 129:45–52.
25. Levine MM, Caplan ES, Waterman D, Cash RA, Hornick RB, Snyder MJ. Diarrhea caused by *Escherichia coli* that produces only heat-stable enterotoxin. Infect Immun 1977; 17:78–82.

26. Gorden J, Small PLC. Acid resistance in enteric bacteria. Infect Immun 1993; 61:364–367.
27. Clerc P, Sansonetti PJ. Entry of *Shigella flexneri* into HeLa cells: Evidence for directed phagocytosis involving actin polymerization and myosin accumulation. Infect Immun 1987; 55:2681–2688.
28. Sansonetti PJ, Rondel J, Canted R, Provost M-C, Huerre M. Infection of rabbit Peyer's patches by *Shigella flexneri*: Effect of adhesive or invasive bacterial phenotypes on follicle-associated epithelium. Infect Immun 1996; 64:2752–2764.
29. Mounier J, Vasselon R, Hellio R, Lesourd M, Sansonetti PJ. *Shigella flexneri* enters human colonic Caco-2 epithelial cells through the basolateral pole. Infect Immun 1992; 60:237–248.
30. Menard R, Sansonetti PJ, Parsot C. Nonpolar mutagenesis of the *ipa* genes defines IpaB, IpaC, and IpaD as effectors of *Shigella flexneri* entry into epithelial cells. J Bacteriol 1993; 175:5899–5906.
31. Menard R, Sansonetti PJ, Parsot C. The secretion of the *Shigella flexneri* Ipa invasins is induced by the epithelial cell and controlled by IpaB and IpaD. EMBO J 1994; 13:5293–5302.
32. Perdomo JJ, Gounon P, Sansonetti. Polymorphonuclear leukocyte transmigration promotes invasion of colonic epithelial monolayer by *Shigella flexneri*. J Clin Invest 1994; 93:633–643.
33. High N, Mounier J, Provost MC, Sansonetti PJ. IpaB of *Shigella flexneri* causes entry into epithelial cells and escape from the phagocytic vacuole. EMBO J 1992; 11:1991–1999.
34. Bernardini M L, Mounier J, D'Hauteville H, Coquis-Rondon M, Sansonetti PJ. Identification of *icsA*, a plasmic locus of *Shigella flexneri* that governs bacterial intra- and intercellular spread through interaction with F-actin. Proc Natl Acad Sci USA 1989; 86:3867–3871.
35. Allaoui A, Mounier J, Pervost MC, Sansonetti PJ, Parsot C. *ics*B: A *Shigella flexneri* virulence gene necessary for the lysis of protrusions during intercellular spread. Mol Microbiol 1992; 6:1605–1616.
36. Sansonetti PJ, Mounier J. Metabolic events mediating early killing of host cells infected by *Shigella flexneri*. Microb Pathog 1987; 3:53–61.
37. Levine MM, Kaper JB, Black RE, Clements ML. New knowledge on pathogenesis of bacterial enteric infections as applied to vaccine development. Microbiol Rev 1983; 47:510–550.
38. Maurelli AT. Regulation of virulence genes in *Shigella*. Mol Biol 1990; 6:425–432.
39. Timakov VD, Petrovskaya VG, Bondarenko VM. Studies of the genetic control of *Shigella* subgroup B type specific antigens. Ann Inst Pasteur 1970; 118:3–9.
40. Kopecko DJ, Washington O, Formal SB. Genetic and physical evidence for plasmid control of *Shigella sonnei* form 1 cell surface antigen. Infect Immun 1980; 29:207–214.
41. Watanabe H, Timmis KN. Small plasmid in *Shigella dysenteriae* 1 specifies one or more functions essential for O antigen production and bacterial virulence. Infect Immun 1984; 43:391–396.

42. Lindberg AA, Karnell A, Weintraub A. The lipopolysaccharide of *Shigella* bacteria as a virulence factor. Rev Infect Dis 1991; 13[Suppl 4]:S279–284.
43. Nassif X, Mazert M-C, Mounier J, Sansonetti PJ. Evaluation with an *iuc*: Tn10 mutant of the role of aerobactin production in the virulence of *Shigella flexneri*. Infect Immun 1987; 55:1963–1969.
44. Lindberg AA, Karnell A, Pal T, Sweiha H, Hultenby K, Stocker BAD. Construction of an auxotrophic *Shigella flexneri* strain for use as a live vaccine. Microbial Pathogen 1990; 8:433–440.
45. DuPont H L, Hornick RB, Dawkins AT, Snyder MJ, Formal SB. The response of man to virulent *Shigella flexneri* 2a. J Infect Dis 1969; 119:296–299.
46. Taylor D, Echeverria P, Pal T, Sethabutr O, Sailborisuth S, Srichamorn S, Rowe B, Cross J. The role of *Shigella* spp., enteroinvasive *Escherichia coli* and other enteropathogens as causes of childhood dysentery in Thailand. J Infect Dis 1986; 153:1132–1138.
47. Kinsey MD, Formal SB, Dammin GJ, Giannella RA. Fluid and electrolyte transport in rhesus monkeys challenged intracecally with *Shigella flexneri* 2a. Infect Immun 1976; 14:368–371.
48. Fasano A, Noriega FR, Maneval DR, Chanasongcram S, Russell R, Guandalini S, Levine M. *Shigella* enterotoxin 1: an enterotoxin of *Shigella flexneri* 2a active in rabbit small intestine in vivo and in vitro. J Clin Invest 1995; 95:2853–2861.
49. Nataro JP, Seriwatant J, Fasano A, Maneval DR, Guers LD, Noriega F, Dubovsky F, Levine MM, Morris JG, Jr. Identification and cloning of a novel plasmid-encoded enterotoxin in enteroinvasive *Escherichia coli* and *Shigella* strains. Infect Immun 1995; 63:4721–4728.
50. Endo Y, Tsurugi K, Yetsudo T, Takeda Y, Ogasawara T, Igarashi K. Site of action of a Vero toxin (VT2) from *Escherichia coli* O157:H7 and of Shiga toxin on eucaryotic ribosomes. Eur J Biochem 1988; 171:45–50.
51. Obrig TG, Louise CB, Lingwook CA, Boyd B, Barley-Maloney L, Daniel TO. Endothelial heterogeneity in Shiga toxin receptors and responses. J Biol Chem 1993; 268:15484–15488.
52. Levine MM, DuPont HL, Formal SB, Hornick RB, Takeuchi A, Gangarosa EJ, Snyder MJ, Libonati JP. Pathogenesis of *Shigella dysenteriae* 1 (Shiga) dysentery. J Infect Dis 1973; 127:261–270.
53. Mathan VI, Mathan MM. Intestinal manifestations of invasive diarrheas and their diagnosis. Rev Infect Dis 1991; 13[Suppl 4]:S311-313.
54. Herrington DA, Van De Verg L, Formal SB, Hale TL, Tall BD, Cruz SJ, Tramont EC, Levine MM. Studies in volunteers to evaluate candidate *Shigella* vaccines: further experience with a bivalent *Salmonella typhi-Shigella sonnei* vaccine and protection conferred by previous *Shigella sonnei* disease. Vaccine 1990; 8:353–357.
55. Kotloff KL, Nataro JP, Losonsky GA, Wasserman SS, Hale TL, Taylor DN, Sadoff JC, Levine MM. A modified *Shigella* volunteer challenge model in which the inoculum is administered with bicarbonate buffer: Clinical experience and implications for *Shigella* infectivity. Vaccine 1995; 13:1488–1494.

56. Huskins WC, Griffiths JK, Faruque ASG, Bennish ML. Shigellosis in neonates and young infants. J Pediatr 1994; 125:14–22.
57. Ashkenazi S, Dinari G, Zevulunov A, Nitzan M. Convulsions in childhood shigellosis. Clinical and laboratory features in 153 children. Am J Dis Child 1987; 141:208–210.
58. Avital A, Maayan C, Goitein J. Incidence of convulsions and encephalopathy in childhood *Shigella* infections. Clin Pediatr 1982; 21:645–648.
59. Koster F, Levin J, Walker L, Tung KSK, Gilman RH, Rahaman MM, Majid MA, Islam S, Williams RC, Jr. Hemolytic-uremic syndrome after shigellosis. Relation to endotoxemia and circulating immune complexes. N Engl J Med 1978; 298:927–933.
60. Rahaman MM, Alam AKMJ, Islam MR, Greenough WB, 3rd, Lindenbaum J. Shiga bacillus dysentery associated with marked leukocytosis and erythrocyte fragmentation. Johns Hopkins Med J 1975; 136:65–70.
61. Altman RL, Li KI, Juster F, Van Horn KG, Schlesinger I, Hetzler T. Hip joint infection caused by *Shigella sonnei* in a one-year-old boy. Ped Infect Dis J 1994; 13:1156–1158.
62. Squires RH, Keating JP, Rosenblum JL, Askin F, Ternberg JL. Splenic abscess and hepatic dysfunction caused by *Shigella flexneri*. J Pediatr 1981; 98:429–430.
63. Rubin HM, Eardley W, Nichols BL. *Shigella sonnei* osteomyelitis and sickle-cell anemia. Am J Dis Child 1968; 116:83–87.
64. Bennish ML. Potentially lethal complications of shigellosis. Rev Infect Dis 1991; 13[Suppl 4]:S319–324.
65. Bennish ML, Azad AK, Rahman O, Phillips RE. Hypoglycemia during childhood diarrhea: Prevalence, pathophysiology, and outcome. N Engl J Med 1990; 322:1357–1363.
66. Bennish ML, Harris JR, Wojtyniak BJ, Struelens M. Death in shigellosis: Incidence and risk factors in hospitalized patients. J Infect Dis 1990; 161:500–506.
67. Struelens MJ, Patte D, Kabir I, Salam A, Nath SK, Butler T. *Shigella* septicemia: Prevalence, presentation, risk factors, and outcome. J Infect Dis 1985; 152:784–790.
68. Nelson MR, Shanson DC, Hawkins DA, Bazzard BG. *Salmonella, Campylobacter,* and *Shigella* in HIV-seropositive patients. AIDS 1992; 6:1495–1498.
69. Henry FJ, Alam N, Aziz KMS, Rahaman MM. Dysentery, not watery diarrhea, is associated with stunting in Bangladeshi children. Human Nutrition: Clinical Nutrition 1987; 41C:243–249.
70. Black RE, Brown KH, Becker S, Alim ARMA, Huq I. Longitudinal studies of infectious diseases and physical growth of children in rural Bangladesh. II. Incidence of diarrhea and association with known pathogens. Am J Epidemiol 1989; 18:964–969.
71. Bennish ML, Salam MA, Wahed MA. Enteric protein loss during shigellosis. Am J Gasteroent 1993; 88:53–57.

72. Sieper J, Braun J, Wu P, Hauer R, Laitko S. The possible role of *Shigella* in sporadic enteric reactive arthritis. Br J Rheumatol 1993; 32:582–585.
73. Finch M, Rodey G, Lawrence D, Blake P. Epidemic Reiter's syndrome following an outbreak of shigellosis. Eur J Epidemiol 1986; 2:26–30.
74. Keat A. Reiter's syndrome and reactive arthritis in perspective. N Engl J Med 1983; 309:1606–1614.
75. Williams KM, Raybourne RB. Demonstration of cross-reactivity between bacterial antigens and class I human leukocyte antigens by using monoclonal antibodies to *Shigella flexneri*. Infect Immun 1990; 58:1774–1781.
76. Stieglitz H, Lipsky P. Association between reactive arthritis and antecedent infection with *Shigella flexneri* carrying a 2-Md plasmid and encoding an HLA-B27 mimetic epitope. Arthritis Rheum 1993; 36:1387–1391.
77. Hermann E, Yu DTY, Meyer zum Buschenfelde K-H, Fleischer B. HLA-B27-restricted CD8 T cells derived from synovial fluids of patients with reactive arthritis and ankylosing spondylitis. Lancet 1993; 342:646–650.
78. Cohen D, Green MS, Block C, Slepon R, Lerman Y. Natural immunity to shigellosis in two groups with different previous risks of exposure to *Shigella* is only partly expressed by serum antibodies to lipopolysaccharide. J Infect Dis [letter] 1992; 165:785–787.
79. Mel DM, Terzin AL, Vuksic L. Studies on vaccination against bacillary dysentery. 3. Effective oral immunization against *Shigella flexneri* 2a in a field trial. Bull WHO 1965; 32:647–655.
80. Cohen D, Green MS, Block C, Slepon R, Ofek I. Prospective study of the association between serum antibodies to lipopolysaccharide O antigen and the attack rate of shigellosis. J Clin Micro 1991; 29:386–389.
81. Black RE, Levine MM, Clements ML Losonsky G, Herrington D, Berman S, Formal S. Prevention of shigellosis by a *Salmonella typhi-Shigella sonnei* bivalent vaccine. J Infect Dis 1987; 155:1260–1265.
82. Oaks EV, Hale TL, Formal SB. Serum immune response to *Shigella* protein antigens in *Rhesus* monkeys and humans infected with *Shigella spp.* Infect Immun 1986; 53:57–63.
83. Tacket CO, Binion SB, Bostwick E. Losonsky G, Roy MJ, Edelman R. Efficacy of bovine milk immunoglobulin concentrate in preventing illness after *Shigella flexneri* challenge. Am J Trop Med Hyg 1992; 47:276–283.
84. Hayani KC, Guerrero ML, Morrow AL, Gomez HF, Winsor DK, Ruiz-Palacios GM, Cleary TG. Concentration of milk secretory immunoglobulin A against *Shigella* virulence plasmid-associated antigens as a predictor of symptom status in *Shigella*-infected breast fed infants. J Pediatr 1992; 121:852–856.
85. Cleary TG, Winsor DK, Reich D, Ruiz-Palacios G, Calva JJ. Human milk immunoglobulin A antibodies to *Shigella* virulence determinants. Infect Immun 1989; 57:1675–1679.
86. Clemens JD, Stanton B, Stoll B, Shahid NS, Banu H, Alauddin Chowdhury AKM. Breast feeding as a determinant of severity in shigellosis. Am J Epidemiol 1986; 123:710–720.

87. Kotloff KL, Losonsky GA, Nataro JP, Wasserman SS, Hale TL, Taylor DN, Newland JW, Sadoff JC, Formal SB, Levine MM. Evaluation of the safety, immunogenicity, and efficacy in adults of four doses of live oral hybrid *Escherichia coli-Shigella flexneri* 2a vaccine strain EcSf2a-2. Vaccine 1995; 13:495–502.
88. Pickering LK, DuPont HL, Olarte J, Conklin R, Ericsson C. Fecal leucocytes in enteric infections. Am J Clin Pathol 1977; 68:562–565.
89. Speelman P, McGlaughlin R, Kabir I, Butler T. Differences in clinical features and stool findings in shigellosis and amoebic dysentery. Trans R Soc Trop Med Hyg 1987; 81:549–551.
90. Adkins JH, Santingo LT. Increased recovery of enteric pathogens by use of both stool and rectal swab specimens. J Clin Microbiol 1987; 25:158–159.
91. Wells JG, Morris GK. Evaluation of transport methods for isolating *Shigella spp.* J Clin Microbiol 1981; 13:789–790.
92. DeWitt TG, Humphrey KF, McCarthy P. Clinical predictors of acute bacterial diarrhea in young children. Pediatrics 1985; 76:551–556.
93. Fan K, Morris AJ, Reller LB. Application of rejection criteria for stool cultures for bacterial enteropathogens. J Clin Microbiol 1993; 31:2233–2235.
94. Varavithya W, Sunthornkachit R, Eampokalap B. Oral rehydration therapy for invasive diarrhea. Rev Infect Dis 1991; 13[Suppl 4]:S325-S331.
95. Formal SB, Abrams GD, Schneider H, Sprinz H. Experimental *Shigella* infections: VI. Role of the small intestine in an experimental infection in guinea pigs. J Bacteriol 1963; 85:119–125.
96. DuPont HL, Hornick RB. Adverse effect of lomotil therapy in shigellosis. JAMA 1973; 226:1525–1528.
97. Minton NA, Smith PG. Loperamide toxicity in a child after a single dose. Br Med J 1987; 294:1383.
98. Chow CB, Li SH, Leung NK. Loperamide associated necrotising enterocolitis. Acta Paediatr Scand 1986; 75:1034–1036.
99. Murphy GS, Bodhidatta L, Echeverria P, Tansuphaswadikul S, Hoge CW, Imlarp S, Tamura K. Ciprofloxacin and loperamide in the treatment of bacillary dysentery. Ann Intern Med 1993; 118:582–586.
100. Salam MA, Bennish ML. Antimicrobial therapy for shigellosis. Rev Infect Dis 1991; 13[Suppl 4]:S332–S341.
101. Haltalin KC, Nelson JD, Hinton LV, Kusmiesz HT, Sladoje M, Comparison of orally absorbable and nonabsorbable antibiotics in shigellosis. A double-blind study with ampicillin and neomycin. J Pediatr 1968; 72:708–720.
102. Haltalin KC, Nelson JD, Kusmiesz HT, Hinton LV. Comparison of intramuscular and oral ampicillin therapy for shigellosis. Pediatr 1968; 73:617–622.
103. Nelson JD, Kusmiesz H. Shelton S. Oral or intravenous trimethoprim-sulfamethoxozole therapy for shigellosis. Rev Infect Dis 1982; 4:546–550.
104. Nelson JD, Haltalin KC. Amoxicillin less effective than ampicillin against *Shigella* in vitro and in vivo: relationship of efficacy to activity in serum. J Infect Dis 1974; 129[Suppl]:S222–227.
105. Salam MA, Seas C, Khan WA, Bennish ML. Treatment of shigellosis: IV.

Cefixime is ineffective in shigellosis in adults. Ann Intern Med 1995; 123:505–508.

106. Orenstein WA, Ross L, Overturf GD, Wilkins J, Redfield Dr, Underman A. Antibiotic treatment of acute shigellosis: failure of cefamandole compared with trimethoprim/sulfamethoxazole and ampicillin. Am J Med Sci 1981; 282:27–33.
107. Varsano I, Eidlitz-Marcus T, Nussinovitch M, Elian I. Comparative efficacy of ceftriaxone and ampicillin for treatment of severe shigellosis in children. J Pediatr 1991; 118:207–215.
108. Tauxe RV, Puhr ND, Wells JG, Hargrett-Bean N, Blake PA. Antimicrobial resistance of *Shigella flexneri* in the USA: The importance of international travelers. J Infect Dis 1990; 162:1107–1111.
109. Ries AA, Wells JG, Olivola D, Ntakibiroro M, Nyandwi S, Ntibakivayo M, Ivey CB, Greene KD, Tenover FC, Wahlquist SP, Griffin PM, Tauxe RV. Epidemic *Shigella dysenteriae* type 1 in Burundi: Panresistance and implications for prevention. J Infect Dis 1994; 169:1035–1041.
110. Bennish ML, Salam MA, Haider R, Barza M. Therapy for shigellosis. II. Randomized double-blind comparison of ciprofloxacin and ampicillin. J Infect Dis 1990; 162:711–716.
111. Bhattacharya SK, Bhattacharya MK, Dutta P, Sen D, Rasaily R, Moitra A, Pal SC. Randomized clinical trial of norfloxacin for shigellosis. J Trop Med Hyg 1991; 45:683–687.
112. De Mol P, Mets T, Lagasse R, Vandepitte J, Mutwewingabo A, Butzler J-P. Treatment of bacillary dysentery: A comparison between enoxacin and nalidixic acid. J Antimicrob Chemother 1987; 19:695–698.
113. Lolekha S, Patanachareon S, Thanangkul B, VIbulbandhitkit S. Norfloxacin versus co-trimoxazole in the treatment of acute bacterial diarrhoea: A placebo controlled study. Scand J Infect Dis 1988; 56[Suppl]:35–45.
114. Bennish ML, Salam MA, Khan WA, Khan AM. Treatment of shigellosis: III. Comparison of one- or two-dose ciprofloxacin with standard 5-day therapy. Ann Intern Med 1992; 117:727–734.
115. Schaad UB. Role of the new quinolones in pediatric practice. Pediatr Infect Dis J 1992; 11:1043–1046.
116. Alam AN, Islam MR, Hossain MS, Mahalanabis D, Hye HKMA. Comparison of pivmecillinam and nalidixic acid in the treatment of acute shigellosis in children. Scand J Gastroenterol 1994; 29:313–317.
117. Prado D, Liu H, Velasquez T, Cleary TG. Comparative efficacy of pivmecillanam and cotrimoxazole in acute shigellosis in children. Scand J Infect Dis 1993; 25:713–719.
118. Khan MU. Interruption of shigellosis by hand washing. Trans R Soc Trop Med Hyg 1982; 76:164–168.
119. Shaughnessy HJ, Olsson RC, Bass K, Friewer F, Levison SO. Experimental human bacillary dysentery: Polyvalent dysentery vaccine in its prevention. JAMA 1946; 132:362–368.
120. Venkatesan M, Fernadez-Prada C, Buysse JM, Formal SB, Hale TL. Virulence

phenotype and genetic characteristics of the T_{32}-ISTRATI *Shigella flexneri* 2a vaccine strain. Vaccine 1991; 9:358–363.

121. Cooperation Group of Dysentery Vaccine and Bing Rui W. Study on the effect of oral immunization of T_{32} strain against bacillary dysentery in field trials. Arch Roumaines Pathol Exp Microbiol 1984; 43:285–289.
122. Formal SB, Oaks EV, Olsen RE, Wingfield-Eggleston M, Snoy PH, Cogan JP. Effect of prior infection with virulent *Shigella flexneri* 2a on the resistance of monkeys to subsequent infection with *Shigella sonnei*. J Infect Dis 1991; 164:533–537.
123. Levine MM, Gangarosa EJ, Barrow WB, Morris GK, Wells JG, Weiss CF. Shigellosis in custodial institutions. IV. In vivo stability and transmissibility of oral attenuated streptomycin-dependent *Shigella* vaccines. J Infect Dis 1975; 131:704–707.
124. Mel DM, Arsic BL, Radovanovic ML, Litvinjenko S. Live oral *Shigella* vaccine: Vaccination schedule and the effect of booster dose. Acta Microbiol Acad Sci Hung 1974; 21:109–114.
125. Kotloff KL, Herrington DA, Hale TL, Newland JW, Van De Verg, L, Cogan JP, Snoy, PJ, Sadoff JC, Formal SB, Levine MM. Safety, immunogenicity, and efficacy in monkeys and humans of invasive *Escherichia coli* K-12 hybrid vaccine candidates expressing *Shigella flexneri* 2a somatic antigen. Infect Immun 1992; 60:2218–2224.
126. Karnell A, Li A, Zhao CR, Karlsson K, Minh NB, Lindberg AA. Safety and immunogenicity study of the auxotrophic *Shigella flexneri* 2a vaccine SFL1070 with a deleted *aro*D gene in adult Swedish volunteers. Vaccine 1995; 13:88–99.
127. Sansonetti PJ, Rondel J. Construction and evaluation of a double mutant of *Shigella flexneri* as a candidate for oral vaccination against shigellosis. Vaccine 1989; 7:443–450.
128. Sansonetti PJ, Rondel J, Fontaine A, d'Hauteville H, Bernardini ML. *OmpB* (osmo-regulation) and *icsA* (cell-to-cell spread) mutants of *Shigella flexneri*: Vaccine candidates and probes to study the pathogenesis of shigellosis. Vaccine 1991; 9:416–422.
129. Noriega FR, Losonsky G, Lauderbaugh C, Liao FM, Wang JY, Levine MM. Engineered ΔguaB-A, Δ*vir*G *Shigella flexneri* 2a strain CVD 1205: Construction, safety, immunogenicity and potential efficacy as a mucosal adjuvant. Infect Immun 1996; 64:3055–3061.
130. Taylor DN, Trofa AC, Sadoff J, Chu CY, Bryla DA, Shiloach J, Cohen D, Ashkenazi S, Lerman Y, Egan W, Schneerson R, Robbins JB. Synthesis, characterization and clinical evaluation of conjugate vaccines composed of the O-specific polysaccharide of *Shigella dysenteriae* type 1, *Shigella flexneri* type 2, *Shigella sonnei (Plesiomonas shigelloides*) bound to bacterial toxoids. Infect Immun 1993; 61:3678–3687.
131. Cohen D, Ashkenazi S, Green M, Gdalevich M, Yavzori M, Slepon R, Robin G, Orr N, Ashkenazi I, Shemer J, Taylor D, Sadoff J, Schneerson R, Robbins

J. Safety, immunogenicity and efficacy of a *Shigella sonnei*-O specific polysaccharide conjugate vaccine in Israeli volunteers (abstr). 35th Interscience Conference on Antimicrobial Agents and Chemotherapy, San Francisco, Sept 17–20, 1995.

10

Clostridium difficile Colitis in Gastrointestinal Infections

JOANNE K. LINEVSKY
Boston University School of Medicine, Boston, Massachusetts

CIARAN P. KELLY
Beth Isreal Deaconess Medical Center and Harvard Medical School, Boston, Massachusetts

I. INTRODUCTION

Clostridium difficile is a gram-positive, spore-forming anaerobic bacillus. It colonizes the human large intestine when the normal colonic flora is disturbed by antibiotic therapy. Pathogenic strains of *C. difficile* release protein exotoxins that cause colonic injury and diarrhea. Individuals colonized by toxigenic *C. difficile* may be asymptomatic, may experience mild diarrhea, or may develop severe pseudomembranous colitis. Diagnosis depends upon demonstrating *C. difficile* toxin in the stool. Metronidazole is the agent of choice for mild or moderately severe diarrhea. Oral vancomycin is used for patients who are intolerant of metronidazole or those with severe colitis. Both agents are highly effective but diarrhea recurs in 20% of patients when therapy is discontinued. Rarely, diarrhea and colitis progress despite therapy and colectomy may be required. Over the past twenty years major advances have been made in understanding the pathogenesis, diagnosis, and treatment of *C. difficile* diarrhea. However, this organism continues to flourish in our hospitals and nursing homes where it is a common cause of infectious diarrhea. Judicious antibiotic use and fundamental infection control measures such as handwashing after patient contact are essential to reduce the prevalence of nosocomial *C. difficile* infection and diarrhea.

II. A Brief History of *C. difficile* Colitis

Pseudomembranous enterocolitis was reported in 1893 (1) but was rare before the advent of antibiotic therapy. *Clostridium difficile* was originally identified in 1935 by Hall and O'Toole who named it "*Bacillus difficilis*" because of the difficulty they experienced in isolating and culturing the organism (2). They noted that cultures of *B. difficilis* produced lethal toxins but since it was isolated from the stools of healthy neonates the pathogenic role of *C. difficile* was not immediately evident.

In the 1950s the use of broad-spectrum antibiotics resulted in an increased incidence of pseudomembranous colitis. For some years *Staphylococcus aureus* was believed to be the causative agent (3). In 1974 Tedesco reported diarrhea and pseudomembranous colitis as a frequent complication of clindamycin therapy (4). However, stool cultures of patients with "clindamycin colitis" did not grow *S. aureus*, suggesting that another, as yet undefined, etiologic agent was responsible. The mystery was solved through studies of antibiotic-associated colitis in animals. Guinea pigs or hamsters treated with antibiotics almost invariably develop a lethal cecitis that resembles fulminant pseudomembranous colitis in humans (5,6). In 1977 Bartlett et al. reported that the ceca of hamsters with antibiotic-associated colitis contained a cytopathic *Clostridial* toxin (7). Similar toxins were identified in the stool of patients with pseudomembranous colitis and *Clostridium difficile* was soon identified as the source of the toxins (8–10).

III. PATHOGENESIS OF *C. DIFFICILE* DIARRHEA

The sequence of events which results in *C. difficile* diarrhea is as follows: 1. disruption of the normal colonic microflora by antibiotic therapy, 2. exposure to and colonization by toxigenic *C. difficile*, and 3. release of *C. difficile* toxins into the colonic lumen resulting in mucosal injury and inflammation (Figure 1). Host susceptibility to *C. difficile* colitis varies considerably. Many infected individuals are asymptomatic carriers whereas others develop severe or recurrent diarrhea and colitis (11).

A. Disruption of the Colonic Microflora by Antibiotics

The normal colonic microflora resists the growth of *C. difficile* (12). The mechanism for this inhibitory effect is not known but healthy adults are seldom colonized by the organism (13). Neonates, in contrast, are frequently colonized by *C. difficile* (2,13,14). This presumably reflects the fact that the infants' colonic bacterial flora are not yet fully established, which provides a temporary opportunity for *C. difficile* growth. In older children and adults antibiotic therapy, particularly with agents that have activity against enteric microbes,

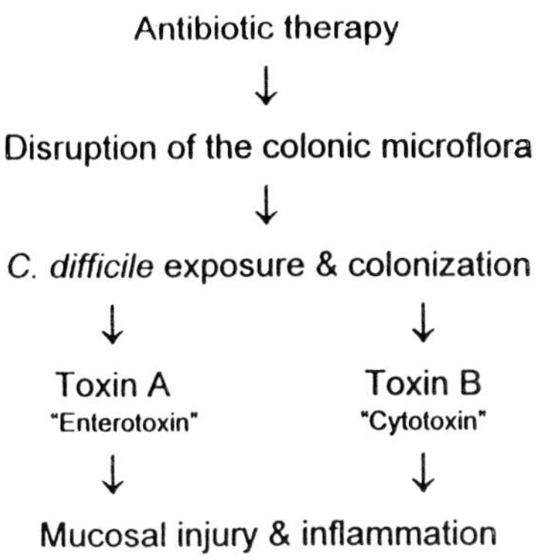

Figure 1 Pathogenesis of *Clostridium difficile* diarrhea.

alters the colonic microenvironment and allows *C. difficile* to flourish (Table 1). Certain antibiotics such as clindamycin and lincomycin are notorious for their propensity to induce pseudomembranous colitis (4). However, ampicillin/amoxicillin and cephalosporins, because of their widespread use, are the agents which most commonly cause *C. difficile* diarrhea in current clinical practice (Table 2) (11,15–17). Interestingly, isolates of *C. difficile* are often sensitive

Table 1 Isolation Rates of Toxigenic *C. Difficile* from the Stool in Various Patient Populations

Subject group	*C. difficile* positive
Pseudomembranous colitis	95–100%
Hospital in-patients	20%
Healthy adults	0–3%
Healthy neonates and infants	25–80%

Table 2 Antimicrobial Agents That Cause *C. Difficile* Diarrhea and Colitis

Frequently	Infrequently	Rarely or never
Ampicillin and amoxicillin	Tetracyclines	Parenteral aminoglycosides
Cephalosporins	Sulfonamides	Bacitracin
Clindamycin	Erythromycin	Metronidazole
	Chloramphenieol	Vancomycin
	Trimethoprim	
	Quinolones	

Source: Ref. 17.

to many antibiotics including agents, such as ampicillin, which cause *C. difficile* diarrhea (18,19). This underscores the fact that *C. difficile* overgrowth results from disruption of the normal colonic bacterial flora rather than resistance of the organism to antibiotic therapy. Chemotherapy for malignancy may also disturb the normal microbial barrier and result in *C. difficile* infection and diarrhea (20).

B. *C. difficile* Exposure and Colonization

After the colon has been "prepared" by antibiotics, exposure to *C. difficile* must occur in order for colonization to take place. *C. difficile* infection and diarrhea is most common in hospital and nursing-home patients. In this setting frequent antibiotic use is combined with heavy environmental contamination by *C. difficile* and ample opportunity for cross-infection (11,16,21–24). Acquisition of *C. difficile* by hospitalized patients may occur by direct patient–patient contact or indirectly through environmental contamination (16,18,22,24–26). Whatever the route of infection, studies have shown that as many as 20% of in-patients are colonized by *C. difficile* at some point during their hospital stay (22,23). Although some develop diarrhea, the majority are asymptomatic carriers. Thus nosocomial *C. difficile* contamination results from shedding of the organism by symptomatic patients and by an even larger hidden reservoir of asymptomatic carriers (22). *C. difficile* can be cultured readily from the hospital environment (18,22,23,25,27,28). Its ability to form spores that may persist for many months and still remain viable makes the task of environmental decontamination especially difficult. Health workers caring for patients with *C. difficile* diarrhea frequently carry the organism on their hands and clothing (22). *C. difficile* diarrhea rarely occurs in such workers but they may represent an important route for cross-infection (29,30). New admissions to hospitals are a further source of *C. difficile* since many of these patients have already been colonized during a prior hospital stay. Their readmission, or transfer to another health care facility serves to perpetuate and extend the cycle of infection (16,22–24,26).

C. difficile diarrhea is an unusual complication of out-patient antibiotic therapy. The organism is ubiquitous and toxigenic strains can be cultured from soil samples and from the feces of animals (31). Nonetheless, the prevalence of *C. difficile* in the general environment is far lower than that evident in health-care facilities. This presumably explains why simple antibiotic-associated diarrhea is common in out-patients whereas *C. difficile* diarrhea and colitis is rare. A recent community-based study found that *C. difficile* diarrhea was diagnosed after only 1 in 15,000 out-patient antibiotic prescriptions. This corresponded to 7.7 identified cases per 100,000 person-years in the study population (32).

C. *C. difficile* Toxins A and B

Pathogenic strains of C. difficile release two protein exotoxins, toxin A and toxin B (Table 3). Both are extremely large with molecular weights of 308 and 269 kDa respectively (33–36). The two toxins show almost 50% homology in their amino acid sequences. The carboxyl end of both molecules contain multiple repeating units and this area is believed to contain the receptor binding domain of the toxins. Toxin A binds to the trisaccharide Galα-1-3Galβ1-4GlcNAc (37). This binding is blocked by a monoclonal antibody directed against an epitope on the carboxyl portion of toxin A (38). This antibody also neutralizes the enterotoxic activity of toxin A in animal studies (39–41). Thus binding of toxin A to cell surface carbohydrate structures is believed important for toxin-A–mediated intestinal injury (42). Although toxin B also has repeating units at its carboxyl end, it does not bind to Galα-1-3Galβ1-4GlcNAc and the nature of its receptor is unknown.

Toxin A is commonly referred to as the "enterotoxin" and toxin B the "cytotoxin." However, these names are misleading since there is considerable overlap in the structure, effects, and mechanisms of action of the two molecules. Tiny quantities of toxin B cause rounding of mammalian cells and this cytotoxic effect is the basis for the tissue culture assay for C. difficile infection (43–46). Toxin A causes an identical cytotoxin effect but at approximately one thousand fold higher concentrations. It is now known that both toxins have the same intracellular mechanism of action and act as enzymes to catalyze the glucosylation of Rho (47–51). Rho proteins are members of the ras-related superfamily of small GTPases and are essential for maintenance of the actin cytoskeleton. *C. difficile* toxins use UDP-glucose as a substrate to glucosylate Rho at a threonine residue in the "effector" domain of the molecule. This modification of Rho causes the disaggregation of actin filaments, cell rounding, and ultimately cell death.

Toxin A acts as an inflammatory enterotoxin and is as potent as cholera toxin in stimulating fluid secretion in animal intestine (44,52,53). However, unlike

Table 3 *Clostridium difficile* Toxins

	Toxin A, Enterotoxin	Toxin B, Cytotoxin
Molecular weight	308 kDa protein	269 kDa protein
Intracellular mechanism of cytotoxicity	Glucosylate Rho proteins	Glucosylate Rho proteins
Cytotoxin	+	+++
Inflammatory enterotoxin	Human and animal intestine	Human colon

cholera toxin, toxin A also causes marked mucosal injury and inflammation (53,54). Toxin B has little, if any, direct enterotoxin effects in animal models (52). However, if the intestinal mucosa is damaged by the effects of toxin A, then toxin B becomes lethal to animals (55). Furthermore, in recent studies using human intestinal tissues, toxin B was even more harmful to the human colon than toxin A (56). Thus both toxins may act in synergy to cause diarrhea and colitis in humans. Toxin A is directly chemotactic to neutrophils and both toxins A and B stimulate cytokine release from monocytes (54,57–60). These proinflammatory effects may account for the marked inflammation and pseudomembrane formation that characterizes *C. difficile* colitis (61).

D. Host Susceptibility to *C. difficile* Diarrhea

C. difficile infection is associated with a wide spectrum of clinical presentation. It is not clear why many individuals colonized by *C. difficile* are asymptomatic whereas others develop severe or recurrent colitis. Differences in virulence between strains of *C. difficile* may account for some of these differences. However, the age of the host and the host's immune status are also important determinants of disease severity.

Toxins A and B are the major, recognized virulence factors of *C. difficile.* Other than toxin production and spore formation, no virulence factors have been defined that clearly effect either the course of disease or the likelihood of cross-infection. With rare exception, pathogenic strains of *C. difficile* release both toxin A and B whereas nonpathogenic strains produce neither (62,63). The amount of toxin produced in vitro varies considerably between different strains but this does not appear to correlate with clinical virulence (13).

Age plays a major role in determining response to *C. difficile* infection. Infants frequently harbor toxigenic *C. difficile* yet seldom develop diarrhea or pseudomembranous colitis (2,13,14,19,64–66). The basis for their decreased susceptibility to *C. difficile* toxin-mediated intestinal injury is unknown. One theory, based upon studies of neonatal rabbits, is that infants have little or no intestinal expression of toxin receptors (67).

The frail and elderly are highly susceptible to *C. difficile* diarrhea and are especially likely to suffer severe or complicated disease. The majority of sporadic and epidemic cases of C. difficile occur in elderly, debilitated hospital patients (11,16,21–23,26,68). Outbreaks of *C. difficile* diarrhea have also been reported in nursing homes (21). Predisposing factors, in addition to age and antibiotic use, include a prolonged hospital stay, sharing a room with a patient infected with *C. difficile*, admission to an intensive care unit, gastrointestinal surgery, and use of antacids or acid antisecretory therapy (22,69–73). Patients suffering from AIDS frequently receive antibiotic therapy. As a result, *C. difficile* is an important, treatable cause of infectious diarrhea and colitis in this patient group (74). There is no difference in response to treatment of *C. difficile* infection in AIDS patients as compared to immunocompetent patients (75).

Failure to mount an appropriate antibody response to *C. difficile* and its toxins may predispose to severe or recurrent *C. difficile* diarrhea and colitis (76). Active or passive immunization of animals against *C. difficile* toxins is protective (40,77–79,80,82). In these animal studies the mechanism of protection appeared to be through toxin neutralization rather than prevention of colonization (80). A similar mechanism may explain the asymptomatic carrier state in humans.

Up to two-thirds of healthy adults have serum antibodies against toxin A and toxin B and a similar proportion have colonic secretory IgA antitoxin (81,82). The antitoxin activity of serum from elderly patients may be lower and a declining antibody response could contribute to the increased rate of symptomatic infection in older, inform individuals (83,84). Human colostrum also contains toxin-neutralizing activity but it is not clear whether maternal antibodies, delivered through the placenta or via breast milk, protect infants from *C. difficile* diarrhea (82,85,86).

Increased anti-*C. difficile* antibody levels and toxin-neutralizing activity have been demonstrated in convalescent sera of patients with *C. difficile* diarrhea (81,87–89). A number of studies have reported that patients suffering from severe or recurrent *C. difficile* diarrhea have lower anti-*C. difficile* antibody levels as compared to individuals with mild disease or healthy controls (76,84,88–92). However, one study found no association between serum or intestinal anti–toxin-A responses and disease course (93). Thus there is considerable but so far inconclusive evidence that antitoxin antibody responses are at least partially protective in humans. The potential therapeutic role of active or passive immunization against *C. difficile* toxins is discussed below.

IV. CLINICAL PRESENTATION

Diarrhea is the cardinal symptom of *C. difficile* colitis. In some instances it is mild and self-limiting; whereas in others, profuse diarrhea occurs resulting in dehydration and marked malaise. Diarrhea usually begins during the course of antibiotic therapy but is sometimes delayed until some days after antibiotics have been stopped. Longer latency periods of several weeks can occur but are unusual. Thus all patients presenting with diarrhea should be questioned regarding previous antibiotic use.

Occult blood may be detectable in the stool but hematochezia is uncommon in *C. difficile* colitis. Fecal leukocyte counts are often increased particularly in patients with more severe colitis. Cramping, abdominal pain, and mild abdominal tenderness may accompany the diarrhea. A low-grade fever and systemic polymorphonuclear leukocytosis are common. Occasionally there may be dramatic increases in peripheral blood neutrophil counts to as high as 70,000 per microliter (94). A protein-losing enteropathy with hypoalbuminemia may also complicate severe *C. difficile* colitis (94).

Diarrhea is a very common side effect of antibiotic use. In most cases *C. difficile* infection is absent and a specific etiologic agent cannot be identified. Agents such as ampicillin and cephalosporins that give rise to *C. difficile* diarrhea also commonly cause "simple" antibiotic-associated diarrhea. However, simple antibiotic-associated diarrhea differs from *C. difficile* diarrhea in a number of important respects. It is usually mild, it is not generally associated with systemic abnormalities such as fever and leukocytosis, and colitis is rarely evident. Some individuals show a propensity to developing diarrhea whenever they use a broad-spectrum antibiotic. Diarrhea may be more frequent and severe when higher antibiotic dosage is used. The severity of *C. difficile* diarrhea is not dose related. As discussed earlier, simple antibiotic-associated diarrhea is common in out-patients while *C. difficile* diarrhea is usually a nosocomial infection. The most important difference between these two disorders is that simple antibiotic-associated diarrhea usually resolves within a few days of stopping antibiotics whereas *C. difficile* infection may progress to severe, even fatal, pseudomembranous colitis even after the inciting antibiotic has been withdrawn.

V. DIAGNOSTIC STUDIES

If *C. difficile* diarrhea is suspected on clinical grounds, a variety of stool tests are available to confirm infection with toxigenic *C. difficile* (Table 4). Endoscopic examination of the colon is seldom indicated but is diagnostic when pseudomembranous colitis is present. Radiographic studies of the abdomen may be abnormal in patients with severe colitis but the changes are not usually specific for *C. difficile* infection.

A. Stool Tests for *C. difficile*

1. *Cytotoxin Assay*

The stool cytotoxin assay is the most sensitive and specific test available for diagnosing *C. difficile* infection. This assay is based upon the ability of *C. difficile* toxin B to produce a characteristic cell-rounding effect on cells growing in culture (45). To perform the test, an aliquot of centrifuged and filtered stool supernatant is added to cells growing in monolayers, usually fibroblasts. The cells are examined after 24 and 48 hours for the cytopathic cell-rounding effect produced by toxin B. The specificity of this effect for toxin B is confirmed by simultaneously performing the assay in the presence of a neutralizing antiserum to toxin B.

Table 4 Diagnostic Tests for *C. difficile* Infection

Test	Detects	Advantages	Disadvantages
Cytotoxin Assay	Toxin B	"Gold standard" Highly sensitive and specific	Requires tissue culture facility Takes 24–48 hours
ELISA[a]	Toxin A or B	Fast (2–6 hours) Easy to perform	Not as sensitive or specific as cytotoxin assay
Latex agglutination assay	Bacterial enzyme (glutamate dehydrogenase)	Fast Inexpensive Easy to perform	Poor sensitivity and specificity
Culture	Toxigenic and nontoxigenic *C. difficile*	Allows strain typing in epidemics Sensitive	Requires aerobic culture Not specific for toxin-producing bacteria Takes 2–5 days

[a]Enzyme-linked immunosorbant assay.

The cytotoxin assay continues to be the "gold standard" for diagnosing infection with toxigenic *C. difficile* because of its remarkable sensitivity in detecting as little as 10 pg of toxin B. The test is positive in 95% of patients with antibiotic-associated pseudomembranous colitis (19). The cytotoxin assay is highly specific for the presence of *C. difficile* toxin but cannot differentiate between patients with *C. difficile* colitis and those who are asymptomatic carriers. The disadvantages to this diagnostic method are that tissue-culture facilities are needed and the assay takes 24 to 48 hours to complete. Thus, if the stool sample is sent to an outside facility for assay the result may not be available for 2 to 3 days. Stool specimens for the assay need to be fresh or kept refrigerated as the potency of the toxin decreases rapidly at room temperature (95). Most laboratories report the results of the cytotoxin assay as either positive or negative. Although patients with pseudomembranous colitis tend to have high toxin levels (Burdon, J. Clin. Path. 1981) there is no clear correlation between the toxin titer and the severity of disease (96).

2. *Toxin ELISA*

Enzyme-linked immunosorbant assays (ELISA) have now been developed to detect *C. difficile* toxin A or toxin B in stool samples (97). The sensitivity of commercially available ELISA test kits are generally greater than 90% but their sensitivities vary (between 70% and 95%) (98–100). The cost of ELISA kits are generally higher than the commercially available cytotoxin assay but this is balanced by lower labor and equipment costs for the ELISA. Although the sensitivities and specificities of ELISA tests are not as high as the tissue-culture cytotoxin assay, ELISA tests do not require tissue-culture facilities and can be performed in only a few hours. Thus most hospital laboratories can perform these assays in-house and provide test results quickly.

3. *Latex Agglutination Test*

The latex agglutination test is rapid, inexpensive, and easy to perform. It was originally reported to detect *C. difficile* toxin A. However, subsequent studies have shown that the agglutinin reacts instead with a bacterial enzyme, glutamate dehydrogenase (101,102). This enzyme is not specific for *C. difficile* nor does it differentiate between toxin-producing and non-toxin-producing strains. The latex agglutination assay has largely been superseded by the ELISA tests, which provide more reliable results.

4. *C. difficile Culture*

C. difficile is difficult to culture on most media but can be grown with relative ease on selective medium containing cycloserine and cefoxitin (103). A major disadvantage of culture is that it does not differentiate between toxigenic and nontoxigenic strains. *C. difficile* cultures must be tested for toxin production since up to a quarter of clinical isolates are nontoxigenic and therefore nonpathogenic. Culture followed by confirmation of toxin production is labor intensive and time consuming and a final result may not be available for 4 to 5 days. These factors limit the clinical utility of *C. difficile* culture. However, stool or rectal swab culture is a valuable epidemiologic tool. It provides a sensitive means of detecting *C. difficile* colonization and isolates may be typed to study patterns of cross-infection.

B. Endoscopy and Biopsy

Endoscopy is seldom required to diagnose *C. difficile* diarrhea. Although the endoscopic appearance of pseudomembranous colitis is distinctive it is not present in all cases of *C. difficile* diarrhea. Many patients have no evident colitis or show only mild and nonspecific inflammatory changes. Sigmoidoscopy or colonoscopy is indicated when the etiology of diarrhea and colitis is not clear from the results of stool tests. Endoscopy may also be helpful in severe or fulminant colitis where the finding of characteristic pseudomembranes would provide an immediate diagnosis. In these circumstances, as in all case of acute colitis, endoscopy should be performed without prior enemas and air insufflation should be kept to a minimum to avoid precipitating toxic dilatation or perforation.

The characteristic findings in pseudomembranous colitis consist of multiple, small (2–5 mm) yellow plaques covering a hyperemic colonic mucosa (Figure 2). The plaques adhere to the underlying mucosa and may coalesce to form larger pseudomembranes. The rectum and sigmoid colon are usually involved allowing for the diagnosis by sigmoidoscopy. However, in a minority of cases, the colitis may be confined to the right side of the colon (104). Biopsies should be taken in cases of suspected *C. difficile* colitis as histologic examination may reveal characteristic "volcano" lesions even in the absence of overt pseudomembranes (61) (Figure 3).

C. Radiographic Studies

The findings on plain abdominal radiographs in pseudomembranous colitis are nonspecific. Colonic distention, loss of haustral markings, and small bowel dilation are often seen in severe colitis (Figure 4a). Colonic edema and thumbprinting are less common (Figure 4b). Barium enema evaluation is not recommended in suspected pseudomembranous colitis because of the risk of causing toxic megacolon or perforation.

Abdominal CT scans are now frequently performed on patients with severe *C. difficile* colitis and may reveal dramatic colonic wall thickening and edema often accompanied by a small amount of ascites. The colonic edema may not

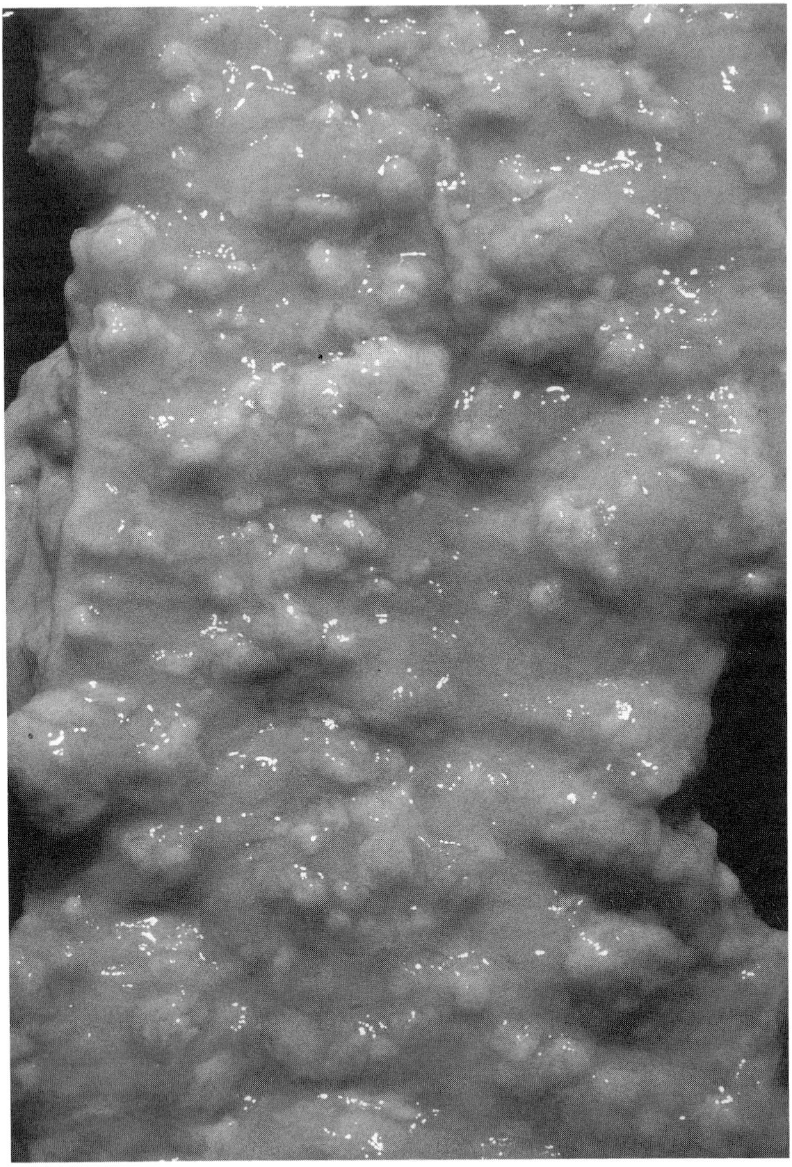

Figure 2 Colectomy specimen from a patient with pseudomembranous colitis. Characteristic raised, adherent, yellow plaques, which vary in size from 2 to 10 mm, are visible on the colonic mucosa. The intervening mucosa is hyperemic but is not ulcerated.

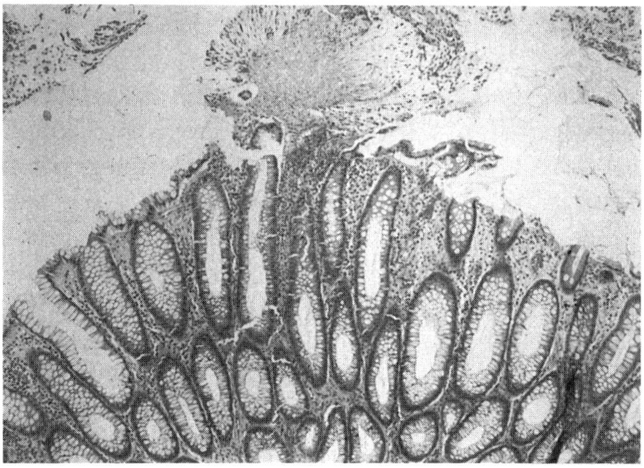

Figure 3 Pseudomembranous colitis with "summit lesion" or "volcano lesion." This endoscopic biopsy shows focal ulceration of the colonic mucosa (center frame) with exudation of a pseudomembrane (arrow) comprised of inflammatory cells, fibrin, and necrotic debris. The adjoining mucosa is intact (hematoxylin and eosin, ×125).

be uniform but rather localized to only one portion of the colon (105). The CT finding of an "accordion pattern" with a series of broad edematous colonic haustral folds is thought to be relatively specific for pseudomembranous colitis (106) (Figure 5).

VI. TREATMENT

A. General Measures

C. difficile diarrhea has a wide range of clinical presentations and therapy should be tailored to the severity of disease. No treatment is indicated for asymptomatic carriers (21). In cases of mild, antibiotic-associated diarrhea in otherwise healthy individuals without fever, significant abdominal pain, or leukocytosis, discontinuation of antibiotics may be all that is needed for symptoms to resolve. This conservative approach allows for reconstitution of the normal colonic microflora and lessens the risk of relapsing diarrhea. Patients with more severe or persisting diarrhea or with other clinical evidence of colitis should receive antimicrobial therapy using metronidazole or vancomycin. Both of these agents are very effective in the short term but relapsing diarrhea is a common problem. In cases in which antibiotic therapy cannot be discontinued, the antimicrobial regimen should be altered, if possible, to employ agents that are less likely to encourage *C. difficile* overgrowth (Table 5). Antidiarrheal agents that reduce colonic motility (e.g. Lomotil, Immodium) should be avoided for fear of worsening toxin-induced colitis and precipitating toxic megacolon.

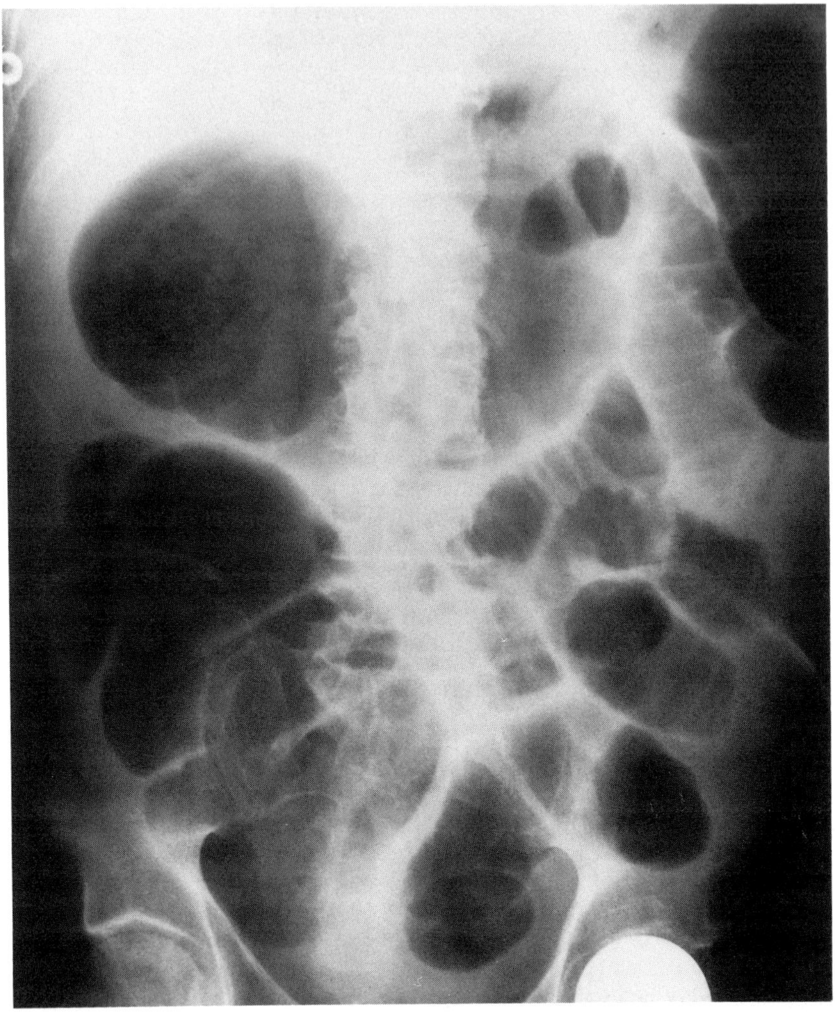

Figure 4 Plain abdominal radiographs demonstrating abnormalities seen in patients with severe pseudomembranous colitis. Colonic dilatation (first panel). Loops of dilated small intestine are also evident indicating a paralytic ileus. Thumbprinting (examples indicated by arrows [second panel]) reflecting marked colonic mucosal edema (courtesy of Joseph T. Ferrucci Jr., MD).

B. Metronidazole or Vancomycin?

Metronidazole, 250 mg four times daily for 10 days, is now considered the drug of choice for mild to moderately severe *C. difficile* diarrhea (71). Response rates are greater than 95%. Most patients report a marked improvement in their diarrhea within two to three days and complete resolution of diarrhea within

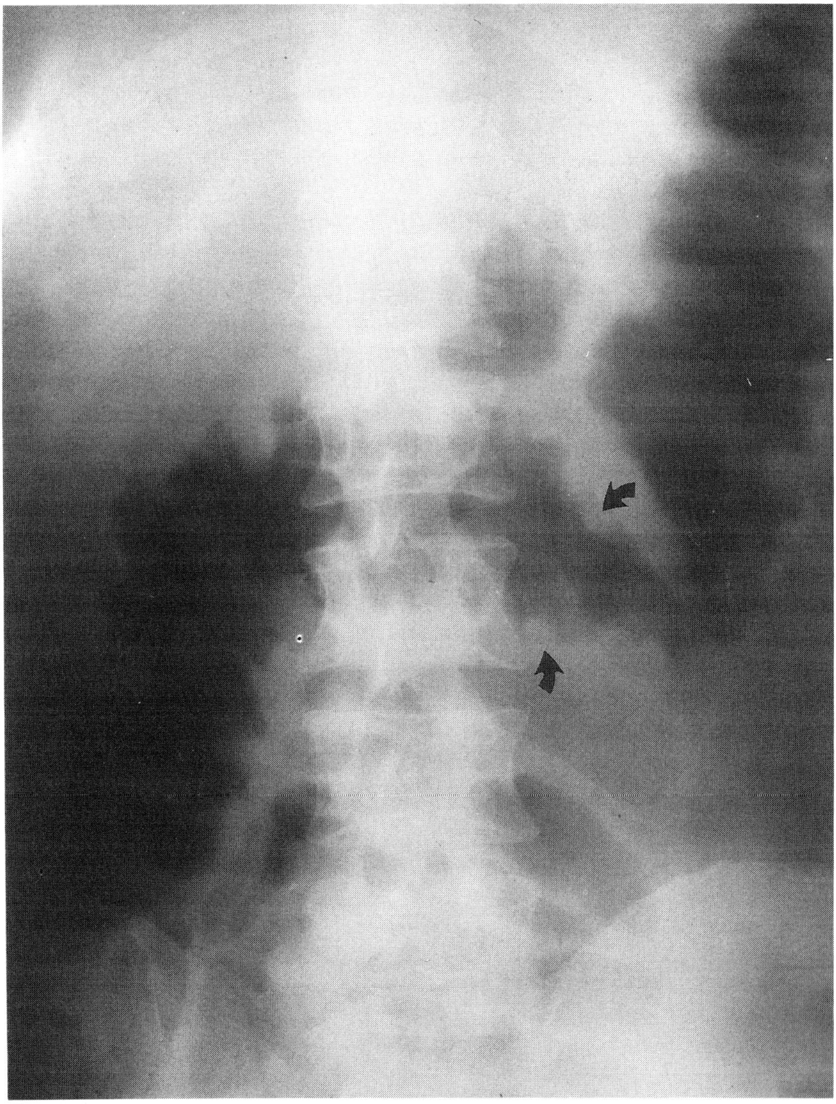

Figure 4 Continued

seven to ten days. Oral metronidazole is well absorbed but therapeutic levels are obtained in the feces via excretion into the bile and exudation across the inflamed colonic mucosa (107). Systemic side effects occur in some patients and include nausea, a metallic taste, and alcohol intolerance.

Vancomycin, 125 mg four times daily for 10 days, is also highly effective in controlling *C. difficile* diarrhea (108). Oral vancomycin is not absorbed,

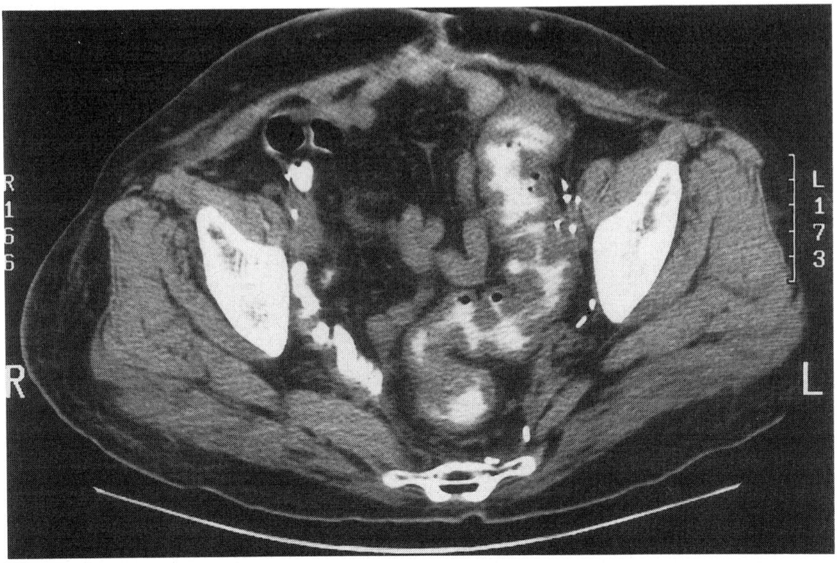

Figure 5 Computerized tomograph of the abdomen in *Clostridium difficile* colitis demonstrating marked thickening of the colonic wall in the sigmoid colon. The "accordion pattern" is evident, produced by a series of broad edematous haustral folds.

resulting in very high fecal concentrations and few, if any, systemic side effects. Thus its bioavailability is ideal for treating *C. difficile* infection. Vancomycin was the first agent used to treat pseudomembranous colitis and is still considered by most to be more potent than metronidazole (109–111). Metronidazole is as effective as vancomycin in treating mild to moderately severe *C. difficile* diarrhea but vancomycin may be more effective in fulminant colitis. Metronidazole is usually preferred, however, because vancomycin is expensive and because of fears that its widespread use will accelerate the spread of nosocomial vancomycin-resistant bacteria. The cost of a standard course of oral vancomycin is $230 compared to $13 for metronidazole. The cost of intravenous vancomycin is much lower for hospital pharmacies and therefore it is far cheaper for in-patients to take the intravenous formulation orally. Following the emergence of vancomycin-resistant enterococci, the Centers for Disease Control have advised against using vancomycin for *C. difficile* infection, except in isolated cases (112). Currently oral vancomycin is indicated for severe or fulminant pseudomembranous colitis, for patients who are intolerant of metronidazole, and for the few patients who fail to respond to metronidazole.

Table 5 Drug Therapy for Pseudomembranous Colitis

Drug	Dosage[a]	Cost[b]	Indications	Percentage effective[c]	Percentage recurrence[c]	Comments
Metronidazole	250 mg po *qid* × 10 days or 500 mg iv q6h	$13.00 $8.80/iv dose	1st line therapy for mild to moderate colitis	98%	7%	Potential for systemic side effects: nausea, vomiting, metallic taste, disulfiram reaction
Vancomycin	125 mg po *qid* × 10 days	$232	Severe or fulminant colitis Metronidazole intolerance Metronidazole treatment failure	96%	18%	No systemic side effects Not recommended as first line therapy due to potential to develop vancomycin-resistant enterococcus

[a]Pediatric Dosage: Metronidazole; 5–7 mg/kg po *tid* × 10 days; Vancomycin: 40 mg/kg po in 3–4 divided doses.
[b]Cost of drug regimen based on current retail price at a Boston pharmacy.
[c]Ref. 145.

C. Other Antimicrobial Agents

Bacitracin is a poorly absorbed antibiotic with good in vitro activity against *C. difficile*. In clinical studies the response rate to bacitracin is approximately 80% and the relapse rate is greater than 30%, which compares unfavorably to either vancomycin or metronidazole (113,114).

Teicoplanin is an antibiotic related to vancomycin which, at an oral dose of 200 mg twice daily for 10 days, shows equal efficacy to vancomycin in treating *C. difficile* diarrhea. Initial clinical studies with teicoplanin report a relapse rate of only 3%, considerably lower than that seen with either metronidazole or vancomycin (115). However, these early results require confirmation in larger trials. Oral teicoplanin is currently not available for clinical use in the United States.

Nonantibiotic therapies for *C. difficile* disease such as toxin-binding agents and biotherapy are discussed below.

VII. FULMINANT *C. DIFFICILE* COLITIS

A. Presentation

A minority of patients with *C. difficile* infection develop severe or fulminant pseudomembranous colitis. Clinical signs include fever, hypotension, diffuse abdominal tenderness, and abdominal distention. A markedly elevated neutrophil count is typical. Life-threatening complications such as colonic perforation, peritonitis, and septicemia may ensue. Diarrhea can be mild or completely absent in severe *C. difficile* colitis (116). This apparent paradox may be explained by the development of toxic dilatation of the colon often accompanied by small bowel ileus (Figure 4). Fulminant colitis may also present with acute abdominal pain without any prior history of diarrhea (68).

B. Medical Therapy

Oral vancomycin is often used in preference to oral metronidazole in severe pseudomembranous colitis. In critically ill patients higher doses of vancomycin (such as 250 mg or 500 mg every 6 hours) may be beneficial, especially in the early stages of therapy. As the patient's condition improves, the dose of vancomycin can be lowered to 125 mg. Unfortunately, many patients with severe *C. difficile* colitis cannot tolerate oral vancomycin therapy because of recent surgery, small bowel ileus, or colonic inertia. In these circumstances metronidazole, 500 mg every 6 hours, should be administered intravenously. Intravenous vancomycin is not effective in treating *C. difficile* colitis as it is not excreted into the gastrointestinal tract. However, intravenous metronidazole can be supplemented by vancomycin administered via nasogastric tube or by enema (500 mg every 4 to 6 hours)(117).

C. Surgical Therapy

A few patients with severe *C. difficile* colitis will not respond to medical therapy. If no improvement is evident within 48 to 72 hours of instituting maximal therapy, or if the patient's condition continues to deteriorate, surgical intervention should be considered (118). Surgery is life-saving in patients with refractory *C. difficile* colitis and in those who suffer colonic perforation. Although various surgical approaches have been advocated, subtotal colectomy with temporary ileostomy is usually effective. This approach has the least morbidity and mortality and can be converted to an ileal-rectal anastomosis at a later date (119). Multiple colonic perforations are often found at surgery. If there is a single perforation and the colitis is focal, a segmental resection may be successful. The overall mortality for surgical interventions in this disease is high (approximately 35%), which reflects the poor clinical condition of patients at the time of emergency surgery. As expected, mortality with a single perforation is considerably less than for multiple perforations (33% vs. 66%) (119).

VIII. RECURRENT *C. DIFFICILE* DIARRHEA

Recurrent diarrhea is the most common complication of *C. difficile* infection and occurs in 10–20% of patients treated for *C. difficile* colitis. Thus patients should be alerted to this possibility. Relapse is often the result of infection with the same strain of organism as in the initial attack (120). It is not clear when this relapse is due to persistent infection or reinfection from a patient's environment that has become contaminated by *C. difficile* and its spores. Ironically, therapy with metronidazole or vancomycin perpetuates disruption of the colonic microflora and therefore may predispose to *C. difficile* colonization and growth. Individuals who suffer one relapse are more likely to suffer another and the relapse rate amongst those who have already suffered two or more relapses is over 60% (109,121). The published record for multiple relapses is a patient with eighteen episodes of *C. difficile* diarrhea (122). It has been suggested that colonic diverticulosis may predispose to recurrent diarrhea by providing a haven for persistence of *C. difficile* spores (123). Another theory, discussed below, is that an inadequate antibody response predisposes to recurrent bouts of *C. difficile* diarrhea.

The clinical presentation of relapse is similar to that of the original attack. Recurrent diarrhea usually begins within 4 weeks of stopping metronidazole or vancomycin (108,124,125). Diagnosis of relapse should include stool analysis for *C. difficile* toxin since transient alterations in bowel habit are common following any episode of acute infectious diarrhea. It should also be noted that some individuals have *C. difficile* toxins in their stools after therapy but do not suffer symptomatic relapse.

There is no treatment that invariably prevents recurrent *C. difficile* diarrhea. If symptoms are mild, further antibiotic therapy may be withheld and this approach, if successful, is very likely to prevent subsequent relapses. The usual treatment for a first relapse is a second 10 to 14 day course of metronidazole or vancomycin (Table 6). Relapses do not indicate the development of antibiotic resistance by *C. difficile*. Hence, the agent used to treat the initial episode can be used again. A wide variety of approaches have been suggested for patients with multiple relapses. A standard course of vancomycin (or metronidazole) followed by a slow taper is often successful. If this also fails, a wide variety of regimens have been proposed including a number of "nonantibiotic" treatments. Many of these therapies are novel and ingenious but, with the exception of *Saccharomyces boulardii* (see below) none are supported by controlled trials to demonstrate efficacy.

IX. CONTROL OF NOSOCOMIAL *C. DIFFICILE* INFECTION

Outbreaks of *C. difficile* diarrhea are frequent in hospitals and nursing homes (16,18,21,24,26,126,127). In fact, *C. difficile* is now the most common cause of infectious diarrhea in hospitalized patients in the developed world (128). As

Table 6 Approach to Recurrent *C. Difficile* Colitis

First relapse
Symptomatic treatment if symptoms are mild
10–14 day course of metronidazole or vancomycin
Second relapse
Vancomycin taper[a]
Further relapse
Saccharomyces boulardii in combination with metronidazole or vancomycin[b]
Vancomycin in tapering dose as above plus cholestyramine 4 g *bid*[c]
Vancomycin 125 mg *qid* and rifampicin 600 mg *bid* for 7 days[d]
Intravenous immunoglobulin therapy[e]
Therapy with microorganisms (see text)

[a]125 mg q6h for 7 days, 125 mg q12h for 7 days, 125 mg qd for 7 days, 125 mg qod for 7 days, 125 mg every 3 days for 7 days. Ref. 123.
[b]Ref. 121.
[c]Ref. 144.
[d]Ref. 153.
[e]Ref. 90.

discussed above, the frequent use of broad spectrum antibiotics, environmental contamination by *C. difficile* and its spores, and the high carriage rates amongst hospitalized patients combine to make control of nosocomial *C. difficile* infection and diarrhea a difficult task. Judicious use of antibiotics and observation of universal infection control measures are the most important means of limiting the prevalence of this iatrogenic disease. Avoiding antibiotic use entirely prevents the disease. When antibiotics are required, narrow spectrum agents that carry a lower risk for *C. difficile* diarrhea should be used whenever appropriate (Table 2).

Early diagnosis of patients with *C. difficile* diarrhea is obviously important. However, the majority of in-patients who are colonized are asymptomatic (22,23). Thus "universal" infection control measures must be applied. These include hand washing between patient contacts and wearing disposable gloves when at risk for contact with body fluids (129). Cohort nursing of infected patients has been employed since direct person-to-person transmission of infection may be important in *C. difficile* epidemics (16,26). Fomites such as commodes or thermometers should also be considered potential routes of cross-infection (18,22,23,25,27,28,130). Thorough cleaning and disinfection of the hospital environmental has been advocated as a means to reduce the burden of *C. difficile* spores (21,26). Treatment of asymptomatic carriers has also been attempted but with disappointing results. Neither metronidazole or vancomycin are effective in reducing long-term carriage rates (131).

In summary, controlling endemic disease and outbreaks of *C. difficile* diarrhea is best achieved by a multifaceted approach that incorporates restriction of antibiotic use, early recognition and treatment of antibiotic-associated diarrhea, education of staff to adherence of fundamental infection-control precautions, regular cleaning and disinfection of the hospital environmental, and in the case of outbreaks, restriction of patient and staff movements.

X. NONANTIBIOTIC THERAPY FOR *C. DIFFICILE* DIARRHEA?

Metronidazole or vancomycin are very effective in treating *C. difficile* diarrhea in the short term. However, they are not effective in preventing recurrent *C. difficile* diarrhea, reducing *C. difficile* carriage rates, or reducing the prevalence of *C. difficile* diarrhea in our hospitals (11,22,23,121,131,132). Certainly, the use of additional antibiotics to treat antibiotic-induced *C. difficile* colitis is counter-intuitive. Metronidazole and vancomycin have considerable activity against the normal colonic bacterial flora and both agents cause lethal *C. difficile* cecitis in hamsters (133). Their effect on the colonic microflora may be instrumental in facilitating recurrent *C. difficile* infection and diarrhea. In fact, there have been some reports of *C. difficile* diarrhea caused by metronidazole therapy (134,135). The absence of similar reports implicating vancomycin may simply be due to the fact that *C. difficile* diarrhea is the sole indication for using oral vancomycin.

The ideal therapeutic agent for *C. difficile* colitis would prevent toxin-mediated diarrhea and colitis while encouraging restitution of the colonic microflora. A normal complement of colonic bacteria are the ultimate protection against *C. difficile* colonization and disease. Nonantibiotic approaches to the treatment of *C. difficile* infection can be divided into three groups: biotherapies, agents that bind *C. difficile* toxins, and immunization.

A. Biotherapy

Saccharomyces boulardii is the most studied and best characterized biotherapy for *C. difficile* disease (128). It is a nonpathogenic yeast originally obtained from moldy lychee fruit. It is not currently marketed as a drug in the United States but is widely used in Europe to prevent antibiotic-associated diarrhea. *S. boulardii* protects animals from experimental *C. difficile* enterocolitis but its mechanism of action is not clear. Various studies have suggested that *S. boulardii* inhibits *C. difficile* growth, inactivates *C. difficile* toxins and reduces toxin-receptor binding (136,137). Clinical trials demonstrate that oral *S. boulardii* taken with antibiotics effectively reduces the incidence of simple, antibiotic-associated diarrhea (138). When *S. boulardii* is administered following standard therapy with metronidazole or vancomycin, it also reduces the incidence of recurrent *C. difficile* diarrhea in patients who have already suffered multiple relapses (121,139). However, *S. boulardii* therapy does not appear to be worthwhile in patients treated for a first episode of *C. difficile* diarrhea (121).

Biotherapies other than *S. boulardii* have not been subject to controlled clinical trial and accounts of their efficacy are largely anecdotal. Most reports relate to treatment of patients with relapsing *C. difficile* diarrhea. Agents which have been administered in the hopes of competing with and eradicating toxigenic *C. difficile* include oral lactobacillus (140), cultures of enteric bacteria by enema (141), cultures of nontoxigenic *C. difficile* via nasogastric tube (142), and even enemas of human feces taken from healthy donors (143).

B. Toxin-binding Agents

Anion-binding resins, in particular cholestyramine, have some efficacy in treating acute *C. difficile* diarrhea and have also been used in relapsing diarrhea (144). Their presumed mechanism of action is to adsorb and thereby neutralize *C. difficile* toxins. Cholestyramine has a cure rate of only 68% when used as initial therapy for *C. difficile* diarrhea (145). This compares poorly with either metronidazole or vancomycin. Cholestyramine has also been used as an adjunct to vancomycin in patients with recurrent *C. difficile* diarrhea (133) (Table 6).

Binding of *C. difficile* toxins by cholestyramine is quite nonspecific. More recently, oligosaccharides containing toxin-A binding sequences have been synthesized and linked to an inert silica-based support (146). These compounds specifically bind to and neutralize toxin A. However, the nature of the *C. difficile* toxin-B receptor is unknown. Thus similar toxin-B neutralizing compounds have not been reported. It is difficult to predict the efficacy of an agent that specifically neutralizes toxin A but not toxin B since, as discussed above, the relative importance of toxins A and B in causing disease in humans is unclear.

C. Antitoxin Antibodies

There is some evidence to suggest that individuals with severe, prolonged, or recurrent *C. difficile* diarrhea may show an inadequate antibody response to *C. difficile* and its toxins (78,84,88–91). If this is indeed true, it is reasonable to propose that either passive or active immunization may be beneficial. In one study, five children with recurrent *C. difficile* diarrhea were found to have low serum anti-toxin-A antibody levels and were treated with intravenous pooled human gamma globulin (90). Since many adults have serum antibodies to *C. difficile* toxins, the pooled gamma globulin preparation contained high levels of antitoxin. All of the children showed a good clinical response and clearance of cytotoxin activity from their stools.

Oral passive immunization is effective in animals and may be a more attractive alternative to intravenously administered gamma globulin (40,80). There is a single report of the use of oral human immunoglobulin A in a boy with recurrent *C. difficile* infection (147). A hyperimmune bovine immunoglobulin concentrate has been prepared from the colostrum of cows immunized against *C. difficile* toxins (148). Similar immunoglobulin preparations, taken orally, have been effective against other enteric pathogens (149–151). The anti-*C. difficile* bovine immunoglobulin concentrate neutralizes the cytotoxicity of toxin A and toxin B and protects against *C. difficile* colitis in animals (148,152). However, its efficacy in treating or preventing *C. difficile* diarrhea and colitis in humans has yet to be determined.

Active immunization against *C. difficile* may provide an effective means of reducing the prevalence and severity of *C. difficile* diarrhea in our hospital population. Formalin-inactivated culture filtrate from toxigenic *C. difficile* or purified inactivated toxins are effective for animal immunization and similar preparations could be developed as human vaccines (78–80,148). Another approach under investigation is the production of a recombinant protein vaccine composed of nontoxic fragments of toxin A and toxin B (40,41,76,101). If an effective vaccine is produced , the prime candidates for immunization will be the elderly and infirm who are at greatest risk for developing nosocomial *C. difficile* infection and diarrhea.

REFERENCES

1. Finney JMT. Gastroenterostomy for cicatrizing ulcer of pylorus. Bull Johns Hopkins Hosp 1893; 4:53.
2. Hall IC, O'Toole E. Intestinal flora in newborn infants with description of a new pathogenic anaerobe, *Bacillus difficilis*. Am J Dis Child 1935; 49:390–402.
3. Hummel RO, Altemeier WA, Hill EO. Iatrogenic staphylococcal enterocolitis. Ann Surg 1964; 160:551.
4. Tedesco FJ, Barton RW, Alpers HD. Clindamycin-associated colitis. Ann Int Med 1974; 81:429–433.
5. Hamre DM, Rake G, McKeet CM, et al. The toxicity of penicillin as prepared for clinical use. Am J Med Sci 1943; 206:642.
6. Green RH. The association of viral activation with penicillin toxicity in guinea pigs and hamsters. Yale J Biol Med 1974; 47:166.
7. Barlett JG, Onderdonk AB, Cisneros AB, et al. Clindamycin-associated colitis due to toxin-producing species of *Clostridium* in hamsters. J Infect Dis 1977; 136:701.
8. Larson HE, Parry FV, Price AB, et al. Underdescribed toxin in pseudomembranous colitis. Br J Med 1977; 1:1246–1248.
9. Bartlett JG, Chang TW, Gurwith M, et al. Antibiotic-associated pseudomembranous colitis due to toxin producing *clostridia*. N Engl J Med 1978; 298:531–534.
10. Larson HE, Price AB, Honour P, Boriello SP. *Clostridium difficile* and the aetiology of pseudomembranous colitis. Lancet 1978; I:1062–1066.
11. Kelly CP, Pothoulakis C, LaMont JT. *Clostridium difficile* colitis. N Eng J Med 1994; 330:257–262.
12. Borriello SP. The influence of the normal flora on *Clostridium difficile* colonization of the gut. Ann Med 1990; 162:678–684.
13. Viscidi R, Willey S, Bartlett JG. Isolation rates and toxigenic potential for *Clostridium difficile* isolates from various patient populations. Gastroenterology 1981; 81:5–9.
14. Larson HE, Barclay FE, Honour P, Hill ID. Epidemiology of *Clostridium difficile* in infants. J Infect Dis 1982; 146:727–733.
15. Silva J, Fekety R, Werk C, et al. Inciting and etiologic agents of colitis. Rev Infect Dis 1984; 6:S214–S221.
16. Nolan NPM, Kelly CP, Humprheys JFH, et al. An epidemic of pseudomembranous colitis: importance of person to person spread. Gut 1987; 28:1467–1473.
17. Kelly CP, LaMong JT. Treatment of *Clostridium difficile* diarrhea and colitis. In: Wolfe MM, ed. Gastrointestinal Pharmacotherapy. Philadelphia:WB Saunders Co, 1993:199–212.
18. Fekety R, Kim K-H, Brown D, et al. Epidemiology of antibiotic-associated colitis. Isolation of *Clostridium difficile* from the hospital environment. Am J Med 1981; 70:906–908.

19. Barlett JG, Taylor NS, Chang TW, Dzink JA. Clinical and laboratory observations in *Clostridium difficile* colitis. Am J Clin Nutr 1981; 33:2521–2526.
20. Kamthan AG, Bruckner HW, Hirschman SZ, Agus SG. *Clostridium difficile* diarrhea induced by cancer chemotherapy. Arch Intern Med 1992; 152:1715–1717.
21. Bender BS, Bennett R, Laughan B, et al. Is *Clostridium difficile* endemic in chronic-care facilities? Lancet 1986; *ii*:11–13.
22. McFarland LV, Mulligan ME, Kwok RYY, et al. Nosocomial acquisition of *Clostridium difficile* infection. N Engl J Med 1989; 320:204–210.
23. Johnson S, Clabots CR, Linn FV, Olson MM, Peterson LR, Gerding DN. Nosocomial *Clostridium difficile* colonisation and disease. Lancet 1990; 336:97–100.
24. Clabots CR, Johnson S, Olson MM, Peterson LR, Gerding DN. Acquisition of *Clostridium difficile* by hospital patients: evidence for colonized new admissions as a source of infection. J Infect Dis 1992; 166:561–567.
25. Kaatz GW, Gitlin SD, Schaberg DR, Wilson KH, Kauffman CA, Seo SM, Fekety R. Acquisition of *Clostridium difficile* from the hospital environment. Am J Epidemiol 1988; 127:1289–1294.
26. Cartmill TD, Panigrahi H, Worsley MA, McCann DC, Nice CN, Keith E. Management and control of a large outbreak of diarrhea due to *Clostridium difficile*. J Hospital Infect 1994; 27:1–15.
27. Mulligan ME, Rolfe RD, Finegold SM, George WL. Contamination of a hospital environment by *Clostridium difficile*. Curr Microbiol 1979; 3:173–175.
28. Kim KH, Fekety R, Batts DH, et al. Isolation of *Clostridium difficile* from the environment and contacts of patients with antibiotic-associated colitis. J Infect Dis 1981; 143:42–50.
29. Strimling MO, Sacho H, Berkowitz I. *Clostridium difficile* infection in health-care workers. Lancet 1989; 1:866–867.
30. Delmee M. *Clostridium difficile* infection in health-care workers. Lancet 1989; 2:1095.
31. Haffiz S. *Clostridium difficile* and its toxins. PhD dissertation, University of Leeds, Leeds, England, 1974.
32. Hirschorn L, Trnka Y, Onderdonk A, Lee M, Platt R. Epidemiology of community-acquired *C. difficile*-associated diarrhea. J Infect Dis 1994; 169:127–33.
33. Barroso LA, Wang SZ, Phelps CJ, Johnson JL, Wilkins TD. Nucleotide sequence of *Clostridium difficile* toxin B gene. Nucleic Acids Res 1990; 18:4004.
34. Dove CH, Wang SZ, Proce SB, Phelps CJ, Lyerly CM, Wilkins TD, Johnson JL. Molecular characterization of the *Clostridium difficile* toxin A gene. Infect Immun 1990; 58:480–488.
35. Von Eichel-Streiber C, Laufenberg-Feldmann R, Sartingen S, Schulze J, Sauerborn M. Cloning of *Clostridium difficile* toxin B gene and demonstration of high N-terminal homology between toxin A and B. Medical Microbiol Immunol 1990; 179:271–279.
36. von Eichel-Streiber C, Laufenberg-Feldmann R, Sartingen S, Schulze J, Sauerborn M. Comparative sequence analysis of the *Clostridium difficile* toxins A and B. Mol Gen Genet 1992; 233:260–268.

37. Krivan HC, Clark GF, Smith DF, Wilkins TD. Cell surface binding site for *Clostridium difficile* enterotoxin: evidence for a glycoconjugate containing the sequence 1-3-Galβ1-4GlcNAc. Infect Immun 1986; 53:573–581.
38. Frey SM, Wilkins TD. Localization of two epitopes recognized by monoclonal antibody PCG-4 on *Clostridium difficile* toxin A. Infect Immun 1992; 60:2488–2492.
39. Lyerly DM, Phelps CJ, Toth J, Wilkins TD. Characterization of toxins A and B of *Clostridium difficile* with monoclonal antibodies. Infect Immun 1986; 54:70–76.
40. Corthier G, Muller MC, Wilkins TD, Lyerly D, L'Haridon R. Protection against experimental pseudomembranous colitis in gnotobiotic mice by use of monoclonal antibodies against *Clostridium difficile* toxin A. Infect Immun 1991; 59:1192–1195.
41. Kamiya S, Yamakawa K, Meng XQ, Ogura H, Nakamura S. Production of a monoclonal antibody to *Clostridium difficile* toxin A which neutralizes enterotoxicity but not haemagglutination activity. FEMS Microbiology Letters 1991; 65:311–315.
42. Pothoulakis C, LaMont JT, Eglow R, Gao N, Rubins JR, Theoharides TC, Dickey BF. Characterization of rabbit ileal receptors for *Clostridium difficile* toxin A: Evidence for a receptor-coupled G protein. J Clin Invest 1991; 88:119–125.
43. Taylor NS, Thorne GM, Bartlett JG. Comparison of two toxins of produced by *Clostridium difficile*. Infect Immun 1981; 34:1036–1043.
44. Lyerly DM, Lockwood DE, Richardson SH, Wilkins TD. Biological activities of toxins A and B of *Clostridium difficile*. Infect Immun 1982; 35:1147–1150.
45. Pothoulakis C, Barone LM, Ely R, Faris B, Clark ME, Franzblau C, LaMont JT. Purification and properties of *Clostridium difficile* cytotoxin B. J Biol Chem 1986; 261:1316–1321.
46. Sullivan NM, Pellet S, Wilkins TD. Purification and characterization of toxins A and B of *Clostridium difficile*. Infect Immun 1982; 35:1032–1040.
47. Just I, Richter H-P, Prepens U, von Eichel-Streiber C, Aktories K. Probing the action of *Clostridium difficile* toxin B in *Xenopus laevis* oocytes. J Cell Science 1994; 107:1653–1659.
48. Just I, Fritz G, Aktories K, Giry M, Popoff MR, Boquet P, Hegenbarth S. von Eichel-Streiber C. *Clostridium difficile* toxin B acts on the GTP-binding protein Rho. J Biol Chem 1994; 269:10706–10712.
49. Just I, Selzer J, von Eichel-Streiber C, Aktories K. The low molecular mass GTP-binding protein Rho is affected by toxin A from *Clostridium difficile*. J Clin Invest 1995; 95:1026–1031.
50. Just I, Selzer J, Wilm M, von Eichel-Streiber C, Mann M, Aktories K. Glucosylation of Rho proteins by *Clostridium difficile* toxin B. Nature 1995; 375:500–503.
51. Just I, Wilm M, Selzer J, Rex G, von Eichel-Streiber C, Mann M, Aktories K. The enterotoxin from Clostridium difficile (ToxA) monoglucosylates the Rho proteins. J Biol Chem 1995; 270:13932–13936.
52. Triadafilopoulos G, Pothoulakis C, O'Brien M, LaMont JT. Differential effects

of *Clostridium difficile* toxins A and B on rabbit ileum. Gastroenterol 1987; 93:273–279.
53. Triadafilopoulos G, Pothoulakis C, Weiss R, Giampaolo C, LaMont JT. Comparative study of *Clostridium difficile* toxin A and cholera toxin in rabbit ileum. Gastroenterology 1989; 97:1186–1192.
54. Kelly CP, Becker S, Linevsky JT, Joshi MA, O'Keane JC, Dickey BF, LaMont JT, Pothoulakis C. Neutrophil recruitment in *Clostridium difficile* toxin A enteritis in the rabbit. J Clin Invest 1994; 93:1257–1265.
55. Lyerly DM, Saum KE, MacDonald D, Wilkins T. Effect of toxins A and B given intragastrically to animals. Infect Immun 1985; 47:349–352.
56. Riegler M, Sedivy R, Pothoulakis C, Hamilton G, Zarcherl J, Bischof G, Cosentini E, Feil W, Schiessel R. LaMont JT, Wenzl E. *Clostridium difficile* toxin B is more potent than toxin A in damaging human colonic epithelium in vitro. J Clin Invest 1995; 95:2004–2011.
57. Pothoulakis C, Sullivan R, Melnick DA, Triadafilopoulos G, Gadenne A-S, Meshulam T, LaMont JT. *Clostridium difficile* toxin A stimulates calcium release and chemotactic response in human granulocytes. J Clin Invest 1988; 81:1741–1745.
58. Flegel WA, Muller F, Daubener W, et al. Cytokine response by human monocytes to *Clostridium difficile* toxin A and B. Infect Immun 1991; 59:3659–3666.
59. Miller PD, Pothoulakis C, Baeker TR, LaMont JT, Rothstein TL. Macrophage-dependent stimulation of T cell-depleted spleen cells by *Clostridium difficile* toxin A and calcium ionophore. Cellular Immunol 1990; 126:155–163.
60. Linevsky JT, Keates S, Pothoulakis C, LaMont JT, Kelly CP. IL-8 release and neutrophil activation by *Clostridium difficile* toxin-exposed monocytes. Gastreoenterology 1995; 108:A863.
61. Price AB, Davies DR. Pseudomembranous colitis. J Clin Pathol 1977; 30:1–12.
62. Lyerly DM, Barroso LA, Wilkins TD, et al. Characterization of a toxin A-negative, toxin-B positive strain of *Clostridium difficile*. Infect Immun 1992; 60:4633–4639.
63. Borriello SP, Wren BW, Hyde S, et al. Molecular, immunological and biological characterization of a toxin A-negative, toxin B-positive strain of *Clostridium difficile*. Infect Immun 1992; 60:4192–4199.
64. Donta TS, Myers MG. *Clostridium difficile* toxin in asymptomatic neonates. Pediatrics 1982; 100:431.
65. Thompson CM, Gilligan PH, Fisher MC, Long SS. *Clostridium difficile* cytotoxin in a pediatric population. Am J Dis Child 1983; 137:271–274.
66. Tullus K, Aronsson B, Marcus S, Mollby R. Intestinal colonization with *Clostridium difficile* in infants up to 18 months of age. Eur J Clin Microbiol Infect Dis 1989; 8:390–393.
67. Eglow R, Pothoulakis C, Itzkowitz S, Israel EJ, O'Keane CJ, Gong D, Gao N, Xu YL, Walker WA, LaMont JT. Diminished *Clostridium difficile* toxin A sensitivity in newborn rabbits is associated with decreased toxin A receptor. J Clin Invest 1992; 90:822–829.

68. Triadafilopoulos G, Hallstone AE. Acutte abdomen as the first presentation of pseudomembranous colitis. Gastroenterol 1991; 101:685–691.
69. McFarland LV, Surawicz CM, Stamm WE. Risk factors for *Clostridium difficile* carriage and *C. difficile*-associated diarrhea in a cohort of hospitalized patients. J Infect Dis 1990; 162:678–684.
70. McFarland LV. Diarrhea acquired in hospital. Gastroenterology Clinics of North America. 19923; 22:563–577.
71. Rolfe RD, Finegold SM, eds. *Clostridium difficile*: Its role in intestinal disease. San Diego, CA: Academic Press, 1988.
72. Bartlett JG. *Clostridium difficile*: Clinical considerations. Reviews Infect Dis 1990; 12:S243–251.
73. Brown E, Talbot GH, Axelrod P, Provencher M, Hoegg C. Risk factors for *Clostridium difficile* toxin-associated diarrhea. Infect Control Hosp Epidemiol 1990; 11:283–290.
74. Cappell MS, Philogene C. *Clostridium difficile* infection is a treatable cause of diarrhea in patients with advanced human immunodeficiency virus infection: A study of seven consecutive patients admitted from 1986 to 1992 to a university teaching hospital. Am J Gastro 1993; 88:891–897.
75. Cozart JC, Kalangi SS, Clench MH, Taylor DR, Borucki MJ, Pollard RB, Soloway RD. *Clostridium difficile* diarrhea in patients with AIDS versus non-AIDS controls. J Clin Gastroenterol 1993; 16:192–194.
76. Kelly CP. Immune response to *Clostridium difficile* infection. Eur J Gastroenterol Hepatol (in press).
77. Allo M, Silvia J, Fekety R, Rifkin GD, Waskin H. Prevention of clindamycin-induced colitis in hamsters by *Clostridium sordellii* antitoxin. Gastroenterology 1979; 76:351–355.
78. Libby JM, Jortner BS, Wilkins TD. Effects of the two toxins of *Clostridium difficile* in antibiotic associated cecitis in hamsters. Infect Immun 1982; 36:822–829.
79. Fernie DS, Thomson RO, Batty I, Walker PD. Active and passive immunization against antibiotic associated caecitis in hamsters. Develop Biol Standard 1983; 53:325–332.
80. Kim PH, Iaconis JP, Rolfe RD. Immunization of adult hamsters against *Clostridium difficile* associated ileocecitis and transfer of protection to infant hamsters. Infect Immun 1987; 55:2984–2992.
81. Viscidi R, Laughon BE, Yolken R, Bo-Linn P, Moench T, Ryder RW, Bartlett JG. Serum antibody response to toxins A and B of *Clostridium difficile*. J Infect Dis 1982; 148:93–100.
82. Kelly CP, Pothoulakis C, Orellana J, JT LaMont. Human colonic aspirates containing IgA antibody to *Clostridium difficile* toxin A inhibit toxin A-receptor binding. Gastroenterol 1992; 102:35–40.
83. Nakamura S, Mikawa M, Nakashio S, Takabatake M, Okado I, Yamakawa K, Serikawa T, Okumura S, Nishida S. Isolation of *Clostridium difficile* from the feces and the antibody in sera of young and elderly adults. Microbiol Immunol 1981; 25:345–351.

84. Bacon AE, Fekety R. Immunoglobulin G directed against toxins A and B of *Clostridium difficile* in the general population and patients with antibiotic-associated diarrhea. Diagn Microbiol Infect Dis 1994; 18:205–209.
85. Wada N, Nishida N, Iwaki S, Ohi H, Miyawaki T, Taniguchi N, Migita S. Neutralizing activity against *Clostridium difficile* toxin in the supernatants of cultured colostral cells. Infect Immun 1980; 29:545–550.
86. Kim K, Pickering LK, DuPont HL, Sullivan N, Wilkins T. In vitro and in vivo neutralizing activity of human colostrum against purified toxins A and B of *Clostridium difficile*. J Infect Dis 1984; 150:57–62.
87. Lishman AH, Al-Jumali IJ, Record CO. Antitoxin production in antibiotic-associated colitis? J Clin Pathol 1981; 34:414–415.
88. Aronsson B, Granstrom M, Mollby R, Nord Ce. Enzyme-linked immunosorbent assay (ELISA) for antibodies to *Clostridium difficile* toxins in patients with pseudomembranous colitis and antibiotic-associated diarrhoea. J Immunol Methods 1983; 60:341–350.
89. Aronsson B, Granstrom M, Mollby R, Nord CE. Serum antibody response to *Clostridium difficile* toxins in patients with *Clostridium difficile* diarrhoea. Infection 1985; 13:97–101.
90. Leung DY, Kelly CP, Boguniewicz M, Pothoulakis C, LaMont JT, Flores A. Treatment with intravenously administered gamma globulin of chronic relapsing colitis induced by *Clostridium difficile* toxin. J Pediatr 1991; 118:633–637.
91. Warny M, Vaerman J-P, Avesani V, Delmee M. Human antibody response to *Clostridium difficile* toxin A in relation to clinical course of infection. Infection Immun 1994; 62:384–389.
92. Mulligan ME, Miller SD, McFarland LV, Fung HK, Kwok RYY. Elevated levels of serum immunoglobulins in asymptomatic carriers of *Clostridium difficile*. Clin Infect Dis 1993; 16:S239–S244.
93. Johnson S, Gerding DN, Janoff EN. Systemic and mucosal antibody response to toxin A in patients with *Clostridium difficile*. J Infect Dis 1992; 166:1287–1294.
94. LaMont JT, Rashid A. Case records of the Massachusetts General Hospital. N Eng J Med 1994; 330:420–426.
95. Bowman RA, Riley TV. Isolation of *Clostridium difficile* from stored specimens and comparative susceptibility of various tissue culture cell lines to cytotoxin. FEMS Microbiol Lett 1986; 34:31–35.
96. Tedesco FJ. Antibiotic-associated pseudomembranous colitis with negative proctosigmoidoscopy examination. Gastroenterology 1979; 77:295–297.
97. DiPesio JR, Varga FJ, Conwell DL, Kraft JA, Kozak K, Willis DH. Development of a rapid enzyme immunoassay for *Clostridium difficile* toxin A and its use in the diagnosis of *C. difficile*-associated disease. J Clin Microbiol 1991; 29:2724–2730
98. Merz CS, Kramer C, Forman M, Gluck L, Mills K, Senft K, Steiman I, Wallace N, Charache P. Comparison of the four commercially available rapid enzyme immunoassays with cytotoxin assay for detection of *Clostridium difficile* toxin(s) from stool specimens. J Clin Microbiol 1994; 32:1142–1147.
99. Whittier S, Shapiro DS, Kelly WF, Walden TP, Wait KJ, McMillon LT, Gilligan

PH. Evaluation of four commercially available enzyme immunoassays for laboratory diagnosis of *Clostridium difficile*-associated diseases. J Clin Microbiol 1993; 31:2861–2865.
100. Barbut F, Kajzer C, Planas N, Petit J-C. Comparison of three enzyme immunoassays, a cytotoxicity assay, and toxigenic culture for diagnosis of *Clostridium difficile*-associated diarrhea. J Clin Microbiol 1993; 31:963–967.
101. Lyerly DM, Wilkins TD. Commercial latex test for *Clostridium difficile* toxin A does not detect toxin A. J Clin Microbiol 1986; 23:622–623.
102. Lyerly DM, Barroso LA, Wilkins TD. Identification of the latex test-reactive protein of *Clostridium difficile* as a glutamate dehydrogenase. J Clin Microbiol 1992; 29:2639–2642.
103. George WL, Sutter VL, Citron D, Finegold SM. Selective and differential medium for isolation of *Clostridium difficile*. J Clin Microbiol 1979; 9:214–219.
104. Tedesco FJ, Corles JK, Brownstein RE. Rectal sparing in antibiotic-associated pseudomembranous colitis: a prospective study. Gastroneterol 1982; 83:1259–1260.
105. Boland GW, Lee MJ, Cats AM, et al. Antibiotic-induced diarrhea: Specificity of abdominal CT for the diagnosis of *Clostridium difficile* disease. Radiology 1994; 191:103–106.
106. Fishman EK, Kavuru MK, Jones BJ, et al. Pseudomembranous colitis: CT evaluation of 26 cases. Radiology 1991; 180:57–60.
107. Bolton RP, Culshaw MA. Faecal metronidazole concentrations during oral and intravenous therapy for antibiotic-associated colitis due to *Clostridium difficile*. Gut 1986; 27:1169–1172.
108. Fekety R, Silva J, Kauffman C, et al. Treatment of antibiotic-associated *Clostridium difficile* colitis with oral vancomycin: Comparison of two dosage regimens. Am J Med 1989; 86:15–19.
109. Barlett JG, Tedesco FJ, Shull S, et al. Symptomatic relapse after oral vancomycin therapy of antibiotic-associated pseudomembranous colitis. Gastroenterology 1980; 78:431–434.
110. Tedesco FJ, Markham R, Gurwith M, et al. Oral vancomycin for antibiotic-associated pseudomembranous colitis. Lancet 1978; 2:226–228.
111. Keighley MRB, Burdon DW, Arabi Y, et al. Randomized controlled trial of vancomycin for pseudomembranous colitis and postoperative diarrhea. Br Med J 1978; 2:1667–1669.
112. Centers for Disease Control and Prevention. Preventing the spread of vancomycin resistance. Federal Register 1994; 59:25758–25763.
113. Dudley MN, McLaughlin JC, Carrington G, et al. Oral bacitracin vs. vancomycin therapy of *Clostridium difficile*-induced diarrhea: a randomized double-blind trial. Arch Intern Med 1986; 146:1101–1104.
114. Young GP, Ward PB, Bayley N, et al. Antibiotic-associated colitis due to *Clostridium difficile*: double blind comparison of vancomycin with bacitracin. Gastroenterology 1985; ;89:1038–1045.
115. DeLalla F, Nicolin R, G, Rinaldi E, et al. Prospective study of oral teicolplanin

vs oral vancomycin for therapy of pseudomembranous colitis and *C. difficile*-associated diarrhea. Antimicrob Agents Chemother 1992; 36:2192–2196.
116. Burke GW, Wilson ME, Mehrez IO. Absence of diarrhea in toxic megacolon complicating *Clostridium difficile* pseudomembranous colitis. Am J Gastro 1988; 83:304–307.
117. Fekety R, Quintiliani R. Current approach to the treatment of antibiotic associated diarrhea. Infect Surg 1982; 9:13–24.
118. Bradley SJ, Weaver DW, Maxwell NT, et al. Surgical management of pseudomembranous colitis. Am Surg 1988; 54:329–332.
119. Morris JB, Zollinger RM, Stellato TA. Role of surgery in antibiotic-induced pseudomembranous enterocolitis. am J Surg 1990; 160:535–539.
120. Tabaqchali S, Holland D, O'Farrell S, et al. Typing scheme for *Clostridium difficile*: Its application in clinical and epidemiological studies. Lancet 1984; 935–938.
121. McFarland LV, Surawicz CM, Greenberg RN, Fekety R, Elmer GW, Moyer KA, Melcher SA, Bowen KE, Cox JL, Noorani Z, Harrington G, Rubin M, Greenwald D. A randomized placebo-controlled trial of *Saccharomyces boulardii* in combination with standard antibiotics for *Clostridium difficile* disease. JAMA 1994; 271:1913–1918.
122. Finegold SM, George WL. Therapy directed against *Clostridium difficile* and its toxins: Complications of therapy. In: Rolfe RD, Finegold SM, eds. *Clostridium difficile*: Its role in intestinal disease. New York: Academic Press, 1988:342–357.
123. Tedesco FJ, Gordon D, Fortson WC. Approach to patients with multiple relapses of antibiotic-associated pseudomembranous colitis. Am J Gastroenterol 1985; 80:867–868.
124. Cherry RD, Portnoy D, Jabbari MM, Daly DS, Kinnear DG, Goresby CA. Metronidazole: an alternative therapy for antibiotic-associated colitis. Gastroenterology 1982; 82:849–851.
125. Teasley DG, Gerding DN, Olson MM, et al. Prospective randomized trial of metronidazole versus vancomycin for *Clostridium difficile*-associated diarrhea and colitis. Lancet 1983; 2:1043–1046.
126. Poxton IR, Aronsson B, Mollby R, Nord CE, Collee JG. Immunochemical fingerprinting of *Clostridium difficile* strains isolated from an outbreak of antibiotic-associated colitis and diarrhoea. J Med Microbiol 1984; 17:317–324.
127. Delmee M, Bulliard G, Simon G. Application of a technique for serogrouping *Clostridium difficile* in an outbreak of antibiotic-associated diarrhoea. J Infect 1986; 13:5–9.
128. McFarland LV, Bernasconi P. *Saccharomyces boulardii*: A review of an innovative biotherapeutic agent. Microbiol Ecology in Health and Disease 1993; 6:157–171.
129. Johnson S, Gerding DN, Olson MM, et al: Prospective, controlled study of vinyl glove use to interrupt *Clostridium difficile* nosocomial transmission. Amer J Med 1990; ;88:137–140.
130. Brooks SE, Veal RO, Kramer M, Dore L, Schupf N, Adachi M. Reduction in

incidence of Clostridium difficile-associated diarrhea in an acute care hospital and a skilled nursing facility following replacement of electronic thermometers with single-use disposables. Infect Cont Hosp Epid 1992; 13:98–103.
131. Johnson S, Homann SR, Bettin KM, Quick JN, Clabots CR, Peterson LR, Gerding DN. Treatment of asymptomatic *Clostridium difficile* carriers (fecal excretors) with vancomycin or metronidazole. Ann Int Med 1992; 117:297–302.
132. Young G, McDonald M. Antibiotic-associated colitis: Why do patients have recurrence? Gastroenterol 1986; 90:1098–1099.
133. Bartlett JG. Treatment of *Clostridium difficile* colitis. Gastroenterology 1985; 89:1192.
134. Thompson G, Clark AH, Hare K, Spilg WGS. Pseudomembranous colitis after treatment with metronidazole. Br Med J 1981; 282:804.
135. Saginur R, Hawley CR, Bartlett JG. Colitis associated with metronidazole therapy. J Infect Dis 1980; 141:772.
136. Toothaker RD, Elmer GW. Prevention of clindamycin-induced mortality in hamsters by *Saccharomyces boulardii*. Antimicrob Agents Chemother 1984; 26:552–556.
137. Pothoulakis C, Kelly CP, Joshi MA, Gao N, O'Keane JC, Castagliuolo I, LaMont JT. *Saccharomyces boulardii* inhibits *Clostridium difficile* toxin A binding and enterotoxicity in rat ileum. Gastroenterology 1993; 104:1108–1115.
138. Surawicz CM, Elmer GW, Speelman P, McFarland LV, Chinn J, Van Bell G. Prevention of antibiotic-associated diarrhea by *Saccharomyces boulardii*: a prospective study. Gastroenterology 1989; 96:981–988.
139. Surawicz CM, McFarland LV, Elmer GW, Chinn J. Treatment of recurrent *C. difficile* colitis with vancomycin and *Saccharomyces boulardii*. Amer J Gastroenterol 1989; 84:1285–1287.
140. Gorbach SL, Chang TW, Goldin B. Successful treatment of relapsing *Clostridium difficile* colitis with *Lactobacillus GG*. Lancet 1987; 2:1519.
141. Tvede M, Rask-Madsen J: Bacteriotherapy for chronic relapsing *Clostridium difficile* diarrhoea in six patients. Lancet 1989; I:1156–1160.
142. Seal D, Borriello SP, Barclay F, et al. Treatment of relapsing *Clostridium difficile* diarrhoea by administration of a non-toxigenic strain. Eur J Clin Microbiol 1987; 6:51–53.
143. Schwann A, Sjolin S, Trottestam U, Aronsson B. Relapsing *Clostridium difficile* enterocolitis cured by rectal infusion of normal feaces. Scand J Infect Dis 1984; 16:211–215.
144. Kreutzer EW, Milligan RD. Treatment of antibiotic-associated pseudomembranous colitis with cholestyramine resin. Johns Hopkins Med J 1978; 147:67–72.
145. Peterson LR, Gerding DN. Antimicrobial agents. In: Rambaud J-C and Ducluzeau R, eds. *Clostridium difficile*-associated intestinal diseases. Paris: Springer-Verlag, 1990:115–127.
146. Heerze LD, Kelm MA, Talbot JA, Armstrong GD. Oligosaccharide sequences attached to an inert support (SYNSORB) as potential therapy for antibiotic-associated diarrhea and pseudomembranous colitis. J Infect Dis 1994; 169:1291–1296.
147. Tjellström B, Stenhammar L, Eriksson S, Magnusson K-E. Oral immunoglobu-

lin A supplementation in treatment of *Clostridium difficile* enteritis. Lancet 1993;341:702.

148. Lyerly DM, Bostwick EF, Binion SB, Wilkins TD. Passive immunization of hamsters against disease caused by *Clostridium difficile* by use of a bovine immunoglobulin G concentrate. Infect Immun 1991; 59:2215–2218.

149. Tacket CO, Losonsky G, Link H, Hoang Y, Guesry P, Hilpert H, Levine MM. Protection by milk immunoglobulin concentrate against oral challenge with enterotoxigenic *Escherichia coli*. N Engl J Med 1988; 318:1240–1243.

150. Davidson GP, Whyte PBD, Daniels E, Franklin K, Nunan H, McCloud PI, Moore AG, Moore DJ. Passive immunization of children with bovine colostrum containing antibodies to human rotavirus. Lancet 1989; ii:709–712.

151. Nord J, Ma P, DiJohn D, Tzipori S, Tacket CO. Treatment of cryptosporidial diarrhoea in AIDS patients with bovine hyperimmune colostrum. AIDS 1990; 4:581–584.

152. Kelly CP, Vavva F, Castagliuolo I, Bostwick E, Keates S, LaMont JT, Pothoulakis C. Bovine immunoglobulin concentrate, a novel approach to *Clostridium difficile* colitis. Am J Gastroenterol 1993; 88:1577.

153. Buggy BP, Fekety R, Silva J. Therapy of relapsing *Clostridium difficile*-associated diarrhea and colitis with the combination of vancomycin and rifampin. J Clin Gastroenterol 1987; 2:155–159.

11

Parasitic Infections of the Intestine

GEORGE TRIADAFILOPOULOS
Palo Alto Veterans Affairs Health Care System and Stanford University School of Medicine, Stanford, California

I. INTRODUCTION

Parasitic infections of the intestine are major clinical problems in both the developing and developed world (1). In the United States these infections can be imported by refugees, immigrants, or travelers returning from the developing-world countries. Domestic infections may occur in the setting of community water-borne epidemics, in residents of daycare centers or long-term nursing facilities, in male homosexuals, in hikers or campers consuming untreated stream water, and in persons who eat undercooked or raw meat or fish (2).

The parasites infecting the intestine can be classified into two main groups, the protozoa and the helminths (3) (see Table 1). Helminths are in turn further classified into nematodes or roundworms, cestodes or tapeworms, and trematodes or flukes.

II. DIAGNOSIS

The diagnosis of a parasitic infection of the intestine should be considered either as part of epidemiologic or public-health screening in asymptomatic individuals, or as part of the evaluation of clinical symptoms, signs, and laboratory findings suggestive of a possible infection (4) (see Table 2).

Table 1 Comparison of Protozoa and Helminths

Feature	Protozoa	Helminths
Structure	Unicellular	Multicellular with organ systems
Replication	Human host	Intermediate host
Eosinophilia	Uncommon	Frequent

A. Epidemiologic Screening

Examination of stools for parasites may be performed in restaurant workers and in childcare providers in order to identify healthy carriers that could potentially serve as the source of an epidemic. Parasitologic examination of the stool should also be considered in individuals who have returned from a trip to an endemic country (5).

B. Evaluation of Clinical Symptoms or Signs

The clinical symptoms or signs that would prompt the physician to consider small-intestinal parasitic infections are diverse and nonspecific. Presenting symptoms may include nonspecific dyspepsia, postprandial epigastric fullness, nausea or vomiting. Abdominal pain is common and may be localized in the epigastrium, mimicking peptic ulcer or gall bladder disease, or the right iliac fossa, simulating appendicitis or inflammatory bowel disease. Abdominal distention is frequent. Diarrhea is usually watery, voluminous and not associated with tenesmus or blood (6). Anal or vulva pruritus suggests the possibility of pinworm (7). Extraintestinal symptoms may include weight loss, asthma, insomnia, or pruritic maculopapular rash.

Table 2 Common Parasitic Infections of the Intestines

Location	Species		Cardinal symptom(s)
Small Bowel	*Protozoa*	Giardiasis	Diarrhea, malabsorption
	Nematodes	Ascariasis	Intestinal obstruction
		Ancylostomiasis	Anemia
		Strongyloidiasis	Hyperinfection syndrome
	Cestodes	Taenia	Asymptomatic
Colon	*Protozoa*	Amebiasis	Colitis, dysentery
	Nematodes	Enterobiasis	Anal pruritus
		Trichuriasis	Asymptomatic
	Trematodes	Schistosomiasis	Diarrhea, portal hypertension

C. Laboratory Clues

Peripheral blood eosinophilia is a frequent laboratory finding that should suggest the possibility of a parasitic infection of the intestine. Hypereosinophila occurs only with helminthic infections and occasionally with protozoa (see Table 3). The degree of hypereosinophilia may vary with time, host, or parasite (8). In general, maximal levels of hypereosinophilia occur prior to the maturation of the parasite, when fecal parasitologic examination is still negative.

III. SPECIFIC INFECTIONS

A. Protozoan Infections

1. Giardiasis

Giardia lamblia, a cosmopolitan parasite with a worldwide prevalence of up to 40%, is the most commonly diagnosed intestinal protozoan in the United States. It localizes and multiplies in the small intestine and may cause acute or chronic diarrhea with malabsorption (9). However, most patients who harbor the parasite are asymptomatic. Communitywide epidemics of giardiasis in the United States are due to poorly filtered water. High incidence of the infection due to contaminated water are also noted in travelers to Eastern Europe, particularly St. Petersburg, and in campers and hikers in the Western United States. *Giardia* may also spread by sexual or close person-to-person contact through fecal-oral contamination. There is an association between giardiasis and dysgammaglobulinemias, particlarly IgA and IgM deficiencies with or without associated nodular lymphoid hyperplasia of the small intestine (10).

Table 3 Causes of Parasitic Eosinophilia (Eosinophil Count > 300/mL)

Prominent in early infection	Schistosomiasis
	Ascariasis
	Ancylostomiasis (hookworm)
	Intestinal flukes
	Taenia saginata
Intermittent	Ascariasis
	Cestodes (tapeworm)
Persistent eosinophilia with negative stool examination	*Strongyloides stercoralis*
	Ancylostomiasis (hookworm)
	Trichinosis
	Anisakiasis

Source: Ref. 8.

Giardia lamblia exists in two forms: the cysts and the vegetative forms, or trophozoites. Humans acquire the infection by ingesting cysts that excyst and multiply in the proximal small bowel where the flagellated trophozoites attack the mucosa and cause inflammation and partial villous atrophy. The pathogenesis of diarrhea and malabsorption in giardiasis is not clearly elucidated and probably multifactorial, with the most pronounced effects on the intestinal microvillous membrane absorptive mechanisms (11).

Symptomatic patients present with recurrent attacks of diarrhea with urgency and upper abdominal bloating and discomfort. Weakness, flatulence, abdominal distention, and nausea occur frequently. There is no tenesmus and fever is rare. There may be severe malabsorption to carbohydrates (D-xylose and lactose), fat, and vitamin B_{12}, with explosive loose pale stools.

The diagnosis of giardiasis is made clinically and treatment is established empirically (12). In travelers, diarrhea usually occurs near the end of the trip and persists upon return, in contrast to other forms of traveler's diarrhea that occur early and resolve rapidly. Giardia cysts and less frequently trophozoites can be seen by light microscopy of stool samples examined either fresh or fixed with formalin and stained with trichrome. Stool examination is the preferred method for the diagnosis of *G. lamblia* and also allows identification of other protozoa or helminths. However, because of variation in cyst excretion, different stool specimens from different days should be examined. Examination of three separate stool specimens increases the diagnostic yield to 85% (13). The motile trophozoites may be detected in duodenal fluid aspirates with a lesser degree of sensitivity but in a complementary fashion to the stool examination. Trophozoites can also be detected by endoscopic brush cytology, by mucosal impression smears of small intestinal biosies, or by routine histopathology. Commercially available enzyme-linked immunosorbent assays (ELISA) that identify *Giardia lamblia* antigens in the stool have sensitivity and specificity ranging from 87% to 100% and may be useful in cases of "microscopy negative" giardiasis (14). Fecal detection assays based on DNA are under development (15). Detection of anti-Giardia IgG antibodies does not distinguish past from present infection; however, anti-Giardia IgM antibodies are only elevated during the acute phase of the infection and fall rapidly after the infection is eradicated.

Metronidazole (Flagyl, 250 mg po *tid* in adults or 5 mg/kg po *tid* in children for 7 days) is the most effective and commonly used drug for giardiasis (16). Although successful in more than 90% of cases, it frequently causes upper abdominal discomfort, nausea, metallic taste, an dark urine. If used with alcohol, it causes disulfuram-like reactions. Tinidazole, a related drug not available in the United States, has the advantage of a single oral dose (2 gm in adults, 75mg/kg in children) and similar efficacy rates. When treatment fails, possibilities include drug resistance or reinfection. A repeat course of metronidazole at higher doses may not be tolerable due to the side effects of the drug. Although quinacrine (Atabrine, 100 mg po *tid* in adults, 2 mg/kg po *tid* in children for 5 days) is a highly effective drug against *G. lamblia* and ideal when metronidazole therapy fails, it is generally unavailable in the United States (17). Side effects with quinacrine include gastrointestinal disturbances, dizziness, headache, nausea, vomiting, and rarely toxic psychosis (18). Furazolidine (Furoxone, 100 mg po *qid* in adults or 2 mg/kg po *tid* in children for 7 days) is more than 80% successful, is available as a suspension for pediatric use, and provides the best alternative for those failing metronidazole therapy. Side effects with furazolidine include nausea, vomiting, fever, rash, and hemolysis in G-6-PD-deficient patients (19). Because none of these drugs is considered safe in pregnancy, paromomycin (Humatin, 500 mg po *tid* for 7 days) is a possible choice since it is poorly absorbed (see Table 4). One month after completion of therapy, repeat stool examination should demonstrate eradication of the parasite. Persistent symptoms and a negative stool examination should raise the possibility of postinfective lactose intolerance or intestinal candidiasis.

Preventive measures against *G. lamblia* include decontamination and monitoring of water supplies and personal hygiene. A vaccine is not available.

2. *Amebiasis*

Among numerous other species of amebae that inhabit the human intestinal tract, *Entamoeba hisolytica* is the only pathogenic one and must be distinguished from other amebae, particularly *Entamoeba hartmanii* and *Entamoeba coli*. *Dientamoeba fragilis,* which resembles an ameba and may occasionally cause mild gastrointestinal infections, is related to flagellates and not to amebae. Two other amebae, of the species *Naegleria* and *Acanthamoeba*, which inhabit polluted water and swimming pools worldwide, may cause fulminant meningitis and encephalitis but not intestinal amebiasis.

Entamoeba histolytica causes amebiasis, an acute and chronic disease with variable manifestations (20). Although the colon is the usual site of initial disease, the infection may spread to other organs, particularly the liver. The worldwide average prevalence of amebiasis is 10%, but in tropical and subtropical regions of close cohabitation and poor sanitation it reaches 80%. In the United States the disease occurs mainly in travelers returning from endemic regions of the world and less than 5% of cases occur as a result of fecal-oral contamination in daycare centers, mental institutions, or during sexual intercourse (21).

The disease is propagated between humans through *E. histolytica* cysts, which are excreted in the feces, survive outside the body, and then are ingested in water or contaminated uncooked food, particularly lettuce. After excystment of mature cysts in the small bowel, free trophozoites survive in the colon and may invade and ulcerate the mucosa causing amebic dysentery (22). Some tro-

Table 4 Common Antiparasitic Drugs, Their Specific Indications, and Side Effects

Drug	Common indication(s)	Common side effect(s)
Emetine	Invasive amebiasis	Cardiac arrythmias
Furazolidone	Giardiasis	Nausea, fever, rash
Iodoquinol	Amebiasis (noninvasive)	Rash, nausea
Mebendazole	Nematodes (roundworm, hookworm, whipworm, pinworm) Cestodes	Diarrhea, abdominal pain
Metronidazole	Invasive amebiasis Giardiasis	Metallic taste, nausea, disulfiram reaction
Niclosamide	*Taenia saginata*, *Hymenolepis nana*	Nausea, abdominal pain
Paromomycin	Amebiasis	Nausea, dyspepsia
Piperazine	Ascariasis, enterobiasis	Nausea
Praziquantel	Intestinal tapeworms (beef, pork, fish, dwarf) Cysticercosis Trematodes (blood, liver, intestinal flukes)	Abdominal pain, nausea, drowsiness, headache
Pyrantel pamoate	Ascariasis Enterobiasis Ancylostomiasis	Dyspepsia
Quinacrine	Giardiasis	Bitter taste, anorexia, dyspepsia, disulfiram reaction
Thiabendazole	Strongyloidiasis Trichinosis	Nausea, dyspepsia, drowsiness, headache
Trimethoprimsulfamethoxazole	Isosporiasis	Rash, hepatitis, blood dyscrasias

phozoites encyst again and mature in the distal colon contributing to fecal contamination and spread. Similarly, in asymptomatic carriers, or patients with mild forms of the disease, nonmotile cysts predominate and are responsible for disease propagation. In amebic dysentery, protozoan invasion results in focal colitis, which is usually maximal in the cecum but may involve the entire colon with flask-shaped ulcers of variable size. Only infrequently, when amebic ulcers penetrate the muscularis, severe intestinal bleeding may occur. Rarely a localized granuloma, or "ameboma," is formed as a discrete cecal mass simulating carcinoma. After penetration of the bowel wall, portal venous invasion may carry the amebae into the liver where they multiply and destroy the parenchyma, causing amebic liver abscess with its characteristic thick, chocolate brown liquid content, often described as anchovy sauce. In widespread disease, especially in patients on corticosteroids, amebae may be found in any organ of the body, such as the skin, brain, lungs, and eyes (23).

Although the precise mechanism of invasion is not clearly understood, it appears that the virulence of *E. histolytica* correlates with increased expression and excretion of cysteine proteinases. Pathogenic *E. histolytica* has a unique proteinase gene, the ACP1 gene, not present in nonpathogenic *E. histolytica*, which is associated with increased proteinase expression, activity, and in vitro cytopathic effect (24).

Entamoeba histolytica causes a spectrum of manifestations ranging from the asymptomatic carrier state to fulminant colitis and generalized widespread infection. Asymptomatic carriers usually only pass cysts in their stool and contribute to disease spread but they are also at risk to develop amebic dysentery. Depending on the location and extent of the intestinal amebiasis, symptomatic patients present with intermittent diarrhea, grumbling abdominal pain, and general malaise. The disease is usually chronic, with waxing and waning mucus diarrhea, sometimes with streaks of blood, alternating with constipation. In contrast to ulcerative colitis, tenesmus is only infrequently present, only when the rectum is involved. The acute, fulminant colitis is clinically indistinguishable from acute ulcerative colitis with crampy abdominal pain and bloody mucus diarrhea, leading to toxic megacolon with fever, dehydration, sepsis, and circulatory shock. Physical examination reveals tenderness that localizes along the colon, particularly over the cecum and the sigmoid colon. Acute right-lower-quadrant pain may simulate acute appendicitis. Abdominal distention, localized guarding and paucity of bowel sounds associated with systemic toxicity suggest toxic colonic dilation. In these instances, amebae may not be readily found in the stool, but it is essential to rule out their presence before treating with corticosteroids for acute idiopathic inflammatory bowel disease. Rarely, cecal perforation or massive bleeding may occur. Colonic narrowing by an ameboma presents with signs and symptoms of intestinal obstruction of intussusception simulating colonic neoplasm (25).

Hepatic amebic abscess is a major extraintestinal manifestation that occurs in about 1% of patients with intestinal amebiasis, particularly in men residing in endemic areas. The clinical features of amebic liver abscess are variable. There is usually no preceeding history of amebiasis or diarrhea and *E. histolytica* is found in the stool in only a minority of patients (26). Early symptoms are insidious right-upper-quadrant discomfort, fever, and malaise. Later, low-grade or spiking fever, sweats, cough, and dull and constant but occasionally sharp, pleuritic right-upper-quadrant pain, radiating to the right shoulder predominate. Anorexia, nausea, weight loss, and general fatigue are common. Jaundice is rare. Physical examination reveals tender, enlarged liver, occasionally bulging on the anterior abdominal wall surface; the right hemidiaphragm is raised and its excursion is diminished. A pleural or hepatic friction rub may be audible. There is neutrophilic leukocytosis. Unless imaging techniques are applied, the less common abscess of the left hepatic lobe may not be diagnosed clinically because of vague and minimal signs and symptoms (27). Rupture of a large amebic abscess through the diaphragm into the lung leads to bronchohepatic fistula manifesting with intermittent cough productive of thick, anchovy-sauce-like material. Rupture into the pleura, the peritoneum, or the pericardium occurs rarely. This may precipitate septic shock or pericardial tamponade with vascular collapse, thus requiring urgent intensive medical therapy and surgical drainage (28).

In more than 90% of cases, the diagnosis of amebiasis is made by microscopic examination of repeated (more than three) fresh feces in a saline wet-mount preparation. However, barium studies, the prior use of mineral oil, or antibiotics may decrease the diagnostic yield for weeks. *E. histolytica* motile trophozoites, 30 microns in diameter, with protruding and retracting pseudopodia and containing ingested red blood cells are characteristic and pathognomonic of acute amebiasis. Concentration techniques and permanent mounts using trichrome stain improve the identification of amebic cysts. An immunodiagnostic assay, based on detection of epitopes of the adhesin present only in pathogenic strains of *E. histolytica*, has 97% sensitivity and 100% specificity (29). Serologic tests, particularly the enzyme immunoassay, are useful in detecting patients with invasive amebiasis, as patients with amebic colitis or amebic liver abscess have high titers while asymptomatic cyst carriers have low or negative titers (30). Because the rectum is less frequently involved than the cecum, sigmoidoscopy is not as useful as it is in idiopathic ulcerative colitis and colonoscopy may be necessary. In contrast to the diffuse nature of ulcerative colitis or bacillary invasive diarrheas, *E. histolytica* causes discrete, flask-shaped ulcers with intervening normal mucosa (Figure 1). In fulminant amebiasis however, the severity of the disease and the rectal involvement make the endoscopic differential diagnosis impossible. If sigmoidoscopy is performed before any therapy and without bowel preparation, aspiration of fecal exudative material from the base of the ulcers and preparation of a wet mount reveals the typical trophozoites occasionaly surrounded by Charcot–Leyden crystals. Mucosal biopsies are not particularly useful as they reveal the nondistinctive features of colitis and trophozoites in less than 50% of cases, despite multiple sections.

Plain abdominal films may reveal colonic dilation, irregularity of the wall, or free air under the diaphragm in cases of severe, fulminant amebic colitis with toxic megacolon or perforation. Barium studies should never precede the repeated collection of stool samples for parasitologic examination, otherwise identification of the amebae is precluded. Barium enema studies may reveal spasm, thumbprinting, loss of haustrae, granularity of the colonic wall, "collar-button" or deep penetrating ulcers, or strictures. The colon is involved segmentally or

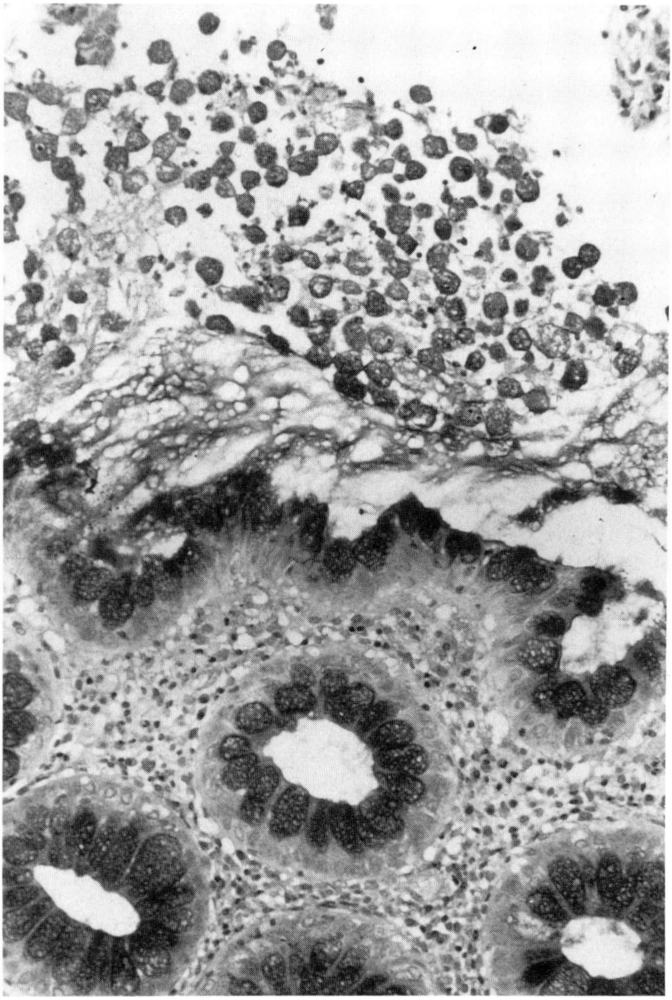

Figure 1 Colonic ulcer containing numerous *E. histolytica.*

entirely, and skip areas are common, mimicking Crohn's colitis. The cecum is affected in more than 90% of cases and may become concentrically narrowed. Narrowing, ulceration, and nodular filling defects may also involve the appendix and the ascending colon but usually spare the ileocecal valve and the terminal ileum. Ultrasonography is the procedure of choice for the diagnosis of amebic liver abscess because it is noninvasive, sensitive, inexpensive, and generally available (31). The finding of round hypoechoic cr anechoic areas in patients with a clinical picture suggestive of amebic abscess and positive serology is generally considered adequate evidence to allow initiation of therapy without performing aspiration. In atypical cases or in cases that fail to respond to amebicidal therapy, computed tomography should be performed. Aspiration of the abscess cavity is currently rarely needed for diagnosis and is reserved for the detection of superimposed bacterial infection and the prevention of rupture of large abscesses (32).

The treatment of choice for both acute amebic dysentery and amebic liver abscess is metronidazole (Flagyl, 750 mg po *tid* in adults or 15 mg/kg po *tid* in children for 10 days). This regimen is highly effective with rapid therapeutic response and very rare failures. In cases of fulminant amebic colitis and in patients who cannot tolerate the drug orally, metronidazole should be given intravenously in order to ensure absorption and tissue penetration. Side effects include upper abdominal discomfort, nausea, metallic taste and, if used with alcohol, disulfuram-like reactions. Upon completion of therapy with metronidazole, follow-up therapy with poorly-absorbed, luminal-active drugs may be initiated in order to eliminate cysts and prevent disease relapse and spread. For this purpose, paromomycin (Humatin, 500 mg po *tid* in adults or 10 mg/kg po *tid* in children for 7 days) or iodoquinol (Yodoxin, 650 mg po *tid* in adults or 13 mg po *tid* in children for 20 days) are used. Paromomycin may precipitate gastrointestinal symptoms but it is safe in pregnancy (see Table 4). Iodoquinol may also cause gastrointestinal distress and rashes and is best avoided during pregnancy. Mild to moderate amebiasis may be treated with lower metronidazole dose (500 mg po *tid* in adults or 10 mg/kg po *tid* in children for 10 days) followed by the luminal-active regimen described above. Asymptomatic cyst carriers should also be treated because they may infect other people and they may themselves eventually develop invasive disease. In such cases, treatment with a luminal-active drug alone is more than 90% successful. Mentronidazole should not be used in this situation.

Although in most patients antiamebic therapy is rapidly effective, fulminant amebic colitis with toxic megacolon and peritoneal signs may necessitate subtotal colectomy. Colonic perforation during the course of amibicidal therapy also requires immediate laparotomy with colostomy, and peritoneal drainage should be performed under continuous amebicidal cover therapy. In cases of colonic narrowing due to ameboma, medical therapy should be initiated first, as it leads to resolution of the obstruction in most cases. Surgical resection should only be considered for the rare failures. Almost all patients with amebic liver abscess respond to medical therapy within 3 days and failures are usually associated with other superinfections or malignancy. In such cases, needle aspiration under ultrasound or CT guidance is used for both diagnosis and therapy. Surgical drainage is only reserved for complicated amebic abscesses and always under amebicidal coverage.

Prevention against *E. histolytica* infection involves correction of unsanitary conditions and avoidance of potentially contaminated water and food, particularly raw vegetables. A vaccine is not available and prophylaxis of travelers to endemic areas with metronidazole or iodoquinol is not recommended.

3. *Dientamebiasis*

Dientamoeba fragilis is an ameba-like flagellate previously considered as a harmless commensal, which is now known to cause chronic infection in humans. It is a noninvasive luminal parasite of the cecum and proximal large intestine that is most likely transmitted by direct fecal-oral route through pinworm eggs that contain the organism. Infection occurs most frequently in children in daycare centers and in institutionalized adults with poor personal hygiene. There is an up to 20-fold higher association between enterobiasis and dientamebiasis than with any other helminthic infections (33).

Although most infections are asymptomatic, the parasite may cause abdominal pain, anorexia, nausea, and diarrhea. The diagnosis of dientamebiasis should always be considered when patients with enterobiasis complain of abdominal pain and diarrhea and inversely, pinworm infection should be considered when patients with *D. fragilis* infection complain of anal pruritus or are found to have peripheral eosinophilia. The diagnosis rests on the identification of *D. fragilis* in either fresh or appropriately preserved stool samples stained with hematoxylin or trichrome. Because of variable excretion of the parasite, several stool samples need to be examined.

The best therapy against symptomatic *Dientamoeba fragilis* is paramomycin (Humatin, 500 mg po *tid* in adults or 10 mg/kg po *tid* in children for 7 days). Less effective alternatives include iodoquinol (Yodoxin, 650 mg po *tid* in adults or 13 mg po *tid* in children for 20 days) or tetracycline (500 mg po *qid* for 10 days).

4. *Cryptosporidiosis*

Cryptosporidium parvum is a small protozoan that may cause diarrhea in both immunocompetent and immunodeficient individuals (34). In clinical practice, it is most frequently encountered as a cause of chronic, watery, debilitating diarrhea in patients with acquired immunodeficiency syndrome (AIDS) and other immunocompromised patients (35). It is also an important cause of waterborne diarrhea in immunocompetent adults (health care workers and daycare center staff) and children worldwide. Daycare outbreaks, nosocomial outbreaks, and sporadic traveler's diarrhea have also been linked to cryptosporidiosis. Domestic and wild animals serve as the reservoirs for most infections by contaminating surface water. Person-to-person, fecal-oral spread, and transmission during male homosexual intercourse are noted mostly in urban settings.

Although most commonly associated with diarrhea, *Cryptosporidium* may be found in asymptomatic, immunocompetent carriers. The prevalence of the infection varies from 1% to 30% worldwide.

The wide clinical spectrum of cryptosporidiosis depends on the immunologic stats of the host on one hand and parasite virulence factors on the other (36). The parasite replicates mainly on the intestinal surface of the jejunum and ileum, leading to villous atrophy and resulting in malabsorption of solutes and water, osmotic changes across the gut wall with fluid release into the lumen, brush border enzyme deficiency, and epithelial barrier dysfunction. In immunocompromized hosts, the biliary and pancreatic ducts may also be involved (37).

The clinical manifestations of *Cryptosporidium* infection in the immunocompromised host are described in a separate chapter. The most common manifestation of the infection in an immunocompetent patient is profuse, watery diarrhea, which is worse postprandially, and associated with abdominal cramps, nausea, vomiting, and constitutional symptoms (38). There is no fever or gastrointestinal bleeding. The diarrhea lasts for 1–2 weeks and resolves spontaneously without recurrences. Weight loss is seen only rarely, in severe and protracted cases.

Identification of oocysts in fecal samples by acid-fast staining is a simple and effective method to establish the diagnosis of *Cryptosporidium* infection. Because of variable oocyst excretion, examination of three or more stool samples is frequently required. Concentrations of the stool samples is usually not needed in patients with severe diarrhea, but may be used in epidemiologic field studies. Fecal leukocytes are typically absent, but other copathogens may be noted. Other more sensitive and specific methods, such as immunofluorescence using fluorescein-labeled monoclonal antibodies or ELISA kits, may be used for the detection of oocysts in stool samples of symptomatic individuals, asymptomatic carriers, or sources of contamination. Newer, more sensitive and specific methods using the polymerase chain reaction are capable of detecting one parasite per stool sample and are expected to dramatically improve out diagnostic yield, particularly in epidemiologic studies. Parasite identification in duodenal fluid aspirates, small-intestinal biopsies and brushings, and electron microscopy of small-intestinal samples may also be diagnostic but are less frequently used today for routine diagnosis (see Figure 2). Serologic tests, detecting IgM or IgG antibodies to *Cryptosporidium* by ELISA or indirect immunofluorescence assay, are not useful in diagnosis because titers persist long after the infection has resolved.

In immunocompetent patients with cryptosporidial diarrhea, supportive therapy with fluid and electrolyte replacement and antidiarrheal drugs is adequate until the infection resolves. However, immunocompromised patients are unlikely

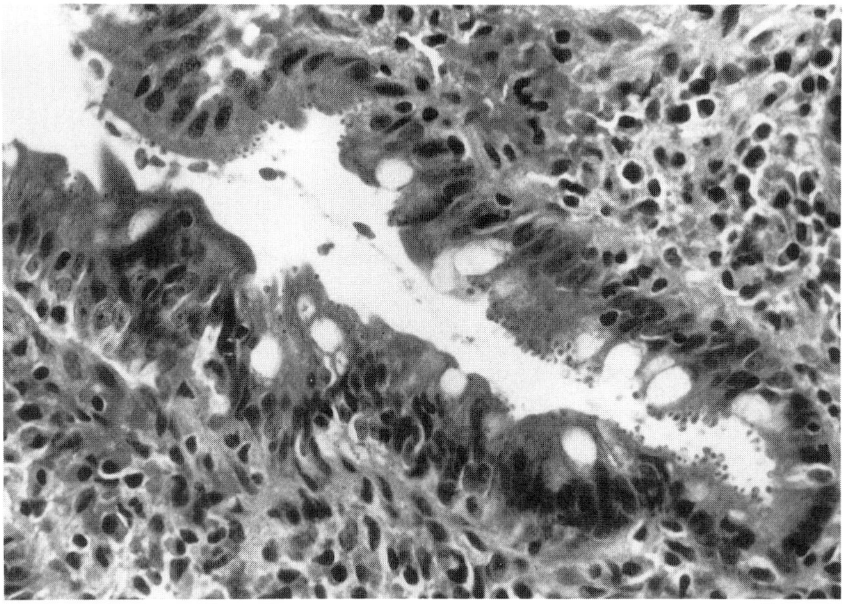

Figure 2 Cryptosporidia attached to the intestinal epithelial surface.

to spontaneously clear the infection and they require specific therapy (39). Unfortunately, no antimicrobial agent has proved to be consistently effective against *Cryptosporidium*. Paromomycin (Humatin, 500 mg po *tid* in adults or 10 mg/kg po *tid* in children for 10 days) is a promising agent (40). Side effects are minor and include nausea and abdominal discomfort (41).

Because patients and asymptomatic carriers are potential reservoirs of *Cryptosporidium*, hand washing and enteric precautions are very important in the prevention of spread. Because *Cryptosporidium* oocysts are very resistant to various disinfection methods, eradication of the parasite from environmental sources remains difficult.

5. *Microsporidiosis*

Microsporidia are intracellular protozoa that may cause infection in both immunocompetent and immunodeficient individuals (42). Microsporidiosis however is an increasingly recognized cause of water diarrhea and malabsorption in AIDS patients and is discussed in a separate chapter (43).

6. *Cyclospora Infection*

Variably classified as *Cryptosporidium*-like oocyst, *Cyanobacterium*-like body, or blue-green alga, this new protozoan parasite causes self-limited, explosive, watery diarrhea in both immunocompetent and immunosuppressed individuals. *Cyclospora* mostly affects children in developing countries, but hospital outbreaks from contaminated water sources have been recently reported in the United States. The parasite damages the small-intestinal surface causing chronic inflammation and villous atrophy. Although it stains variably on acid-fast stain, *Cyclospora* autofluoresce under ultraviolet light like neon-blue circles. The infection may respond successfully to co-trimoxazole therapy.

7. *Isospora belli* Infection

Isospora belli, an intracellular coccidian protozoan related to Cryptosporidia, is an important cause of watery, protracted diarrhea in immunocompromised host, and, in particular, patients with AIDS (see Chapter) (35). Isosporiasis may nevertheless affect immunocompetent individuals and it may be the cause of sporadic traveler's diarrhea or daycare-center outbreaks. The clinical presentation of acute, explosive, watery diarrhea and abdominal cramps is indistinguishable from cryptosporidiosis. In immunocompetent patients, symptoms universally resolve spontaneously within a few weeks. The diagnosis is best made by demonstrating the bright red, elliptical oocysts on modified acid-fast stain of several stool samples collected daily. Occasionally the parasite may be found in small-intestinal biopsy samples obtained at endoscopy. The infection responds promptly to therapy with trimethoprim-sulfamethoxazole (Bactrim 160/800 mg po *qid* for 10 days). Pyrimethamine may aso be used (44).

8. *Blastocystis hominis* Infection

Blastocystis hominis is a common protozoan of the human gastrointestinal tract, particularly the colon, but its pathogenic role currently remains controversial (45). *B. hominis* has been identified in both sporadic and epidemic diarrhea throughout the world, but it is more prevalent in tropical and subtropical regions. It is increasingly recognized in both immunocompetent and immunocompromised hosts, with prevalence rates ranging from 3% in the former group to 52% in the latter. Coinfection with other parasites may occur in up to 50% of cases. The agent is presumably transmitted through a fecal-oral route and although animals may be infected, it is not known if they serve as reservoirs for human infection.

B. hominis infection may cause variable symptoms or remain asymptomatic (46). Watery, nonbloody diarrhea, abdominal cramps, bloating, nausea, fever, and malaise may last from a few hours to several days or years, occasionally leading to significant dehydration.

Colonoscopy, biopsy, and barium studies of the small and large intestine are normal. There is no peripheral blood eosinophilia and the stool does not reveal fecal leukocytes. The diagnosis therefore is based upon the demonstration of *B. hominis* in fecal smears preferably stained with hematoxylin or trichrome, which reveal the typical vacuolated form of the parasite. Diarrheal stools containing more than five *B. hominis* organisms per high-power field in the absence of other pathogens imply significant infection requiring therapy.

Although no drug has been shown to be clearly effective, metronidazole (Flagyl, 500 mg po *tid* in adults or 5 mg/kg po *tid* in children for 7 days) is most commonly prescribed. Alternative drugs include iodoquinol (Yodoxin, 650 mg po *tid* in adults, or 13 mg/kg po *tid* in children for 20 days) or furazolidine (Furoxone, 100 mg po *qid* in adults or 1.25 mg/kg suspension po *qid* in children for 7 days). Treatment of asymptomatic carriers is not recommended.

9. Nonpathogenic Protozoa

Nonpathogenic protozoa, such as *Enteromonas hominis, Entamoeba hartmanii, Entamoeba coli, Endolimax nana, Trichomonas hominis, Retortamonas intestinalis,* and *Chylomastix mesnili* can be frequently found on stool examination, either isolated or in conjunction with other organisms. Even when found in diarrheal stools, these agents should not be regarded as the cause of the patient's abdominal complaints and further search for the responsible pathogen is warranted.

B. Helminthic Infections

Intestinal helminthiases are among the most prevalent chronic infections in humans. Helminths are classified into two groups: Nemathelminths, which include nematodes (roundworms), and Platyhelminths, which include cestodes (tapeworms) and trematodes (flukes).

1. Nematodes

Human infections due to nematodes may be classified in three categories: 1. intestinal nematodes, 2. tissue-invasive nematodes, and 3. other-animal nematodes that may cause ectopic infection in humans.

The major intestinal nematodes are *Ascaris lubricoides, Enterobius vermicularis, Trichuris trichiura, Necator americanus, Ancylostoma duodenale, Strongyloides stercoralis,* and *Capillaria phillippinensis*. They are cylindrical worms with lengths that vary from millimeters to several centimeters and have a uniform body. Adult female worms live in the intestinal lumen without causing tissue invasion and pass their eggs or larvae in the stool. They may cause cough, fever, and eosinophilia during the stage of larval invasion (47).

Common tissue invasive nematodes are *Wuchereria bancrofti, Loa loa, Brugia malayi,* and *Onchocerca volvulus*. They cause disease either by their adult forms or their microfilariae, which migrate into the bloodstream and invade tissues causing eosinophilia.

The most important animal nematodes that may affect humans are *Toxocara canis, Trichinella spiralis, Anisakis marina, Ancylostoma brasiliensis, Angiostrongylus cantonensis,* and *Gnathostoma spinigerum.* These nematodes cause disease by their larvae, which become trapped in a particular organ, evoking inflammation and eosinophilic granuloma formation (48).

2. *Ascariasis (Roundworm)*

Ascaris lubricoides (roundworm) is a large, yellow, round worm 20–30 cm long that causes infection worldwide, in both temperate and tropical climates. Ascariasis is the most common helminthic infection globally, second only in prevalence to enterobiasis in the United States, and affects mainly children between the ages of 5–10 years.

Humans are the main hosts and are infected by ingesting food containing mature ova (49). Larvae are released from ova in the proximal intestine, enter the circulation, and ultimately reach the pulmonary alveoli where they develop further. Such larval migration through the lungs may cause pneumonitis with cough and hemoptysis, usually associated with allergic manifestations and eosinophilia (Loeffler's syndrome). Larvae then ascend into the tracheobronchial tree, are swallowed, and enter the duodenum where they mature into adult worms. In the small intestine, worms may cause no symptoms or may induce nausea, vomiting, colicky abdominal pain, and diarrhea. Occasionally worms may be regurgitated or passed rectally. In severe infections, a mass of worms may cause strangulation or intestinal obstruction. Blockage of the bile duct, pancreatic duct, and the appendix may occur with resulting jaundice, epigastric or right-upper-quadrant pain, cholangitis, appendicitis or peritonitis (50). In children, severe infections cause growth retardation and cachexia.

The diagnosis of ascariasis is made by finding the adult worms, larvae, or eggs expelled spontaneously through the mouth, nose, or rectum, or detected radiologically, endoscopically or at a surgery (see Figure 3). Eggs are detected by microscopic examination of two or three separate smears. Marked eosinophilia may be detected during the larval migration phase but is not associated with adult infection. Serologic methods for the detection of IgM antibodies have limited specificity and sensitivity and are of no practical value. Barium studies of small or large bowel may reveal the presence of single or multiple radiolucent filling defects.

Ascariasis should always be treated to prevent complications. The drug of choice is mebendazole (Vermox, 100 mg po *bid* for 3 days in both adults and children); it is almost 100% effective with only rare diarrhea or abdominal discomfort as side effects. Mebendazole is contraindicated in pregnancy. Alternatively, a single dose of pyrantel pamoate (Antiminth, suspension, 11 mg/kg po to a maximum of 1 gm in both adults and children) is over 90% effective with only mild and transient gastrointestinal side effects (see Table 4). If

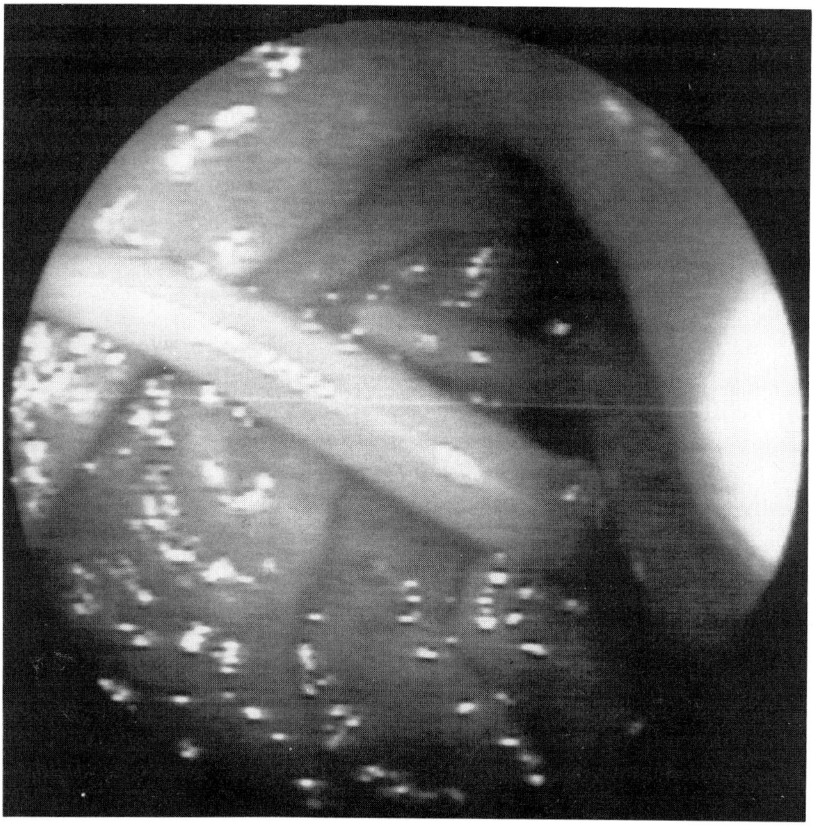

Figure 3 *Ascaris lubricoides* in the upper small intestine as visualized during endoscopy.

a mixed infection with hookworm is present, treatment should be continued for 3 days. If ascariasis causes incomplete intestinal obstruction, pyrantel pamoate can be used through the nasogastric tube. For complete intestinal obstruction or strangulation, surgery is necessary to remove the worm and/or the ischemic bowel. Biliary or pancreatic ascariasis responds to therapy with antihelminthic drugs and removal of the worm by ERCP. Supportive therapy suffices for the pulmonary phase of ascariasis; steroids are required only for severe cases.

Preventive measures against ascariasis can be applied individually (personal hygiene, hand washing, water boiling, and improved sanitation) and on a community-wide basis (mass or targeted chemotherapy) in areas of high prevalence and poor socioeconomic level.

3. *Enterobiasis (Pinworm)*

Enterobius vermicularis (formerly *Oxyuris*) is a large-bowel nematode 0.5–1 cm long that affects all socioeconomic and age groups worldwide but more commonly in temperate than tropical climates. Because of its morphology, it is frequently called pinworm or threadworm. Enterobiasis is the most common helminthic infection in the United States and affects particularly small children, in whom infection rates range from 10%–50%. Because physical proximity and overcrowding facilitate transmission, enterobiasis is also particularly prevalent in institutionalized individuals, male homosexuals, and members of the same household (51).

Humans are the only hosts of the infection. Upon egg ingestion, larvae hatch in the proximal small bowel, and develop into adult forms in the cecum. Adult worms are found predominantly in the colon (52). After mating, gravid female worms traverse the colon and lay their eggs on the perianal skin and cause intense itching, especially at night. The ova are then often carried to the mouth on fecally contaminated fingers of the infected individual causing reinfection. In female patients, the genitalia may be invaded.

Most infected individuals are asymptomatic. The main symptom, perianal pruritus, is present in 30% of patients. Because of its intensity, pruritus is often associated with insomnia, irritability, perianal excoriations, and secondary perianal skin infections and abscesses. Some children experience anorexia and weight loss. Vulvovaginitis and other pelvic infections result from genital invasion. Young girls with enterobiasis may present with enuresis or recurrent urinary-tract infections. Diarrhea, abdominal pain, or eosinophilia are notably absent. When present, these symptoms should prompt the search for coinfection, particularly with *Dientameba fragilis*, a large-bowel protozoan that is transmitted within pinworm eggs in up to 50% of cases.

Demonstration of adult worms or eggs in the stool, the perianal skin, or the fingers by inspection or proctoscopy confirms the diagnosis. The most reliable test is the cellulose acetate (adhesive) test. Three examinations performed on consecutive nights or upon awakening in the morning have 90% sensitivity; seven tests increase the sensitivity to 100%. For the test, a wooden tongue depressor draped with the sticky side of scotch tape facing outwards is pressed against the perianal skin. The tape is then placed on a glass slide and examined under a microscope for eggs. Stool examination for eggs has a very low yield—less than 5%—but is important to rule out other coinfections particularly with *Dientameba fragilis*.

Treatment is necessary for both symptomatic and asymptomatic individuals in order to eliminate the risk of transmission to others. All members of the household should be treated simultaneously to prevent reinfection. Personal hygienic measures, such as frequently changing of linen and underwear, handwashing, and bathing should be enforced. Single-dose treatment with mebendazole (Vermox, 100 mg in both adults and children), is 90–100% effective with only rare diarrhea or abdominal discomfort as side effects (53). Mebendazole is contraindicated in pregnancy. Alternatively, a single dose of pyrantel pamoate (Antiminth, suspension, 11 mg/kg po to a maximum of 1 gm in both adults and children) is over 90% effective with only mild and transient gastrointestinal side effects (see Table 4). Since both these drugs are more effective against pinworms and less so against their larvae or eggs, treatment should be repeated once in 2 weeks.

Prevention against enterobiasis involves identification and treatment of index cases in schools, families, or institutions, personal hygienic measures, and mass chemotherapy.

4. Trichuriasis (Whipworm)

Trichuris trichiura is a large-bowel nematode, 3–5 cm in length, which causes endemic infections mainly in tropical regions, but also in temperate climates. Because of the morphology of the adult worm, *T. trichiura* is commonly called whipworm. As with ascariasis, trichuriasis affects mainly children between ages 5 and 10 who live in areas of poor sanitation. Although humans are the primary host for *T. trichiura*, person-to-person transmission does not occur because the eggs require 3 weeks in the soil to become infective. Ingested fertilized eggs hatch their larvae in the small intestine but the mature worms develop and penetrate in the cecum and proximal colon causing focal colitis (54).

Mild infections are asymptomatic. Moderate infections cause a nonspecific chronic colitis with abdominal pain and diarrhea (55). Severe infections—mainly in children of the tropics—commonly manifest with crampy diarrhea, occasionally with mucus and blood, tenesmus, anal pruritus, and rectal prolapse. In these children, malnutrition, growth retardation, anemia, and impairment of cognitive function may occur.

The diagnosis is based on the demonstration of adult worms, or the typical barrel-shaped eggs of *T. trichiura* in the stool. Barium enema may reveal linear filling defects attached to the colonic wall. At colonoscopy, the adult worms may be seen protruding into the lumen, surrounded by mucosal changes of chronic colitis (56). Iron deficiency anemia, eosinophilia, mild hypoalbuminemia are seen only in severe infections.

Mild or asymptomatic infections are self-limited and do not require therapy. Treatment of moderate-to-severe infections with mebendazole (Vermox, 100 mg po *bid* in adults and children for 3 days) is curative in 80% of cases with rare side effects of nausea and diarrhea (57). A single dose of oxantel pamoate, 15 mg/kg orally, is also highly effective and particularly useful for mass chemotherapy programs. Because the immature worms of *T. trichiura* are less susceptible to antihelminthic drugs, retreatment may be necessary.

Personal hygiene, washing of fruits and vegetables, and proper sanitation are the best means for disease prevention. Mass chemotherapy may also prevent transmission by reducing worm burden.

5. *Strongyloidiasis*

Strongyloides stercoralis is a small-intestinal nematode that causes infection worldwide but it is especially prevalent in the Far East and other tropical and subtropical climates. Because of its ability to replicate within its host, *S. stercoralis* may cause potentially fatal opportunistic infections in immunocompromised patients, particularly those receiving corticosteroids (58).

Humans are the natural host of the infection (59). Filariform larvae of *S. stercoralis* penetrate intact skin and, through venous or lymphatic channels, are transported to the lungs. After breaking into the alveoli, they migrate up the trachea, mature, and they are expectorated and swallowed, in a similar way to hookworms. In the proximal small intestine parasitic adult females penetrate the lamina propria, deposit their eggs, and cause infection and malabsorption. After the eggs hatch in the bowel, some larvae develop into filariform larvae that penetrate the mucosa or the perianal skin causing autoinfection persisting for many years (60). Other rhabditiform larvae eventually pass with the feces to contaminate the environment where, under the appropriate conditions of temperature and humidity, molt into filariform larvae capable of reinitiating the cycle. Immunosuppression, particularly with corticosteroids, disrupts the usually well-regulated autoinfection leading to an increase in the number of adult forms (hyperinfection) and dissemination of larvae throughout the body, eliciting severe inflammatory response that is nearly always fatal (61). The majority of infected individuals are either asymptomatic or have mild nonspecific symptoms of abdominal pain, bloating, and mild intermittent diarrhea. Heavy infections may be associated with malabsorption and weight loss. In contrast, disseminated strongyloidiasis is usually heralded by severe, profuse, bloody diarrhea that results from larval invasion of the intestinal and colonic mucosa (62). Changes in the colonic mucosal permeability eventually lead to larval and polymicrobial sepsis and systemic microabscess formation. The most common event in such patients is diffuse and frequently lethal bronchopneumonia and pulmonary hemorrhage. Gram-negative polymicrobial meningitis, cerebral abscess formation, and generalized cutaneous purpura may also occur.

Stool examination is the primary method for the diagnosis of strongyloidiasis. Because the sensitivity of a single stool examination for *Strongyloides* ranges from 30–50%, serial stool samples should be examined using concentration techniques (63). Although rhabditiform larvae are most commonly identified, filariform larvae and eggs may be detected. If the diagnosis is strongly suspected and repeat stool examinations are negative, sampling of duodenal contents either by aspiration or by the Enterotest string test, may reveal larvae

(64). In cases of hyperinfection, *Strongyloides* larvae may be found not only in stool but also in other fluids, such as sputum and cerebrospinal fluid. Several immunoassays are commercially available for the detection of serum antibodies against filariform larvae and their antigens. An especially useful test is an enzyme-linked immunosorbent assay (ELISA), which detects parasite-specific IgG antibodies with a sensitivity and specificity of 90% (65). Eosinophilia, usually 5–15% of the total white cell count, is variable in patients with chronic infection but is absent in the hyperinfection syndrome. Total serum immunoglobulin E (IgE) elevation occurs in 50–70% of patients with strongyloidiasis.

Because of the potential for fatal superinfection, strongyloidiasis should always be treated. The drug of choice is thiabendazole (Mintezol 25 mg/kg/day po in two divided doses for 2 days, maximum dose 3 gm/day, in both adults and children). Thiabendazole is 90% effective but is associated with frequent side effects, such as nausea, vomiting, and dizziness (66) (see Table 4). In rare instances multiple courses are necessary to eradicate the infection. In disseminated strongyloidiasis, higher doses (50mg/kg/day) for longer periods (5 days or more) are required. Ivermectin and albendazole are also effective agents but are not approved for use in the United States (67). Weeks or months after therapy, serial stool examination should be performed to confirm eradication of the infection.

Prevention of the disease is best achieved by public health measures aimed at proper waste disposal. Patients from endemic areas who are candidates for immunosuppression or corticosteroid therapy should be screened for asymptomatic strongyloidiasis in order to prevent hyperinfection.

6. Ancylostomiasis (Hookworm Infection)

Intestinal hookworm infection, or ancylostomiasis, is caused by *Ancylostoma duodenale* or *Necator americanus*, two species that have similar life cycles and cause widespread disease in areas of poor sanitation of the tropics and subtropics. Humans are the only hosts to the adult hookworm, a whitish nematode, 1 cm long, which attaches to the mucosa of the duodenum and proximal jejunum in large numbers. Hookworm eggs excreted in feces hatch in warm, moist soil releasing larvae that develop and reach the filariform infective stage. Human contact with contaminated soil allows larval penetration into the skin, which is the main mode of infection, although larvae of *A. duodenale* may enter through the mouth. Individuals at risk are children and adults in frequent contact with soil, such as gardeners or plumbers (68). At the site of penetration, the larvae may cause allergic inflammatory response with pruritic, maculopapular rash, and, sometimes, serpiginous tracts, similar to cutaneous larva migrans. From the skin, hookworm larvae are carried to the lungs through the bloodstream, enter the alveoli, ascend the bronchi to the pharynx, are swallowed and develop in the proximal small intestine. The passage through the lungs may cause transient eosinophilia and pulmonary eosinophilic pneumonitis. In the small bowel, the worms attach to the mucosa and withdraw blood. Because each adult worm may ingest 0.1 to 0.4 mL of blood, significant iron and protein deficiency may ensue, but the infection does not cause malabsorption (69).

Mild, established infections in a well-nourished adult may be asymptomatic. Hookworm dermatitis (ground itch), characterized by itchy erythema, papules, or pustules is usually found on the feet during the phase of larval penetration of the skin (70). The transpulmonary larval passage may cause paroxysmal cough, hemoptysis, and focal pulmonary infiltrates. Hookworms in the intestinal tract may cause nausea, vomiting, postprandial epigastric pain, flatulence, and diarrhea, mimicking duodenal ulcer, giardiasis, or celiac sprue. Malnourished individuals may present with severe iron deficiency anemia and hypoproteinemia, leading to facial and peripheral edema, ascites, and heart failure. Children may develop mental and physical growth retardation.

The diagnosis is made by recognizing the characteristic eggs in the stool. Direct fecal smears are usually sufficient, but concentration techniques are necessary in light infections. Hookworm eggs of different species are very similar, but they may contain larvae at variable stages of differentiation. When recovered in duodenal contents, the distinction between *A. duodenale* and *N. americanus* is based on the anatomy of the buccal capsule, which contains ventral teeth in the former and semilunar plates in the latter. Iron deficiency anemia and mild-to-moderate peripheral eosinophilia are common. Small-intestinal biopsies may range from normal mucosa to severely affected flat mucosa, but such changes are not diagnostic of the infection and represent the severe malabsorption that coexists in some patients. Similarly, the findings on small-bowel barium studies are nonspecific thickening of the mucosal folds, barium segmentation, and enhanced peristalsis. In cases of eosinophilic pneumonitis, larvae may be detected in respiratory secretions, and stools may be negative because the pulmonary phase occurs weeks or months before the worms mature in the intestine to release their eggs. A positive stool examination during the course of eosinophilic pneumonitis in turn indicates a longstanding parasitic infection.

Mebendazole (Vermox, 100 mg po *bid* for 3 days in both adults and children) is the treatment of choice (71) (see Table 4). Although a single dose of pyrantel pamoate (Antiminth suspension 11 mg/kg po, maximum 1 gm, in both adults and children) is effective against *A. duodenale*, it must be repeated for 3 days in cases of *N. americanus*. Stools should be reexamined two weeks after therapy and retreatment may be necessary. Although the anemia of hookworm infection responds well to oral iron therapy, it may be severe enough to require transfusions. Because of the coexistent hypoproteinemia in such cases, diuretic therapy may be required to prevent pulmonary edema.

7. *Trichostrongyliasis*

Trichostrongyliasis is common in Asia. Several species of *Trichostrongylus* may infect humans consuming foods that contain infective larvae. Adult worms attach to the proximal small-intestinal mucosa but rarely cause symptoms. On stool examination *Trichostrongylus* eggs may be mistaken for hookworm eggs, but they are larger and less rounded. Treatment is highly effective and involves either thiabendazole 25 mg/kg po twice daily for two days) or pyrantel pamoate (11mg/kg po once, maximum dose 1 gm).

8. *Capillariasis*

Intestinal capillariasis is mostly caused by *Capillaria philippinensis*, primarily found in the Philippines and Southeast Asia (72). Humans become infected by consuming raw, small, freshwater fish, snails, or crustaceans. The adult worms are small (3–4 mm long) and dwell in the jejunum causing anorexia, nausea, vomiting, and large-volume diarrhea. With chronic or severe infections, protein-losing enteropathy, steatorrhea, edema, and muscle wasting may occur (73). Untreated sub-acute *C. phillipinensis* infection has a mortality of up to 10%.

The diagnosis is based on egg identification in the stool. The treatment of choice is mebendazole (Vermox, 200 mg orally twice daily for 20 days, in both adults and children) (74). In severe cases, fluid and electrolyte replacement and antidiarrheal drugs may be needed. Prevention of capillariasis can be achieved by avoiding ingestion of undercooked freshwater fish, snails, or crustaceans.

9. *Anisakiasis*

Anisakiasis should be considered wherever raw saltwater fish is consumed. *Anisakis* species are present in the muscle of mackerel, salmon, and herring. A related parasite, *Pseudoterranova* species, are present in cod, halibut, Pacific red snapper, and flatfish. The infection is becoming increasingly recognized worldwide, although most cases are seen in Japan, Holland, and the Pacific coast of South America. Humans become infected by eating raw fish dishes, such as sushi, sashimi, herring, and ceviche that contain *Anisakis* species (see Table 5).

Table 5 Parasites Acquired by Eating Raw Fish

Anisakis species	Mackerel, herring, salmon, cod, pollack, halibut, flatfish, greenling, Pacific red snapper, squid
Diphyllobothrium latum	Trout, salmon, pike, walleye
Intestinal fluke	Salmon
Eustrongylides	Sushi, sashimi, minnows

Source: Schantz PM. The dangers of eating raw fish. N Engl J Med 1989; 320:1143–5.

The clinical manifestations of the infection depend on the species involved. Infection with *Pseudoterranova* species in the United States rarely causes severe illness. Patients present with mild epigastric pain and a sense of the worm in their esophagus or pharynx. They typically expectorate the live worm within 2 days after ingesting raw fish. In contrast, in Japan codworm anisakiasis causes severe symptoms. Within a few hours after raw-fish ingestion, patients experience severe, recurring, epigastric pain, nausea, vomiting, and a tingling sensation in the throat. If endoscopy is performed, larvae may be seen invading the posterior wall of the stomach, which appears edematous and hemorrhagic. Similar clinical manifestations may be noted with *Anisakis* invasion of the stomach. If the larvae invade the small bowel, crampy abdominal pain, nausea, vomiting, fever, and diarrhea may occur. Such clinical presentation may mimic acute appendicitits, peritonitis, or Crohn's disease. Ulceration, abscess formation, eosinophilic granuloma formation of the intestinal wall and intestinal perforation may occur.

The diagnosis is frequently suspected by careful history of recent ingestion of raw saltwater fish. Eosinophilia is frequently present. Upper endoscopy provides the definitive diagnosis by revealing the invading larvae in the stomach or proximal small intestine. *Pseudoterranova* larvae appear as thick yellow strings whereas *Anisakis* larvae are white and thin (75). Endoscopic removal is curative. Although not diagnostic, upper gastrointestinal barium series may detect larvae or reveal thickening of the small intestine.

Typically anisakiasis is a self-limited illness. Treatment with thiabendazole may be tried but is not of proven value. Emergency laparotomy is frequently performed for presumed appendicitis or peritonitis. If the correct diagnosis is made, resection is not necessary. Anisakiasis can be prevented by proper handling of saltwater fish. Cooking for at least 10 min at 60°C, freezing to –20°C for 3 days, or commercial blast freezing are effective methods. Salting, marinating, or cold smoking however are not effective in killing either *Anisakis* or *Pseudoterranova* species.

10. Cestodes (Tapeworms)

Cestodes are ribbon-like worms that consist of a series of segments (proglottids) and attach to the surface of the small intestine through an anterior end, or scolex. They may vary in length from 30 mm to 30 m. Cestodes lack a true alimentary tract and absorb all nutrients through a surface membrane that attaches to the intestinal villi of the host. Humans acquire the infection by eating undercooked beef meat infected with *Cysticercus bovis*, the larva of *Taenia saginata* (beef tapeworm); undercooked pork meat infected with *Cysticercus cellulosae* (pork tapeworm), the larva of *Taenia solium* (pork tapeworm); or undercooked fish infected with larvae of *Diphyllobothrium latum* (fish tapeworm). *Hymenolepsis nana* (dwarf tapeworm) may also cause significant human disease.

11. Taenia Saginata

The beef tapeworm, *Taenia saginata*, is one of the largest human parasites with lengths up to 30 m. It is highly endemic in Africa and Latin America, particularly in areas where the consumption of undercooked or raw beef is common (76). Humans serve as the host for the adult tapeworm, which attaches its scolex to the small intestinal mucosa and grows by segment (proglottid) formation. After cross fertilization between the segments the distal end of the adult parasite sheds gravid proglottids with eggs that pass through the bowel in the open environment where they may be ingested by cattle, the intermediate host. Larvae, liberated from the ingested eggs, pass into the tissues of the intermediate host where they serve as sources of human reinfection.

The majority of infected patients remain asymptomatic until they notice the passage of tapeworms in the stool or their underclothing. Rarely postprandial bloating, nausea. or anal pruritus are noted. Malabsorption or weight loss are rare. Peripheral eosinophilia is only present initially and is not a feature of established infection. The diagnosis is made by identifying proglottids in the stool. By pressing the proglottids between two microscope slides and then injecting india ink through the sides one can count the number of lateral uterine branches and thus distinguish *Taenia saginata* (more than 12 branches) from *Taenia solium* (less than 10 branches). Alternatively the diagnosis can be made using the adhesive-tape test to collect eggs deposited in the perianal area. However, the eggs of *T. saginata* and *T. solium* are indistinguishable and are not frequently present in the stool. An ELISA examination of fecal samples may be of value (77).

Praziquantel (Biltricide 15–20 mg/kg po once, in both adults and children) is 100% effective (78) (see Table 4). Alternatively, niclosamide single 2-g dose in adults or 1–1.5 g in children may be used. Soon after effective therapy and for several days thereafter, intact or disintegrating segments of the parasite containing eggs pass per rectum either spontaneously or as a result of a purge. If recovery of the scolex is desired in order to ensure than the parasite will not regenerate, stool should be collected and examined for at least 3 days after a purge. Otherwise, cure can be confirmed by reexamining the stool for proglottids 3 months after completion of antihelminthic therapy. Preventive measures against *Taenia saginata* infection include through cooking of beef, public education against the consumption of raw meat, sanitary disposal of human feces, and regional mass chemotherapy.

12. Taenia Solium (Cysticercosis)

Taenia solium, or pork tapeworm, is particularly endemic in Central and South American and Southeast Asia where pig raising is common (79). Depending on the stage of the parasite that is ingested, *T. solium* causes either taeniasis, if cysticerci in inadequately cooked pork are ingested and the adult worm develops in the intestine, or cysticercosis, if *T. solium* eggs are ingested, hatched in the proximal intestine, and the resulting larvae penetrate various tissues leading to inflammation and ultimately necrosis and calcification.

The adult worm of *T. solium* is found only in humans following the ingestion of undercooked pork containing larvae (cysticerci). Human disease results from ingestion of ova that release larvae in the stomach. From there, larvae penetrate the intestinal wall and invade many parts of the body causing infection of the central nervous system (neurocysticercosis), subcutaneous tissues and muscle, skin, the heart, and other viscera. Pigs, the intermediate hosts, ingest eggs or adult worms contained in human feces and develop cysticercosis of the muscles, subcutaneous tissues, and viscera, thereby completing the cycle.

Patients with *T. solium* infection are mostly asymptomatic; rarely they may notice abdominal pain, weight loss, or proglottid segments passing in their stool. Infiltration of the skin by cysticerci may be palpable as pea-like bodies and lead to urticaria. Early infections are associated with eosinophilia. After many months or years of infection, the larvae die in the muscles and the cysts calcify, leading to their radiographic recognition. Similar reactions in the brain may lead to a multitude of focal or diffuse neurologic syndromes, hydrocephalus, and particularly epilepsy (80). In endemic areas, the most common cause of seizures is cysticercosis.

The diagnosis is made by recognition of the proglottids or eggs in the stool. Because their eggs are indistinguishable, differentiation between *T. saginata* and *T. solium* depends on the recovery of mature proglottids in the stool. Serodiagnosis with indirect hemagglutination antibody ELISA may be useful for disseminated cysticercosis.

Treatment of *T. solium* is similar to *T. saginata* and can be effectively achieved with either praziquantel (Biltricide, 15-20 mg/kg po once, in both adults and children) or niclosamide (2 g po as one dose of four chewable tablets) (81). A purgative is usually given several hours later in order to reduce the likelihood of regurgitation of *T. solium* eggs. Stools should be reexamined several months after therapy to confirm eradication. Prevention of the disease relies on cooking pork well before eating it and controlling human fecal contamination of drinking water and food.

13. Diphyllobothrium latum Infection

Infection by *D. latum* is found in areas where freshwater fish, such as trout and salmon, are regularly consumed (see Table 5). Such areas include the western United States, the Great Lakes region, Canada, Alaska, the lake areas of western Europe, Russia, and Scandinavia, and some areas in Asia and Central Africa.

The life cycle of *D. latum* requires two intermediate hosts, a crustacean and a freshwater fish. Parasite eggs develop in freshwater and hatch into coracidia, which are ingested by small crustaceans within which they develop into larvae.

Upon ingestion of the crustacean by a freshwater fish, the larvae migrate from the intestinal lumen of the fish to the muscle where they develop into infective plerocercoids. The fish is then ingested by a large carnivorous fish which is in turn ingested by humans. Within the human intestine larvae develop into adult worms which attach to the mucosa and lay eggs (82).

Most infected humans are asymptomatic but vague abdominal pain, nausea, and diarrhea may occur. A significant complication of *D. latum* infection is megaloblastic anemia that is due to competition between the worm and the host for vitamin B_{12} (83). Identification of *D. latum* eggs in the feces leads to effective therapy with praziquantel (Biltricide, 15–20 mg/kg po once, in both adults and children). Vitamin B_{12} replacement therapy is required for megaloblastic anemia. Prevention is achieved by adequate cooking of freshwater fish.

14. Hymenolepsis nana (Dwarf Tapeworm)

Infection by *Hymenolepsis nana* or the dwarf tapeworm occurs most commony in children of tropical and subtropical areas with poor sanitation. *H. nana* eggs are ingested from contaminated soil and develop into cysticercoids that attach to the small intestinal mucosa and mature into adult worms. Eggs may either mature into adult worms in the small intestine or pass through the feces and contaminate the soil.

Most *H. nana* infections are asymptomatic, although heavy infections may lead to vague abdominal pain, nausea, diarrhea, and weight loss. The diagnosis is based on the identification of typical eggs in the feces. A single dose of praziquantel (Biltricide, 15–20 mg/kg po once, in both adults and children) is curative (84). Prevention is achieved by personal hygiene and improvement of sanitary conditions.

15. Trematodes (Flukes)

Trematodes or flukes are flatworms that cause significant morbidity worldwide. In particular, schistosomiasis, a chronic human infection represents a major health problem worldwide. Other intestinal flukes that can cause significant human disease include *Fasciolopsis buski, Heterophyes heterphyes,* and *Metagonimus yokogawi* but these are all very rare in the United States.

16. Schistosomiasis (Bilharziasis)

Schistosomiasis is a chronic trematode infection that affects more than 200 million people worldwide (85). Humans are infected by three major species: *Schistosoma mansoni*, found in Africa, the Arabian peninsula, South America, and Caribbean; *Schistosoma japonicum*, found in Japan, China, and the Philippines; and *Schistosoma haemotobium*, found in Africa and the Middle East. Humans acquire the infection through exposure to contaminated fresh water containing a specific snail that serves as the necessary intermediate host. Schistosomal eggs contaminating fresh water hatch into schistosomal miracidia, enter snails and emerge as free-swimming cercaria. Cercaria may penetrate the human-host skin, enter blood vessels, mature and mate in the portal vein system, and then migrate to various body locations. *S. mansoni* and *S. japonicum* lodge in the intestine and excrete eggs in the feces; *S. haematobium* invades the blood vessels of the urinary bladder and excretes eggs in the urine. Eggs may also be transported through the portal vein into the liver. Because of the absence of the specific freshwater snail in the United States the disease is not transmitted but it may be encountered in travelers or immigrants from endemic areas.

The severity of disease varies depending on the geography, the specific organism, the path of exposure, worm burden, and host defenses. Egg deposition in the intestinal submucosa leads to inflammation, hyperemia, hemorrhages, ulcers, and polyp formation. Such patchy mucosal involvement may lead to a sandpaper appearance. Necrosis, obstruction, and fistulization may occur. *Schistosoma* eggs from the intestine may access the portal vein and become entrapped in the portal areas of the liver. Here they may cause progressive portal and periportal granulomatous inflammation and fibrosis that spares the liver parenchyma and leads to presinusoidal portal hypertension. From the liver, eggs may also be shunted into the lungs, which leads to pulmonary hypertension.

The clinical presentation of schistosomiasis may be distinguished in three stages (86). The first stage (schistosomal dermatitis) develops acutely upon cercarial penetration of the skin and is characterized by papular pruritic rash. The second stage of acute schistosomiasis develops one to two months after a heavy primary infection and is characterized by spiking fevers, myalgias, crampy abdominal pain, bloody diarrhea, fatigue, urticaria, hepatosplenomegaly, and peripheral blood eosinophilia. With *S. japonicum* in Japan, this severe reaction is called Katayama fever. The third stage of chronic schistosomiasis is caused by heavy deposition of eggs in the intestine, liver, or urinary bladder. With *S. mansoni* or *S. japonicum* infection, fever, abdominal pain, bloody diarrhea, and hepatosplenomegaly are the cardinal manifestations. Portal hypertension with variceal bleeding may occur but hepatic encephalopathy is very rare. With *S. hematobium* infection, bladder involvement leads to frequency, dysuria, and hematuria. In longstanding infections, intestinal polyps and bladder carcinoma may occur.

During acute schistosomiasis, ova of all species may be identified on parasitologic examination of freshly passed, concentrated stool. For *S. hematobium*, urine samples need to be obtained in the late morning hours for higher yield. Because ova of all species are present in the rectal mucosa of most patients, rectal biopsies are diagnostic. For optimal results, a rectal mucosal sample is obtained, compressed with a drop of warm saline solution between the slide and its coverslip and examined for schistosomal eggs under the microscope. Serologic tests generally should not be relied upon for the diagnosis of schistosomiasis because of significant false-positive and false-negative results (87). Computed tomography or magnetic resonance imaging may reveal changes of periportal fibrosis or colonic-wall calcifications or pericolic abscesses. Colonoscopy reveals edematous colonic mucosa, microulcerations, and multiple polyps.

Praziquantel (Biltricide, two oral doses of 20 mg/kg in one day for *S. haematobium* and *S. mansoni*; three oral doses of 20 mg/kg in one day for *S. japonicum*, in both adults and children) is highly effective and well tolerated. Side effects may include headache, drowsiness, malaise, bitter taste, and vomiting (88). (see Table 4). Patients with schistosomal portal hypertension tolerate variceal bleeding better than patients with cirrhosis and should generally be treated conservatively. Portal decompressive surgery should only be considered in patients with recurrent bleeding because it carries the risk of postoperative hepatic encephalopathy.

17. Fasciolopsiasis

Fasciolopsis buski (giant intestinal fluke), a common parasite in many parts of Asia, infects humans and pigs. Humans acquire the infection by ingesting water plants such as water chestnut, water bamboo, or water lotus, which contain metacercariae of the parasite. Larvae excyst in the proximal small intestine and develop into adult worms, which attach to the mucosal surface causing inflammation and ulceration. Large numbers of parasites may lead to intestinal obstruction.

The majority of infected patients are asymptomatic; those with heavy worm load may develop crampy abdominal pain, nonbloody diarrhea, facial and peripheral edema, ascites, and intestinal obstruction. Anemia and peripheral eosinophilia are common. The diagnosis is made by stool examination for either adult worms or typical *F. buski* eggs.

The treatment of choice is praziquantel (Biltricide, 75 mg/kg in three oral doses over one day, in both adults and children). Prevention of the infection is achieved by boiling of freshwater nuts and vegetables before consumption.

18. Other Intestinal Flukes

Humans may be infected by two other small intestinal flukes, *Metagonimus yokogawai* (Southeast Asia) and *Heterophyes heterophyes* (Northern Africa, Southeast Asia) by eating raw fish that contains metacercariae (see Table 5). The metacercariae mature into adult, 2–3 cm long flukes that attach to the proximal small-intestinal mucosa. Although mostly asymptomatic, these infections can cause abdominal pain and diarrhea. Finding of the typical eggs in the host feces leads to therapy with praziquantel, 25 mg/kg orally three times in one day.

REFERENCES

1. Jernigan J, Guerrant RC, Pearson RD. Parasitic infections of the small intestine. Gut 1994; 35:289–293.
2. Warren KS. Helminthic diseases endemic in the United States. Am J Trop Med Hyg 1974; 23:723–730.
3. Mahmoud AAF. Parasitic protozoa and helminths: Biological and immunological challenges. Science 1989; 246:1015–1022.
4. Tanowitz HB, Weiss LM, Wittner M. Diagnosis and treatment of intestinal helminths. Gastroenterology 1993; 101:265–273.
5. Strickland GT. Hunter's Tropical Medicine. 7th ed. Philadelphia; W.B. Saunders, 1991.
6. Genta RM. Diarrhea in helminthic infections. Clin Infect Dis 1993; 16(suppl 2):S122–129.
7. Russell L. The pinworm, *Enterobius vermicularis*. Prim Care 1991; 18:13–23.
8. Wellet PF. Eosinophilia in travelers. Med Clin North Am 1992; 76:1413–1432.
9. Smith JW. Giardiasis. Ann Rev Med 1980; 31:373–380.
10. Flannagan PA. *Giardia*: Diagnosis, clinical course and epidemiology. A review. Epidemiol Infect 1992; 109:1–22.
11. Adam RD. The biology of *Giardia spp*. Microbiol Rev 1991; 55:706–732.
12. Jones JE. Giardiasis. Primary Care. 1991; 18:43–52.
13. Goka AKJ, Rolston DDK, Mathan VI, Farthing MJG. The relative merits of faecal and duodenal juice microscopy in the diagnosis of giardiasis. Trans R Soc Trop Med Hyg 1990; 84:66–67.
14. Addiss DG, Mathews HM, Stewart JM, et al. Evaluation of a commercially available enzyme-linked immunosorbent assay for *Giardia lamblia* antigen in stool. J Clin Microbiol 1991; 29:1137–1142.
15. Char S, Farthing MJG. DNA probes for diagnosis of enteric infection. Gut 1991; 32:1–3.
16. Farthing MJ. Giardia comes of age: Progress in epidemiology, immunology, and chemotherapy. J Antimicrob Chemother 1992; 30:563–566.
17. Bassily S, et al. The treatment of *Giardia lamblia* with mepacrine, metronidazole, and furazolidine. J Trop Med Hyg 1970; 73:15–18.
18. Davidson RA. Issues in clinical parasitology: the treatment of giardiasis. Am J Gastroenterol 1984; 79:256–261.
19. Murphy TV, Nelson JD. Five versus ten days of therapy with furazolidone for giardiasis. Am J Dis Child 1983; 137:267–271.
20. Reed SL. Amebiasis: An update. Clin Infect Dis 1992; 14:385–391.
21. Bruckner DA. Amebiasis. Clin Microbiol Rev 1992; 5:356–369.
22. Reed S, Bouvier J, Pollak AS, et al. Cloning of a virulence factor of *Entamoeba histolytica*. Pathogenic strains possess a unique cysteine proteinase gene. J Clin Invest 1993; 92:1532–1540.
23. Ahmed M, McAdam KP, Sturm AW, et al. Systemic manifestations of invasive amebiasis. Clin Infec Dis 1992; 15:974–982.

24. Reed S, Bouvier J, Pollack AS, et al. Cloning of a virulence factor of *Entamoeba histolytica* protein. Pathogenic strains possess a unique cysteine proteinase gene. J Clin Invest 1993; 91:1532–1540.
25. Adams EB, McLeod IN. Invasive amebiasis. I. Amebic dysentery and its complications. Medicine 1977; 56:315–323.
26. Irusen EM, Jackson TF, Simjee AE. Asymptomatic intestinal colonization by pathogenic *Entamoeba histolytica* in amebic liver abscess: Prevalence, response to therapy, and pathogenic potential. Clin Infect Dis 1992; 14:889–893.
27. Missalek W. Ultrasonography in the diagnosis of amoebic liver abscess and its complications. Trop Doct 1992; 22:59–64.
28. Adams EB, McLeod IN. Invasive amebiasis. II. Amebic liver abscess and its complications. Medicine 1977; 56:324–334.
29. Haque R, Kress K, Wood S, et al. Diagnosis of pathogenic *Entamoeba histolytica* infection using a stool ELISA based on monoclonal antibodies to the galactose-specific adhesin. J Infect Dis 1993; 167:247–249.
30. Lotter H, Mannweiler E, Schreiber M, et al. Sensitive and specific serodiagnosis of invasive amebiasis by using a recombinant surface protein of pathogenic *Entamoeba histolytica*. J Clin Microbiol 1992; 30:3163–3167.
31. Juimo AG, Gervez F, Angwafo FF. Extraintestinal amebiasis. Radiology 1992; 182:181–183.
32. Katzenstein D, et al. New concepts of amebic liver abscess derived from hepatic imaging, serodiagnosis, and hepatic enzymes in 67 consecutive cases in San Diego. Medicine 1982; 61:237–246.
33. Spencer MJ, Chapin MR, Garcia LS. *Dientamoeba fragilis*: a gastrointestinal protozoan infection in adults. Am J Gastroenterol 1982; 77:565–569.
34. Soave R. Cryptosporidiosis and isosporiasis in patients with AIDS. Infect Dis Clin North Am 1988; 2:485–494.
35. Wittner M, Tanowitz HB, Weiss LM. Parasitic infections in AIDS patients. Cryptosporidiosis, isosporiasis, microsporidiosis, and cyclosporiasis. Infect Dis Clin North Am 1993; 7:569–586.
36. McGowan I, Hawkins AS, Weller IV. The natural history of cryptosporidial diarrhoea in HIV-infected patients. AIDS 1993; 7:349–354.
37. Blanshard C, Jackson AM, Shanson DC, Francis N, Gazzard B. Cryptosporidiosis in HIV-seropositive patients. Q J Med 1992; 85:813–823.
38. Wolfson JS, et al. Cryptosporidiosis in immunocompetent patients. N Engl J Med 1985; 312:1278–1282.
39. Gellin BG, Soave R. Coccidian infections in AIDS. Toxoplasmosis, cryptosporidiosis, and isosporiasis. Med Clin North Am 1992; 76:205–234.
40. Fichtenbaum CJ, Ritchie DJ, Powderly WG. Use of paromomycin for treatment of cryptosporidiosis in patients with AIDS. Clin Inf Dis 1993; 16:298–300.
41. Armitage K, et al. Treatment of cryptosporidiosis with paromomycin. Arch Int Med 1992; 152:2497–2499.

42. Sun T. Microsporidiosis in the aquired immunodeficiency syndrome. Infect Dis Newsletter 1993; 12:20–22.
43. Curry A, Canning EU. Human microsporidiosis. J Infect Dis 1993; 27:229–236.
44. Weiss LM, et al. *Isospora belli* infection: Treatment with pyrimethamine. Ann Int Med 1988; 109:474–475.
45. Zierdt CH. *Blastocystis hominis*-past and future. Clin Microbiol Rev 1991; 4:61–79.
46. Udkow MP, Markell EK. *Blastocystis hominis*: prevalence in asymptomatic *versus* symptomatic hosts. J Infect Dis 1993; 168:242–244.
47. Markell EK. Intestinal nematode infections. Pediatr Clin North Am. 1985; 32:971–986.
48. Landry SM, et al. Trichinosis: Common source outbreak related to commercial pork. South Med J 1992; 85:428–429.
49. Hall A, Anwar KS, Tomkins AM. Intensity of reinfection with *Ascaris lubricoides* and its implications for parasite control. Lancet 1992; 339:1253–1257.
50. Khuroo MS, Zarger SA, Mahajan R. Heptaobiliary and pancreatic ascariasis in India. Lancet 1990; 335:1503–1506.
51. Cook CG. *Enterobius vermicularis* infection. Lancet 1994; 35:1159–1162.
52. Goldenberg SP, Marignani P. The endoscopic appearance of colonic enterobiasis. Gastrointest Endosc 1990; 36:309–310.
53. Drugs for parasitic infections. Med Lett Drugs Ther 1995; 35:111–122.
54. Zachary PE, Cooke AR. Endoscopic diagnosis of whipworm. Am J Gastroenterol 1994; 89:461.
55. Sandler M. Whipworm infestation in the colon and rectum simulating Crohn's colitis. Lancet 1981; 2:210.
56. Okamura S, Washida Y, Iesaki K, Hayashi S. Colonoscopic diagnosis of whipworm infection. Gastrointest Endosc 1993; 39:215–216.
57. Scragg JN, Proctor EM. Further experience with mebendazole in the treatment of symptomatic trichuriasis in children. Am J Trop Med Hyg 1978; 27:255–257.
58. Igra-Seigman Y, Kapila R, Sen P. Syndrome of hyperinfection with *Strongyloides stercoralis*. Rev Infect Dis 1981; 3:397–407.
59. Genta RM, Weesner R, Douce RW, et al. Strongyloidiasis in US veterans of the Vietnam and other wars. JAMA 1987; 258:49–52.
60. Corsini AC. Strongyloidiasis and chronic urticaria. Postgrad Med J 1982; 58:247–248.
61. Dwork KG, Jaffe JR, Lieberman HD. Strongyloidiasis with massive hyperinfection. N Y State J Med 1975; 75:1230–1234.
62. Stoopack PM, Raufman JP. Aphtoid ulceration of the colon in strongyloidiasis. Am J Gastroenterol 1991; 86:639–642.
63. Nielsen PB, Mojon M. Improved diagnosis of *Strongyloides stercoralis* by seven consecutive stool specimens. Zentralbl Bakteriol Mikrobiol Hyg (A) 1987; 263:616–618.
64. Koga K, Kasuya S, Khamboonruang C. A modified agar plate method for the detection of *Strongyloides stercoralis*. Am J Trop Med Hyg 1991; 45:518–521.

65. Genta RM. Predictive value of an enzyme-linked immunosorbent assay (ELISA) for the serodiagnosis of strongyloidiasis. Am J Clin Pathol 1988; 89:391–394.
66. Grove DI. Treatment of strongyloidiasis with thiabendazole: man analysis of toxicity and effectiveness. Trans R Soc Trop Med Hyg 1982; 76:114–118.
67. Shikiya K, Kinjo N, Uehara T, et al. Efficacy of ivermectin against *S. stercoralis*. Intern Med 1992; 31:310–312.
68. Hotez PJ. Hookworm disease in children. Pediatr Infect Dis J 1989; 516–520.
69. Variyam E, Banwell J. Hookworm disease: Nutritional implications. Rev Infect Dis 1982; 4:830–833.
70. Hotez PJ, Narashimhan S, Haggerty J, et al. Hyaluronidase from infective *Ancylostoma* hookworm larvae and its possible functions in tissue invasion and ecdysis. Infect Immun 1992; 60:1018–1023.
71. Biddulph J. Mebendazole and albendazole for infants. Pediatr Infect Dis J 1990; 9:9.
72. Chicino G, Bernuzzi AM, Bruno A, et al. Intestinal capillariasis acquired in Indonesia: A case report. Am J Trop Med Hyg 1992; 47:10–12.
73. Dronda F, Chaves F, Sanz A, et al. Human intestinal capillariasis in an area of nenendemicity: Case report and review. Clin Infect Dis 1993; 17:909–912.
74. Cross JH. Intestinal capillariasis. Clin Microbiol Rev 1992; 5:120–129.
75. Ikeda K, Kumoshiro R, Kifune T. Nine cases of acute gastric anisakiasis. Gastrointest Endosc 1989; 35:304–308.
76. Schultz MG, Hermos JA, Steele JH. Epidemiology of beef tapeworm infection in United States. Public Health Rep 1970; 85:169–176.
77. Deplazes P, Eckert J, Pawlowski ZS, et al. An enzyme-linked immunosorbent assay for the diagnostic detection of *Taenia saginata* copro-antigens in humans. Transact R Soc Trop Med Hyg 1991; 85:391–396.
78. King CH, Mahmoud AAF. Drugs five years later: Praziquantel. Ann Int Med 1989; 110:290–296.
79. Pawlowski ZS. Perspectives on the control of *Taenia solium*. Parasitol Today 1990; 6:371–375.
80. Schantz PM, Moore AC, Munoz JL, et al. Neurocysticercosis in an orthodox Jewish community in New York City. N Engl J Med 1992; 327:692–695.
81. Webbe G. Treatment of cestode infections. Taeniasis and cysticercosis. Med Chir Dig 1985; 14:497–503.
82. Kyronseppa H. The occurrence of human intestinal parasites in Finland. Scand J Infect Dis 1993; 25:671–673.
83. Von Bornsdorff B. *Diphyllobothrium latum* as a cause of pernicious anemia. Parasitology 1957; 5:207–210.
84. Schenone H. Praziquantel in the treatment of *Hymenolepsis nana* infections in children. Am J Trop Med Hyg 1980; 29:320–321.
85. Nash TE. Schistome infection in humans: perspectives and recent findings. Ann Int Med 1982; 97:740–754.
86. Hiatt RA, Sotomayor ZR, Sanchez G, et al. Factors in the pathogenesis of acute schistosomiasis mansoni. J Infect Dis 1979; 139:659–666.

87. Rossi CL, Tsang VCW, Pilcher JB. Rapid, low-technology field-applicable and laboratory applicable enzyme-linked immunosorbent assays for immunodiagnosis of *Schistosoma mansoni*. J Clin Microbiol 1991; 29:1836–1841.
88. Butterworth AE, Sturrock RF, Ouma JH, et al. Comparison of different chemotherapy strategies against *Schistosoma mansoni* in Machakos District, Kenya: effects on human infection and morbidity. Parasitology 1991; 103:339–355.

12

Hepatobiliary and Pancreatic Infections in the Acquired Immunodeficiency Syndrome

ANDREW P. KEAVENY, MICHAEL S. KARASIK, and NEZAM H. AFDHAL
Boston University School of Medicine, Boston, Massachusetts

I. INTRODUCTION

The liver and biliary tract are frequent sites of human immunodeficiency virus (HIV) related disease, presenting with a diverse clinical and pathological spectrum that can prove challenging for both diagnosis and management. Primary hepatic infection is unusual; more commonly the liver is involved as part of multisystemic diseases associated with the immunocompromised patient. In this chapter we will focus on the initial clinical features of HIV infection in the liver, biliary tract, and pancreas prior to discussing some specific infective pathogens.

II. GENERAL GUIDELINES FOR THE EVALUATION OF THE AIDS PATIENT WITH ABNORMAL LIVER FUNCTION

A. Epidemiology

Abnormal liver function is seen in over 90% of patients with HIV infection at least once in the course of their illness. The major modes of transmission of HIV are sexual contact (both hetero- and homosexual) and intravenous (IV) drug usage. Since this is also the major mode of transmission of hepatitis B (HBV), hepatitis C (HCV) and hepatitis D (HDV), these viruses are almost endemic in the HIV population (1). We will discuss these viral hepatitides briefly and also describe the hepatic infections that are unique to the immunosupressed patient. Hepatobiliary manifestations of AIDS are seen in the latter stages of disease when the CD4 cell count is less than 100/mm^3 and the patient is profoundly immunosuppressed.

B. Clinical Features

Significant hepatobiliary disease occurs in up to 70% of patients during the course of HIV infection (2,3). Clinical assessment should include a detailed history with special attention to the stage of progression of HIV infection (CD4 count), presence of opportunistic infections involving other organ systems, concomitant drug usage, and the presenting clinical features. The majority of patients present with mildly abnormal liver function tests and nonspecific right upper quadrant (RUQ) pain. Fever and chills are suggestive of a systemic infection such as an abscess or ascending cholangitis. Progressive liver disease with jaundice and features of liver failure is most commonly seen in patients with preexisting liver disease. Hepatomegaly is a common but nonspecific clinical finding. Examination of other organ systems is important for identifying patients with suspected systemic infections or neoplasms with liver involvement.

Liver blood tests are a useful guide to the underlying etiology of the liver disease. As in non-HIV positive patients, it is helpful to classify patients into those with cholestatic liver disease and predominately canalicular enzyme elevation (increased alkaline phosphatase and gamma glutamyltransferase) or hepatitis where raised serum transaminases (alanine aminotransferase and aspartate aminotransferase) imply hepatocellular necrosis. A mixed picture may also be found. Table 1 shows the biopsy-proven diagnosis of 25 consecutive patients seen at Boston City Hospital with HIV and abnormal liver function or hepatomegaly and fever. Patients were divided into three groups: (1) hepatitis (ALT > 100 IU/L), (2) cholestasis (alkaline phosphatase > 3 times normal) and (3) hepatomegaly and fever. In group 1, an elevated ALT was able to distinguish viral and nonspecific hepatitis from opportunistic infections. However, in Groups 2 and 3, the etiologies of abnormal LFTs were much broader and included chronic liver disease from alcohol, infections, and both intrahepatic and extrahepatic cholestasis.

The differential diagnosis of abnormal LFTs in AIDS is extensive and the most important causes include drug toxicity, infections, and hepatic neoplasms (see Table 2). An algorithm for the evaluation of a patient with symptoms and abnormal LFT's is given in Figure 1.

Table 1 Liver Function Tests in AIDS Patients—Boston City Hospital Experience

Hepatitis			Cholestasis			FUO + Hepatomegaly		
Liver Bx	ALT	AlkPhos	Liver Bx	ALT	AlkPhos	Liver Bx	ALT	AlkPhos
MAI	600	326	CAH- C	259	863	MAI	34	3820
CAH- C	396	100	CAH- C	68	1700	MAI	66	280
CAH- C	237	73	MAI	34	3820	Cirrhosis	38	109
CAH- C	259	178	MTB	210	1327	Alc. Hep	56	352
CAH- B	400	117	CMV	195	984	CAH- C	68	1700
CAH- B	549	126	Cholangitis	99	1370	Steatosis	352	182
NSH	223	170	Cholangitis	67	1657	Cholangitis	66	1430
NSH	334	134	VBDS	85	1810	NSH	75	124
Steatosis	292	152	VBDS	80	896			
			VBDS	83	617			

Liver biopsy and LFTs in 25 consecutive patients with AIDS presenting with hepatitis, cholestasis, or FUO and hepatomegaly. NSH, nonspecific hepatitis; VBDS, vanishing bile duct syndrome; CAH-C, chronic hepatitis C; MTB, mycobacterium tuberculosis; MAI, mycobacterium avium intracellulare.

Table 2 Differential Diagnosis of Abnormal LFTS in the Patient with AIDS

Drug Induced	Infections	Neoplasms
Ketoconazole	Viral	Kaposis sarcoma
Fluconazole	Hepatitis B,C,D	Lymphoma, B-cell
Trimepthoprim-sulfamethoxazole	Cytomegalovirus	
Rifampin	Herpes	
Isoniazid	Epstein–Barr	
DDI		
Pentamidine	Fungal	
Pyrimethamine	Candida	
Dapsone	Cryptococcosis	
	Coccidia	
	Histoplasmosis	
	Mycobacterial	
	Tuberculosis	
	Avium Intracellulare	
	Protozoan	
	Pneumocystis	
	Toxoplasmosis	
	Microsporidia	
	Cryptosporidium	

C. Imaging Studies

Imaging of the liver plays a critical role, particularly in patients with cholestasis or hepatomegaly (4). Ultrasound can often differentiate between intrahepatic mass lesions or extrahepatic cholestasis with dilated intrahepatic ducts. Evaluation of the liver parenchyma for infiltrative processes is much less satisfactory. In many instances maximal information concerning the liver and the extrahepatic abdomen and pelvis can be obtained by a total abdomino-pelvic computerized tomography (CT) scan with IV and oral contrast. A CT scan has the advantage of identifying retroperitoneal lymph nodes that may be enlarged in disseminated infections such as *Mycobacterium avium* complex (MAC) or lymphoma. Endoscopic retrograde cholangiopancreatography (ERCP) should be performed in all patients with dilated extra- and/or intrahepatic bile ducts. It permits interventions such as sphincterotomy and stent placement as well as allowing bile and tissue sampling. Magnetic resonance cholangiopancreatography (MRCP) may prove to be a useful noninvasive method of assessing the

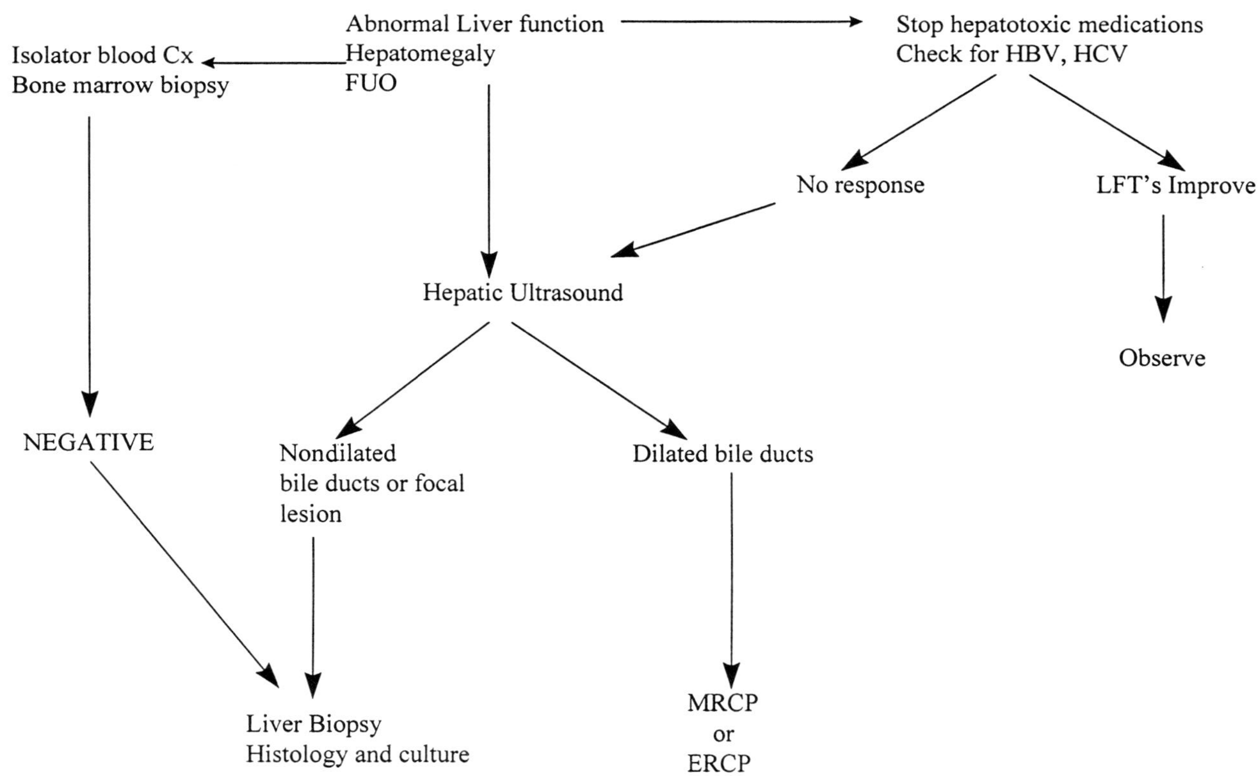

Figure 1 Algorithm for evaluation of hepatic disease in symptomatic AIDS patients.

biliary tree. The MRCP technique may be as sensitive and specific as ERCP in the diagnosis of common hepatobiliary and pancreatic disorders and has the potential to replace ERCP as an initial diagnostic modality (5). Hepatobiliary scintigraphy using technitium-99m diisopropylphenylcarbamoylmethyl iminodiacetic acid has previously been employed in investigating AIDS-related biliary disease (6) but is less sensitive than ERCP. Recently, laparoscopy was used to investigate clinical or biochemical liver abnormalities and had no procedure-related mortality. Findings included peritoneal involvement, massive adhesions, focal liver and splenic lesions due to opportunistic infections, or neoplasms (7). This approach may have some value in the assessment of abdominal pain in patients with AIDS.

D. Role of Liver Biopsy

The diagnostic yield of liver biopsies varies from 24–80%, the value increasing with the duration of AIDS, the number of different prior opportunistic infections, and a higher serum level of alkaline phosphatase at the time of biopsy (8,9). The most common histological findings include macrosteatosis, nonspecific portal inflammation, and granulomas (10). In patients with CD4 counts less than 200/mm^3, liver biopsies should be processed for viral, fungal, and mycobacterial culture in addition to routine histology. The use of special stains, including modified Ziehl–Nielsen for acid-fast bacilli (AFB) can be diagnostic. Table 3 lists liver biopsy findings with their differential diagnosis.

Table 3 Common Pathological Findings in the Liver in AIDS

Pathological Lesion	Etiology
Steatosis-macrovesicular	HIV malnutrition
	Hepatitis C
Steatosis-microvesicular	Drug induced
Sinusoidal dilation	HIV malnutrition
	Tumor-associated
	Peliosis hepatitis
Granulomatous hepatitis	MAI (poorly formed)
	MTB
	Fungal infections
	Histoplasmosis
	Candida
	Hepatitis C
	Drug-induced, sulfonamides
Bile duct sclerosis	CMV
	Idiopathic vanishing bile duct syndrome

Since this procedure is not without significant morbidity in AIDS patients (11), we prefer to use other biopsy sites such as bone marrow in the routine evaluation of fever of unknown origin. Bone marrow biopsy has an 80% yield for disseminated cytomegalovirus (CMV) and MAC infections but if negative we will proceed to liver biopsy. However, in two recent series where a total of 84 liver biopsies were performed, there was no postprocedure mortality, suggesting that this test can be safely utilized to establish a diagnosis when less invasive investigations are negative (12,13). A microbiological diagnosis may be made within 3 days if appropriate tests are applied to the biopsy specimen (13). The value of routine liver biopsy to evaluate abnormal LFTs alone is questionable since the diagnostic yield is low and chronic liver disease or cirrhosis is seldom treated aggressively in a patient with AIDS.

Applying these guidelines to the AIDS patient with liver disease should aid in the choice of the appropriate diagnostic tests that will identify most hepatobiliary pathogens.

III. HEPATIC INFECTIONS

A. Bacterial Infections

Bacterial infections of the liver are uncommon in patients with AIDS. However immunosuppressed individuals are predisposed to bacterial pathogens including *Shigella* and *Salmonella*, which often result in bacteremia as well as colitis (2). Liver abscess has not been reported as occurring more frequently in AIDS patients, but prolonged therapy for enteric bacterial infections with IV antibiotics such as ampicillin and trimethoprim/sulfamethoxazole is recommended to prevent relapse (2). Liver abscesses should be treated with long-term antibiotics and percutaneous drainage for larger collections.

B. Viral Infections

The hepatotrophic viruses B, C, and D, cytomegalovirus (CMV), herpes simplex (HSV), and HIV can all cause hepatitis in AIDS patients. The clinical sequelae of multiple viral infections in HIV patients is variable and ranges from the carrier state to fulminant hepatitis with liver failure. The major determinant appears to be the host's ability to respond to hepatic infection although there is some debate that certain viruses such as HCV are more virulent when there is HIV co-infection. The degree of immunosupression at the time of hepatitis infection will often determine the patient's clinical course.

1. Hepatitis B

Since both HIV and HBV are transmitted by parenteral exposure or sexual contact, 90% of HIV-infected individuals have serological evidence of current or past exposure to HBV (14). However only 10–15% of these HIV patients with HBV markers have detectable hepatitis B surface antigen (HBsAg) and markers of active viral replication such as HBeAg or HBV DNA (15,16).

The clinical manifestations of HBV with active hepatitis require an intact host immune response. Therefore the virological and clinical response to HBV infection is dependent upon the time of HBV infection with respect to the underlying HIV infection. Clinically since HBV is more infective than HIV, most patients with risk factors for the two infections have contracted HBV prior to HIV. In these patients the clinical course of HBV infection is the same as in the immunocompetent with 5–10% progressing to either chronic hepatitis B or becoming HBV carriers. Patients with AIDS who subsequently develop acute HBV infection have increased HBV viremia (17) and are approximately three times more likely to become chronic carriers (1,2,17,18). Measurement of HBV viral DNA levels often shows very active viral replication with serological evidence of HBeAg. Despite this active viremia, serum transaminases are low and histological evidence of active hepatitis is unusual, making the disease less severe than in immunocompetent patients with chronic hepatitis B (19,20). Another potential explanation for the elevated markers of HBV replication seen in AIDS patients may be the shorter duration of HBV infection, rather than immunosupression itself (21).

There is evidence to suggest that HBV may directly increase HIV replication (22–26). Furthermore, it has also been suggested that HBV may alter the host's response to HIV resulting in a reduction of the latent period of HIV infection (1,18). However despite these concerns, there is no convincing evidence from clinical studies that HBV plays a significant role in AIDS progression (27).

Hepatitis B reactivation, defined as either reappearance of HBeAg or as reappearance or rising titers of HBV DNA, has been described in HIV patients. Reactivation remains uncommon and is usually symptomatic (28,29). In patients with chronic HBV contracted prior to significant immunosuppression, severe liver damage may be present with chronic active hepatitis or even cirrhosis (16). Acute liver failure, histologically closely resembling fibrosing cholestatic hepatitis seen in patients posttransplantation for HBV, has also been reported in AIDS patients. This injury is probably related to uncontrolled viral replication within hepatocytes resulting in direct cytotoxicity (30).

Patients with HBV and HIV coinfection respond poorly to interferon therapy (31,32). Epidemiological studies earlier in the HIV epidemic suggested that HBV infection usually preceded that of HIV but recently there is an increased likelihood of HIV infection occurring before or concurrent with HBV (17). Risk-factor modification and effective vaccination programs have been suggested as measures to reduce HBV infection rates in HIV-positive individuals. However, responses to both plasma-derived and recombinant HBV vaccines are poor, which is primarily related to CD4 cell loss (16,33–36). In one study there was no response to recombinant HBV vaccine amongst 11 patients with a CD4 cell count less than 700/mm^3 and only a 50 percent response rate in those with CD4 cell counts over 700/mm^3 (36). Vaccination at the time of new HBV infection has been associated with increased risk of chronic HBV carriage (17). In addition, immunological memory is impaired as loss of HBsAg occurs more frequently in HIV-positive than in HIV-negative patients (37).

Combination antiviral therapy with Zidovudine and interferon alpha-2b was given to 11 patients with chronic active hepatitis due to HBV, HDV, and HCV infections or a combination of the three. Combination antiviral therapy reduced serum alanine aminotransferase, increased CD4 count, and promoted HBeAg seroconversion (38). Our current recommendation is that antiviral therapy should be reserved for patients with severe progressive liver disease and CD4 cell counts greater than 200/mm^3. However great caution must be exercised in administering interferon to patients with cirrhosis as treatment is associated with significant side effects (39). The newer antiviral agents, famcyclovir and lamivudine have been successfully used in liver-transplant patients and may be useful, either alone or in combination, in treating selected HIV-positive patients (40).

2. *Hepatitis C*

Hepatitis C (HCV) is the commonest cause of chronic liver disease in the United States with an estimated prevalence of 3.5 million cases and an incidence of 150,000 new infections annually (41,42). The major modes of transmission of HCV are IV drug use (40%), sporadic, community acquired infection with vertical spread (40%), and sexual transmission, probably accounting for the remaining 20%. In mothers who are HIV positive, there is an increased risk of vertical maternal-fetal transmission of HCV (43). Unlike the immunocompetent where HCV antibodies are seen in greater than 95% of infected patients, only 70% of patients infected with HIV and HCV have HCV antibodies. This loss of HCV antibody response increases with the degree of immunodeficiency, giving rise to a false negative HCV ELISA (44,45). Polymerase chain reaction (PCR) for HCV RNA is therefore the best diagnostic means of identifying active HCV infection in patients with HIV.

The clinical significance of infection with both HCV and HIV is unclear. There is evidence to suggest that increased HCV viremia occurs in patients coinfected with HIV (46). As compared to the HIV-seronegative population, in whom it takes as long as 30 years to develop complications of chronic HCV infection, patients coinfected with HIV may progress more rapidly (47,48). In one prospective cohort study of 97 hemophiliacs who were both anti-HIV and anti-HCV positive, the cumulative incidence of liver failure was 17% ten years after HIV infection (47). In contrast, a study of predominately non-IV drug using male homosexuals showed that HCV infection did not appear to adversely influence survival in patients with HIV (49). The differences in the two studies may be related to the duration of HCV infection prior to the acquisition of HIV. No prospective predictor currently available can identify those patients with both infections who will develop accelerated liver disease. In addition, for those coinfected individuals who survive 10 years, the cumulative risk of developing AIDS is almost twice that of liver failure (47). Therefore, given the natural history of HIV infection, there are no definitive guidelines in selecting patients for treatment of HCV. Sustained response rates (10–15%) to alpha-interferon are no different in HIV-positive patients with CD4 counts greater than 400/mm^3 patients compared to immunocompetent chronic HCV patients (50–52). However, more significant side effects, particularly bone marrow suppression, are seen in HIV patients (53). In our practice, we reserve treatment for those patients who have symptomatic liver disease, regardless of CD4 cell count, or for those patients who have high CD4 cell counts and moderate to severe hepatitis on liver biopsy. The goals of therapy in this subgroup are different from the immunocompetent and long-term sustained response with loss of HCV RNA and normalization of transaminases is probably neither achievable or necessary in this subgroup. We prefer to consider therapy successful if active hepatitis is reduced and symptoms are improved. We have treated a number of patients who presented with cholestatic symptoms (54), abdominal pain, and weight loss but later achieved excellent clinical response. Symptoms have resolved and HCV has disappeared as tested by RT-PCR while patients are on interferon. Further research is required to define the role of anti-HCV treatment in patients with HIV.

3. Hepatitis D

Hepatitis D is a small defective RNA virus that depends upon either coinfection or previous infection (superinfection) with hepatitis B. Overall hepatitis D virus infection is found in about 5% of all HBsAg-positive patients and hence is in a similar proportion of HBsAg positive HIV-infected individuals. The highest incidence is in intravenous drug abusers with lower rates in hemophiliacs and homosexuals (55).

Both coinfection and superinfection of HDV in the immunosuppressed patient would be expected to have a higher rate of progression to chronic disease given the significantly lower incidence of hepatitis B clearance (1,2,18). Chronic coinfection with HDV, the predominant clinical form of the disease, is normally associated with a more rapid and progressive downhill course than in patients with HBV infection alone. Because of this a significant proportion of HDV and HIV coinfected patients will develop liver failure prior to succumbing to HIV-related diseases. The aggressive course has been attributed to the direct cytopathic effect of HDV. Immune suppression related to HIV has been shown to increase the levels of expression of HDV (1,56–58).

The diagnosis of HDV infection is more difficult in HIV-seropositive individuals. Progressive immune suppression may lead to loss of a detectable antibody response so that these patients may be anti-HDV negative (59,60). Confirmation of infection is thus dependent upon demonstration of either hepatitis D antigen or HDV RNA in the serum or on liver biopsy. Detection of HDV RNA in serum is performed by either dot blot or PCR-based methods; the latter is significantly more sensitive and appears to correlate well with HDAg demonstrated in liver biopsy tissue (61). Hepatitis D can suppress HBV replication such that there is loss of the normal hepatitis B markers including HBsAg, reappearing only after resolution of the acute HDV infection. These patients may therefore be diagnosed incorrectly as having a non-A-E hepatitis unless HDV antigen or RNA assays are used. Resolution of infection is marked by loss of HDV antigens and RNA as well as by development of anti-HDV of the IgM class.

Treatment of HDV with alpha interferon has generally been disappointing (62). Suppression of HDV replication with improvement in hepatic histology during therapy has been achieved but sustained responses are seen only in patients who lose HBsAg during therapy (63,64). One small study has reported successful treatment of hepatitis D in 2 of 5 HIV-positive patients with asymptomatic HIV infection (65). Given the high relapse rate in non-HIV-positive patients and the poor response of hepatitis B to interferon (IFN), it is difficult to recommend routine IFN therapy in immunosuppressed patients with HDV infection.

4. *Cytomegalovirus and Herpes Simplex Hepatitis*

Both of these viruses have been associated with severe clinical hepatitis in HIV patients with markedly elevated serum transaminases. Hepatitis is usually only seen in immunosuppressed patients with CD4 counts less than $100/mm^3$ and is part of overwhelming systemic infection.

The liver biopsy features of CMV hepatitis are large intranuclear and cytoplasmic inclusions within bile duct epithelium, endothelial cells, or hepatocytes. Polymorphonuclear aggregates may also be seen. Herpes simplex hepatitis is characterized by inflammation and hepatocellular necrosis, multinucleated hepatocytes, and intranuclear inclusion bodies (66,67). For a specific diagnosis, immunohistochemistry, electron microscopy, and viral culture of the liver biopsy may be performed.

Therapy of CMV infection is dealt with in Chapter 9. Since CMV or herpes hepatitis is rarely the only clinical manifestations of these infections, patients are often also being treated with antiviral agents. Cytomegalovirus can be effectively treated with intravenous gancyclovir or foscarnet and herpes hepatitis responds to intravenous acyclovir. Since hepatitis with these viruses is both a manifestation of severe immunocompromise and multisystem infection, the prognosis is usually very poor with greater than 50% mortality despite therapy.

C. Mycobacterial Infections

1. Mycobacterium-Avium Complex

a. Epidemiology. Mycobacterium-avium complex is the most commonly reported hepatic opportunistic infection, usually seen in patients who already have had multiple previous opportunistic infections (2,10). As many as 50% of HIV-antibody-positive individuals develop mycobacterial infections at some time during their illness, usually when the CD4 cell count falls below 100/mm^3 (68). Up to 40% of liver biopsy or postmortem livers from AIDS patients contain *Mycobacterium-avium* complex (MAC) or *Mycobacterium tuberculosis* (MTB) (8,10,69).

b. Clinical Features. Fever, malaise, anorexia, weight loss, abdominal pain, and diarrhea are typically present and often associated with hepatosplenomegaly. Jaundice is rare (2,70). Leukopenia, anemia, and thrombocytopenia may be present. The usual liver-function test profile is of mildly elevated serum transaminases with marked alkaline phosphatase levels and GGT. Minimal alkaline phosphatase elevation is possibly due to bone marrow involvement as well as obstruction of the terminal branches of the biliary tree by the granulomatous infiltration (2,10). Liver ultrasound or CT scan are unhelpful as hepatic abnormalities are variable and nonspecific, the commonest being a diffusely hyperechoic liver or "bright liver" (71).

c. Diagnosis. Blood culture using special isolator tubes is the most useful diagnostic procedure in evaluating MAC infection (70,72). Negative bronchopulmonary culture does not exclude dissemination of mycobacteria (73). Bone marrow examination and culture may be useful diagnostically, especially if granuloma are seen—these have been shown to correlate with MAC infections in 80% of cases in a series of 314 patients (74).

If the above investigations are negative, liver biopsy may reveal noncaseating, often poorly formed granulomas, with large foamy macrophages, a paucity of lymphocytes and abundant AFB on staining (67). Culture of liver tissue should always be performed and will identify *Mycobacterium* even when no AFB or granuloma are demonstrated by histology (75). However, this may take several months. Amplification and sequencing of mycobacterial ribosomal RNA genes from blood or tissue specimens may permit earlier diagnosis of MAC (76).

d. Treatment. The specific treatment of MAC infection is discussed in Chapter 7. Treatment for MAI may result in symptomatic improvement of pain and fever and can be associated with a decrease in circulating MAI load. When MTB is in the differential, antituberculous therapy should be commenced pending culture results and may provide symptomatic relief (15). The prognosis for disseminated MAC infection is poor, with a reported median survival of 8 months in patients who received treatment (77).

2. *Mycobacterium Tuberculosis*

a. Epidemiology. The incidence of *Mycobacterium tuberculosis* (MTB) is increasing in the HIV community with an overall prevalence rate in HIV-infected patients ranging from 5 to 35%. Infected individuals are more likely to be male, African-American, Haitian, or Latino (77). As MTB is more virulent than nontuberculous mycobacteria and other opportunistic pathogens, active infection tends to occur at higher peripheral CD4 cell counts, often greater than $200/mm^3$ (78). Patients infected with HIV are predisposed to activation of latent MTB, to the acquisition of new infection, and may become reinfected with a second tuberculous strain (79). There has been a disproportionate rise in the incidence of extrapulmonary, as opposed to pulmonary, MTB during the HIV epidemic, from 3% of cases in 1984 to 20% in 1990 (78). Between 35 to 65% of patients with TB and AIDS have extrapulmonary involvement and 16 to 23% have isolated extrapulmonary disease (77).

b. Clinical Features. The onset of infection is frequently insidious and patients may present with constitutional symptoms of fever, night sweats, malaise, and weight loss. Extrapulmonary disease is more common in the later stages of AIDS (77). Hepatosplenomegaly may be found on examination. Hepatic abscesses can develop in the severely immunocompromised, as a result of rapid mycobacterial growth.

c. Diagnosis. The presence of MTB may be established by culturing blood, urine, sputum, liver, lymph node, or bone marrow for AFB. Blood cultures using a lysis-centrifugation system are positive in 26–42% of HIV-infected patients with MTB and are recommended whenever disseminated disease is suspected (77). Since *M. tuberculosis* infection often occurs with higher CD4 counts than MAC, granulomas tend to be better formed in tissue specimens. In contrast to MAC, *Mycobacterium tuberculosis* infection is usually associated with few if any AFB on staining of the liver biopsy.

d. Treatment. Combination therapy with rifampin, isoniazid, ethambutol, and/or pyrazinamide should be commenced whenever a patient is suspected of having MTB or if AFB are found in a specimen from an HIV-infected individual. Deoxyribonucleic acid probes help distinguish MTB from other mycobacteria but if clincial parameters favor MAC, additional therapy with either clofazimine or ciprofloxacin is appropriate. Drug therapy should be adjusted once culture results are available. Isoniazid-resistant strains of MTB have been reported and should be considered in nonresponders to traditional 4-drug regimes (77). The optimal duration of therapy is unknown but should be at least one year. Liver function tests need to be carefully monitored during treatment. The response to treatment in HIV-positive patients is proportional to the CD4 count and is typically good especially when immunosupression is not severe.

D. Fungal Infections

Acquired-immunodeficiency-syndrome-associated mycoses affecting the liver usually present in a nonspecific fashion reflecting disseminated disease (80).

1. *Candida*

a. Epidemiology and Definition. Candida esophagitis is an AIDS-defining diagnosis and is commonly seen in the esophagus of 80% of patients during the course of HIV infection. Oro-esophageal AIDS is seen without severe immunocompromise but disseminated disease is unusual since empiric antifungal therapy and prophylaxis with fluconazole are widely used.

b. Clinical Features. Symptoms of hepatic candidiasis include right-sided abdominal pain, nausea, and vomiting. Signs are an unremitting fever despite broad spectrum antibiotic therapy, hepatomegaly, and right hypochondrial tenderness. Some patients may have a history of previous esophageal candidiasis with symptoms of dysphagia and/or odonyphagia (2). Neutropenia and elevated alkaline phosphatase are the usual laboratory abnormalities. Patients with AIDS may have cutaneous anergy. Radiological investigations may reveal the classic "bull's eye" or uniformly hyperechoic lesions on liver ultrasound (81). Computerized tomography findings include multiple radiolucent hepatic and splenic lesions.

c. Diagnosis. Blood and urine cultures may be positive for candida suggesting systemic disease. Histology of liver or esophagus will demonstrate tissue-invasive mycelia with silver stains and Candida can be confirmed by culture of these tissues.

d. Treatment. Most patients who have had a previous episode of Candida infection are on maintenance prophylaxis with either ketoconazole or fluconazole. In disseminated, life-threatening infection, IV amphotericin is the treatment of choice (2,82). The optimal duration of therapy is unknown.

2. *Cryptococcus Neoformans*

a. Epidemiology. Cryptococcus neoformans is a ubiquitous fungus and the second most commonly isolated fungal pathogen in AIDS (83). Meningitis is the most serious manifestation of this infection.

b. Clinical Features. Hepatic involvement usually presents with hepatomegaly and modestly elevated liver-function tests. Poorly formed granulomas may develop in the liver along with Kupffer cell hyperplasia and sinusoidal and portal tract inflammation. Hepatitis has been reported from hematogenous dissemination; however, the dominant clinical features relate to central nervous system or lung involvement. Hepatic infection has been found in 5% of AIDS patients at autopsy (84).

c. Diagnosis. *Cryptococcus* may be found in cerebrospinal fluid (CSF), lungs, skin, blood, and urine, as well as in the liver. India ink, Gomori's silver stain, or nigrosin wet-mount preparation demonstrate the organism. We recommend culture as well as India ink stains since *Cryptococcus* readily grows in standard blood-culture media and on blood agar (83). Cryptococcal antigen latex agglutination test for cryptococcal polysaccharide in serum or CSF is useful and should be performed in all suspected cases.

d. Treatment. In severely ill patients, we recommend intravenous amphotericin B as the preferred treatment (83). For less severely ill patients, fluconazole administered as a single oral dose is effective and it may be combined with flucytosine for initial treatment. Optimal duration of therapy is unclear and we recommend up to 10 weeks with repeat cultures to confirm eradication of *Cryptococcus* prior to stopping treatment. There is a high risk of relapse so indefinite maintenance therapy with fluconazole is recommended. Relapsing infection may be treated by increasing the dose of fluconazole or changing to amphotericin B. The role of itraconazole in primary treatment is unclear but it may be used as an alternate maintenance agent (80,83,85).

3. Coccidioides Immitis

A prospective study has indicated that each year 10% of people infected with HIV living in areas where the fungus is endemic, such as the Southwestern United States, will contract active coccidioidomycosis infections (86). Primary infection and reactivation occur in HIV-positive individuals, patients typically presenting with a subacute illness manifested by pulmonary involvement (84). Hepatic involvement is usually in the context of disseminated disease and is characterized histologically by a granulomatous response.

Diagnosis is by histological or cytological examination of sputum or tissue specimens, especially of bronchoscopy washings. The fungus may be cultured from infected material. Mature cultures are highly infectious and should only be handled in appropriately equipped laboratories (86). Serum IgM antibodies are detected temporarily in 75% of people with primary infection.

Treatment is with long-term intravenous amphotericin-B. Limited noncomparative trials have suggested that the triazoles are also effective in coccidiomycosis (85,86).

4. *Histoplasma Capsulatum*

Similar to other opportunistic pathogens, hepatic histoplasmosis usually develops as part of a progressively disseminated infection. Endemic areas for this organism include the Ohio and Mississippi River Valleys and Central and South America where it frequently is the initial opportunistic infection in HIV-positive individuals (87). Reactivation of a quiescent infection can also occur and fulminant illness has been described.

In disseminated disease, constitutional features of fever, night sweats, and weight loss occur along with lymphadenopathy, hepatosplenomegaly, and abnormal liver-function tests.

The best diagnostic yield is from bone marrow, blood, or lung stained with periodic acid-Schiff, Wright's, or Giemsa stain for *H. capsulatum* (84). In the liver, histoplasmosis may give rise to poorly formed granuloma that are nonspecific and culture is necessary for definitive diagnosis (Figure 2).

Therapy with intravenous amphotericin-B is effective but relapse is common after treatment is stopped, necessitating subsequent maintenance therapy. Itraconazole is the only triazole effective against *H. capsulatum* (85).

E. Protozoal and Miscellaneous Parenchymal Infections

Protozoa are frequent causes of infection in AIDS but parenchymal liver involvement is rare.

1. *Pneumocystis carinii*

Extra-pulmonary *Pneumocystis carinii* may present with liver infiltration noted on liver biochemistry as elevated serum transaminases and mild increases in the canalicular enzymes (88). These cases may arise from failure of prophylactic inhaled pentamidine to treat extrapulmonic sites (67,89–92). Morphological changes in the liver include nodules in the hepatic lobule and hepatic sinusoidal distension with foamy eosinophilic material that stains positive for *P. carinii* with a methenamine silver stain (67,93). Hepatic calcification on CT is suggestive of *P. carinii* infection (94,95). One case report described a patient with persistently elevated canalicular enzymes, normal ultrasound, CT, ERCP, and involvement of portal triads with *P. carinii*, but showing a spared liver parenchyma (96). Treatment is with intravenous trimethoprim/sulfamethoxazole or pentamidine.

2. *Microsporidia*

A Microsporidia species, *Encephalitozoon cuniculi*, has been reported as the cause of fatal hepatocellular necrosis in 1 patient with AIDS (97). Liver histology showed suppurative necrosis and granulomatous change, predominately involving the portal tracts. The diagnosis is based principally on electron mi-

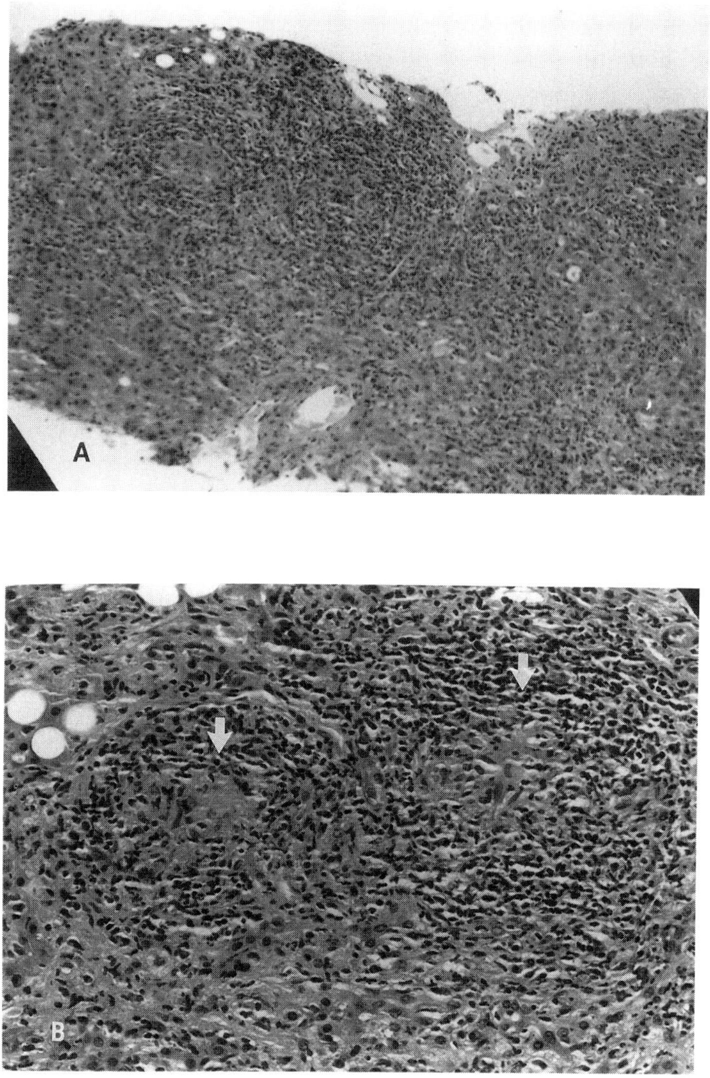

Figure 2 (A) Low-power view of liver biopsy in a 26-year-old man with AIDS and fever. Note increase of inflammatory cells throughout the liver with normal hepatic architecture. (B) High-power micrograph showing 2 well-formed granulomas (arrows) without caseation or giant cells and with no visible organisms. Culture of biopsy grew histoplasma.

croscopic identification of the protozoa spores, which also are Gram-stain positive. Treatment of Microsporidia is discussed in Chapter 7.

3. *Toxoplasma gondii*

This organism infrequently involves the liver. Diagnosis is by culture or microscopic examination of Wright–Giemsa-stained specimens. Treatment is with pyrimethamine and sulphadiazine (98).

4. *Leishmania donovani*

Leishmania donovani invasion of the liver has been noted (13). Careful examination of biopsy specimens is necessary to detect the small basophilic organisms that are either May–Grünwald- or Giemsa-stain positive. Liver Kupffer cells are typically hypertrophied and the portal tracts are infiltrated with histiocytes, lymphocytes, and plasma cells. Treatment is with a pentavalent antimonial using either sodium stibogluconate or meglumine antimoniate (99).

5. *Helminths*

Strongyloides stercoralis, a helminth of the nematode family, causes a hyperinfection syndrome in the immunocompromised patient (100). The liver is usually involved by hematogenous spread of the larvae from the gastrointestinal tract. *S. stercoralis* was the cause of 2 focal hepatic lesions in a patient with hyperinfection syndrome and stool examination was positive for the organism (101). Demonstration of the larvae in duodenal or small-bowel biopsies is diagnostic. Therapy is with thiabendazole but relapses are common (102).

F. Peliosis Hepatitis

1. *Definition*

This condition is characterized by multiple blood-filled cysts of variable size occurring throughout the liver and was initially described in patients dying of tuberculosis or other wasting diseases (103).

2. *Clinical Features*

Peliosis hepatitis can present focally on liver biopsy without any major clinical disease or can present with hepatomegaly, liver failure, and portal hypertension. Systemic features include fever and anemia. A severe consumptive coagulopathy complicated by intraabdominal bleeding with hemoperitoneum may occur (104). Other organs may be involved, including the spleen. The biochemical abnormalities seen are elevations in the serum transaminases, bilirubin, alkaline phosphatase, and a raised prothrombin time.

3. *Pathophysiology and Diagnosis*

Peliosis in AIDS patients is described as a bacillary angiomatosis, similar to bartonellis (105). *Rochalimaea henselae*, in the order Rickettsiales, has been cultivated from 2 immunocompromised patients (one with HIV infection) with peliosis hepatitis after Warthin–Starry stain revealed numerous bacillary organisms in the affected areas of the liver (105,106). Careful attempts at demonstrating the organism by this stain in tissue specimens are essential for diagnosis. It is transmitted by the fleas of infested cats (107).

4. *Treatment*

Symptomatic improvement was obtained after the administration of erythromycin in 1 case and of erythromycin followed by norfloxacin in the other. As *R. henselae* is slow growing and potentially capable of intracellular localization, treatment of at least 1 month in the immunocompromised host has been recommended, using agents with good intranuclear penetration such as erythromycin, doxycycline, or chloramphenicol (105). One patient with peliosis complicated by severe anemia, massive hepatomegaly, and pyrexia responded rapidly to zidovudine and ampicillin/sulbactam, possibly indicating some role for the HIV virus itself in damaging liver endothelial cells (104).

IV. BILIARY TRACT INFECTIONS

A. Cholecystitis

While gallstones are the commonest cause of cholecystitis in non-HIV infected patients, acalculous cholecystitis is more common in patients with AIDS. Acalculous cholecystitis was originally described in severely ill patients with multisystem dysfunction after trauma and severe burns (108–110). Patients positive for HIV can develop this condition when severely immunosuppressed and debilitated without precipitating stresses. The diagnosis of acalculous cholecystitis should be considered where there are unexplained findings such as fever, peritonitis, and leukocytosis (111–113). However no history may be available from profoundly debilitated individuals and the presentation may be nonspecific. Physical examination usually demonstrates abdominal tenderness in the RUQ and the presence of a palpable gallbladder has been reported (114). The risk of perforation with the development of peritonitis is high (2).

1. *Pathophysiology*

The immunosuppressed state of the patient with AIDS seems to predispose to gallbladder inflammation and secondary invasion by opportunistic pathogens (111). A number of different pathogens have been implicated in the etiology of acalculous cholecystitis including Cytomegalovirus, *Cryptosporidium*, Candida and *Campylobacter* (2,115,116). In 50% of cases no obvious pathogen is identified. The gallbladder is inflamed, edematous, and ulcerated, particularly in CMV-associated cases where ischemic vasculitis is present (3). An antecedent history of diarrhea is frequently present, especially if *Cryptosporidium* is subsequently isolated from the gastrointestinal tract.

2. *Diagnosis*

There is no specific test for diagnosing acalculous cholecystitis other than laparotomy. Gallbladder wall thickening and pericholecystic fluid in the absence of gallstones may be seen on ultrasound but these findings are nonspecific and of no prognostic value (113,117). Air within the gallbladder wall may be seen if necrosis has occurred (3). Radionuclide scintigraphy (HIDA scan) and oral cholecystogram may be diagnostic, demonstrating a nonfunctioning gallbladder. However false-positive HIDA scans can occur in patients who are not eating.

3. *Treatment*

Urgent cholecystectomy is necessary to prevent gallbladder rupture, and peritonitis (15). When cholecystectomy is not an option, percutaneous CT or ultrasound guided cholecystotomy can be used to decompress the gallbladder and prevent rupture.

4. *Prognosis*

Delay in clinical diagnosis is common and gallbladder gangrene and microperforation are frequently present at laparotomy. The overall prognosis in patients developing acalculous cholecystitis is poor as it reflects a severely immunocompromised state.

B. AIDS-Cholangiopathy

A chronic stricturing disease of the biliary tract, AIDS-cholangiopathy is associated with infections and malignancies. It produces a diagnostic triad of RUQ pain, elevated serum alkaline phosphatase, and morphological abnormalities in the biliary tree identical to primary sclerosing cholangitis (118). Cholangiopathy usually occurs in patients whose CD4 cell count is less than $50/mm^3$.

The radiological changes in AIDS-cholangiopathy include stricturing, irregularities, and filling defects of the intrahepatic and extrahepatic bile ducts (Figure 3). The common bile duct (CBD) may have a "beaded" mucosal pattern (119,120). Papillary stenosis, a stenosis of the terminal CBD with proximal dilatation can also be found (118,119) (see Figure 4). Papillary stenosis can also affect the pancreas by causing juxtaampullary pancreatic duct strictures (120,121). Very rarely only the medium-sized intrahepatic lobular ducts are affected leading to a progressive sclerotic destruction of bile ducts. Liver biopsy shows loss of intrahepatic small and medium size bile ducts, a so-called vanishing bile duct syndrome.

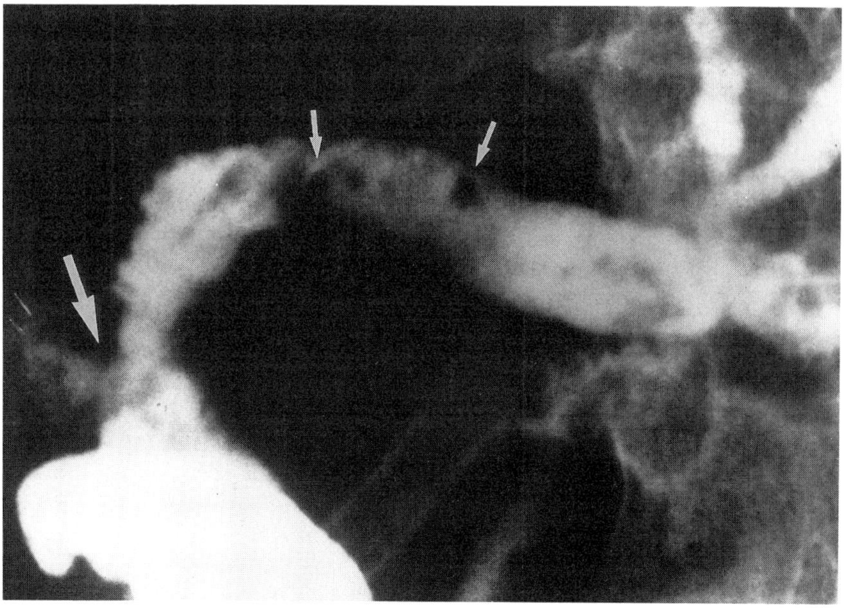

Figure 3 AIDS Sclerosing Cholangitis: ERCP showing highly irregular left and right hepatic ducts, which form a common hepatic duct at their junction (small arrow). Left intrahepatic ducts shows a beaded appearance with multiple filling defects (small arrows).

1. Etiology and Pathophysiology

Originally AIDS-cholangiopathy was associated with CMV and *Cryptosporidium* infection (122,123). However multiple other organisms have been identified on biopsy or culture of the biliary system ante- or postmortem including MAC, microsporidia, and herpes simplex virus (119–121,124). In up to 50% of cases, no infectious agent may be isolated from the biliary tree (119,120). Chronic inflammation secondary to colonization by the pathogens may explain HIV-cholangiopathy (113,119). Mucosal squamous metaplasia of the bile duct epithelium, possibly due to chronic *Cryptosporidium* infection, has been reported (127).

Male homosexuality has been identified as a major risk in some series (118,121). However this may be a result of selection bias from the respective HIV populations or alternatively, relate to the higher rate of gut pathogen carriage occurring in homosexuals (121). There is no evidence for direct HIV infection of the biliary epithelium, although vasculitis secondary to HIV might lead to ischemic injury of the biliary system. Alternatively HIV may induce

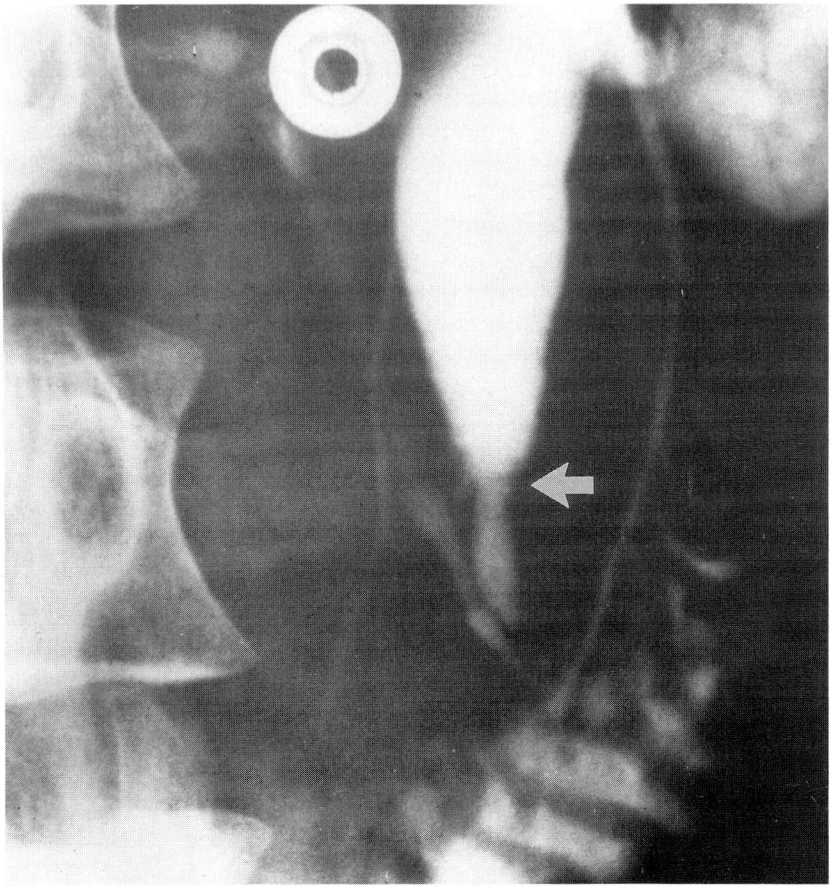

Figure 4 AIDS Papillary Stenosis: ERCP in a 32-year-old female with AIDS and CD4 count of $60/mm^3$ complaining of RUQ pain and fever. Note stenosis of the common bile duct (CBD) at the level of ampulla of Vater (arrow) with proximal dilation of CBD. Biopsy of ampulla showed intranuclear inclusion bodies consistent with CMV.

HLA antigen presentation by the biliary epithelium predisposing to immune-mediated injury of bile ducts (128,129). Another possible explanation for the findings in AIDS-cholangiopathy is that the persistent portal bacteremia in AIDS patients leads to a sclerotic inflammatory injury of bile ducts (119).

2. *Clinical Features*

The commonest presenting feature is right-upper-quadrant pain. Other symptoms include fever, nausea, and vomiting, while jaundice is rare as obstruction is usually incomplete (3,118,130). We recommend ultrasound in all patients with advanced AIDS and RUQ pain. Occasionally cholangitis is the first presentation of AIDS or HIV infection (121,131).

3. *Diagnosis*

Liver-function tests reveal a markedly elevated serum alkaline phosphatase and gamma-glutamyt transferase, mildly elevated bilirubin and only a minimal rise in the transaminases. A dilated CBD and/or intrahepatic ducts are seen on ultrasound or CT scan. It has been reported that ultrasound may show a hyperechoic nodule in the distal CBD corresponding to edema of the papilla of Vater, when 500 mL of water is given orally (132). Endoscopic ultrasound has been used to study the CBD and papilla, proving more sensitivity than transabdominal sonography in detecting abnormalities (118). Computerized tomography may help to exclude extrinsic compression of the CBD (3). Cholangiography, preferably endoscopic, is the gold standard in assessing the biliary tree since it may demonstrate abnormal ducts in the presence of normal ultrasound scans (119). The most frequent pattern of radiological abnormality seen is that of distal CBD stenosis with diffusely irregular intrahepatic bile ducts (Figure 4) (118–121). In addition, when done endoscopically, biopsies and therapeutic intervention can be performed if appropriate. Magnetic resonance cholangiopancreatography is a novel and sensitive technique for noninvasive evaluation of the biliary tree (133).

Multiple duodenal and papillary biopsies sent for both microbiological and histological analysis are most likely to identify pathogenic organisms (121). Intraductal biopsies can be safely obtained at ERCP using a biopsy forceps passed through the duodenoscope into the mid and high portions of the CBD (127) (see Figure 5). We routinely attempt to biopsy both strictures and filling defects in the common bile duct. The diagnostic accuracy of bile culture is poor (134). Precise identification of organisms such as microsporidia is often difficult, requiring careful analysis of the biopsy specimens using special stains, light, and electron microscopy.

4. *Treatment*

Sphincterotomy relieves the pain associated with papillary stenosis in only about 50% of patients. Serum biochemical values may also improve although the distorted appearances of the intrahepatic tree remain (118–120,134). The ERCP procedure appears to be well tolerated without increased morbidity in AIDS patients. If ERCP is unsuccessful, transhepatic cholangiography should be attempted, surgical sphincteroplasty being reserved for symptomatic patients with whom other approaches have failed (3). In patients with biliary strictures, secondary bacterial cholangitis is a risk, and we advocate endoscopic stenting of focal strictures.

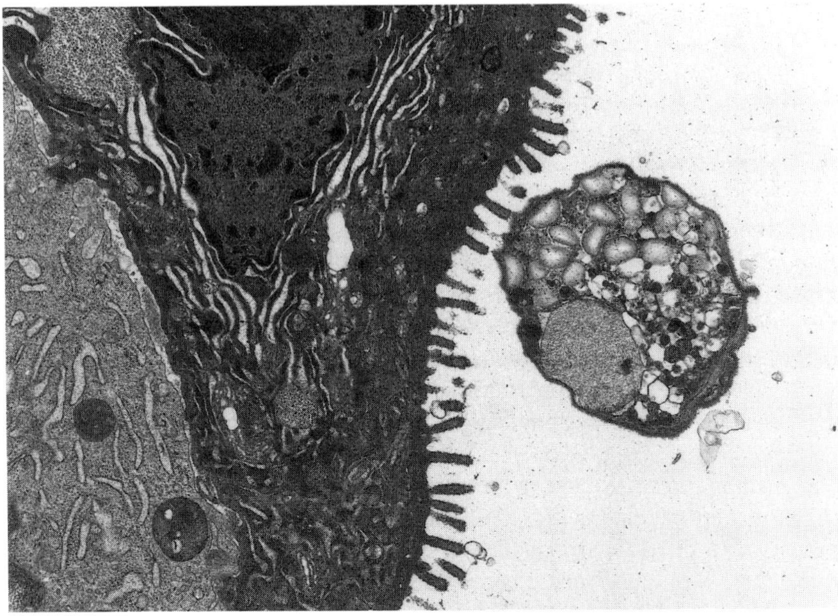

Figure 5 Biliary Cryptosporidium: Electron micrograph of intraductal bile duct biopsy from patient in Figure 4. Note large Cryptosporidium adjacent to bile duct epithelium.

There is no specific effective treatment for *Cryptosporidium* or microsporidia infection (125,126). Ganciclovir and foscarnet have been used against CMV, eradicating the organism from the duodenum but cholangiograms remained unaltered (118,131). Ganciclovir's lack of efficacy may be related to drug resistance (135) or inadequate biliary levels as it is primarily excreted via the kidneys (126).

Ursodeoxycholic acid, a hydrophilic bile acid, has been used in chronic cholestatic conditions of the liver (136). We have noted symptomatic improvement in HIV-positive patients with recurrent abdominal pain, abnormal canalicular enzymes, and intrahepatic biliary strictures when this treatment is employed.

5. *Prognosis*

The prognosis for AIDS-cholangiopathy is poor, with a twelve month survival of 14% in one series (121). Progression of AIDS rather than biliary-tract-related diseases is the usual cause of death (131).

V. PANCREATIC INFECTIONS

A. Epidemiology

The incidence of acute pancreatitis in HIV-infected individuals is between 5 and 22% (137–139). Pancreatitis has been reported in 9 (17%) of 53 pediatric patients with AIDS who were followed during a 6-year period (140). It is unclear how many cases are the result of pancreatic infections. Pancreatic infection is rarely found antemortem but autopsy studies have revealed opportunistic infections of the pancreas in 24% of 81 AIDS patients (139). These autopsy findings may falsely increase the prevalence rate since they include nonspecific features such as acinar dilatation, which also occurs with similar frequency in immunocompetent controls (139,141,142).

The prevalence of hyperamylasemia in patients with AIDS has been estimated to be 54% (143). However, its value as a diagnostic test in pancreatitis is diminished as hyperamylasemia is frequently of salivary gland origin or due to macroamylasemia (143,144). Increased serum amylase and lipase values were detected in 16 (16%) of 100 consecutive AIDS patients, being associated with abdominal pain in 6 patients and enteric opportunistic infections in 10 (145). Six patients had evidence of cryptosporidiosis, 4 of microsporidiosis, and 1 patient had evidence of CMV. The level of amylase had no correlation with clinical outcome.

B. Etiology

While opportunistic infections and medications are more often associated with acute pancreatitis in HIV-seropositive than seronegative patients, the etiology is frequently multifactorial. Commonly identified pathogens include CMV, *Pneumocystis carinii*, MAC, and *Cryptosporidium* (137–139,146,147). Drugs implicated in pancreatitis include pentamidine, 2′, 3′-dideoxyinosine, and trimethoprime-sulfamethoxazole (137–139). In children, pentamidine exposure, especially when the CD4 cell count is less than 100/mm^3, has a particularly strong association with the development of pancreatitis (140).

C. Pathophysiology

Ascending infection, similar to that seen in the biliary tree, causes inflammation and destruction of the pancreatic parenchyma and probably accounts for clinically significant pancreatitis (139). Interstitial edema and a mixed inflammatory cell infiltrate have been demonstrated around the pancreatic duct, which may explain the development of pancreatic duct strictures in patients with AIDS-cholangiopathy (113,119,120,132). *Cryptosporidium* colonization of the pancreatic ducts is associated with transformation of pancreatic ductal epithelium to stratified squamous epithelium (127).

D. Clinical Features

Of 45 HIV-positive patients with acute pancreatitis, 60% had a moderately severe acute pancreatitis and 40% had mild disease, as assessed by Ranson's criteria (137,148). Common clinical findings include abdominal pain and vomiting (138,140). Although patients with HIV and acute pancreatitis are more likely to have greater anemia, hypoalbuminemia, leukopenia, fever, diarrhea, and hepatomegaly than non-HIV infected individuals, these differences are most likely attributable to HIV-associated immunosuppression and malnutrition rather than pancreatitis itself (138). The presentation may be atypical and pancreatitis may remain unsuspected until an abdominal CT scan is performed in the investigation of abdominal pain. We recommend considering pancreatitis in the differential diagnosis of patients who have deteriorated in the absence of typical clinical features, such as severe abdominal pain (149). A case of biliary obstruction secondary to acute pancreatitis in an AIDS patient has been reported (149).

E. Treatment

As for non-HIV related pancreatitis, the primary treatment is supportive. Medications associated with pancreatitis should be stopped if possible. Antemortem identification of opportunistic pancreatic pathogens is difficult and often there is no effective therapy available when an organism is identified. In the presence of known systemic CMV, associated pancreatitis should be treated with intravenous ganciclovir or foscarnet.

REFERENCES

1. Horvath J, Raffanti SP. Clinical aspects of the interactions between human immunodeficiency virus and the hepatotrophic viruses. Clin Infect Dis 1994; 18:339–347.
2. Cappell MS. Hepatobiliary manifestations of the acquired immune deficiency syndrome. Am J Gastroenterol 1991; 86:1–15.
3. Schneiderman DJ. Hepatobiliary abnormalities of AIDS. Gastroenterol Clin North Am 1988; 17:615–630.
4. Grumbach K, Coleman BG, Gal AA, Arger PH, Mintz MC, Arenson RL, Aquino L. Hepatic and biliary tract abnormalities in patients with AIDS. J Ultrasound Med 1989; 8:247–254.
5. Barish MA, Yucel EK, Soto JA, Chuttani R, Ferrucci JT. MR cholangiopancreatography: efficacy of three dimensional turbo spin echo technique. Am J Roentgenol 1995; 165:295–300.

6. Quinn D, Pocock N, Freund J, Kelleher A, Penny R, Brew B. Radionuclide hepatobiliary scanning in patients with AIDS-related sclerosing cholangitis. Clinical Nucl Med 1992; 18:417–422.
7. Jeffers LJ, Alzate I, Aguilar H, Reddy KR, Idrovo V, Cheinquer H, Hasan FA, Parker T, et al. Laparoscopic and histologic findings in patients with the human immunodeficiency virus. Gastrointestinal Endoscopy 1994; 40:160–164.
8. Cappell MS, Schwartz MS, Biempica L. Clinical utility of liver biopsy in patients with serum antibodies to the human immunodeficiency virus. Am J Med 1990; 88:123–130.
9. Prüfer-Krämer L, Krämer A, Weigel R, Rögler G, Fleige B, Krause PH, Hahn EG, et al. Hepatic involvement in patients with human immunodeficiency virus infection: discrepancies between AIDS patients and those with earlier stages of infection. J Infect Dis 1991; 163:866-869.
10. Schneiderman DJ, Arenson DM, Cello JP, Margaretten W, Weber TE. Hepatic disease in patients with the acquired immune deficiency syndrome (AIDS). Hepatology 1987; 7:925–930.
11. Gordon SC, McFadden RF, Reddy KR, Schiff ER. Major hemorrhage after percutaneous liver biopsy in patients with AIDS (letter). Gastroenterology 1991;100:1787.
12. Marano BJ, Bonanno CA. Liver biopsy in patients with the acquired immunodeficiency syndrome (letter). Am J Gastroenterol 1993; 88:2139–2140.
13. Cavicchi M, Pialoux G, Carnot F, Offredo C, Romana C, Deslandes P, Dupont B, Berthelot P, Pol S. Value of liver biopsy for the rapid diagnosis of infection in human immunodeficiency virus-infected patients who have unexplained fever and elevated serum levels of alkaline phosphatase or gamma-glutamyl transferase. Clin Infect Dis 1995; 20:606–610.
14. Lebovics E, Dworkin BM, Heier SK, Rosenthal WS. The hepatobiliary manifestations of human immunodeficiency virus infection. Am J Gastroenterol 1988; 83:1–7.
15. Karasik MS, Afdhal NH. Gastrointestinal manifestations. In: Libman H, Witzburg RA, eds. HIV infection: A Primary Care Manual. 3d ed. Boston: Little, Brown, 1995:165–180.
16. Lichtenstein DR, Makadon HJ, Chopra S. Fulminant hepatitis B and delta virus coinfection in AIDS. Am J Gastroenterol 1992; 87:1643–1647.
17. Hadler SC, Judson FN, O'Malley, PM, Altman NL, Penley K, Buchbinder S, Schable CA, Coleman PJ, et al. Outcome of hepatitis B virus infection in homosexual men and its relation to prior human immunodeficiency virus infection. J Infect Dis 1991; 163:454–459.
18. McNair ANB, Main J, Thomas HC. Interactions of the human immunodeficiency virus and the hepatotropic viruses. Semin Liver Dis 1992; 12:188–196.
19. Bodsworth N, Donovan B, Nightingale BN. The effect of concurrent human immunodcficiency virus infection on chronic hepatitis B: a study of 150 homosexual men. J Infect Dis 1989; 160:577–582.
20. Rustgi VK, Hoofnagle JH, Gerin JL, Gelmann EP, Reichert CM, Cooper JN, Macher AM. Hepatitis B virus infection in the acquired immunodeficiency syndrome. Ann Intern Med 1984; 101:795–797.

21. Koblin BA, Taylor PE, Rubinstein P, Stevens CE. Effect of duration of hepatitis B virus infection on the association between human immunodeficiency virus type-1 and hepatitis B viral replication. Hepatology 1992; 15:590–592.
22. Romet-Lemonne J-LM, McLlane MF, Elfassi E, Haseltine WA, Azocar J, Essex M. Hepatitis B infection in cultured lymphoblastoid cells. Science 1983; 221:667–669.
23. Laure F, Zagury D, Saimot AG, Gallo RC, Hahn BH, Brecht C. Hepatitis B virus DNA sequences in lymphoid cells from patients with AIDS and AIDS-related complex. Science 1985; 229:561–563.
24. Maguire HF, Hoeffler JP, Siddiqui A. HBV X protein alters the DNA binding specificity of CREB and ATF-2 by protein-protein interactions. Science 1991; 252:842–844.
25. Twu JS, Robinson WS. Hepatitis B virus X gene can transactivate heterologous viral sequences. Proc Natl Acad Sci USA 1989; 86:2046–2050.
26. Seto E, Yen TSB, Peterlin BM, Ou JH. Trans-activation of the human immunodeficiency virus long terminal repeat by the hepatitis B virus X protein. Proc Natl Acad Sci USA 1988; 85:8286–8290.
27. Solomon RE, VanRaden M, Kaslow RA, Lyter D, Visscher B, Farzadegan H, Phair J. Association of hepatitis B surface antigen and core antibody with acquisition and manifestations of human immunodeficiency virus type 1, (HIV-1) infection. Am J Public Health 1990; 80:1475–1478.
28. Levy P, Marcellin P, Martinot-Peignoux M, Degott C, Nataf J, Benhamou J-P. Clinical course of spontaneous reactivation of hepatitis B virus infection in patients with chronic hepatitis B. Hepatology 1990; 12:570–574.
29. Homan C, Krogsgaard K, Pedersen C, Andersson P, Nielsen JO. High incidence of hepatitis B infection and evolution of chronic hepatitis B infection in patients with advanced HIV infection. J AIDS 1991; 4:416–420.
30. Fang JWS, Wright TL, Lau JYN. Fibrosing cholestatic hepatitis in patient with HIV and hepatitis B (letter). Lancet 1993; 342:1175.
31. McDonald JA, Caruso L, Karayiannis P, Scully LJ, Harris JR, Forster GE, Thomas HC. Diminished responsiveness of male homosexual chronic hepatitis B virus carriers with HTLV-III antibodies to recombinant interferon. Hepatology 1987; 7:719–723.
32. Brook MG, Chan G, Yap I, Karayiannis P, Lever AM, Jacyna M, Main J, Thomas HC. Randomised controlled trial of lymphoblastoid interferon alfa in European men with chronic hepatitis B virus infection. Br Med J 1989; 299:652–656.
33. Odaka N, Eldred L, Cohn S, Munoz A, Fields HA, Fox R, Solomon R, Kaslow R, Polk BF. Comparative immunogenicity of plasma and recombinant hepatitis B virus vaccines in homosexual men. JAMA 1988; 269:3635–3637.
34. Collier AC, Corey L, Murphy VL, Handsfield HH. Antibody to human immunodeficiency virus (HIV) and suboptimal response to hepatitis B vaccination. Ann Intern Med 1988; 109:101–105.
35. Loke RHT, Murray-Lyon IM, Coleman JC, Evans BA, Zuckerman AJ. Diminished response to recombinant hepatitis B vaccine in homosexual men with HIV antibody: an indicator of poor prognosis. J Med Virol 1990; 31:109–111.

36. Bruguera M, Cremades M, Salinas R, Costa J, Grau M, Sans J. Impaired response to recombinant hepatitis B vaccine in HIV-infected persons. J Clin Gastroenterol 1992; 14:27–30.
37. Biggar RJ, Goedert JJ, Hoofnagle JH. Accelerated loss of antibody to hepatitis B surface antigen among immunodeficient homosexual men infected with HIV (letter). N Engl J Med 1987; 316:630–631.
38. Visco G, Alba L, Grisetti S, Guarascio P, Narciso P, Sette P, Struglia C, Tossini G, Tozzi V. Zidovudine plus interferon alfa-2b treatment in patients with HIV and chronic active viral hepatitis. Gut 1993; (suppl):S107–S108.
39. DiBisceglie AM. Long-term outcome of interferon-alpha therapy for chronic hepatitis B. J Hepatol 1995; 22(suppl 1):65–67.
40. Benhamou Y, Dohin E, Lunel-Fabiani F, Poynard T, Huraux JM, Katlama C, Opolon P, Gentilini M. Efficacy of lamivudine on replication of hepatitis B virus in HIV-infected patients (letter). Lancet 1995; 345:396–397.
41. Terrault N, Wright T. Interferon and hepatitis C. N Engl J Med 1995; 332:1509–1511.
42. Alter MJ. Epidemiology of hepatitis C in the West. Seminars Liver Dis 1995; 15:5–14.
43. Giovannini M, Tagger A, Ribero ML, Zuccotti G, Pogliani L, Grossi A, Ferroni P, Fiocchi A. Maternal-infant transmission of hepatitis C and HIV infections; a possible interaction (letter). Lancet 1990; 335:1166.
44. Chirianni A, Abrescia N, Tullio-Cataldo P. Anti-HCV prevalence in HIV infected patients (abstract no. WB87). In: Program and abstracts of the VII International Conference on AIDS (Florence). Florence: Instituto Superiore di Sanità, 1991.
45. Chamot E, Herschel B, Wintsch J, Robert CF, Gabriel V, Deglon JJ, Yerly S, Perrin L. Loss of antibodies against hepatitis C virus in HIV-seropositive intravenous drug users. AIDS 1990; 4:1275–1277.
46. Sherman KE, O'Brien J, Gutierrez AG, Harrison S, Urdea M, Neuwald P, Wilber J. Quantitative evaluation of hepatitis C virus RNA in patients with concurrent human immunodeficiency virus infections. J Clin Microbiol 1993; 31:2679–2682.
47. Eyster ME, Diamondstone LS, Lien J-M, Ehmann WC, Quan S, Goedert JJ for the Multicenter Hemophilia Cohort Study. Natural history of hepatitis C virus infection in multitransfused hemophiliacs: effect of coinfection with human immunodeficiency virus. J AIDS 1993; 6:602–610.
48. Martin P, DiBisceglie AM, Kassianides C, Lisker-Melman M, Hoofnagle JH. Rapidly progressive non-A, non-B hepatitis in patients with human immunodeficiency virus infection. Gastroenterology 1989; 97:1559–1561.
49. Wright TL, Hollander H, Pu X, Held MJ, Lipson P, Quan S, Polito A, Thaler MM, et al. Hepatitis C in HIV-infected patients with and without AIDS: prevalence and relationship to patient survival. Hepatology 1994; 20:1152–1155.
50. Boyer N, Marcellin P, Degott C, Degos F, Saimot AG, Erlinger S, Benhamou JP. Recombinant interferon-alpha for chronic hepatitis C in patients positive for antibody to human immunodeficiency virus. J Infect Dis 1995; 15:723–724.
51. Marriott E, Navas S, del Romero J, Garcia S, Castillo I, Quiroga JA, Carreno V.

Treatment with recombinant alpha-interferon of chronic hepatitis C in anti-HIV positive patients. J Med Virol 1993; 40:107–111.
52. Mauss S, Heintges T, Albrecht H, Niederau C, Jablonowski H. Treatment of chronic hepatitis C with interferon-α in patients infected with the human immunodeficiency virus 1 (abstract). Gastroenterology 1995; 108:A873.
53. Fried MW, Hoofnagle, JH. Therapy of hepatitis C. Seminars Liver Dis 1995; 15:82–91.
54. Rockstroh JK, Spengler U, Raab P, Hammerstein U, Oldenburg J, Brackmann HH, Sauerbruch T. Does development of cholestatic liver disease in HIV and hepatitis C coinfected hemophiliacs indicate an unfavorable prognosis? (abstract). Gastroenterology 1995; 108:A905.
55. Troisi CL, Hollinger FB, Hoots WK, et al. A multicenter study of viral hepatitis in a United States hemophiliac population. Blood 1993; 81:412–418.
56. Buti M, Esteban R, Espanol MT, Malagelada A, Jardi R, Rodriquez-Frias F, Roget M, Guardia J. Influence of human immunodeficiency virus infection on cell mediated immunity in chronic D hepatitis. J Infect Dis 1991; 163:1351–1353.
57. Eyster ME, Sanders JC, Battegay M, Di Bisceglie AM. Suppression of hepatitis C virus (HCV) replication by hepatitis D virus (HDV) in HIV-infected hemophiliacs with chronic hepatitis B and C. Dig Dis Sci 1995; 40:1583.
58. de Pouplana M, Soriano V, Samaniego JG, Enriquez A, Munoz F, Gonzalez-Lahoz J. More severe course of delta hepatitis in HIV infected patients. Genitourin Med 1995; 71:132–133.
59. Shattock AG, Finlay H, Hillary IB. Possible reactivation of hepatitis D with chronic δ antigenaemia by human immunodeficiency virus. B Med J 1987; 294:1656–1657.
60. Grippon P, Ribiers O, Cadranel JF, Pelletier S, Pillot B, Emerit J, Opolon P. Long-term delta antigenaemia without appearance of delta antibody in two immunodeficient patients. Lanncet 1987; 1:1031.
61. Jardi R, Buti M, Cotrina M, Rodriquez F, Allende H, Esteban R, Guardia J. Determination of hepatitis delta virus RNA by polymerase chain reaction in acute and chronic delta infection. Hepatology 1995; 21:25–29.
62. Madejon A, Cotonat T, Bartolome J, Castillo I, Carreno V. Treatment of chronic hepatitis D virus infection with low and high doses of interferon-alpha 2a: utility of polymerase chain reaction in monitoring the antiviral response. Hepatology 1994; 19:1331–1336.
63. Farci P, Mandas A, Coiana A, Lai ME, Desmet V, Van Eyken P, Gibo Y, et al. Treatment of chronic hepatitis D with interferon alfa-2a. N Engl J Med 1994; 330:88–94.
64. Gaudin JL, Faure P, Godinot H, Gerard F, Trepo C. The French experience of treatment of chronic type D hepatitis with a 12 month course of interferon alpha-2b: results of a randomized controlled trial. Liver 1995; 15:45–52.
65. Buti M, Esteban R, Jardi R, Rodriguez-Fria F, Allende H, Cotrina M, Guardia J. Treatment of chronic type D hepatitis and concomitant human immunodeficiency infection with alpha interferon. J Hepatology 1992; 14:412–413.
66. Rizzetto M. Systemic virosis producing hepatitis occasionally, or as an opportu-

nistic infection in the immunocompromised host. In: McIntyre N, Benhamou J-P, Bircher J, Rizzetto M, Rodes J, eds. Oxford Textbook of Hepatology. Oxford: Oxford University Press, 1991:635–638.
67. Bach N, Theise ND, Schaffner F. Hepatic histopathology in the acquired immunodeficiency syndrome. Semin Liver Dis 1992; 12:205–212.
68. Collins FM. Mycobacterial disease, immunosuppression and acquired immunodeficiency syndrome. Clinical Microbiology Reviews 1989; 2:360–377.
69. Wilkins MJ, Lindley R, Dourakis SP, Golden RD. Surgical pathology of the liver in HIV infection. Histopathology 1991; 18:459–464.
70. MacDonell KB, Glassroth J. *Mycobacterium avium* complex and other nontuberculous mycobacteria in patients with HIV infection. Semin Respir Infect 1989; 4:123–132.
71. Wetton CWN, McCarthy M, Tomlinson D, Rosbotham J, Crofton ME. Ultrasound findings in hepatic mycobacterial infections in patients with acquired immune deficiency syndrome (AIDS). Clin Radiology 1993; 47:36–38.
72. Kiehn TE, Edwards FF, Brannon P, Tsang AY, Maio M, Gold JW, Whimbey E, Wong B, McClatchy JK, Armstrong D. Infections caused by *Mycobactrium avium* complex in immunocompromised patients: diagnosis by blood culture and fecal examination, antimicrobial susceptibility tests, and morphological and seroagglutination characteristics. J Clin Microbiology 1985; 21:168–173.
73. Tenholder MF, Moser RJ 3d, Tellis CJ. Mycobacteria other than tuberculosis: pulmonary involvement in patients with acquired immunodeficiency syndrome. Arch Int Med 1988; 148:953–955.
74. Nichols L, Florentine B, Lewis W, Sattler F, Rarick MU, Brynes RK. Bone marow examination for the diagnosis of mycobacterial and fungal infections in the acquired immunodeficiency syndrome. Arch Path and Lab Med 1991; 115:1125–1132.
75. Prego V, Glatt AE, Roy V, Thelmo W, Dincsoy H, Raufman JP. Comparative analysis of blood culture for fungi and mycobacteria, liver biopsy and bone marrow biopsy in the diagnosis of fever of undetermined origin in human immunodeficiency virus-infected patients. Arch Intern Med 1990: 150:333–336.
76. Emler S, Bottger EC, Broers B, Cassis I, Perrin L, Hirschel B. Growth-deficient mycobacteria in patients with AIDS: diagnosis by analysis of DNA amplified from blood or tissue. Clin Infect Dis 1995; 20:772–775.
77. Farber HW, Barber TW. Mycobacterial Infections. In: Libman H, Witzburg RA, eds. HIV Infection: A Primary Care Manual. 3d ed. Boston: Little Brown, 1995:309–324.
78. Pitchenik AE, Fertel D. Tuberculosis and nontuberculosis mycobacterial disease. In: White DA, Gold JWM, eds. Medical Management of AIDS patients. Med Clin North Am 1992; 76:121–171.
79. Small PM, Shafer RW, Hopewell PC, Singh SP, Murphy MJ, Desmond E, Sierra MF, Schoolnik GK. Exogenous reinfection with multidrug-resistant *Mycobacterium tuberculosis* in patients with advanced HIV infection. N Engl J Med 1993; 328:1137–1144.

80. Diamond RD. The growing problem of mycoses in patients infected with the human immnodeficiency virus. Rev Infect Dis 1991; 13:480–486.
81. Pastakia B, Shawker TH, Thaler M, O'Leary T, Pizzo PA. Hepatosplenic candidiasis: wheels within wheels. Radiology 1988; 2:417–421.
82. Sulis CA. Candidiasis. In: Libman H, Witzburg RA, eds. HIV Infection: A Primary Care Manual. 3d ed. Boston: Little, Brown, 1995:399–407.
83. Suga AM, Saunders CA. Cryptococcosis. In: Libman H, Witzburg RA, eds. HIV Infection: A Primary Care Manual. 3d ed. Boston: Little, Brown, 1995:325–335.
84. Daar ES, Meyèr RD. Bacterial and fungal infections. In: White DA, Gold JWM, eds. Medical Management of AIDS patients. Med Clin North Am 1992; 76:173–203.
85. Viviani MA. Opportunistic fungal infections in patients with acquired immune deficiency syndrome. Chemotherapy 1992; 38(suppl 1):35–42.
86. Stevens DA. Coccidioidomycosis. N Engl J Med 1995; 332:1077–1082.
87. Johnson PC, Khardori N, Najjar AF, Butt F, Mansell PW, Sarosi GA. Progressive disseminated histoplasmosis in patients with acquired immunodeficiency syndrome. Am J Med 1988; 85:152–158.
88. Viner BL. *Pneumocystis* Pneumonia. In: Libman H, Witzburg RA, eds. HIV Infection: A Primary Care Manual. 3d ed. Boston: Little, Brown, 1995:275–308.
89. Sachs JR, Greenfield SM, Sohn M, Turner JL. Disseminated *Pneumocystis carinii* infection in a patient with the acquired immune deficiency syndrome. Am J Gastroenterol 1991; 86:82–85.
90. Hagopian WA, Huseby JS. *Pneumocystis* hepatitis and choroiditis despite successful aerosolized pentamidine pulmonary prophylaxis. Chest 1989; 96:949–951.
91. Grimes MM, LaPook JD, Bar MH, Wasserman HS, Dwork A. Disseminated *Pneumocystis carinii* infection in a patient with immunodeficiency syndrome. Hum Path 1987; 18:307–308.
92. Raviglione MC, Mariuz P, Sugar J, Mullen MP. Extrapulmonary *Pnenumocystis* infection (letter). Ann Int Med 1989; 111:339.
93. Richie JL, Yamaguchi E, Virani N, Quinn BD, Chaisson RE. Extrapulmonary *Pneumocystis* infection (letter). Ann Int Med 1989; 111:339–340.
94. Fishman EK, Magid D, Kuhlman JE. *Pneumocystis carinii* involvement of the liver and spleen: CT demonstration. J Comput Assist Tomogr 1990; 14:146–148.
95. Lubat E, Megibow AJ, Balthazar EJ, Goldenberg AS, Birnbaum BA, Bosniak MA. Extrapulmonary *Pneumocystis carinii* infection in AIDS: CT findings. Radiology 1990; 174:157–160.
96. Merkel IS, Good CB, Nalesnik M, Roseman SR. Chronic *Pneumocystis carinii* infection of the liver: A case report and review of the literature. J Clin Gastroenterol 1992; 15:55–58.
97. Terada S, Reddy KR, Jeffers LJ, Cali A, Schiff ER. Microsporidian hepatitis in the acquired immunodeficiency syndrome. Ann Int Med 1987; 107:61–62.
98. Currier JS, Sulis CA. Toxoplasmosis. In: Libman H, Witzburg RA, eds. HIV Infection: A Primary Care Manual. 3d ed. Boston: Little, Brown, 1995:337–347.
99. Bryceson ADM. Visceral leishmaniasis. In: McIntyre N, Benhamou J-P, Bircher

J, Rizzetto M, Rodes J, eds. Oxford Textbook of Hepatology. Oxford: Oxford University Press, 1991:707–711.

100. Cook GC. *Strongyloides stercoralis* hyperinfection syndrome: how often is it missed? Q J Med 1987; 64:625–629.
101. Rawat B, Simons ME. *Strongyloides stercoralis* hyperinfestation: another cause of focal hepatic lesions. Clinical Imaging 1993; 17:274–275.
102. Treadwell TL. Gastrointestinal parasites. In: Libman H, Witzburg RA, eds. HIV Infection: A Primary Care Manual. 3d ed. Boston: Little, Brown, 1995:409–417.
103. Zak FG. Peliosis hepatis. Am J Pathol 1950; 26:1–15.
104. Garcia-Tsao G, Panzini L, Yoselevitz M, West AB. Bacillary peliosis hepatis as a cause of acute anemia in a patient with the acquired immunodeficiency syndrome. Gastroenterology 1992; 102:1065–1070.
105. Slater LN, Welch DF, Min K-W. *Rochalimaea henselae* causes bacillary angiomatosis and peliosis hepatis. Arch Int Med 1992; 152:602–606.
106. Steeper TA, Rosenstein H, Weiser J, Inampudi S, Snover DC. Bacillary epithelioid angiomatosis involving the liver, spleen, and skin in an AIDS patient with concurrent Kaposi's sarcoma. Am J Clin Pathol 1992; 97:713–718.
107. Koehler JE, Glaser CA, Tappero JW. *Rochalimaea henselae* infection: a new zoonosis with the domestic cat as reservoir. JAMA 1994; 271:531–535.
108. Munster AM, Brown JR. Acalculous choleycystitis. Am J Surg 1967; 113:730–734
109. Long TN, Heimbach DM, Carrico CJ. Acalculous choleycystitis in critically ill patients. Am J Surg 1978; 136:31–36.
110. Howard RJ. Acute acalculous choleycystitis. Am J Surg 1981; 141:194–198.
111. Blumberg RS, Kelsey P, Perrone T, Dickersin R, Laquaglia M, Ferruci J. Cytomegalovirus- and cryptosporidium-associated acalculous gangrenous choleycystitis. Am J Med 1984; 76:1118–1123.
112. Kavin H, Jonas RB, Chowdhury L, Kabins S. Acalculous choleycystitis and cytomegalovirus infection in the acquired immunodeficiency syndrome. Ann Int Med 1986; 104:53–54.
113. Teixidor HS, Godwin TA, Ramirez EA. Cryptosporidiosis of the biliary tract in AIDS. Radiology 1991; 180:51–56.
114. Fournier AM, Michel J. Curvoisier's sign revisited: two patients with palpable gallbladder. Southern Med J 1992; 85:548–550.
115. Cervia JS, Murray HW. Fungal cholecystitis and AIDS (letter). J Infect Dis 1990; 161:358.
116. Wheeler AP, Gregg CR. Campylobacter bacteremia, cholecystitis and the acquired immunodeficiency syndrome (letter). Ann Int Med 1986; 105:804.
117. Romano AJ, vanSonnenberg E, Casola G, Gosink BB, Withers CE, McCutchan JA, Leopold GR. Gallbladder and bile duct abnormalities in AIDS: sonographic findings in eight patients. Am J Roentgenol 1988; 150:123–127.
118. Benhamou Y, Caumes E, Gerosa Y, Cadranel JF, Dohin E, Katlama C, Amouyal P, Canard JM, et al. AIDS-related cholangiopathy: critical analysis of a prospective series of 26 patients. Dig Dis Sci 1993; 38:1113–1118.

119. Cello JP. Human immunodeficiency virus-associated biliary tract disease. Semin Liver Dis 1992; 12:213–218.
120. Farman J, Brunetti J, Baer JW, Freiman H, Comer GM, Scholz FJ, Koehler RE, Laffey K, et al. AIDS-related cholangiopancreatographic changes. Abdom Imaging 1994; 19:417–422.
121. Bouche H, Housset C, Dumont J-L, Carnot Y, Menu Y, Aveline B, Belghiti J, Boboc B, et al. AIDS-related cholangitis: diagnostic features and course in 15 patients. J Hepatol 1993; 17:34–39.
122. Pitlik SD, Fainstein V, Garza D, Guarda L, Bolivar R, Rios A, Hopfer RL, Mansell PA. Human cryptosporidiosis: spectrum of disease. Arch Int Med 1983; 143:2269–2275.
123. Margulis SJ, Honig CL, Soave R, Govoni AF, Mouradian JA, Jacobson IM. Biliary tract obstruction in the acquired immunodeficiency syndrome. Ann Int Med 1986; 105:207–210.
124. Pol S, Romana C, Richard S, Carnot F, Dumont J-L, Bouche H, Pialoux G, Stern M, et al. *Enterocytozoon bieneusi* infection in acquired immunodeficiency syndrome-related sclerosing cholangitis. Gastroenterology 1992; 102:1778–1781.
125. Pol S, Romana CA, Richard S, Amouyal P, Desportes-Livage I, Carnot F, Pays J-J, Berthelot P. Microsporidia infection in patients with the human immunodeficiency virus and unexplained cholangitis. N Engl J Med 1993; 328:95–99.
126. Willson R, Harrington R, Stewart B, Fritsche T. Human immunodeficiency virus 1-associated necrotizing cholangitis caused by infection with *Septata intestinalis*. Gastroenterology 1995; 108:247–251.
127. Kline TJ, De Las Morenas T, O'Brien M, Smith BF, Afdhal NH. Squamous metaplasia of extrahepatic biliary system in an AIDS patient with cryptosporidia and cholangitis. Dig Dis Sci 1993; 38:960–962.
128. McKeating J, Griffiths PD, Weiss R. HIV susceptibility conferred to human fibroblasts by cytomegalovirus-induced Fc receptor. Nature 1990; 343:659–661.
129. Sieratzki J, Thung SN, Gerber MA. Major histocompatibility antigen expression in the liver in the acquired immunodeficiency syndrome. Arch Pathol Lab Med 1987; 111:1045–1049.
130. Cello JP. Acquired immunodeficiency syndrome cholangiopathy: spectrum of disease. Am J Med 1989; 86:539–546.
131. Forbes A, Blansard C, Gazzard. Natural history of AIDS related sclerosing cholangitis: a study of 20 cases. Gut 1993; 34:116–121.
132. Da Silva F, Boudghene F, Lecomte I, Delage Y, Grange J-D, Bigot J-M. Sonography in AIDS-related cholangitis: prevalence and cause of an echogenic nodule in the distal end of the common bile duct. Am J Roengtenol 1993; 160:1205–1207.
133. Barkum AN. Endoscopy and gallstones. In: Cotton PB, Tytgat GNJ, Williams CB, eds. Annual of Gastrointestinal Endoscopy. London: Churchill Livingstone 1995:89–99.
134. Urbain D, Jeanmart J, Lemone M, Kiromera A, Muls V, Arendt V, Dewit S. Cholestasis in patients with the acquired immune deficiency syndrome: comparison between ultrasonographic and cholangiographic findings. Am J Gastroenterol 1991; 86:574–576.

135. Erice A, Chou S, Biron KK, Stanat SC, Balfour HH, Jordan MC. Progressive disease due to ganciclovir-resistant cytomegalovirus in immunosuppressed patients. N Engl J Med 1989; 320:289–293.
136. Luketic VA, Sanyal AJ. The current status of ursodeoxycholate in the treatment of chronic cholestatic liver disease. The Gastroenterologist 1994; 2:74–79.
137. Ting CD, Gradon J, Dutta SK. Study of prevalence, severity and etiological factors associated with acute pancreatitis in patients infected with human immunodeficiency virus (abstract). Gastroenterology 1995; 108:A396.
138. Marks M, Cappell MS. A multicenter, multiyear, case-controlled study of 44 consecutive HIV seropositive patients with acute pancreatitis (abstract). Gastroenterology 1994; 106:A730.
139. Dowell SF, Moore GW, Hutchins GM. The spectrum of pancreatic pathology in patients with AIDS. Modern Path 1990; 3:49–53.
140. Miller TL, Winter HS, Luginbuhl LM, Orav EJ, McIntosh K. Pancreatitis in pediatric human immunodeficiency virus infection. J Pediatr 1992; 12:223–227.
141. Brivet FG, Naveau SH, Lemaigre GF, Dormont J. Pancreatic lesions in HIV-infected patients. Baillieres Clin Endocrinol Meta 1994; 8:859–877.
142. Kahn E, Anderson VM, Greco MA, Magid M. Pancreatic disorders in pediatric acquired immune deficiency syndrome. Hum Pathol 1995; 26:765–770.
143. Murthy UK, DeGregorio F, Oates RP, Blair DC. Hyperamylasemia in patients with the acquired immunodeficiency syndrome. Am J Gastroenterol 1992; 87:332–336.
144. Greenberg RE, Bank S, Singer C. Macroamylasemia in association with the acquired immunodeficiency syndrome. Postgrad Med J 1987; 63:677–679.
145. Benhamou Y, Sayegh MH, Dohin E, Gentilini M, Opolon P. AIDS related hyperamylasemia: results of a study of 100 consecutive patients. Gastroenterology 1994; 106:A652.
146. Brivet F, Coffin B, Bedossa P, Naveau S, Petitpretz P, Delfraissy JF, Dormont J. Pancreatic lesions in AIDS (letter). Lancet 1987; 2:570–571.
147. Bricaire F, Marche C, Zoubi D, Saimot AG, Regnier B. HIV and the pancreas (letter). Lancet 1988; 1:65–66.
148. Ranson JHC, Rifkind KM, Turner JW. Prognostic signs and nonoperative peritoneal lavage in acute pancreatitis. Surg Gynecol Obstet 1976; 143:209–219.
149. Wilcox CM, Forsmark CE, Grendell JH, Darragh TM, Cello JP. Cytomegalovirus-associated acute pancreatic disease in patients with acquired immunodeficiency syndrome. Gastroenterology 1990; 99:263–267.

13

Intra-abdominal Abscesses

DORI F. ZALEZNIK
Harvard Medical School and Beth Israel Deaconess Medical Center, Boston, Massachusetts

DENNIS L. KASPER
Harvard Medical School and Brigham and Women's Hospital, Boston, Massachusetts

I. INTRODUCTION

The clinical course and treatment of intra-abdominal infection varies according to the cause of the disease. Intra-abdominal infection can arise from disruption of a normal anatomic barrier, a ruptured appendix, a perforated diverticulum, a necrotizing tumor, or direct trauma. Infection can spread contiguously from a nearby focus, most commonly the gall bladder. Intra-abdominal abscesses, particularly visceral collections, also can result from bacteremia. Regardless of the initiating event, if organisms that colonize the intestine invade the normally sterile peritoneal cavity, they cause inflammation and a predictable series of events. Intra-abdominal infections, as studied both from experimental models and clinical observation, develop in two stages: peritonitis and, if untreated, abscess formation. The predominant microorganisms in each stage of infection are primarily responsible for the pathogenic process.

II. PERITONITIS

Peritonitis can occur as a primary or secondary event. In adults primary peritonitis usually is synonymous with spontaneous bacterial peritonitis, which is seen almost exclusively in patients with alcoholic cirrhosis and preexisting ascites (1). Secondary peritonitis develops when bacteria contaminate the peritoneum as a result of spillage from a viscus. Multiple etiologic organisms almost always are found, but aerobic gram-negative bacilli and anaerobes predominate, especially when the ruptured or leaking viscus is in the colon (2). Following contamination, the first finding is a free-flowing exudate with polymorphonuclear leukocytes (PMNs), the predominant inflammatory cells. Mortality at this stage of infection is appreciable due to gram-negative bacilli in the bloodstream and the resulting endotoxemia. The most common bloodstream isolates are gram-negative bacilli especially *Escherichia coli* and *Klebsiella* sp., but the anaerobic organism, *Bacteroides fragilis*, frequently causes bacteremia as well. The course and clinical symptoms (including abdominal pain) depend on the initial inciting events for secondary peritonitis. Radiologic and laboratory tests are required to determine the source of infection.

Treatment for secondary peritonitis includes early administration of antibiotics targeted particularly at aerobic gram-negative bacilli and anaerobes. Secondary peritonitis generally requires both surgical intervention to correct the inciting event and antibiotic administration. Antibiotics usually are effective in early bacteremia; they help to decrease the likelihood of abscess formation and wound infection and keep the infection from spreading to other sites.

III. INTRA-ABDOMINAL ABSCESSES

A. Pathogenesis

Abscesses are common sequelae of untreated peritonitis and may be found as intraperitoneal or visceral collections. In experimental models of abscess formation, mixed aerobic and anaerobic organisms have been implanted intraperitoneally in rats and mice (3,4). Unless therapy directed at anaerobes is used, animals predictably form intra-abdominal abscesses. As in clinical infections, these experimental abscesses may stud the peritoneal cavity, be found within the omentum or mesentery, or form on the surface of or within viscera, particularly the liver.

Unique virulence factors have been established for the formation of intra-abdominal abscesses. Abscesses are distinct pathologic entities that are neither wholly disease nor wholly host response but in a sense a combination of both. On one hand, an abscess is an infection in which PMNs and viable bacteria coexist within a fibrous capsule; on the other hand, the organisms in an abscess are contained, thereby preventing their systemic or metastatic spread. Research has defined some of the host cells and key virulence factors responsible for abscess formation due to the anaerobic organism, *B. fragilis* (5,6).

Among anaerobic bacteria, *B. fragilis* appears uniquely virulent. The organism is the anaerobe most commonly isolated from intra-abdominal abscess contents as well as the most common isolate in anaerobic bacteremia, though it constitutes only 0.5% of the normal colonic flora (7). In animal models of intra-abdominal sepsis, *B. fragilis* alone can produce abscesses in contrast to other *Bacteroides* species that require an accompanying facultative organism (3). The most important virulence factor in *B. fragilis* is the capsular polysaccharide complex (CPC), composed of two distinct polysaccharides, PS A and PS B, localized to the surface of the organism (6). Structural analysis of PS A and PS B in the CPC has demonstrated an unusual motif of oppositely charged sugars. Polysaccharides containing oppositely charged sugars are able to provoke a host to respond by localizing bacteria into abscesses within the peritoneal cavity (8). The CPC stimulates a population of T lymphocytes, which are critical for the induction of abscesses. These T cells are both CD4 and CD8+; mice depleted of these cells are unable to form abscesses. Other host factors important to the formation of abscesses include the alternative complement pathway and fibrinogen (9,10).

B. Immunity

The production of antibodies to CPC is not essential for protection against abscesses but does facilitate clearance of *B. fragilis* from the bloodstream (11). On the other hand, *B. fragilis* PS A has been shown to stimulate a population of T cells to inhibit abscess induction (12). Subcutaneous administration of PS A in experimental animals can prevent abscess formation after intraperitoneal challenge by either *B. fragilis* or mixed cecal flora.

C. Clinical Presentation

About three-fourths of intraabdominal abscesses are not associated with a specific organ but are found in the peritoneal or retroperitoneal spaces (13). They usually form within days to a few weeks of the development of peritonitis. Abscesses arise in a variety of locations ranging from compartments—such as the subphrenic space, pelvis, or Morrison's pouch—to omentum, psoas muscles, or deeper viscera such as the liver.

Abscesses originate from a variety of infectious processes. Besides fecal spillage from the colon, common inciting events are infections of the female genital tract and pancreatitis. *B. fragilis* is not a common constituent of normal vaginal flora. However, when abscesses arise in the female genital tract—such as a tuboovarian abscess—or extend from the female genital tract into the pelvis or peritoneal cavity, *B. fragilis*, as well as other *Bacteriodes* sp., are often isolated. Without an associated abscess, *B. fragilis* is rarely encountered in pelvic infections such as pelvic inflammatory disease or endometritis (14). In pancreatitis the inciting event for inflammation is leakage of pancreatic enzymes. Infectious complications of pancreatitis, such as pancreatic abscess or intra-abdominal collections of pus, are difficult to distinguish from pancreatitis itself on clinical grounds because fever, leukocytosis, and even abdominal pain are features of both. Some authors favor early needle aspiration of pancreatic collections under computed tomographic (CT) guidance to differentiate pseudocyst from abscess, but this procedure is associated with some hazard, and the recovery of organisms is not of clear significance (15).

Another location in which abscesses are encountered is the psoas muscle. These abscesses result from hematogenous or contiguous spread either from an intra-abdominal or pelvic process or from nearby vertebral bone. Osteomyelitis is commonly associated with psoas abscess, but not with other peritoneal or retroperitoneal collections, and may arise from the spread of infection from muscle to bone or vice versa (16). When Pott's disease was common, *Mycobacterium tuberculosis* was one of the most common causes of psoas abscess. Currently in the United States, *Staphylococcus aureus* or a mixture of enteric organisms including aerobic gram-negative bacilli are most commonly isolated from psoas abscesses (17). When hematogenous spread or a contiguous focus of osteomyelitis is observed, *S. aureus* is the organism most likely to be found. When psoas abscess has an intraabdominal or pelvic source, a mixed enteric flora is most likely to be isolated.

D. Diagnosis

The ability to diagnose intra-abdominal abscesses has improved greatly with scanning techniques, particularly CT scans. Abdominal CT scans probably have the highest yield, but ultrasonography is particularly useful for the right upper quadrant, kidneys, and pelvis. Both gallium- and indium-labeled white blood cells (WBCs) localize in abscesses and may assist in detecting a collection. Since gallium is taken up in the bowel, indium-labeled WBCs may have a slightly greater yield for finding abscesses near the bowel. Since neither of these scans can make a definitive diagnosis, however, other more specific studies, such as CT, need to be performed if an area of abnormality is identified. Abscesses contiguous with or contained within outpouchings of bowel are particularly difficult to detect with scans. Occasionally, a barium enema may detect a diverticular abscess not otherwise diagnosed. Gastrograffin should be injected instead of barium if a free perforation is suspected. In addition, if one study is negative, sometimes an alternative procedure reveals a collection. Although on rare occasions, exploratory laparotomy must still be undertaken if an abscess is strongly suspected, CT scans have largely replaced diagnostic exploratory laparotomy.

E. Treatment

The treatment of intra-abdominal infections involves targeting the inciting focus of infection, administering broad-spectrum antibiotics to cover organisms involved in the associated infection or present as normal flora in the area, and performing a drainage procedure if one or more definitive abscesses have formed. It cannot be overemphasized that, in general, antimicrobial therapy is adjunctive to drainage of the collection(s) and/or surgical correction of an underlying process. An exception to the need to surgically remedy an underlying process is usually found with rupture of a diverticulum. Diverticular rupture most often walls off with the abscess contiguous to the diverticulum instead of leaking organisms freely into the peritoneum. This infection usually responds to antibiotics alone.

A number of regimens are useful in treating intra-abdominal sepsis (18,19,20). The hallmark of treatment is coverage of both gram-negative bacilli and anaerobes. Since mortality in intra-abdominal sepsis is linked to gram-negative bacteremia and endotoxin release, empiric therapy for intra-abdominal infection, particularly early in the disease course, must include adequate gram-negative coverage. Aminoglycosides and second- and third-generation cephalosporins are the agents most widely used to cover these organisms in intra-abdominal processes. Newer antibiotics such as aztreonam, imipenem, piperacillin/tazobactam, ticarcillin/clavulanic acid, and quinolones (e.g. ciprofloxacin) provide excellent coverage of gram-negative bacilli as well, but at a higher cost. Second-generation cephalosporins, such as cefoxitin or cefotetan, do not cover aerobic gram-negative species as broadly as the other agents. Aztreonam, ciprofloxacin, aminoglycosides, and most of the third-generation cephalosporins are not active against anaerobes and therefore need to be used in combination with another antibiotic. There are conflicting studies in the literature about the anaerobic activity of ceftizoxime, a third-generation cephalosporin. Since a number of agents have substantial activity against both anaerobes and gram-negative organisms, third-generation cephalosporins should generally not be considered for treatment of anaerobic infections.

The most active and cost-effective antibiotic for anaerobic coverage currently is metronidazole. Other traditional first-line agents include cefoxitin and clindamycin. Since neither metronidazole nor clindamycin covers aerobic gram-negative bacilli, an additional agent must be used. The clinical importance of resistance among anaerobes to antimicrobial agents is uncertain. Susceptibility testing is not performed routinely in clinical laboratories, but several reference laboratories track resistance rates in different geographic sites over time. A recent report of susceptibility patterns and resistance rates among *Bacteroides* isolates in ten distinct geographic locations in the United States over a five-year period shows three drugs to have the most consistent activity: metronidazole, imipenem, and piperacillin/tazobactam (21). Resistance rates to these drugs were 0, 0.1, and 0.2% respectively, in contrast to resistance rates of 14% for clindamycin and 6% for cefoxitin among 2800 isolates tested. Of the cephamycins, cefoxitin was more active than cefotetan or cefmetazole; these latter agents had high resistance rates among *Bacteroides* species other than *B. fragilis*. The overall resistance rates for these two drugs were 27% and 20% respectively.

Despite statistics that resistance rates are climbing for some drugs, there are only scattered case reports of clinical treatment failures. One very recent case report describes a bacteremic strain of *B. fragilis* that was initially resistant to metronidazole and had reduced susceptibility to imipenem and amoxicillin/clavulanic acid (22). Following treatment of the patient with imipenem, the isolate became resistant to both imipenem and amoxicillin/clavulanic acid. Despite isolated reports such as this one, the relative absence of clinical data on treatment failures for anaerobes compared with aerobic gram-negative bacilli makes interpretation of the clinical importance of resistance rates problematic. Newer agents such as imipenem, ticarcillin/clavulanic acid, piperacillin/tazobactam, meropenem, and ampicillin/sulbactam are highly active against anaerobes. Chloramphenicol, which exhibits strong activity against *B. fragilis* in vitro, nevertheless should probably not be considered a first-line drug for anaerobes because failures of treatment have been documented in both experimental and clinical intra-abdominal infections.

F. Visceral Abscesses

1. Liver Abscesses

The liver is the intra-abdominal organ that most commonly harbors abscesses. In the best known case series, Altemeier et al. reviewed 540 cases of intra-abdominal abscess during a 12-year period (13). Visceral abscesses accounted for 26% of these abscesses. Liver abscesses accounted for 48% of the visceral abscesses and for 13% of the total number of intra-abdominal abscesses. Liver abscesses may occur as single or multiple collections. They may result from hematogenous spread of bacteria or from local spread from contiguous infections within the peritoneal cavity. In the past, appendicitis with rupture leading to peritonitis was the most common route for formation of liver abscess. However, at present biliary tract etiology is the most common. Suppurative pylephlebitis, which usually arises from infection in the female genital tract but may result from infection elsewhere in the peritoneal cavity, is another common source for bacterial seeding of the liver (2).

Clinical symptoms and signs may vary in liver abscess. Nonspecific symptoms such as chills, anorexia, weight loss, nausea, and vomiting may be reported. Fever is the most common sign at presentation. Patients, particularly those with active disease of the bilary tract, may have symptoms and signs localized to the right upper quadrant, including pain, guarding, punch tenderness, and even rebound tenderness. But the absence of right-upper-quadrant findings does not exclude a liver abscess. Only 50% of patients with liver abscesses have hepatomegaly, right-upper-quadrant tenderness, or jaundice; thus half of patients have no symptoms or signs that would direct attention to the liver (23). Particularly in the elderly with liver abscess, fever of unknown origin (FUO) may be the presenting complaint. Thus, diagnostic studies of the right upper quadrant and the abdomen should be part of any FUO workup. The single most reliable laboratory abnormality for liver abscess is an elevated serum alkaline phosphatase level found in 90% of patients (23). Other tests of liver function may be normal, but 50% of patients exhibit elevated bilirubin and 48% exhibit elevated levels of serum aspartate aminotransferase. Other laboratory findings include leukocytosis in 77% of patients, anemia (usually normochromic, normocytic) in 50%, and hypoalbuminemia in 33%. At the time of diagnosis of liver abscess, one-third of patients are bacteremic. Occasionally a chest radiograph may cause suspicion of a liver abscess, especially if a new elevation of the right hemidiaphragm is observed. A right basilar infiltrate and a unilateral pleural effusion may accompany these findings as well.

The most reliable methods for diagnosing liver abscesses include ultrasonography and CT scan. Gallium- or indium-labeled WBC scans and even magnetic resonance imaging may lead to a diagnosis as well. Occasionally, more than one imaging study may be needed. Organisms recovered from liver abscesses depend on the inciting etiology. When the biliary tree is the source, enteric gram-negative aerobic bacilli and enterococci are common isolates. Unless previous surgery on the biliary tree has been performed, anaerobes are not generally involved in liver abscesses arising from biliary infections since anaerobes are not common constituents of the gallbladder. In contrast, in liver abscesses arising from pelvic and other intraperitoneal sources, the organisms found in abscess contents are similar to those found in nonvisceral intra-abdominal abscesses: mixed flora including aerobic and anaerobic species (especially *B. fragilis*). With hematogenous spread of infection, a single organism is most commonly isolated including *S. aureus* or a streptococcal species such as *Streptococcus milleri*.

Liver abscesses caused by *Candida* species usually occur in patients receiving chemotherapy for cancer, as neutrophils return after a period of neutropenia, with or without documented fungemia (24). Treatment of candidal liver abscesses usually requires administration of amphotericin B for an extended period, although recent reports have described successful maintenance therapy with fluconazole after an initial course of amphotericin (25).

Amebic liver abscesses also are important to consider in patients who are from or have traveled to an endemic area within the past six months. The clinical course and appearance may be indistinguishable from pyogenic liver abscesses. Amebic serology is positive in more than 95% of cases; thus a negative result assists in excluding this diagnosis. Diagnostic aspiration of a suspected amebic abscess may be helpful in excluding a pyogenic process but it is uncommon to find parasites in the abscess contents (26). It is not necessary to drain an amebic abscess, as it will respond to therapy with high-dose metronidazole.

Echinococcal infection causes slowly enlarging cysts in the liver and elsewhere, especially the lungs (27). Symptoms and signs arising from the mass effect include pain, symptoms of biliary obstruction, and mass in the right upper quadrant. Rupture or leakage of a hydatid cyst causes fever, eosinophilia, pruritis, and fatal anaphylaxis. Echinococcal infection should be considered in patients who have lived for long periods of time in an endemic area; it is not an infection acquired with transient exposure. Calcification is frequently seen by radiographic studies. Ultrasound studies or CT scans demonstrate cysts, possibly with daughter cysts visualized inside. Contrast usually distinguishes cysts from abscesses. Diagnostic aspiration is not recommended because of concern about fluid leakage that may promote dissemination or anaphylactic reactions. Some centers are reporting successful CT-guided diagnostic aspirations with simultaneous ethanol instillation. Definitive treatment, however, is principally by surgical resection. Frequently, albendazole is given as adjunctive therapy.

Percutaneous and, more rarely, surgical drainage remains the mainstay of therapy for intraabdominal abscesses (including liver abscesses) (28). However, the literature documents growing interest in medical management alone for pyogenic liver abscesses (29). While success is reported, cases treated without definitive drainage generally require longer courses of antibiotics. When percutaneous drainage was compared with open surgical drainage, the average length of hospital stay for the former was almost double that for the latter, although both the time required for fever to resolve and mortality were the same for the two groups (30). Mortality was considerable, averaging 15%, despite treatment. Several factors assist in predicting failure of percutaneous drainage with a pigtail catheter left in place including the presence of multiple, sizable abscesses; viscous abscess contents that tend to plug the catheter; and associated disease (e.g. of the biliary tract) that requires surgery. Primary surgical intervention may be more suitable in these situations. Surgery also may be considered when there appears to be no clinical response to percutaneous drainage in 4–7 days.

2. *Splenic Abscesses*

Splenic abscesses are significantly less common than liver abscesses. In fact, no splenic abscesses were found in Altemeier's large series of intraabdominal abscesses (13). In several autopsy series, the incidence of splenic abscesses has ranged from 0.14% to 0.7% (31,32). There are important differences between splenic and liver abscesses. The presentation of splenic abscesses is subtle, and the diagnosis is frequently made after death, even with current technology. Even in the most recently published series, the diagnosis was missed in 37% of cases and had to be established at autopsy (33). Splenic abscess should be strongly considered in cases of endocarditis, since if untreated, the mortality rate is high. In contrast to liver abscesses, splenic abscesses usually develop from hematogenous spread. Bacterial endocarditis is the most common associated infection. Patients who have received extensive immunosuppressive therapy (particularly those who have malignancy involving the spleen) and patients with hemoglobinopathies or other hematologic disorders (especially sickle cell anemia) also have a propensity for splenic abscesses. Splenic abscesses also may arise occasionally from contiguous spread of infection from intraperitoneal sites or from direct trauma to the spleen.

Approximately 50% of patients with splenic abscesses have abdominal pain, which makes it a more common symptom than for liver abscesses (33). However, only half of patients with this symptom show the pain localized in the left upper quadrant. Splenomegaly is detected in approximately 50% of patients. Fever and leukocytosis generally are found. Fever preceded diagnosis by an average of 20 days in a recent series (33). Other findings include abnormal auscultation of the left chest, and in these cases, chest radiographs may reveal an infiltrate or an isolated left pleural effusion. The most sensitive diagnostic tool for suspected splenic abscess has been CT scan of the abdomen. While ultrasonography also can detect these abscesses, cases have been missed with this modality. Liver-spleen scan or gallium scan also may be useful.

Streptococcal species are the most common bacterial isolates from splenic abscesses; *S. aureus* is the next most common organism, which is likely a reflection of the frequency of associated endocarditis in which these bacteria are common pathogens (33). When gram-negative aerobic organisms are recovered from splenic abscesses, a urinary tract focus (with associated bacteremia) or another intraabdominal source should be considered. In recent series, gram-negative organisms have been reported more often than in older series. *Salmonella* species figure as common pathogens in these series as well, especially in patients with sickle cell hemoglobinopathy. Anaerobic species accounted for only 5% of isolates in the largest collected series (33). However, a category of "sterile abscesses" may mean that techniques for isolating anaerobes were suboptimal.

Because of the high mortality figures reported for splenic abscesses, the treatment of choice is splenectomy with adjunctive antibiotics. Percutaneous drainage also has been employed successfully. The most important determinant for successful outcome in splenic abscesses is early recognition of the process.

3. *Perinephric and Renal Abscesses*

The other major visceral intra-abdominal abscesses to consider are perinephric and renal abscesses, which—like splenic abscesses—are not common. Perinephric abscess was encountered in only 0.02% of hospital admissions and renal abscesses in only 0.2% in Altemeier's series (34,13). Perinephric and renal abscesses usually arise from a different pathogenic mechanism than either liver or splenic abscesses. Before the wide availability of antibiotics, the majority of renal and perinephric abscesses were hematogenous in origin, with *S. aureus* the most common organism. At present, however, more than 75% of perinephric and renal abscesses arise from an initial urinary tract infection (34). Pyelonephritis occurs first after organisms ascend the ureter from the bladder. Bacteria may directly invade the renal parenchyma from medulla to cortex or local vascular channels within the kidney may facilitate the transport of organisms. Intraparenchymal abscess may rupture into the perinephric space.

When abscesses extend into the perinephric space, additional tracking may occur through Gerota's fascia, which can spread into the psoas or transversalis muscles, into the anterior peritoneal cavity, to the subdiaphragmatic space, or down to the pelvis. The most important identified risk factor for the development of perinephric abscesses is concomitant nephrolithiasis, which obstructs urinary flow: 20% to 60% of patients with perinephric abscess have associated renal stones (35). Other risk factors include other structural abnormalities of the urinary tract, a history of urologic surgery, trauma, and diabetes mellitus.

The organisms most frequently encountered in perinephric and renal abscesses are *E. coli, Proteus* sp., and *Klebsiella* sp., which are the three groups of organisms that most commonly cause urinary tract infections. *E. coli*, the most common aerobic species in the colonic flora, has unique virulence properties in the urinary tract, including factors that promote adherence to uroepithelial cells. The urease of *Proteus* sp. splits urea, which creates an alkaline environment hospitable to bacterial growth. *Proteus* sp. also are found frequently in association with large struvite stones caused by the precipitation of magnesium ammonium sulfate in an alkaline environment. While a single bacterial species usually is recovered from a perinephric or renal abscess, multiple species also may be isolated. If a urine culture not contaminated with periurethral flora yields multiple organisms, especially on more than one occasion, a perinephric abscess or renal abscess should be considered in the differential diagnosis.

Candida sp. are another group of organisms that cause renal abscesses. Fungi may spread to the kidney by ascension from the bladder or hematogenously. In the former, ureteral obstruction with large fungal balls is common.

The presentation of perinephric and renal abscesses is nonspecific (34). Flank and abdominal pain are common, and at least 50% of patients are febrile. Pain may be referred to the groin or leg, particularly when infection tracks outside of the kidney into nearby muscles. The diagnosis of perinephric abscess is frequently delayed, as with splenic abscess. Mortality in some series is appreciable but decreasing in frequency and not as high as that for splenic abscesses (34). Perinephric or renal abscess should be most seriously considered when a patient presents with symptoms and signs of pyelonephritis and remains febrile after 4 or 5 days of antibiotic treatment.

Renal ultrasonography and abdominal CT scan are the most useful diagnostic modalities. If a renal abscess or perinephric abscess is diagnosed, associated nephrolithiasis should be sought. Treatment for perinephric or renal abscesses includes drainage of pus and antibiotic therapy directed at the organism(s) recovered. For perinephric abscesses, percutaneous drainage usually is successful.

REFERENCES

1. Levisohn ME, Bush LM. Peritonitis and other intra-abdominal infections. In: Mandell GL, Douglas RG, Bennett JE, eds. Principles and Practice of Infectious Diseases. 4th ed. New York: Churchill Livingstone, 1995:705–740.
2. Zaleznik DF, Kasper DL. Intra-abdominal infections and abscesses. In: Fauci AS, Braunwald E, Isselbacher KJ, Wilson JD, Martin JB, Kasper DL, Hauser SL, Longo DL, eds. Harrison's Principles of Internal Medicine. 14th ed. New York: McGraw-Hill. In press.
3. Onderdonk AB, Kasper DL, Cisneros RL, Bartlett JG. The capsular polysaccharide of Bacteroides fragilis as a virulence factor: comparison of the pathogenic potential of encapsulated and unencapsulated strains. J Infect Dis 1977; 136:82–89.
4. Shapiro ME, Onderdonk AB, Kasper DL, Finberg RW. Cellular immunity to Bacteroides fragilis capsular polysaccharide. J Exp Med 1982; 154:1188–1197.
5. Shapiro ME, Kasper DL, Zaleznik DF, Spriggs S, Onderdonk AB, Finberg RW. Cellular control of abscess formation: role of T cells in the regulation of abscesses formed in response to Bacteroides fragilis. J Immunol 1986; 137:341–346.
6. Tzianabos AO, Pantosti A, Baumann H, Brisson JR, Jennings HJ, Kasper DL. The capsular polysaccharide of Bacteroides fragilis comprises two ironically linked polysaccharides. J Biol Chem 1992; 267:18230–18235.
7. Moore WEC. Anaerobes as normal flora: gastrointestinal tract. In: Finegold SM, ed. Proceedings International Metronidazole Conference Montreal, Quebec, Canada. Princeton: Excerpta Med, 1977:222–228.
8. Tsianabos AO, Onderdonk AB, Rosner B, Cisneros RL, Kasper DL. Structural features of polysaccharides that induce intraabdominal abscesses. Science 1993; 262:416–419.
9. Joiner KA, Gelfand JA, Onderdonk AB, Bartlett JG, Gorbach SL. Host factors in the formation of abscesses. J Infect Dis 1980; 142:40–49.
10. McRitchie DI, Girotti MJ, Glynn MFX, Goldberg JM, Rotstein OD. Effect of systemic fibrinogen depletion on intraabdominal abscess formation. J Lab Clin Med 1991; 118:48–55.
11. Onderdonk AB, Markham RB, Zaleznik DF, Cisneros RL, Kasper DL. Evidence for T cell-dependent immunity to Bacteroides fragilis in an intraabdominal abscess model. J Clin Invest 1982; 69:9–16.
12. Tsianabos AO, Kasper DL, Cisneros RL, Smith RS, Onderdonk AB. Polysaccha-

ride-mediated protection against abscess formation in experimental intra-abdominal sepsis. J Clin Invest 1995; 96:2727–2731.
13. Altemeier WA, Culbertson WR, Fullen WD, Shook CD. Intra-abdominal abscesses. Am J Surg 1973; 125:70–78.
14. Gorbach SL, Bartlett JG. Medical progress: anaerobic infections. N Eng J Med 1974; 290:1177–1184, 1237–1245, 1289–1294.
15. London NJ, Neoptolemos JP, Lavelle J, Bailey I, James D. Serial computed tomography scanning in acute pancreatitis: a prospective study. Gut 1989; 30:397–403.
16. Gordin F, Stamler C, Mills J. Pyogenic psoas abscesses: noninvasive diagnostic techniques and review of the literature. Rev Infect Dis 1983; 5:1003–1011.
17. Ricci MA, Rose FB, Meyer KK. Pyogenic psoas abscess: worldwide variations in etiology. World J Surg 1986; 10:834–843.
18. Solomkin JS, Dellinger EP, Christou NV, Busuttil RW. Results of a multicenter trial comparing impenem/cilastatin to tobramycin/clindamycin for intra-abdominal infections. Ann Surg 1990; 212:581–591.
19. Barboza E, del Castillo M, Tu A, Gotuzzo E. Clindamycin plus amikacin versus clindamycin plus azetreonam in established intraabdominal infections. Surgery 1994; 116:28–35.
20. Investigators of the Piperacillin/Tazobactam intra-abdominal infection study group. Results of the North American trial of piperacillin/tazobactam compared with clindamycin and gentamicin in the treatment of severe intra-abdominal infections. Eur J Surg 1994; 573:S61–66.
21. Aldridge KE, Gelfand M, Reller LB, Ayers LW, Pierson CL, Schoenknecht F, Tilton RC, Wilkins J, Henderberg A, Schiro DD. A five-year multicenter study of the susceptibility of the Bacteroides fragilis group isolates to cephalosporins, cephamycins, penicillins, clindamycin, and metronidazole in the United States. Diagn Microbiol Infect Dis 1994; 18:235–241.
22. Turner P, Edwards R, Weston V, Gazis A, Ispahani P, Greenwood D. Simultaneous resistance to metronidazole, co-amoxiclav, and imipenem in clinical isolate of Bacteroides fragilis. Lancet 1995; 345:1275–1277.
23. Rubin RH, Swartz MN, Malt R. Hepatic abscess: changes in clinical bacteriologic and therapeutic aspects. Am J Med 1974; 57:601–610.
24. Thaler M, Pastakia B, Shawker T, O'Leary T, Pizzo P. Hepatic candidiasis in cancer patients: the evolving picture of the syndrome. Ann Intern Med 1988; 108:88–100.
25. Kauffmann CA, Bradley SF, Ross SC, Weber DR. Hepatosplenic candidiasis: successful treatement with fluconazole. Am J Med 1991; 91:137–141.
26. Reed SL. Amebiasis: an update. Clin Infect Dis 1992; 14:385–393.
27. Nutman TB, Weller PF. Cestodes. In: Fauci AS, Braunwald E, Isselbacher KJ, Wilson JD, Martin JB, Kasper DL, Hauser SL, Longo DL, eds. Harrison's Principles of Internal Medicine. 14th ed. New York: McGraw-Hill. In press.
28. Gerzof SC, Robbins Ah, Johnson WC, Birkett HD, Nabseth DC. Percutaneous catheter drainage of abdominal abscesses. New Engl J Med 1981; 305:653–657.
29. Maher JA, Reynolds TB, Yellin AE. Successful medical treatment of pyogenic liver abscess. Gastroenterol 1979; 77:618–622.

30. Bertel CK, van Heerden JA, Sheedy PF. Treatment of pyogenic hepatic abscesses: surgical vs percutaneous drainage. Ach Surg 1986; 121:554–558.
31. Chulay JD, Lankerani MN. Splenic abscess. Am J Med 1976; 61:513–522.
32. Chun CH, Raff MJ, Contreras L, Varghese R, Waterman N, Daffner R, Melo JC. Splenic abscess. Medicine 1980; 59:50–65.
33. Linos DA, Nagorney DM, McIlrath DC. Splenic abscess—the importance of early diagnosis. Mayo Clin Proc 1983; 58:261–264.
34. Hutchinson FN, Kaysen GA. Perinephric abscess: the missed diagnosis. Med Clin North Am 1988; 72:993–1013.
35. Edelstein H, McCabe RE. Perinephric abscess: modern diagnosis and treatment. Medicine 1988; 67:118–131.

14

Sexually Transmitted Anorectal Infections

LAURENCE S. BAILEN and MARK A. PEPPERCORN
Beth Israel Hospital and Harvard Medical School, Boston, Massachusetts

I. INTRODUCTION

The anorectum is the portal of entry for many sexually transmitted diseases (STD). Bacterial, viral, fungal, protozoal, and helminthic organisms all may cause infectious and neoplastic complications in the anorectum. Anal intercourse and other sexual practices involving the anorectum are well-known mechanisms for transmission of sexually transmitted diseases. Since the early 1980s, with the evolution of the Acquired Immunodeficiency Syndrome (AIDS) epidemic, sexual behavior has changed among homosexual and heterosexual populations and rates of gonorrhea and syphilis, for example, have decreased.

Unfortunately, education on the prevention of sexually transmitted disease has not reached all people. Many in the United States engage in unsafe sexual practices: adolescents and people of all ethnic backrounds. It has been estimated that 10% of sexually active Americans practice anal intercourse. This is a conservative estimate as several population-based surveys document rates of 5–30% of heterosexual men and women practice anal intercourse (1–7). Many heterosexual men and women are unaware of the need for condom use. Approximately 90% of the men and women in one study did not know that men should wear condoms during anal intercourse (7). Therefore, there remains a large body of the American population unaware of situations in which measures should be used to prevent sexually transmitted diseases.

The AIDS epidemic has brought drastic changes to sexual behavior amongst homosexual men (8,9). Because of widespread international and national education on high-risk sexual practices that enhance the transmission of the human immunodeficiency virus, rates of rectal gonorrhea and syphilis dropped in the 1980s (10,11). However, despite this early success many homosexual men lapse into unprotected sexual behaviors including anal intercourse without a condom and anilingus. Most commonly men attribute being in a steady relationship, being unprepared, and other psychosocial factors as reasons for engaging in unprotected high-risk sexual practices (12–14). Thus, it is important for the clinician to take a detailed sexual history including practices engaged in and whether or not the patient utilized adequate protection.

After a detailed sexual history and an evaluation of the patient's symptoms, the examination of the anorectal area must be performed carefully. Pain and exquisite tenderness may accompany many sexually transmitted anorectal infections. Therefore, after careful inspection and palpation of the perianal area, anoscopy and proctoscopy may need to be performed under anesthesia. By optimizing patient comfort the clinician is better able to visualize the anorectum as well as obtain adequate cultures and biopsies.

This chapter will review the epidemiology, clinical presentation, diagnosis, and treatment of bacterial, viral, and parasitic infections of the anorectum and also comment upon neoplastic, traumatic, and idiopathic disorders of this area. Special attention will be addressed to specific issues regarding AIDS and Human Immunodeficiency Virus (HIV) positive patients. Table 1 summarizes the symptoms, endoscopic findings, diagnosis and treatment of several major sexually transmitted anorectal diseases discussed in detail in the text.

II. BACTERIAL INFECTIONS

A. Gonorrhea

1. Epidemiology

Gonorrhea has been described since ancient times. The incidence of gonorrhea increased dramatically in the 1960s and 1970s in the United States then leveled off in the early 1980s and has been declining. There were 172 cases of gonorrhea per 100,000 population in 1993 (15). Much of the decline is attributed to safer sexual practices in the setting of the AIDS epidemic. Gonorrhea is still a major problem among blacks and hispanics where prevalence rates of gonorrhea are up to ten times higher than other ethnic groups. Furthermore, gonorrhea has become more prevalent in heterosexual urban poor in association with higher rates of prostitution and drug use. Within the HIV population and among homosexual men, Neisseria gonorrhea has been cultured from the rectum in up to 16% of symptomatic patients presenting to screening clinics or involved in surveillance studies (16–18).

Table 1 Major Sexually Transmitted Anorectal Diseases

Organism	Symptoms	Endoscopy/Anoscopy	Laboratory Evaluation	Treatment
Gonorrhea	Rectal discharge, pain Tenesmus, constipation	Proctitis with mucus discharge anal canal not involved	Gram stain and culture on Thayer–Martin media	Ceftriaxone 125 mg IM × 1 or ciprofloxacin 500 mg po × 1
Chlamydia	Anorectal pain, tenesmus Rectal discharge Rectal strictures	Friable, ulcerating mucosa Nodular/cobblestone	Culture Direct immunofluorescence Enzyme immunoassay	Doxycycline 100 mg po *bid* × 7 d or azithromycin 1 g po × 1 Alt: ofloxacin 300 mg po *bid* × 7 d
Syphilis	Rectal pain Painful defecation Purulent discharge	Primary: ulcer with firm cartilagenous borders Secondary: proctitis condyloma lata	Dark-field exam of fresh scrapings RPR Serology[a] FTA-ABS[b]	Penicillin G 2.4 million units IM In HIV: additional doses weekly for three weeks up to total 7.2 million units
Herpes simplex virus	Anorectal pain Pruritus ani Anal discharge Hematochezia	Vesicles, ulcer Friable, erythematous or diffusely ulcerated mucosa	Tzanck test of ulcer base Viral culture Serology	Sitz baths, lidocaine ointment Acyclovir 400 mg 5×/day
Human papillomavirus	Asymptomatic or pruritus, hematochezia	Warts found in moist areas, clusters of pedunculating lesions that bleed easily on contact	Exclude syphilis Biopsy	Podofilox topical therapy Cryotherapy with liquid nitrogen Trichloroacetic acid
CMV[c]	Rectal pain Hematochezia	Anal and perianal ulcerations	Biopsy Serology; CMV antigenemia PCR[d]	Ganciclovir Foscarnet
Entamoeba histolytica	Asymptomatic, diarrhea, or ulcerations	Friable, edematous mucosa Ulcer: flask-shaped with clean base	Three separate stool specimens for amebic cysts Serology	Metronidazole 750 mg *TID* for 5–10 days Luminal agents (see text)

[a](RPR) Rapid plasma reagin.
[b](FTA-ABS) Fluorescent treponemal antibody absorption test.
[c]Cytomeglovirus (CMV).
[d]Polymerase Chain Reaction (PCR).

2. *Microbiology*

Neisseria gonorrhea is a gram-negative nonmotile diplococcus that does not form spores and characteristically grows in pairs. It is capable of infecting a variety of mucosal surfaces such as columnar or transitional epithelium including the columnar epithelium of the rectum proximal to the anorectal line. Gonococci cause tissue damage by producing enzymatic extracellular products that damage host cells and resist host defenses by complex mechanisms of resistance and genetic transformation (19–21).

Humans are the only reservoirs for Neisseria gonorrhea. To produce rectal infection the gonococcus is transmitted by anilingus, anoreceptive intercourse, perineal contamination, and by local spread of infected cervical secretions in women (22). Therefore, rectal infection is primarily seen in women and homosexual men. After exposure, the gonococcus has an incubation period of 1–14 days with an average of 3–5 days.

3. *Clinical Presentation*

The presentation of rectal gonorrhea may be different in men and women. In women, rectal gonorrhea is predominantly asymptomatic and usually is associated with gonococcal cervicitis (23). In symptomatic men and women, symptoms include constipation, anorectal pain, tenesmus, and a mucopurulent or bloody discharge. Patients may only notice strands of mucus in the stool. This discharge results in perirectal and perianal skin irritation, which may cause secondary rectal pruritus and perirectal erythema. Less common symptoms include diarrhea, fever, and malaise (24,25).

4. *Diagnosis*

Physical exam must be performed carefully on symptomatic patients as denuded perianal and rectal mucosa is exquisitely tender (26). External exam may reveal only perianal erythema due to skin irritation from the discharge. For proctoscopy, one should lubricate the anoscope with water only as other lubricants occasionally contain antibacterial agents (26). Classically the anal canal is not involved in gonorrheal infection and endoscopic findings are nonspecific and usually limited to the distal rectum. These include mucosal friability, erythema, ulceration, and yellowish mucus discharge. Involved areas, primarily near the anorectal junction at the site of the anal crypts and columns of Morgagni, may demonstrate easily induced bleeding. Furthermore, mucus and pus may be expressed from the anal crypts by gentle external pressure. Ulcerations are rarely seen in rectal gonorrhea (27). One study reported that anorectal ulcerations and fissures may be associated with gonorrhea but ulcerations were not correlated with positive cultures (27). In addition, radiologic changes associated with anorectal gonorrhea as seen on barium enema include edematous mucosa with small ulcerations and evidence for limited distensability (28). These findings are also not specific for gonorrhea but may be seen in other forms of proctitis.

Definitive diagnosis is made by gram stain and culture of the mucosal exudate obtained by anoscopy in symptomatic individuals. Exudate obtained at anoscopy for gram stain and culture is more sensitive than if obtained via blind insertion of a sterile cotton swab. In one study, the sensitivity was 79% by anoscopy vs. 53% by blind insertion of a cotton swab (accomplished by inserting a sterile cotton swab 2–3 cm and rotating for ten seconds) (29). If the exudate is contaminated by feces, the procedure should be repeated. Gram-negative intracellular diplococci may be seen in a positive gram-stain smear. Therapy is begun at this point while awaiting results of culture on selective media (Thayer–Martin). Several serologic tests for *N. gonorrhea* are available but not used routinely for diagnosis.

Neisseria meningitidis may be cultured from rectal exudates in approximately 2% of men who have had homosexual contact (30,31). It is unclear what clinical significance *N. meningitidis* has in the anorectum. However, in one series the isolation of only the meningococcus in a symptomatic patient and a clear response to therapy suggest a pathogenic role.

5. *Pathology*

Acute inflammation is the most common finding with infiltration of neutrophils throughout the lamina propria and evidence for crypt abscesses (32). In addition, chronic inflammation with plasma cells and lymphocytes may also be seen but is more commonly associated with chlamydia, syphilis, and herpes simplex II infection. In one study analyzing the spectrum of rectal biopsy abnormalities in homosexual men, many of the biopsy specimens were normal even when *Neisseria gonorrhea* was cultured (33).

6. *Treatment*

The treatment of rectal gonorrhea should be based on several factors: the prevalence of penicillin-resistant and other antibiotic-resistant strains in a particular area, the potential for concurrent infection with other anorectal sexually transmitted diseases, and patient compliance. In the 1970s pencillinase-producing strains of *N. gonorrhea* were first identified. Prior to this discovery, penicillin (PCN) was the mainstay for therapy. Initially, the response to penicillin correlated with the minimum inhibitory concentration of penicillin for the organism. However, this resulted in use of increasing doses of PCN. Antibiotic resistance by the gonococcus is mediated by plasmid or chromosomal factors. Penicillin resistance is plasmid mediated where a new plasmid acquires genes for the production of beta-lactamase. The Gonococcal Isolate Surveillance Project has followed antimicrobial susceptibility patterns since 1986. Since that time there have been no trends towards decreased susceptibility of the gonococcus to the third-generation cephalosporins or quinolones (34).

The Centers for Disease Control recently made new recomendations for single-dose treatment of gonorrhea based on a review of the efficacy, safety, and pharmacokinetics in randomized controlled trials. Single doses of cefixime 400 mg. ciprofloxacin 500 mg, or ofloxacin 400 mg orally are recommended treatment for gonorrhea (35,36). The intramuscular dose of ceftriaxone was reduced to 125 mg based on trials showing that dose to be efficacious (35). Recently single-dose azithromycin has been shown to be efficacious in the treatment of gonorrhea (37). It is not yet clear what the best combined therapy should be for patients with coexistent gonorrheal and chlamydial anorectal infections but patients with possible concomitant chlamydial infection should be treated with doxycycline (38). Ceftriaxone is more effective for concomitant pharyngeal and rectal gonorrhea, a common finding in homosexual men. It is important to document clearance of infection by repeating cultures after treatment and to advise patients to abstain from sexual contact until the infection is cleared. Documented clearance is important especially in areas where resistance may be a problem and in patients with asymptomatic infections.

B. Chlamydia Trachomatis: LGV and Non-LGV Infection

1. Epidemiology

Two different serotypes of chlamydia trachomatis, lymphogranuloma venereum (LGV) and non-LGV, have been isolated from rectal cultures in women and both homosexual and heterosexual men. Lymphogranuloma is rare in the United States: in 1993 there were 279 cases reported to the CDC (15). Approximately 16% of symptomatic HIV patients had positive rectal cultures for chlamydia in one study (16). Similarly, up to 15% of asymptomatic homosexual men have positive rectal cultures (39). In another study 8.3% of homosexual men and 21% of heterosexual women presenting to an STD clinic had positive rectal cultures for chlamydia (40). Again, chlamydial rectal infection is often coexistent with other STDs, particularly gonorrhea.

2. Microbiology

Chlamydia trachomatis exclusively infects humans. It is an obligate intracellular bacteria with a dichotomous life cycle: an elementary body stage and a reticulate body stage. During the elementary body stage the organism maintains a cell wall enabling it to survive extra-cellularly but is metabolically inactive. In the reticulate body stage the organism loses the cell wall and is metabolically active. By endocytosis the organism enters the host cell and utilizes the by-products of the host cell for its own metabolism (41,42).

Chlamydia trachomatis has seventeen immunotypes based on outer membrane protein antigenic differences. Types L_1, L_2, L_3 are responsible for lymphogranuloma venereum. Types A–K and especially D–K are responsible for the majority of rectal infections in the United States (43). The LGV serotypes differ biologically from the other serotypes as they grow easily in culture.

3. *Clinical presentation*

The LGV serotypes produce more virulent disease in humans than the other serotypes but both are transmitted sexually by anoreceptive activity.

After an incubation period of 3–14 days, rectal infection by lymphogranuloma venereum is marked by fever, rectal pain, tenesmus, and a mucoid or bloody discharge. Initially, a small tender vesicle develops then ulcerates and subsequently disappears. Inguinal adenopathy may develop and nodes may coalesce into a large mass. In up to one-third of cases the nodes may be found above and below the inguinal ligament on physical exam producing a pathognomonic "groove sign." The nodes are usually exquisitely tender and may become so large that they obstruct lymphatic drainage and cause lymphedema of the external genitalia. Furthermore, perirectal fistulas, perirectal abscesses, or cryptitis may develop (44,45).

The less virulent and less invasive immunotypes of *Chlamydia trachomatis* (non-LGV) cause a mild proctitis that is manifested by anorectal pain, tenesmus, and rectal discharge (46,47). Many individuals may be asymptomatic as they harbor subclinical infection. In persistent disease, rectal strictures may cause constipation, straining at defecation, and narrow stools.

4. *Diagnosis*

Endoscopic findings in LGV and chlamydial proctitis are varied and may be confused with those seen in inflammatory bowel disease, especially Crohn's disease. The rectal mucosa may appear nodular or cobblestoned with severe mucosal erythema, friability, and ulceration (39,48). The rectal mucosa may also appear normal or rarely it may present as a tumor-like mass (49). In chronic LGV infection the rectal mucosa may show granularity with rectal strictures.

The histopathological findings include crypt abscesses, granulomata, and giant cells, findings similar to those seen in Crohn's disease. In non-LGV strains, neutrophils and chronic inflammatory cells are seen within the lamina propria (33).

The radiological features of LGV by barium enema include loss of haustration and poor distensibility, findings also seen in patients with ulcerative colitis. Barium enema may also assess the presence and severity of rectal strictures. Multiple strictures with intervening normal segments of bowel have been described in LGV proctocolitis (50).

Definitive diagnosis of rectal chlamydial infection is made by immunofluorescence, culture, and serology. Rectal biopsies should be transported in sucrose phosphate media on ice and placed in tissue culture. However, *C. trachomatis* does not grow well in vitro and the multiple steps required to obtain, transport, and maintain chlamydial specimens makes this form of diagnosis not practical. Furthermore, there is a 6–7 day delay in the reporting of final culture results. A complement fixation titer is another method of detecting chlamydial infection. Titers of greater than 1:16 to LGV strains are considered positive for LGV infection. Much higher titers are often observed in non-LGV chlamydia.

The most rapid diagnostic tests for establishing the presence of chlamydia are direct immunofluorescence-staining techniques (51,52). These tests also obviate the difficulties inherent in traditional cell-culture techniques of rectal specimens. These tests detect *C. trachomatis* elementary bodies by direct immunofluorescent staining of rectal secretions by monoclonal antibodies conjugated to fluorescein isothiocyanate (53). A rectal swab is rolled over a slide and the slide is fixed, refrigerated, and transported to the laboratory. The slides are then incubated with the fluorescein-conjugated monoclonal antibody to *C. trachomatis* and then examined for typical *C. trachomatis* elementary bodies. This test is extremely dependent on the skill of the microscopist (53). In one study, the test was approximately 90% sensitive and nearly 100% specific for *C. trachomatis*. In general, the sensitivity ranges from 70–90% and the specificity from 96–99% (54). The CDC recommends use of this test only in experienced laboratories (35).

The enzyme immunoassay test (EIA) is also used to test for *C. trachomatis*. This test employs polyclonal or monoclonal antibodies to the lipopolysaccharide membrane of the chlamydial elementary bodies. However, the CDC currently does not recommend the use of this test for rectal specimens. Other tests still under investigation include nucleic acid hybridization probes and polymerase chain reaction (PCR).

5. *Treatment*

Formerly, doxycycline 100 mg orally two times daily for seven days was the treatment of choice. Recently, single one-gram oral-dose azithromycin has been shown to have similar efficacy as the seven-day course of doxycycline (35). Azithromycin is currently recommended as acceptible therapy. The disadvantage of azithromycin is its high cost versus the convenience of the single-dose regimen. Ofloxacin (300 mg orally two times daily for seven days) is also effective (35).

C. Syphilis

1. *Epidemiology*

In the early 20th century syphilis was a major public health problem. By the mid 1950s the incidence of the disease declined due to the combination of public health measures and the development of penicillin as an effective means of therapy. Syphilis has become more common in the past ten years particularly in association with HIV. The incidence of syphilis has varied in recent years. After rising since 1985, the incidence peaked in 1990 at 20 cases of both primary and secondary syphilis per 100,000 population. In 1993 that value dropped to 10 per 100,000 (16).

The epidemiology of syphilis has been affected by AIDS. From the mid 1970s until the mid 1980s syphilis was extremely common in the male homosexual population. However, the AIDS epidemic has altered sexual behavior among homosexual men. Greater adherence to safe sexual practices has resulted in a decline in the incidence of syphilis in this population. From 1985–1990 there was also a marked rise in the incidence of syphilis among the heterosexual population (55). This increase was especially prominent in the inner city minority population reflecting poor communication of preventive measures. As a result, physicians must consider syphilis in the differential diagnosis of anorectal ulcers and proctitis in both homosexual and heterosexual men and women.

2. *Microbiology*

Syphilis is caused by the spirochete *Treponema pallidum*. The thin, elongated bacterium is not easily visualized under direct light microscopy but is easily seen by dark-field microscopy (56).

3. *Clinical Presentation*

As with other sexually transmitted anorectal infections, the transmission of syphilis is facilitated by minor trauma of the anorectal mucosa during anoreceptive intercourse. Health care workers may be inoculated if gloves are not worn while touching oral or anal lesions or by handling specimens and soiled equipment. Transmission is most effective if the infected partner is in the early stages of syphilis as opposed to the latent phase. Symptoms and signs of infection occur after an incubation period ranging from as short as 10 days up to 90 days after exposure, with an average of three weeks.

Primary syphilis is manifested by a chancre that classically begins as a painless papule that quickly erodes to form an ulcer with a smooth base and firm, cartilagenous-like raised edges (see Figure 1). However, chancres may have variable presentations: macules, ulcers, excoriations, and fissures have been described (57). Furthermore, the lesion may be painful if located at the anal margin or canal. Multiple chancres can be confused with hemorhoids, fissures, fistulas, abscesses, polyps, or lobulated rectal masses (58). Patients may complain of painful defecation, hematochezia, or purulent discharge (59). Tender inguinal adenopathy is a common feature of anorectal syphilis. Rectal syphilis may also mimic lymphoma given that both may have inguinal adenopathy and rectal abnormalities (60,61).

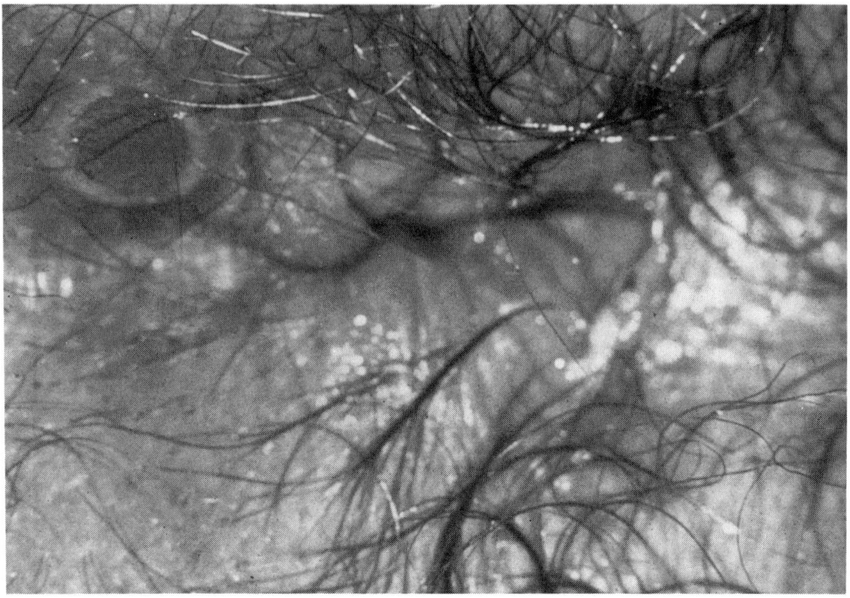

Figure 1 Perianal syphilitic chancre.

Secondary syphilis associated with systemic signs and symptoms may occur two to six months after the primary lesion. Fever, malaise, rash, and generalized lymphadenopathy may develop. In addition, proctitis with rectal discharge and anal burning and pain has also been described. Condyloma lata may also occur in patients with secondary syphilis. These are moist, smooth, perianal lesions with a grayish, raised, verrucous appearance (see Figure 2) (62–64). They usually secrete mucus resulting in a foul discharge and pruritus ani. Condyloma lata are extemely infectious as the lesions and discharge have a large burden of spirochetes.

The presentation, clinical course, and response to therapy for syphilis in HIV-infected patients may be different than the non-HIV-infected population (56,65–69). The interaction of HIV infection on the natural history of syphilis and response to treatment is still unclear. The concern over this issue is based on the observation in some HIV patients who developed neurosyphilis after apparently appropriate initial treatment of syphilis. Several small studies have suggested that patients coinfected with HIV and syphilis have an accelerated, more aggressive course of syphilis (70–73). Patients attending a Baltimore STD clinic with syphilis and concurrent HIV infection and homosexual men with HIV infection attending a Mexico City clinic presented with secondary syphilis and

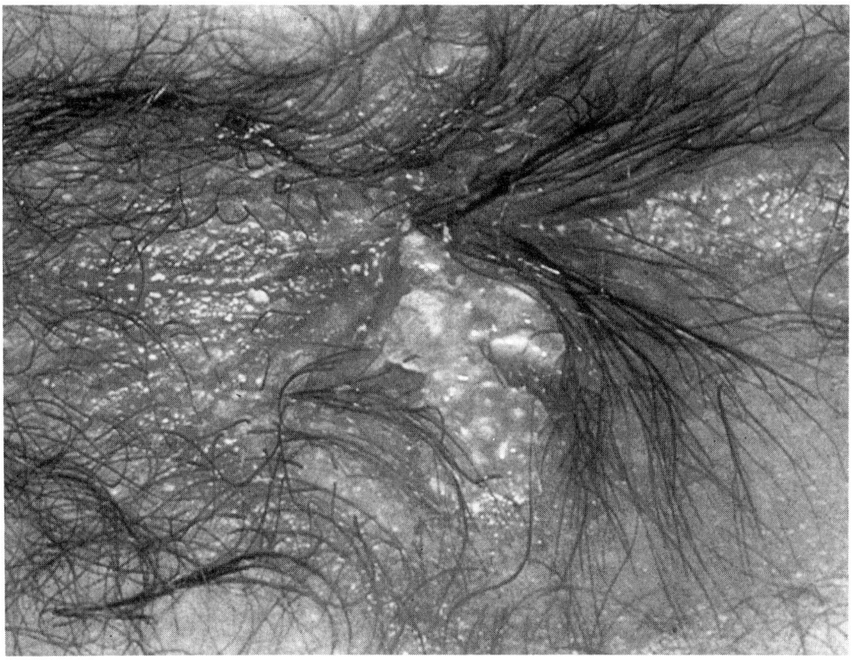

Figure 2 Condyloma lata lesion of perianal syphilis.

persistent chancres (65,67) more often than expected. However, another small study of intravenous drug users with syphilis revealed that the stage at presentation, clinical course, and serologic manifestations of syphilis were not different between HIV positive and negative patients (74).

4. *Diagnosis*

On physical exam, primary chancres may be seen in the perianal area or felt on digital rectal exam. In addition, condyloma lata of secondary syphilis may be appreciated in moist areas such as the anus. On proctoscopy, anal or rectal ulceration may be observed in addition to diffuse involvement of the rectum up to 20 cm with a nonspecific proctitis. Condyloma acuminatum or anorectal warts caused by Human Papillomavirus (HPV), are differentiated from condyloma latum by their more dessicated and keratinized appearance (75).

The histopathology of condyloma lata shows infiltrates of mononuclear cells, predominantly plasma cells and lymphocytes, within the submucosa and lamina propria. On radiologic evaluation nonspecific findings of mucosal nodularity, a narrow rectal lumen, and widening of the presacral space all have been described in association with syphilitic proctitis (76).

Dark-field microscopy is the most direct method to detect the presence of *T. pallidum*. The serous transudate from a moist chancre or condyloma latum when examined under dark-field microscopy reveals *T. pallidum* with a typical corkscrew appearance and spiral motion.

Fluorescent microscopy with monoclonal or polyclonal antibodies to *T. pallidum* is a useful alternative to dark-field exam. Currently, fluorescent microscopy is not widely used despite its superior specificity and ease of interpretation compared to dark-field exam, which may be marred by false negative results due to concurrent antibiotic or local antiseptic use (77). In addition, *T. pallidum* may be demonstrated in tissues and exudates by silver-impregnated staining but this method has a high false positive rate (77).

The most widely used tests to diagnose anorectal syphilitic infection are serologic studies of which there are two types: nontreponemal and treponemal tests. The nontreponemal tests, Venereal Disease Research Laboratory (VDRL) and rapid-plasma-reagin (RPR), utilize a cardiolipin antigen to detect antibodies to *T. pallidum*. These tests are useful in screening large numbers of patients or in following the course of the disease and response to therapy (78,79). For example, these tests have been used to screen HIV populations (80). The titers become positive approximately 1–3 weeks after the development of a primary chancre and will rise to a peak level, in untreated syphilis, during secondary syphilis or early latent disease. If therapy is started shortly after onset of symptoms, the RPR and VDRL will become negative after 1–2 years. A persistently positive VDRL may indicate inadequate treatment or reinfection especially if the titer is greater than 1:4. The major drawback of nontreponemal serologic studies is the high incidence of false positive tests that occur in patients with pneumococcal pneumonia, bacterial endocarditis, tuberculosis, viral hepatitis, rickettsial disease, and noninfectious conditions such as pregnancy, chronic liver disease, and multiple myeloma.

Reactive nontreponemal serologic tests must be confirmed by more sensitive treponemal studies. The most widely used antitreponemal test is the fluorescent treponemal antibody absorption test (FTA-ABS). Other antitreponemal tests include the microhemagglutination assay for *T. pallidum* (MHA-TP) and the hemagglutination treponemal test. The FTA-ABS is an indirect immunofluorescence test utilizing a commercially available antigen that is added to the patient's serum to attract antibodies to treponemes. Antibodies bound to treponemes are then labeled and visualized under fluorescent microscopy. This test is expensive and not used as a screening measure (56). However, the FTA-ABS is first to become positive in primary syphilis and may be useful in patients with suspected syphilis in whom the nontreponemal tests may not yet be reactive. The FTA-ABS will remain positive indefinitely, although in some patients treated very early, titers may fall after 2–3 years (35). False-positive FTA-ABS tests may occur in other infectious diseases, such as Lyme disease, infectious mononucleosis, and malaria, and in noninfectious diseases such as systemic lupus erythematosus. Sequential use of the RPR or VDRL and the FTA-ABS enhances the diagnostic certainty of syphilis when both are reactive.

Patients positive for HIV may have confusing results on serologic testing for syphilis. Titers may be unusually high or low early in the disease and false-negative tests may occur (81). However, nontreponemal tests combined with the treponemal studies are usually accurate in diagnosing syphilis in HIV patients, but more vigorous follow-up testing is necessary.

5. *Treatment*

Intramuscular penicillin G is the preferred treatment for all stages of syphilis. There have been no randomized controlled studies comparing penicillin to other drug therapies given the strong historical evidence by case series, open clinical trials, and experience attesting to penicillin's value. For primary and secondary syphilis benzathine penicillin G (2.4 million units IM in a single dose) is recommended. Alternative treatments are doxycycline (100 mg twice daily orally for two weeks) or tetracycline (500 mg orally four times daily for two weeks) (35). Patients should be reevaluated clinically and serologically at 3 and 6 month intervals to assess response to therapy. Furthermore, patients who present with syphilis without known HIV infection should be tested for HIV as syphilis may enhance the transmission and acquisition of HIV (82).

In patients with HIV infection, additional doses of benzathine penicillin G to a total of 7.2 million units (administered as 2.4 million units weekly for three doses) is suggested based on preliminary results of an ongoing study (83). It had previously been observed that treatment failures with resultant neurosyphilis or ocular syphilis occured in HIV patients who apparently received appropriate initial therapy. Even with additional penicillin treatment, the CDC still recommends cerebrospinal fluid (CSF) be analyzed in HIV patients to rule out neurosyphilis. Patients positive for HIV and allergic to penicillin should undergo a penicillin desensitization rather than treatment with alternative antibiotics. These patients should also be followed clinically and serologically more frequently (1, 2, 3, 6, 9, and 12 months) after therapy. Longitudinal studies have reported variable serologic responses in HIV patients following treatment (84, 85).

D. Other Sexually Transmitted Bacterial Anorectal Pathogens

1. *Chancroid*

The genital ulcerative disease caused by the gram-negative bacillus *Hemophilus ducreyi* is primarily found in Africa and developing countries. However, the disease has been documented on the east coast of the United States in immigrants from the Caribbean and on the west coast in immigrants from Mexico and Southeast Asia. In 1993 approximately 1400 cases of chancroid were reported (16). Chancroid is transmitted sexually and local outbreaks among prostitutes have been reported. A high rate of chancroid has also been observed in patients with HIV.

After an incubation period of 4–7 days, the genital ulcer usually begins as a tender papule with surrounding erythema. Soon thereafter it becomes pustular and ulcerates and becomes quite painful. The typical chancroid ulcer has irregular borders without erythema or induration and with a yellowish mucupurulent exudate overlying a necrotic base. Occasionally, single ulcers may coalesce to form giant ulcers (>2 cm) and rectovaginal fistulas have been reported as a complication of chancroid. Painful inguinal adenopathy is reported in up to 50% of the cases (86).

Diagnosis of chancroid is made by culturing *H. ducreyi* from exudates from the ulcer base using vancomycin-enriched chocolate agar media. Sensitivity of this method is only 80%. Serologic tests include enzyme immunoassays and direct immunofluorescence using a monoclonal antibody directed against *H. ducreyi* (87).

Currently recommended treatments for chancroid include two single-dose regimens: azithromycin 1 gram orally in a single dose, ceftriaxone 250 mg IM in a single dose, or erythromycin 500 mg orally four times daily for 7 days. Alternative regimens include amoxicillin 500 mg plus clavulanate 125 mg orally three times daily for 7 days or ciprofloxacin 500 mg orally two times daily for 3 days (35).

2. *Granuloma Inguinale*

Granuloma inguinale is a chronic granulomatous disease found primarily in tropical or subtropical areas and rarely in the United States. There were 19 cases reported in the United States in 1993 (16). The infection is caused by the gram-negative rod *Calymmatobacterium granulomatis*. Donovanosis is transmitted sexually although it is thought that the vagina may be autoinoculated from the rectum. The genitalia are the primary sites of involvement however the anal region is involved in up to 10% of the cases. After a potentially long incubation period of 8–80 days a beefy red papule develops that enlarges to a nodule then breaks down to form a irregularly shaped ulcer. The area may bleed and secondary infections have been reported. The lesion spreads along warm, moist skin folds to the anal region. Inguinal lymphatics may be involved forming a subcutaneous granuloma (88).

Diagnosis is made by demonstrating Donovan bodies in smears of lesions stained with the Wright or Giemsa stain. Donovan bodies are clusters of blue- or black-staining organisms shaped like safety pins found in the cytoplasm of large mononuclear cells. Antibiotic treatment includes one of the following regimens: tetracycline 500 mg orally four times daily for 14 days, doxycycline 100 mg orally twice daily for 14 days, erythromycin 500 mg orally four times daily for 14 days, or trimethoprim-sulfamethoxazole one double-strength tablet orally two times daily for 14 days (89).

3. *Campylobacter, Shigella, and Salmonella*

The inflammation in *campylobacter, shigella*, and *salmonella* induced enteritis and colitis may extend to the rectum. These organisms are transmitted primarily by the fecal-oral route. However, they have been implicated in sexual transmission by direct or indirect oral-anal contact (90).

Shigellosis is caused by the enteric gram-negative rod *Shigella sonnei* or *Shigella flexneri*. *S. flexneri* has been the species primarily observed among homosexuals in whom the disease may be transmitted sexually.

Shigella commonly infects the distal portion of the bowel including the rectum in orally acquired disease. Oral infection may be accomplished sexually by practicing fellatio after anal intercourse or alternatively shigella may be transmitted by direct inoculation into the rectal mucosa during anal intercourse. Clinically, patients present with the abrupt onset of fever, nausea, and diarrhea, which may be watery or bloody. There is crampy abdominal pain and occasionally mucus or pus in the diarrhea. Endoscopy usually reveals nonspecific mucosal inflammation with friability. Biopsy reveals an extensive acute inflammatory reaction involving the submucosa and muscularis. The diagnosis is made by culturing *shigella* from a stool specimen. Treatment is primarily supportive to prevent dehydration. Antibiotic therapy with ciprofloxacin (500 mg orally twice daily for seven days), trimethoprim-sulfamethoxazole (one double-strength tablet orally twice daily for seven days), or ampicillin (500 mg orally four times daily for five days) is beneficial as a public health concern in these patients when sexual transmission is suspected.

Although salmonellosis is not typically transmitted sexually, typhoid fever has been reported in sexual partners of asymptomatic carriers who shared no food or housing (91). Salmonella bacteremia has also been reported in AIDS patients (17).

Diagnosis of salmonellosis is made by stool culture and treatment is generally supportive. However, given the high rate of bacteremia in the AIDS patient population antibiotic treatment is warranted. Amoxicillin (1 gm orally three times daily or 3–14 days), trimethoprim-sulfamethoxazole (one double-strength tablet orally twice daily for 14 days), or ciprofloxacin (500 mg orally twice daily for 7 days) may be used.

Campylobacter jejuni and other *campylobacter*-like organisms(CLO) may cause proctitis (92) but usually these pathogens are associated with intestinal mucosal inflammation above 15 cm. Of the symptomatic men presenting to a STD clinic in Seattle, *C. jejuni* was isolated from 7% and CLOs from 18%

(90). Diagnosis is confirmed by observing fecal leukocytes and by culturing the organism on selective media. Treatment with erythomycin (500 mg orally four times daily for 7 days) or ciprofloxacin (500 mg orally twice daily for seven days) is recommended for severe *C. jejuni* infections.

4. *Mycoplasma*

Rarely, mycoplasma hominis is found in the anorectum of women (93). It may be associated with proctitis in women (94) but has not been a predominant pathogen in HIV and non-HIV associated anorectal disease.

5. *Streptococcus*

Group B streptococci has been cultured from the rectal area of women (95). There have been no desciptions of clinical proctitis due to the streptococcus. Perianal cellulitis due to Group A beta-hemolytic streptococci has been described in children (96,97).

III. VIRAL INFECTIONS

A. Herpes Simplex Virus (HSV)

1. *Epidemiology*

Herpes simplex virus infections are common in both normal and immunocompromised hosts in whom it can cause anal and perianal ulcers or diffuse proctitis. The CDC estimates that 250,000 cases of anogenital HSV infection occur yearly. In patients presenting to STD clinics with anorectal symptoms, HSV accounts for 20–50% of the cases (15,90). However, herpes proctitis is difficult to diagnose and is probably underdiagnosed. In some studies, up to one-third of HSV-infected patients have coinfections with other pathogenic organisms (98). Of the two HSV serotypes, HSV-1 and HSV-2, HSV-2 is more commonly associated with anorectal disease. The etiology of approximately 10% of anal infections is HSV-1, which is likely a result of oral-anal contact with an individual with HSV-1 around the mouth and lips. Many patients with HSV-2 may be asymptomatic. A recent seroepidemiologic study of 4000 men and women over age 30 revealed that 20% of white men, 25% of white women, 40% of black men, and 60% of black women had positive tests to HSV-2 antibody. These high rates suggest a subclinical course in most patients.

2. *Microbiology*

Herpes simplex virus is a DNA-enveloped virus that replicates in the skin or mucous membrane at the initial site of infection. The typical vesicle contains serous fluid with abundant HSV viral particles. Once the vesicle ruptures, the virus is liberated and able to infect others during sexual contact. The virus has a characteristic latent phase that is not completely understood. After initial contact, the virus will migrate along peripheral sensory nerves and enter sensory or autonomic nerve-root ganglia, and HSV-2 remains latent in lumbar and sacral ganglia. Reactivation from the latent phase may occur following trauma, stress, fever, or immunologic deficiency.

3. *Clinical Presentation*

Many HSV-infected patients are asymptomatic but still shed the virus (99,100). After an incubation period of 2–10 days symptoms of anorectal burning and pruritus ani may precede the development of erythema and clusters of small vesicles at the affected area. Other symptoms include tenesmus, anal discharge, constipation, hematochezia, malaise, and fever. A unique syndrome in patients with HSV proctitis is manifested by neurologic deficits attributable to the affected sacral ganglion. Symptoms of this sacral radiculomyelopathy include urinary retention and difficulty initiating stream, lower abdominal pain, posterior thigh pain, paresthesias of the buttock or perineal region, or impotence (99–103). This constellation of symptoms may be seen in over one-half of patients presenting with HSV proctitis, usually follows rectal symptoms by 2–14 days, and may persist after resolution of the proctitis (100).

On physical exam, single, or more commonly, clusters of vesicles are seen on the perianal skin, the anal canal, or both. The lesions usually ulcerate and become confluent forming a large, irregular ulcer circumscribed by an edematous and erythematous border (see Figure 3). Occasionally, lesions that extend along the gluteal crease to involve the sacrum may be confused with decubitus ulcers. Sigmoidoscopy, which may require local or general anesthesia, may reveal focal or diffuse friability, erythema, mucosal congestion, or diffuse ulceration of the rectal mucosa (100,104,105). Biopsy of herpetic rectal mucosa shows crypt abscesses, neutrophils in the lamina propria, multinucleated cells, or intranuclear inclusions (100,106).

4. *Diagnosis*

The diagnosis of HSV infection is considered with the above symptoms and physical exam, especially with neurologic findings consistent with a sacral radiculopathy. Radiographic findings on barium enema include aphthous ulcers, plaquelike erosions, and deep collar-button ulcerations (107). A Tzanck test, an inexpensive and rapid test of the ulcer base or involved rectal mucosa, will reveal multinucleated giant cells or intranuclear inclusion bodies typical of herpes. The test is performed by scraping the ulcer base with a wooden spatula or scalpel blade and spreading the specimen on a slide, which is then fixed and stained like a PAP smear. Viral isolation in culture is the most sensitive and specific method of diagnosis. Herpes simplex virus usually appears rapidly, within 1–4 days, in tissue culture.

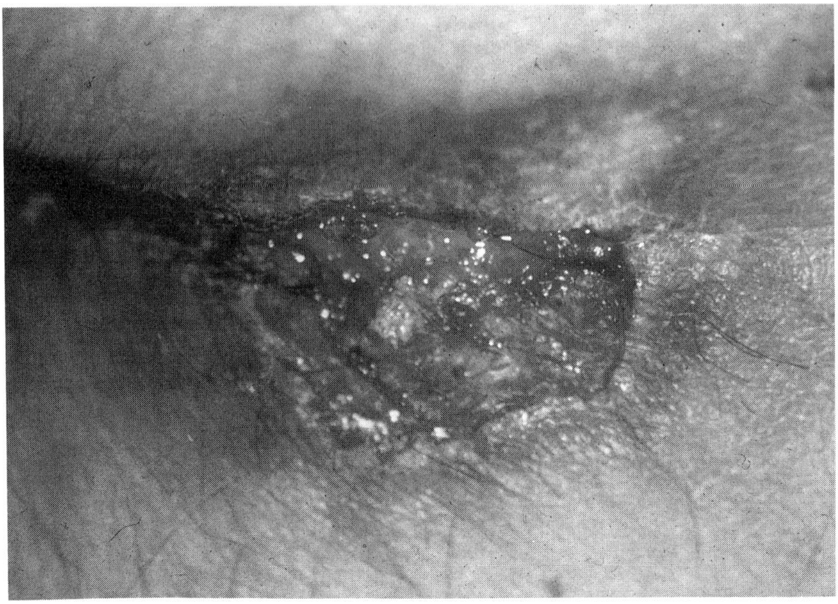

Figure 3 Perianal ulceration of herpes simplex.

Serologic tests for HSV antibodies using immunofluourescence, complement fixation, radioimmunoassays, enzyme-linked immunosorbent assays (ELISA), and others have limited utility. However, new type-specific methods using Western blot assays may become useful in diagnosing subclinical HSV-2 infections that remain underdiagnosed (108,109). Serologic assays are useful in diagnosing past HSV infection but acute and convalescent sera are necessary to retrospectively determine the first-episode infection. These assays are not useful in determining or predicting disease recurrence or transmission. In addition, many of these tests report a quantitative titer. However, this titer is generally not useful in assessing which patients are protected from recrudescent disease and which are not protected as higher titers are associated with more frequent recurrences (110,111).

5. *Treatment*

The clinical course of the disease is usually self-limited in a normal host with resolution after 2–3 weeks. Immunocompromised patients may have a more severe or protracted course. Treatment includes symptomatic management with sitz baths, lidocaine ointment to facilitate painless passage of stool, and analgesics. Some physicians have recommended concurrent antibiotic therapy to treat potential bacterial superinfection although the incidence of coinfection has not been determined (112). Acyclovir is the cornerstone in the pharmacotherapy of anorectal herpes. The recommended dosage for herpes proctitis is 400 mg orally 5 times daily for at least 10 days or until clinical resolution (35,113). Recurrent episodes may be treated with either 200 mg orally 5 times daily for 5 days, 400 mg orally 3 times daily for 5 days, or 800 mg orally two times daily for 5 days. In patients with six recurrences or more in a year, chronic daily suppressive therapy will reduce recurrences by 75%. Daily acyclovir therapy does not eliminate asymptomatic viral shedding and may lead to the development of acyclovir-resistant strains. The acyclovir dose for suppressive HSV therapy is 400 mg orally two times daily.

In patients coinfected with HSV and HIV the initial treatment is the same. However, in more severe disease, initial intravenous therapy (at a dose of 5–10 mg/kg every 8 hours) has been shown to be effective and is recommended by the CDC (35,114). Acyclovir-resistant strains may cause severe, intractable disease in HIV patients. These strains have been treated successfully with high-dose continuous infusion acyclovir for six weeks (115) or with foscarnet (116, 117).

B. Human Papillomavirus, Condyloma Acuminatum, and Anal Warts

1. Epidemiology

Human papillomavirus (HPV) infection produces a spectrum of disease manifestations: condyloma acuminata (anogenital warts), subtle verrucous changes, subclinical infection, or anal dysplasia and cancer. In the United Kingdom where anogenital warts are a reportable disease, a 1986 surveillance study (118) reported the incidence of anogenital warts at nearly 70,000 cases. The infection was more prominent in men than women, possibly due to HIV. Although in the United States anogenital warts (condyloma acuminatum) are not reportable, the incidence in sexually transmitted disease, gastroenterology, and primary care clinics has risen dramatically in the past 10 years.

Anal warts more commonly develop in homosexual men and in those practicing anoreceptive intercourse. However, anal warts are observed in heterosexual men and women with no history of anal coitus (119). Occasionally, condyloma acuminatum from the vulva and perineal area will extend to the perianal and anal area. Many patients are unaware of anal or perianal warts as they are largely asymptomatic (120).

Anal HPV infection is more common in patients with HIV because of sexual behavior patterns as well as the increased frequency of immunosuppression (121). Anal warts are more common than penile warts in HIV positive and negative homosexual men (122). Furthermore, anal cancer has become more common in the HIV population due to the rise in HPV infection. A recent study that presented data linking cancer registries with AIDS databases, reported that anal cancer was nearly forty times more common in patients recently diagnosed with AIDS than in the general population (123).

2. *Microbiology*

Human papillomavirus is a DNA virus that is difficult to grow in culture and serotypes have not been identified. The HPVs are categorized based on their differential genomic material analyzed by molecular hybridization techniques. There are currently more than 70 different genotypes of HPV. Different HPV genotypes have tropism for particular anatomical areas and certain genotypes are more commonly associated with malignant transformation than others. The HPV types 6, 11, 16, 18, 40–45, and 51 are associated with anogenital condyloma acuminata. Types 6 and 11 are most commonly associated with benign condyloma acuminata whereas types 16 and 18 are more commonly associated with malignant change. Types 31, 33, and 35 represent an intermediate risk for progression to malignancy (124–129).

To completely replicate, HPV requires the differentiation of keratinocytes in squamous epithelium. Infectious virions of HPV are only found in more superficial epithelium despite the presence of HPV DNA within more basal cells (130). Local trauma during sexual activity may be a prerequisite to HPV replication as the virus seems to require access to basal cells of the epithelium.

3. *Clinical Presentation*

After an incubation period of, on average, four months (range of 1–20 months), anal HPV infection may present with a variety of clinical pictures. Patients may be entirely asymptomatic and anal warts may be discovered incidently on physical examination or in the setting of genital HPV. On the other hand, patients may complain of pruritus or bleeding due to minor trauma on defecation. Rarely, condyloma acuminata may coalesce and cause very large lesions that cause fecal obstruction and possibly colonization with bacteria resulting in a foul discharge.

The physical appearance of condyloma acuminata may take several forms. The classic condyloma acuminata is found predominantly in moist areas. The warts are red, pink, or gray in color, and may be singular, but more commonly are present in clusters of pedunculating lesions with villous projections resembling a cauliflower (see Figure 4). Rounded papular warts predominate on the drier skin of the perianal area and are usually lighter in color due to being more keratinized. The warts bleed easily on contact. Many patients with external warts may have internal warts; therefore, anoscopy is important in identifying other potential lesions.

The identification of subclinical HPV infection may be a crucial factor in the development of anal cancer. Subclinical infection may be identified by examining the anal and perianal epithelium after soaking with acetic acid and view-

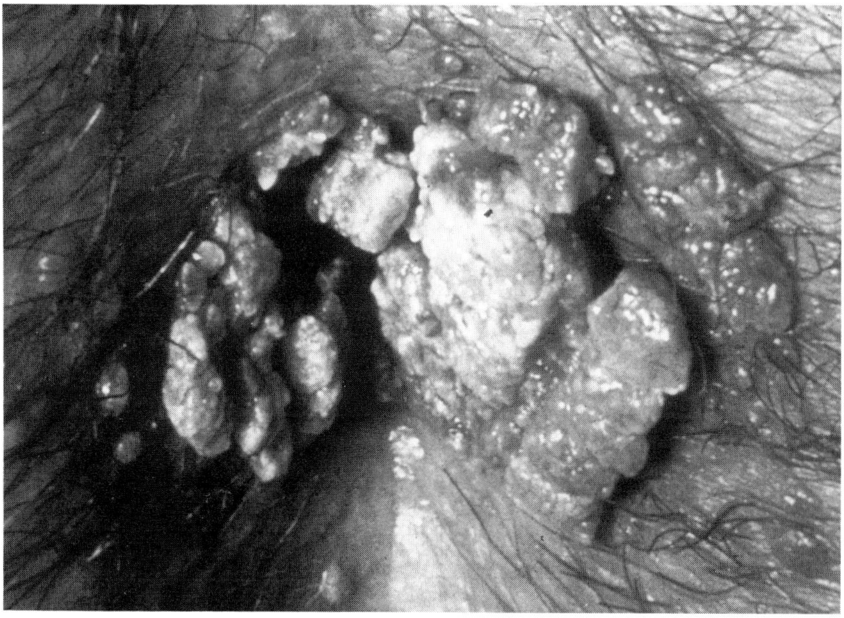

Figure 4 Condyloma acuminata.

ing under magnification. Areas of HPV subclinical infection will appear as white epithelium (131).

4. Diagnosis

Anal warts need to first be differentiated from other lesions such as condyloma lata of secondary syphilis. Condyloma lata are more rounded and dark-field exam and serologic studies should be positive. Biopsies are required to differentiate benign condyloma acuminata from malignant or premalignant lesions. Infection with HPV results in elongation of dermal papillae, acanthosis, and a sharply demarcated border with the dermis. A cytopathic effect of HPV appears as large squamous cells with enlarged and often multiple nuclei (132,133).

The laboratory diagnosis of HPV is limited by the inability to culture the virus and the lack of a validated serologic test. The only way to detect and type HPV infection is by DNA hybridization. As noted earlier, certain HPV types are associated with malignant change. However, how the practitioner uses this information clinically is not clearly defined. The definitive knowledge that a patient has HPV infection is helpful in being certain of the appropriate therapy. However, do patients with HPV 16 or 18 require intensive screening for anal cancer? Do all patients with anal warts require screening for cancer? The answers to these questions are still not clear. Further studies assessing the accuracy and utility of anal cytology and any subsequent therapy for precancerous lesions need to be performed. Some authors currently recommend routine screening of HIV-positive patients practicing anal intercourse, with or without a history of anal warts, for squamous cell anal cancer (131,134).

5. *Treatment*

The treatment of HPV infection is aimed at easing symptoms rather than eradicating HPV. The treatment of HPV infection can be frustrating as recurrences are common, necessitating multiple rounds of therapy. Recurrences may be due to the observation that HPV DNA may be present in normal tissue adjacent to obviously infected areas (135). The reasons to treat are many: cosmetic, to reduce viral shedding, to ameliorate symptoms of bleeding, and to possibly reduce the risk of malignant transformation. There is currently no specific antimicrobial agent to eliminate HPV infection; therefore, therapy utilizes nonspecific superficial modalities.

Podofilox (podophyllotoxin) 0.5% solution is a patient-administered treatment. Podophyllotoxin is one of the active compounds of podophyllin, which causes necrosis of visible wart tissue by its antimetabolic action. Podofilox is a pure compound and does not need to be washed off after use as podophyllin does. The precise mechanism of action is unknown. Use of this medication is limited to warts that are clearly seen by the patient.

Podophyllin therapy is administered by the physician and is relatively inexpensive and safe. It may not be as efficacious as podofilox. As with podofilox, side effects include mild pain and local irritation. The use of these medications is contraindicated in pregnancy. In randomized trials, podofilox was effective in clearing warts in 45–88% of patients with a recurrence rate of 33–60%. Podophyllin was 32–79% effective with 27–65% of patients experiencing recurrences (136,137,138).

For anal warts, cryotherapy with liquid nitrogen is the preferred method of treatment. Cryotherapy does not require anesthesia and usually does not result in postprocedure scarring. Patients experience mild to moderate pain during and after the procedure. Cryotherapy is 63–88% effective with recurrences in 21–39% necessitating further therapy (139).

Other options for therapy of anal warts include surgical removal or application of trichloroacetic acid (TCA) 80–90% to the lesions. Trichloroacetic acid is applied directly to the warts and talc or sodium bicarbonate is powdered on afterwards to remove unreacted acid. These applications are repeated weekly up to six times. If there is no improvement after six treatments other therapies should be considered. During therapy patients should be counseled that they are contagious to noninfected partners and should take appropriate preventive measures. Recent studies analyzing the safety and effectiveness of combination therapy with subcutaneous interferons and cyrotherapy or interferons and podophyllin have not shown any significant benefit to either cyrotherapy or podophyllin alone (140–142).

C. Cytomegalovirus

1. Epidemiology

Cytomegalovirus (CMV) infection is ubiquitous. Depending on the population surveyed, seroprevalence of CMV ranges from 30–100%. Antibody to CMV is present in approximately 95% of homosexual men, many of whom have active disease (143). Most disease in AIDS patients is due to reactivation of CMV rather than primary infection, which accounts for the high seroprevalence in this population (144). Although CMV is more common in immunosuppressed populations, immunocompetent individuals may also be affected.

Cytomegalovirus is transmitted during intimate person-to-person contact via oropharyngeal, vaginal, and cervical secretions as well as urine, breast milk, semen, and blood (145–148). Approximately 30% of homosexual men will harbor the virus in semen. As with other sexually transmitted diseases, trauma associated with vaginal or anal intercourse provides a conduit for the transmission of the virus. Acute infection is usually asymptomatic but there is lifelong latency of the virus that can lead to reactivation.

Cytomegalovirus has become the most common viral opportunistic infection in the HIV-positive population (149). It has been estimated that 20% of patients with AIDS will develop gastrointestinal disease associated with CMV, and CMV may cause disease anywhere from esophagus to rectum. Within the anorectal area, 25% of cultures in one study were positive for CMV (15).

2. Clinical Presentation

Cytomegalovirus may cause a variety of lesions throughout the gastrointestinal tract from esophagus to rectum. Infections of the anorectal area may cause ulcerative lesions, perforations, lesions mimicking neoplasia, solitary ulcers, or diffuse proctocolitis (150–154). Patients may complain of rectal pain, hematochezia, fever, weight loss, and abdominal pain. On anorectal examination, anal and perianal ulcers may be seen. Typically CMV doe not infect keratinized squamous epithelium. However, several reports have documented CMV as the probable etiology of perianal ulcerations and anal fissures in AIDS patients (155–157). On endoscopy, an inflammatory colitis or ulcerative lesions may be seen.

Cytomegalovirus may infect the immunocompetent or the immunosuppressed population. In addition, CMV may be a superinfection in patients with an underlying diseased rectum. Within the immunocompetent population CMV infection is rare but reported. Usually after anal-receptive intercourse a proctocolitis has been described that follows a self-limited course (158,159).

3. *Pathogenesis*

Within the immunocompetent and immunosuppressed patient populations the pathogenesis of CMV infection is unclear. Some have suggested that CMV induces an immunosuppressive action itself by invading host lymphoid cells thereby causing a breakdown in immune reactivity (160). Cytomegalovirus may cause a progressive local vasculitis leading to focal ischemic necrosis and ulcer formation (161).

4. *Diagnosis*

The diagnosis of CMV infection may require several tests. The pathognomonic finding on light microscopy is the presence of intranuclear inclusion bodies within endothelial cells, histiocytes, and macrophages, giving the hallmark "owl's eye" appearance (see Figure 5) (162,163). These histopathologic findings have a sensitivity of approximately 92% in the diagnosis of CMV (163). Atypical CMV inclusions have been described, especially in the AIDS population (164). Thus, one should employ other diagnostic modalities if the diagnosis is unclear from the biopsy specimen.

Serology to detect antibodies to CMV is helpful to assess acute or chronic infection. An elevated IgM titer or a rising IgG titer suggest current infection. However, the presence of IgG antibody to CMV does not imply active infection as CMV may be latent.

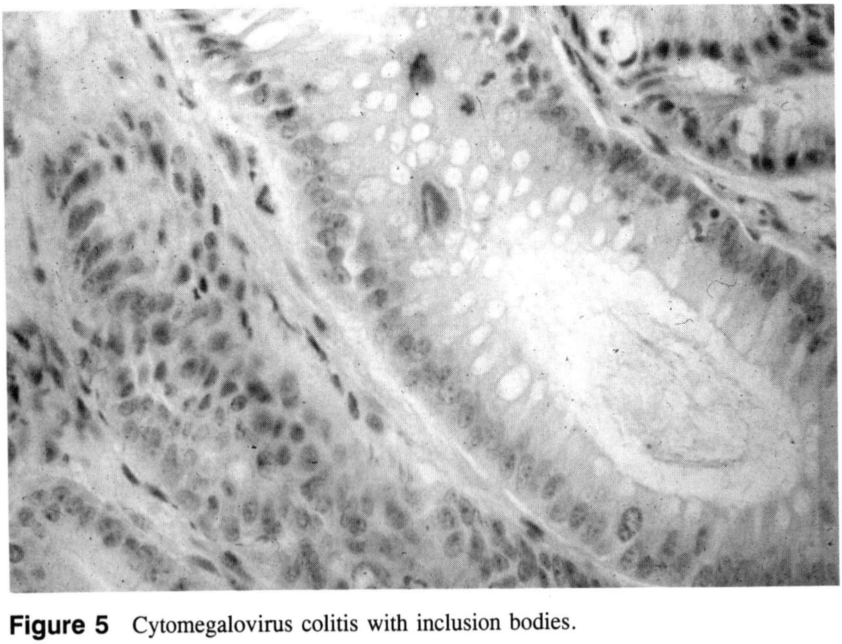

Figure 5 Cytomegalovirus colitis with inclusion bodies.

Viral culture on human fibroblasts is another diagnostic modality, but if viral burden is low in the specimen it may take up to six weeks to see a cytopathic effect consistent with CMV. Therefore, viral culture is not practical if one needs to know the diagnosis quickly.

A more rapid method to assess active CMV infection is CMV antigenemia Monoclonal antibodies are used to detect CMV particles within blood leucocytes. This method is most useful in the early stages of infection when CMV viremia is more common (165).

The polymerase chain reaction (PCR) is a rapid and highly sensitive test to detect the presence of CMV nucleic acid. Since CMV may remain for long periods in tissues it invades, the mere presence of CMV DNA in a blood or any other tissue sample does not imply pathogenicity. How PCR will be used to assess the etiology of a particular anorectal lesion is unclear.

5. *Treatment*

In immunocompetent hosts, anorectal CMV is usually self-limited and therefore only supportive therapy is necessary. Patients rendered transiently immunodeficient by chemotherapy may have spontaneous remissions of CMV infection once immunosuppressive therapy is complete. However, in patients with persistent immunodeficiency, such as AIDS patients, antiviral therapy is needed due to the high mortality of progressive disease.

Several studies have demonstrated clinical, endoscopic, and virologic improvement after therapy of CMV proctitis with ganciclovir, a nucleoside analog that inhibits viral DNA synthesis (166–168). Ganciclovir must be given intravenously and is occasionally associated with neutropenia, thrombocytopenia, and hypotension. The initial induction dose is 10–15 mg/kg in three divided doses daily over three weeks followed by 5 mg/kg maintenance phase. There is a high relapse rate as CMV infection is suppressed, not cured, and there is a rising prevalence of ganciclovir-resistent CMV (169,170). Foscarnet, an inhibitor of DNA synthesis that inhibits viral DNA polymerase, has provided clinical and endoscopic improvement in patients who failed to improve with ganciclovir (171,172). Side effects include renal failure, seizures, headache, and metabolic abnormalities. Thus, close monitoring and inpatient administration is required during foscarnet therapy.

IV. PARASITIC INFECTIONS

A. Protozoal Infections

1. *Amebiasis*

a. Epidemiology. Amebiasis is caused by the protozoan *Entamoeba histolytica*. In addition to fecal-oral spread, particularly in lower socioeconomic classes where sanitation is poor, oral-anal sexual practices are recognized as a mode of transmission of *E. histolytica* (173). During oral-anal contact amebic cysts may be ingested directly. Furthermore, cysts may be carried by the fingers of one partner after touching the other partner's anal or perianal area. Approximately 10% of the world's population harbor the parasite. *E. histolytica* is endemic in areas of India, Africa, Mexico, South and Central America, and Asia. Groups at high risk in the United States for invasive amebiasis are recent immigrants, institutionalized patients, and AIDS patients. Approximately 30–40% of patients with AIDS are infected with amoeba, but most of these amebic strains are nonpathogenic (174,175). Several genetic and epidemiologic studies have confirmed the presence of distinct pathogenic and nonpathogenic strains of *E. histolytica* (176–180).

b. Clinical Manifestations and Diagnosis. Amebiasis may present as aymptomatic infection (passage of cysts), diarrhea, chronic colitis, or ulcerations. Symptoms include rectal pain, tenesmus, abdominal cramps, fever, malaise, and bloody diarrhea. On anoscopy and protoscopy the mucosa may range from normal to very friable and edematous. Ulcerations caused by *E. histolytica* appear as flask-shaped lesions with a clean base that eventually may develop a necrotic base. The endoscopic appearance can be indistinguishable from inflammatory bowel disease and other infectious enteridides (181).

Definitive diagnosis is based on identifying trophozoites or cysts of *E. histolytica* in stool specimens or in a wet mount of a rectal biopsy. Trophozoites are easily killed by antibiotics, antidiarrheal agents, barium, and tap water. Fresh stool specimens should be examined ideally within 20 minutes for motile trophozoites. Three separate stool specimens need to be examined by skilled personnel to achieve a sensitivity of 90%. The false-positive rate for stool microscopy is high in many laboratories due to the misidentification of fecal leukocytes as amoebas. Culture of *E. histolytica* is a more sensitive marker of amebiasis but this technique is not available in most laboratories. Indirect hemagglutin assays are useful in diagnosing acute proctocolitis but the results may remain positive for up to 10 years after acute infection.

Serology by agar gel diffusion, counterimmunoelectrophoresis, or ELISA is positive in 85–95% of patients with invasive disease (182). In general, asymptomatic cyst passers are seronegative; these patients are usually infected with a nonpathogenic strain of *E. histolytica*. Positive serology tests generally become negative within 6–12 months (183,184).

c. Treatment. The recommended therapy for acute amebiasis is 5–10 days of metronidazole at a dose of 750 mg three times daily. Treatment with luminal agents is important in cyst passers as metronidazole is not effective against cysts, and reinfection may occur if luminal agents are not used. Diloxanide furoate (a luminal agent) is only available from the Centers for Disease Control in Atlanta, Georgia and is over 90% efficacious at a dosage of 500 mg three times daily for ten days. Other agents include iodoquinol 650 mg three times daily for twenty days or paromomycin 500 mg three times daily for 10 days. The effectiveness of paromomycin is less than diloxanide furoate and loose stools are a common side effect.

Asymptomatic cyst passers may be treated with any one of the luminal agents alone. However, there is still much debate on whether or not to treat asymptomatic cyst passers. Some argue for routine treatment (185–187) and others against (174,188–190). One study (191) reported that 95% of subjects with culture-positive *E. histolytica* who were untreated, had eradicated the infection spontaneously at one year. Patients positive for HIV have a high rate of carriage of *E. histolytica* and spontaneous reinfection due to continued oral-anal sexual practices. The ability to isolate pathogenic and nonpathogenic strains by zymodeme analysis is not yet available clinically; therefore, given the potential for active disease in immunosuppressed patients, asymptomatic HIV patients should be treated at least two separate times. If this treatment does not eradicate the infection and the patient remains asymptomatic then escalating doses or continued therapy is not warranted.

2. *Giardiasis*

Giardia lamblia is an intestinal parasite that occasionally may be transmitted by oral-anal sexual contact. The parasite has been identified in up to 14% of homosexual men (90). *Giardia* has a predilection for the duodenum and rarely causes symptoms of proctitis. However, *Giardia* trophozoites may be carried to the colon by the rapid transit of diarrhea but do not colonize the rectal mucosa. There has been only one case of Giardia lamblia proctitis described in the literature (192), without any evidence to support an etiologic role of the parasite. Diagnosis is based on finding trophozoites or cysts in stool specimens. Treatment is with metronidazole or quinacrine.

B. Helminthic Infections

1. *Enterobius Vermicularis*

Enterobiasis or pinworm disease (threadworm in the United Kingdom) is caused by the nematode *Enterobius vermicularis*. The infection is most prevalent in children but high rates of infection acquired through anilingus have been documented in homosexual men (193,194). *Enterobius vermicularis* eggs are ingested and then develop into infectious larvae in the colon. The female pinworm migrates to the perianal skin at nightime and deposits her eggs. Reinfection may occur when the area is scratched and then fingers are brought to the mouth. The primary symptom is pruritus ani. Bacterial superinfection is common due to irritation from the pruritus.

Diagnosis is made by history and by microscopic exam of cellophane tape that is pressed against the unwashed perianal skin looking for pinworm eggs.

Repeat testing on separate days will give a higher yield of positive results (195). Eggs are not as reliably found in stool specimens.

Recommended treatment is with mebendazole 100 mg orally in a single dose with a repeat dose one week later. Mebendazole was high luminal concentrations and no serious side effects. Alternative agents include albendazole, piperazine, pyrantel embonate, and vipyrinium embonate. Antipruritic ointment or cream can provide symptomatic relief. Reinfection must be prevented during treatment. This includes abstinence from anilingus, careful handwashing, and cleaning of bedcovers and sleeping garments.

V. NEOPLASTIC LESIONS

Anorectal neoplasms may cause symptoms similar to an acute infectious process including anorectal pain, tenesmus, pruritus, or hematochezia. Symptoms such as incontinence, change in bowel habits, or rectovaginal fistula suggest malignant infiltration of tumor. Since many neoplasms can simulate infection it is important to obtain biopsies of suspicious lesions to rule out neoplastic disease.

A. Kaposi's Sarcoma

Originally described in elderly men of Mediterranean descent, Kaposi's sarcoma (KS) has become a prominent complication of AIDS. It is the most common AIDS-related malignancy and usually involves the skin including the anal and perianal area but may also involve the gastrointestinal tract. Because KS is more common among homosexual men who acquired HIV through sexual contact and who practice high-risk sexual behavior, it is felt that there may be an unidentified sexually transmitted agent or cofactor, in addition to HIV, responsible for KS (196–201).

The clinical presentation of KS in AIDS is varied. Classically, the KS lesion appears as a purplish nodular, papular, or macular lesion. Occasionally, lesions will coalesce and fungate or ulcerate. Rarely, KS may present as a solitary rectal ulcer (202). Although the pathophysiology of KS lesions is not completely understood it is felt that cytokines, such as IL-6, oncostatin M, and basic fibroblast growth factor (b-FGF) play important roles (203,204). Presumptive diagnosis is made by physical exam but biopsy provides a definitive answer. Moreover, it is important to obtain cultures from the anorectum as KS may coexist with other sexually transmitted pathogens such as anal warts and HSV (205).

Topical liquid nitrogen is helpful for patients with small KS lesions in a limited anal or perianal area. The chemotherapeutic agent vinblastine has been injected intralesionally for larger (more than 1 cm) lesions. Alpha-interferon is used intramuscularly or subcutaneously over a three-week period. The best results have been seen in patients with CD4 counts greater than 200. Concurrent administration of alpha-interferon in patients on zidovudine (AZT) has led to more pronounced neutropenia. Other modalities include laser, radiation, and systemic chemotherapy (adriamycin, bleomycin, and vincristine/vinblastine or etoposide alone).

B. Lymphoma

Non-Hodgkin's B-cell lymphomas are also associated with HIV infection (206,207). Epstein–Barr virus (EBV), primarily transmitted through saliva, is associated with the pathogenesis of this tumor (208). Diagnosis is made by biopsy and treatment involves radiation or chemotherapy.

C. Epidermoid Carcinoma of the Anus

Squamous-cell anal cancer is more common in HIV-positive patients and those who practice anoreceptive intercourse. Human papillomavirus (HPV) type 16 is associated with up to 80% of squamous-cell anal cancer while HPV 18 is associated with approximately 8%. Anal cancer is diagnosed by histopathology and treatment must be tailored to the individual patient but will involve a combination of chemotherapy, radiation therapy, and surgery (209).

VI. TRAUMATIC AND IDIOPATHIC DISORDERS

The skin of perianal area and the mucosa of the anus and rectum are prone to trauma from foreign objects used during anal sexual activity. Objects such as vibrators, bottles, and flashlights in addition to manual manipulation may cause a traumatic inflammatory process that is difficult to distinguish from an infectious process. In addition, these objects may be found on physical and diagnostic examination as retained foreign bodies in the rectum, which may account for the patient's symptoms. These objects injure the mucosa, breaking down defenses from infectious agents. The possibility of finding foreign objects highlights the importance of a detailed sexual history.

Occasionally no etiologic agent is found in HIV-associated anorectal ulcers or episodes of proctitis. In several case studies a nonspecific proctitis or anorectal ulceration in HIV patients did not have a clear infectious or neoplastic etiology (210–213). These lesions could be due to an inflammatory response of the bowel epithelium to HIV itself (214).

REFERENCES

1. Seidman SN, Rieder RO. A review of sexual behavior in the United States. Am J Psychiatry 1994; 151:330–41.

2. MacDonald NE, Wells GA, Fisher WA, et al. High risk STD/HIV behavior among college students. JAMA 1990; 263:3155–9.
3. Kotloff KL, Tacket CO, Wasserman SS, et al. A voluntary serosurvey and behavioral risk assessment for human immunodeficiency virus infection among college students. Sex Transm Dis 1991; 18:223–7.
4. Billy JO, Tanfer K, Grady WR, Klepinger DH. The sexual behavior of men in the United States. Fam Plann Perspect 1993; 25:52–60.
5. Masters WH, Johnson VE, Kolodny RC. Crisis: Heterosexual behavior in the age of AIDS. New York: Grove Press, 1988: 58–62.
6. Reinisch JM, Sanders SA, Hill CA, Ziemba-Davis M. High-risk sexual behavior among heterosexual undergraduates at a mid-western university. Fam Plann Perspect 1992; 24:116–21.
7. O'Donnell L, San Doval A, Vornfett R, O'Donnell CR. STD prevention and the challenge of gender and cultural diversity: knowledge, attitudes, and risk behaviors among black and hispanic inner-city STD clinic patients. Sex Transm Dis 1994; 21:137–48.
8. Centers for Disease Control and Prevention. Self reported changes in sexual behaviors among homosexual and bisexual men from the San Francisco City Clinic Cohort. MMWR 1987; 36:187.
9. McKusick L, Coates TJ, Morin SF, Pollack L, Hoff C. Longitudinal predictors of reductions in unprotected anal intercourse among gay men in San Francisco: the AIDS Behavioral Research Project. Am J Public Health 1990; 80:978–83.
10. Centers for Disease Control. Declining rates of rectal and pharyngeal gonorrhea among males—New York City. MMWR 1984; 33:295.
11. Handsfield HH. Decreasing incidence of gonorrhea in homosexually active men—minimal effect on the risk of AIDS. Western J Med 1985; 143:469.
12. Rubb SR, Palenicek JG, Hoover D, Selnes OA, Saah AJ. Psychosocial factors related to unprotected anal intercourse in a cohort of homosexual men. Int Conf AIDS 1993; 9:819.
13. Valleroy L, O'Reilly K, Rolfs R. Predictors of lapse to unprotected anal intercourse in a cohort of homosexual and bisexual men in the U.S.A. Int Conf AIDS 1993; 9:745.
14. Ross MW. Reasons for non-use of condoms by homosexually active men during anal intercourse. Int J STD AIDS 1990; 1:432–4.
15. Centers for Disease Control and Prevention. Summary of Notifiable Diseases, United States, 1993. MMWR 1994; 42:1–65.
16. Goldberg GS, Orkin BA, Smith LE. Microbiology of human immunodeficiency virus anorectal disease. Dis Colon Rectum 1994; 37:439–43.
17. Laughon BE, Druckman DA, Vernon A, et al. Prevalence of enteric pathogens in homosexual men with and without acquired immunodeficiency syndrome. Gastroenterology 1988; 94:984–93.
18. Janda WM, Bohnoff M, Morello JA, Lerner SA. Prevalence and site-pathogen studies of Neisseria meningitidis and Neisseria gonorrhea in homosexual men. JAMA 1980; 244:2060–4.

19. Stern A, Meyer TF. Common mechanism controlling phase and antigenic variation in pathogenic Neisseriae. Mol Microbiol 1987; 1:5–12.
20. Goodman SD, Scocca JJ. Identification and arrangement of the DNA sequence recognized in specific transformation of Neisseria gonorrhoeae. Proc Natl Acad Sci USA 1988; 85:6982.
21. Cannon JG, Sparling PF. The genetics of the gonococcus. Ann Rev Microbiol 1984; 38:111.
22. Bhattacharyya MN, Jephcott AE. Diagnosis of gonorrhea in women. Br J Vener Dis 1974; 50:109–112.
23. Coghill DV, Young H. Genital gonorrhea in women: a serovar correlation with concomitant rectal infection. J Infect 1989; 18:131–41.
24. Hook EW 3rd, Holmes KK. Gonococcal infections. Ann Intern Med 1985; 102:229–43.
25. Pariser H, Marino AF. Gonorrhea: frequency of unrecognized reservoirs. South Med J 1970; 63:198–202.
26. Schecter WP. Examination of the anus and rectum in the HIV infected patient. In: Allen-Mersh TG, Gottesman L, eds. Anorectal Disease in AIDS. Great Britain: Edward Arnold. 1991:75–86.
27. Lebedeff DA, Hochman EB. Rectal gonorrhea in men: diagnosis and treatment. Ann Int Med 1980; 92:463–6.
28. Goodman KJ. Radiologic findings in anorectal gonorrhea. Gastrointestinal Radiology 1978; 3:223–41.
29. Deheragoda P. Diagnosis of anorectal gonorrhea by blind anorectal swabs compared with direct vision swabs taken by proctoscope. Br J Vener Dis 1977; 53:311–14.
30. Judson FN, Ehret JM, Eickhoff TC. Anogenital infection with N. meningitidis in homosexual men. J Infect Dis 1978; 137:458–63.
31. Chapel TA, Gatewood C, Keane MB. Neisseria meningitidis in the anal canal of homosexual men. J Infect Dis 1977; 136:810.
32. McMillan A, McNeillage G, Gilmour HM, Lee FD. Histology of rectal gonorrhea in men, with a note on anorectal infection with Neisseria meningitidis. J Clin Pathol 1983; 36:511–14.
33. Surawicz CM, Goodell SE, Quinn TC, et al. Spectrum of rectal biopsy abnormalities in homosexual men with intestinal symptoms. Gastroenterology 1986; 91:651–9.
34. Gorwitz RJ, Nakashima AK, Moran JS, Knapp JS. Sentinel surveillance for antimicrobial resistance in Neisseria gonorrhoeae—United States, 1988-1991. The Gonococcal Isolate Surveillance Project Study Group. MMWR CDC Surveill Summ 1993; 42:29–39.
35. Centers for Disease Control and Prevention. 1993 Sexually Transmitted Diseases Treatment Guidelines MMWR 1993; 42:56–61.
36. Coker DM, Ahmed-Jushuf I, Arya OP, Chessbrough JS, Pratt BC. Evaluation of single dose ciprofloxacin in the treatment of rectal and pharyngeal gonorrhoea. J Antimicrob Chemother 1989; 24:271–2.

37. Waugh MA. Open study of the safety and efficacy of a single dose of azithromycin for the treatment of uncomplicated gonorrhoea in men and women. J Antimicrob Chemother 1993; 31(suppl E):193–8.
38. Corcoran GD, Ridgway GL. Antibiotic chemotherapy of bacterial sexually transmitted diseases in adults: a review. International Journal of STD and AIDS 1994; 5:165–71.
39. Quinn TC, Goodell SE, Mkrtichian EE, et al. Chlamydia trachomoatis proctitis. N Engl J Med 1981; 305:195–200.
40. Stamm WE, et al. Chlamydia trachomatis proctitis in homosexual men and heterosexual women. In: Mardh PA, Holmes KK, Oriel DJ, Piot P. Schacter J, eds. Chlamydial infections. Amsterdam: Elsevier Biomedical, 1982: 111–114.
41. Moulder JW. Looking at Chlamydia without looking at their hosts. Am Soc Microbiol News 1984; 50:353.
42. Ward ME. Outstanding problems in Chlamydial cell biology. In: Oriel DJ, Ridgway G, Schacter J, et al, eds. Chlamydial infections. Cambridge, England: Cambridge University Press, 1986: 3–14.
43. Barnes RC, Rompalo AM, Stamm WE. Comparision of Chlamydia trachomatis serovars causing rectal and cervical infections. J Infect Dis 1987; 156:953–8.
44. Ghinsberg RC, Firsteter-Gilburd E, Mates A, Nitzan Y. Rectal lymphogranuloma venereum in a bisexual patient. Microbiologica 1991; 14:161–4.
45. Scieux C, Barnes R, Bianchi A, Casin I, Morel P, Perol Y. Lymphogranuloma venereum: 27 cases in Paris. J Infect Dis 1989; 160:662–8.
46. Wexner SD. Sexually transmitted diseases of the colon, rectum, and anus: the challenge of the nineties. Dis Colon Rectum 1990; 33:1048–62.
47. Thompson CI, MacAulay AJ, Smith IW. Chlamydia trachomatis infections in the female rectums. Genitourin Med 1989: 65:269–73.
48. Quinn TC, Goodell SE, Mkrtichian EE, et al. Chlamydia trachomatis proctitis. N Engl J Med 1981; 305:195–200.
49. Ruther U, Rupp W, Muller HA, Jipp P, Schroter G. Rectal pseudotumor due to Chlamydia trachomatis in a male homosexual. Endoscopy 1990; 22:237–8.
50. Sider L, Mintzer RA, Mendelson EB, et al. Radiographic findings of infectious proctitis in homosexual men. Am J Roentgenol 1982; 139:667–71.
51. Stamm WE, Harrison HR, Alexander ER, et al. Diagnosis of Chlamydia trachomatis infections by direct immunofluorescence staining of genital secretions. Ann Intern Med 1984; 101:638–41.
52. Tam MR, Stamm WE, Handsfield HH, et al. Culture-independent diagnosis of Chlamydia trachomatis using monoclonal antibodies. N Engl J Med 1984; 310:1146–50.
53. Rompalo AM, Suchland RJ, Price CB, Stamm WE. Rapid diagnosis of Chlamydia trachomatis rectal infection by direct immunofluorescence staining. J Infect Dis 1987; 155:1075–6.
54. Centers for Disease Control and Prevention. Recommendations for the prevention and management of Chlamydia trachomatis infections. MMWR 1993; 42(RR-12):1–36.

55. Centers for Disease Control. Continuing increase in infectious syphilis—United States. MMWR 1988; 37:35–8.
56. Hook EW, Marra CM. Acquired syphilis in adults. N Engl J Med 1992; 326:1060–9.
57. Chapel TA. The variability of syphilitic chancres. Sex Transm Dis 1978; 5:68.
58. Quinn TC, Lukehart SA, Goodell S, Mkrtichian EE, Schuffler MD, Holmes KK. Rectal mass caused by Treponema pallidum: confirmation by immunofluorescence staining. Gastroenterology 1982; 82:135–9.
59. Akdamar K, Martin RJ, Ichinose H. Syphilitic proctitis. Am J Dig Dis 1977; 22:701–4.
60. Drusin LM, Singer C, Valenti AJ, Armstrong D. Infectious syphilis mimicking neoplastic disease. Arch Intern Med 1977; 137:156–60.
61. Faris MR, Perry JJ, Westermeier TG, Redmond J III. Rectal syphilis mimicking histiocytic lymphoma. Am J Clin Pathol 1983; 80:719–21.
62. Anderson J, Mindel A, Tovey SJ, Williams P. Primary and secondary syphilis, 20 years experience. Genitourin Med 1989; 65:239–43.
63. Hira SK, Patel JS, Bhat SG, Chilikima K, Mooney N. Clinical manifestations of secondary syphilis. Int J Dermatol 1987; 26:103–7.
64. Chapel TA. The signs and symptoms of secondary syphilis. Sex Transm Dis 1980; 7:161–4.
65. Hutchinson CM, Hook EW III, Shepherd M, Verley J, Rompalo AM. Altered clinical presentation of early syphilis in patients with human immunodeficiency virus infection. Ann Intern Med 1994; 121:94–100.
66. Tramont EC. Syphilis in HIV-infected persons. AIDS Clin Rev 1993-94; 61–72.
67. Cruz Palacios C, Garcia ML, Lopez A, et al. HIV modified syphilis: secondary rash and chancre in HIV+ patients. Int Conf AIDS 1994; 10:54.
68. Potekayev N, Potekayev S, Gruzdev B. Peculiarities of clinical manifestations and course of syphilis in HIV-infected patients. Int Conf AIDS 1994; 10:263.
69. Mussini C, Mongiardo N, Manicardi G, Zoboli G, De Rienzo B. Clinical course of syphilis in HIV patients: a prospective study. Int Conf AIDS 1993; 9:393.
70. Musher DM, Hamill RJ, Baughn RE. Effect of human immunodeficiency virus (HIV) infection on the course of syphilis and on the response to treatment. Ann Intern Med 1990; 113:872–81.
71. Hook EW. Syphilis and HIV infection. J Infect Dis 1989; 160:530–4.
72. Darrow WW, Echenberg DF, Jaffe HW, et al. Risk factors for human immunodeficiency virus (HIV) infections in homosexual men. Am J Public Health 1987; 77:479–83.
73. Radolf JD, Kaplan RP. Unusual manifestations of secondary syphilis and abnormal humoral immune response to Treponema pallidum antigens in a homosexual man with asymptomatic human immunodeficiency virus infection. J Am Acad Dermatol 1989; 18:(suppl):423–8.
74. Gourevitch MN, Selwyn PA, Davenny K, et al. Effects of HIV infection on the serologic manifestations and response to treatment of syphilis in intravenous drug users. Ann Intern Med 1993; 118:350–5.

75. Rock B, Shah KV, Farmer ER. A morphologic, pathologic, and virologic study of anogenital warts in men. Arch Dermatol 1992; 128:495–500.
76. Singcharoen T, Praisontarangkul OA. The radiological findings in syphilitic proctitis. Br J Radiol 1987; 60:1137–8.
77. Lowhagen GB. Syphilis: Test procedures and therapeutic strategies. Sem in Dermatol 1990; 9:152–9.
78. Larsen SA, Steiner BM, Rudolph AH. Laboratory diagnosis and interpretation of tests for syphilis. Clin Microbiol Rev 1995; 8:1–21.
79. Johnson PC, Farnie MA. Testing for syphilis. Dermatol Clin 1994; 12:9–17.
80. Soler ME, Gottesman L. Anal and rectal ulceration. In: Allen-Mersh TG, Gottesman L, eds. Anorectal Disease in AIDS. Great Britain: Edward Arnold, 1991:107–10.
81. Sergei P, Potekayev N, Yurin O, Gorbacheva E, Gruzdev B, Pokrovsky VV. The influence of the human immunodeficiency virus infection on the serological manifestations of syphilis. Int Conf AIDS 1993; 9:389.
82. Quinn TC, Classer D, Cannon R, et al. The association of syphilis with risk of human immunodeficiency virus infection in patients attending sexually transmitted diseases clinics. Arch Intern Med 1990; 150:1297.
83. Rolfs RT, Hindershot E, Hackett K, et al. Treatment of early syphilis in HIV infected and HIV uninfected patients. Preliminary results of the Syphilis and HIV study. Presented at the Tenth International Meeting of the International Society for STD Research, Helsinki, Finland, August 29-September 1, 1993.
84. Hass JS, Bolan G, Larsen SA, Clement MJ, Bachetti P, Moss AR. Sensitivity of treponemal tests for detecting prior treated syphilis during human immunodeficiency virus infection. J Infect Dis 1990; 162:862–6.
85. Johnson PDR, Graves SR, Stewart L, Warren R, Dwyer B, Lucas CR. Specific syphilis serologic tests may become negative in HIV infection. AIDS 1991; 5:419–23.
86. Hammond GW, Slutchuk M, Scatliff J, Sherman E, Wilt JC, Ronald AR. Clinical, epidemiological, laboratory, and therapeutic features of an urban outbreak of chancroid in North America. Rev Infect Dis 1980; 2:867–79.
87. Museyi K, Van Dyck E, Vervoort T, Taylor D, Hoge C, Piot P. Use of an enzyme immunoassay to detect serum IgG antibodies to Haemophilus decreyi. J Infect Dis 1988; 157:1039–43.
88. Bassa AGH, Hoosen AA, Moodley J, Bramdev A. Granuloma inguinal (donovanosis) in women. Sex Trans Dis 1993; 20:164–7.
89. Richens J. The diagnosis and treatment of donovanosis (granuloma inguinale). Genitourin Med 1991; 67:441–52.
90. Quinn TC, Stamm WE, Goodell SE, et al. The polymicrobial origin of intestinal infections in homosexual men. N Engl J Med 1983; 309:576–82.
91. Dritz SK, Braff EH. Sexually transmitted typhoid fever. N Engl J Med 1977; 296:1359.
92. Quinn TC, Corey L, Chaffee RG, Schuffler MD, Holmes KK. Campylobacter proctitis in a homosexual man. Ann Int Med 1980; 93:458–9.
93. Munday PE, Furr PM, Taylor-Robinson D. The prevalence of Ureaplasma

urealyticum and Mycoplasman hominis in the cervix and anal canal of women. J Infect 1981; 253–7.
94. Dunlop EMC, Hare MJ, Jones BR, Taylor-Robinson D. Mycoplasmas and "non-specific" genital infections. Clinical aspects. Br J Vener Dis 1969; 45:274.
95. Philipson EH, Palermino DA, Robinson A. Enhanced antenatal detection of group B streptococcus colonization. Obstet Gynecol 1995; 85:437–9.
96. Hirschfield AJ. Two family outbreaks of perianal cellulitis associated with group A beta-hemolytic streptococci. Pediatrics 1970; 46:799:802.
97. Wright JE, Butt HL. Perianal infection with beta-haemolytic streptococcus. Arch Dis Child 1994; 70:145–6.
98. Goodell SE, Quinn TC, Mkrtichian EE, et al. Herpes Simplex Virus: an important cause of acute proctitis in homosexual men. Gastroenterology 1981; 80:1159.
99. Samartasinghe PL, Oates JK, MacLennan IPB. Herpetic proctitis and sacral radiomyelopathy - a hazard for homosexual men. Br Med J 1979; 2:365.
100. Goodell SE, Quinn TC, Mkrtichian EE, Schuffler MD, Holmes KK, Corey L. Herpes simplex virus proctitis in homosexual men: clinical, sigmoidoscopic, and histopathological features. N Engl J Med 1983; 308:868–71.
101. Atia W, Sonnex C. Retention of urine in occult anorectal herpes. Br Med J 1986; 292:39.
102. Oates JK, Greenhouse PR. Retention of urine in anogenital herpetic infection. Lancet 1971; 691–2.
103. White WB, Hanna M, Stewart JA. Systemic herpes simplex virus type 2 infection. Arch Intern Med 1984; 144:826–7.
104. Baker RW, Peppercorn MA. Gastrointestinal ailments of homosexual men. Medicine 1982; 61:390–405.
105. McMillan A, Lee FD. Sigmoidoscopic and microscopic appearance of the rectal mucosa in homosexual men. Gut 1981; 22:1035–41.
106. Goldmeier D. Herpetic proctitis and sacral radiculopathy in homosexual men (letter). Br Med J 1979; 2:549.
107. Shah SJ, Scholz FJ. Anorectal herpes: radiographic findings. Radiology 1983; 147:81–2.
108. Cohen PR. Tests for detecting herpes simplex virus and varicella-zoster virus infections. Dermatol Clin 1994; 12:51–68.
109. Ashley RL. Laboratory techniques in the diagnosis of herpes simplex infection. Genitourin Med 1993; 69:174–83.
110. Reeves WC, et al. Risk of recurrence after first episodes of genital herpes: relation to HSV type and antibody response. N Engl J Med 1981; 305–15.
111. Devillechabrolle A, Hugues-Dorin F, Fortier B, Catalan F. Prevalence of serum antibodies to herpes simplex virus types 1 and 2: application of ELISA technique to 100 cases of anogenital herpes. Sex Transm Dis 1985; 12:40–3.
112. Waugh MA. Herpesvirus hominis infection in men. J Amer Vener Dis Assoc 1976; 3:68.
113. Rompalo AM, Mertz GJ, Davis LG, et al. Oral acyclovir of treatment of first-episode herpes simplex virus proctitis. JAMA 1988; 259:2879–81.

114. Fletcher CV. Treatment of herpes virus infections in HIV-infected individuals. Ann Pharmacother 1992; 26:955–62.
115. Engel JP, Englund JA, Fletcher CV, Hill EL. Treatment of resistant herpes simplex virus with continuous-infusion acyclovir. JAMA 1990; 263:1662–4.
116. Hardy WD. Foscarnet treatment of acyclovir-resistant herpes simplex virus infection in patients with acquired immunodeficiency syndrome: preliminary results of a controlled, randomized, regimen-comparative trial. Am J Med 1992; 92:30s–35s.
117. Erlich KS, Jacobson MA, Koehler JE, et al. Foscarnet therapy for severe acyclovir-resistant herpes simplex virus type-2 infections in patients with acquired immunodeficiency syndrome (AIDS). An uncontrolled trial. Ann Intern Med 1989; 110:710–3.
118. Communicable Disease Surveillance Centre. Sexually transmitted disease surveillance in Britain 1984. Br Med J 1986; 296:942–3.
119. Goorney BP, Waugh MA, Clarke J. Anal warts in heterosexual men. Genitourin Med 1987; 63:216.
120. Sonnex C, Scholefield JH, Kocjan G, et al. Anal human papillomavirus infection in heterosexuals with genital warts: prevalence and relation with sexual behavior. BMJ 1991; 303:1243.
121. Kent C, Samuel M, Winkelstein J. The role of anal/genital warts in HIV infection. JAMA 1987; 258:3385–6.
122. Kiviat N, Rompalo AM, Bowden R, et al. Anal human papillomavirus infection among human immunodeficiency virus seropositive and seronegative men. J Infect Dis 1990; 162:358–61.
123. Melbye M, Cote TR, Kessler L, Gail M, Bigger RJ. High incidence of anal cancer among AIDS patients. The AIDS/Cancer Working Group. Lancet 1994; 343:636–9.
124. Beckmann AM, Daling JR, Sherman KJ, et al. Human papillomavirus infection and anal cancer. Int J Cancer 1989; 43:1042–9.
125. Palmer JG, Scholefield JH, Coates PJ, et al. Anal cancer and human papillomavirus. Dis Colon Rectum 1989; 32:1016–22.
126. Gal AA, Saul SH, Stoler MH. In situ hybridization analysis of human papillomavirus in anal squamous cell carcinoma. Mod Pathol 1989; 2:439–443.
127. Palefsky JM, Holly EA, Gonzales J, Berline J, Ahn DK, Greenspan JS. Detection of human papillomavirus DNA in anal intraepithelial neoplasia and anal cancer. Cancer Res 1991; 51:1014–9.
128. Scholefield JH, Kerr IB, Shepherd NA, Miller KJ, Bloomfield R, Northover JM. Human papillomavirus type 16 DNA in anal cancers from six different countries. Gut 1991; 32:674–6.
129. Zaki SR, Judd R, Coffield LM, Greer P, Rolston F, Evatt BL. Human papillomavirus infection and anal carcinoma. Retrospective analysis by in situ hybridization and the polymerase chain reaction. Am J Pathol 1992; 140:1345–55.
130. Taichman LB, Reilley SS, LaPorta RF. The role of keratinocyte differentiation in the expression of epitheliotropic viruses. J Invest Dermatol 1983; 81:137s–140s.

131. Palefsky JM. Anal human papillomavirus infection and anal cancer in HIV-positive individuals: an emerging problem. AIDS 1994; 8:283–95.
132. Rock B, Shah KV, Farmer ER. A morphologic, pathologic, and virologic study of anogenital warts in men. Arch Dermatol 1992; 128:495–500.
133. Fenger C. Anal neoplasia and its precursors: facts and controversies. Semin Diagn Pathol 1991; 8:190–201.
134. Volberding P. Clinical management of HIV-related malignancies. Annu Conf Australias Soc HIV Med 1993; 5:23.
135. Ferenczy A, Mitao M, Nagai N, Silverstein SJ, Crum CP. Latent papillomavirus and recurring genital warts. N Engl J Med 1985; 313:784–8.
136. Bonnez W, Elswick RK Jr, Bailey-Farchione A, et al. Efficacy and safety of 0.5% podofilox solution in the treatment and suppression of anogenital warts. Am J Med 1994; 96:420–5.
137. Syed TA, Lundin S, Ahmad SA. Topical 0.3% and 0.5% podophyllotoxin cream for self-treatment of condylomata acuminata in women. A placebo-controlled, double-blind study. Dermatology 1994; 189:142–5.
138. Mohanty KC. The cost-effectiveness of treatment of genital warts with podophyllotoxin. Int J STD AIDS 1994; 5:253–6.
139. Dodi G, Infantino A, Moretti R, Scalco G, Lise M. Cryotherapy of anorectal warts and condylomata. Cryobiology 1982; 19:287–8.
140. Bonnez W, Oakes D, Bailey-Farchione A, et al. A randomized, double-blind, placebo-controlled trial of systemically administered interferon-alpha, -beta, or -gamma in combination with cryotherapy for the treatment of condyloma acuminatum. J Infect Dis 1995; 171:1081–9.
141. Handley JM, Horner T, Maw RD, Lawther H, Dinsmore WW. Subcutaneous interferon alpha 2a combined with cryotherapy vs cryotherapy alone in the treatment of primary anogenital warts: a randomized observer blind placebo controlled study. Genitourin Med 1991; 67:297–302.
142. Armstrong DK, Maw RD, Dinsmore WW, et al. A randomised, double-blind, parallel group study to compare subcutaneous interferon alpha 2a plus podophyllin with placebo plus podophyllin in the treatment of primary condyloma acuminatum. Genitourin Med 1994; 70:389–93.
143. Jacobson MA, Mills J. Serious cytomegalovirus disease in the acquired immunodeficiency syndrome: Clinical findings, diagnosis, and treatment. Ann Intern Med 1988; 108–585.
144. Drew WL. Cytomegalovirus infection in patients with AIDS. J Infect Dis 1988; 158:449.
145. Collier AC, Meyers JD, et al. Cytomegalovirus infection in homosexual men: relationship to sexual practices, antibody to human immunodeficiency virus, and cell-mediated immunity. Am J Med 1987; 82:593–601.
146. Drew WL, Mintz L, Miner RC, Sands M, Ketterer B. Prevalence of cytomegalovirus in homosexual men. J Infect Dis 1981; 143:188–92.
147. Chandler SH, Holmes KK, Wentworth BD, et al. the epidemiology of cytomegalovirus infection in women attending a sexually transmitted disease clinic. J Infect Dis 1985; 152:587–605.

148. Handsfield HH, Chandler SH, Caine VA, et al. Cytomegalovirus infection in sex partners: evidence for sexual transmission. J Infect Dis 1985; 151:344–8.
149. Gallant JE, Moore RD, Richman DD, et al. Zidovudine Epidemiology Study Group. Incidence and natural history of cytomegalovirus disease in patients with advanced HIV disease treated with zidovudine. J Infect Dis 1992; 166:1223.
150. Bennett MR, Fine AP, Hanlon JT. Cytomegalovirus hemorrhagic colitis in a non-transplant patient. Postgrad Med J 1985; 77:227–9.
151. Knapp AB, Horst DA, Eliopoulos G, Gramm HF, Gaber LW, Falchuk KR, et al. Widespread cytomegalovirus gastroenterocolitis in a patient with acquired immunodeficiency syndrome. Gastroenterology 1983; 85:1399–1402.
152. Cunningham M, Cantoni L, Humair L. Cytomegalovirus primo-infection in a patient with idiopathic proctitis. Am J Gastroenterol 1986; 81:586–8.
153. Diepersloot RJ, Kroes AC, Visser W, Jiwa NM, Rothbarth PH. Acute ulcerative proctocolitis associated with primary cytomegalovirus infection. Arch Intern Med 1990; 150:1749–51.
154. Lewis-Jones HG, Ward RG, Garvey C. Cytomegalovirus infection masquerading as colonic neoplasia. Br J Radiol 1990; 63:573–4.
155. Puy-Montbrun T, Ganansia R, Lemarchand N, Delechenault P, Denis J. Anal ulcerations due to cytomegalovirus in patients with AIDS: Report of six cases. Dis Colon Rectum 1990; 33:1041–3.
156. Kamel PL. Cytomegalovirus-associated perianal ulceration in AIDS. J Clin Gastroenterol 1992; 14:105–8.
157. Horn TD, Hood AF. Cytomegalovirus is predictably present in perianal ulcers in immunosuppressed patients. Arch Dermatol 1990; 126:642–4.
158. Surawicz CM, Myerson D. Self-limited cytomegalovirus colitis in immunocompetent individuals. Gastroenterology 1988; 94:194–9.
159. Maignan M, Wahl D, Thiaucourt D, Bach D, De Korwin JD, Vaillant G, Paille F, Schmitt J. Self-limited primary cytomegalovirus colitis in an immunocompetent individual. J Intern Med 1992; 232:357–9.
160. Grundy JE. Virologic and pathogenic aspects of cytomegalovirus infection. Rev Infect Dis 1990; 12:S711-9.
161. Frank D, Raicht R. Intestinal perforation associated with cytomegalovirus infection in patients with acquired immunodeficiency syndrome. Am J Gastroenterol 1984; 79:201–5.
162. Hinnant HL, Rotterdam HZ, Bell ET, Tapper ML. Cytomegalovirus infection of the alimentary tract: a clinicopathologic correlation. Am J Gastroenterol 1986; 81:944-50.
163. Cuipepper-Morgan JA, Kotler DP, Scholes JV, Tierney AR. Evaluation of diagnostic criteria for mucosal cytomegalic inclusion disease in the acquired immunodeficiency syndrome. Am J Gastroenterol 1987; 82:1264–70.
164. Schwartz DA, Wilcox CM. Atypical cytomegalovirus inclusions in gastrointestinal biopsy specimens from patients with the acquired immunodeficiency syndrome: diagnostic role of in situ nucleic acid hybridization. Hum Pathol 1992; 23:1019–26.
165. van der Bij W, Torensma R, van Son WJ, Anema J, Schim J, Tagzess AM, et

al. Rapid immunodiagnosis of active cytomegalovirus infection by monoclonal antibody staining of blood leucocytes. J Med Virol 1988; 25:179–88.
166. Chachoua A, Dieterich DT, Krasinski K, et al. Ganciclovir in the treatment of cytomegalovirus gastrointestinal disease with the acquired immunodeficiency syndrome. Ann Intern Med 1987; 107:133–7.
167. Dieterich DT, Kotler DP, Busch DF, et al. Ganciclovir treatment of cytomegalovirus colitis in AIDS: a randomized, double blinded, placebo controlled multicenter study. J Infect Dis 1993; 167:278–92.
168. Reed EC, Wolford JL, Kopecky KJ, Lilleby KE, Dandidker PS, Todaro JL, et al. Ganciclovir for the treatment of cytomegalovirus gastroenteritis in bone marrow transplant patients: A randomized placebo controlled trial. Ann Intern Med 1990; 112:505–10.
169. Erice A, Chou S, Biron KK, Stanat SC, Balfour HH Jr, Jordan MC. Progressive disease due to ganciclovir resistant cytomegalovirus in immunocompromised hosts. N Engl J Med 1989; 320:289–93.
170. Drew WL, Miner RC, Busch DF, Follansbee SE, Gulett J, Mehalko SG, et al. Prevalence of resistance in patients receiving ganciclovir for serious cytomegalovirus infections. J Infect Dis 1991; 163:716–9.
171. Nelson MR, Connolly GM, Hawkins DA, Gazzard BG. Foscarnet in the treatment of CMV infection of the esophagus and colon in patients with AIDS. Amer J Gastro 1991; 86:876–81.
172. Dieterich DT, Poles MA, Dicker M, Tepper R, Lew E. Foscarnet treatment of CMV gastrointestinal infections in AIDS patients who have failed ganciclovir induction. Amer J Gastro 1993; 88:542–8.
173. Phillips SC, Mildvan D, William DC, Gelb AM, White MC. Sexual transmission of enteric protozoa and helminths in a venereal disease clinic population. N Engl J Med 1981; 305:603–6.
174. Allason-Jones E, Mindel A, Sargeaunt PG, Williams P. Entamoeba histolytica as a commensal intestinal parasite in homosexual men. N Engl J Med 1986; 315:353–6.
175. Pearce RB, Abrahms DI. Entamoeba histolytica in homosexual men. N Engl J Med 1987; 316:691–2.
176. Sargeaunt PG, Williams JE, Grene JD. The differentiation of invasive and non-invasive Entamoeba histolytica by isoenzyme electrophoresis. Trans R Soc Trop Med Hyg 1978; 72:519–21.
177. Petri WA Jr, Jackson TFHG, Gathiram V, et al. Pathogenic and nonpathogenic strains of Entamoeba histolytica can be differentiated by monoclonal antibodies to the galactose-specific adherence lectin. Infect Immun 1990; 58:1802–6.
178. Tannich E, Horstmann RD, Knobloch J, et al. Genomic DNA differences between pathogenic and nonpathogenic Entamoeba histolytica. Proc Natl Acad Sci USA 1989; 86:5118–22.
179. Gathiram V, Jackson TFHG. Frequency distribution of E. histolytica zymodemes in a rural South African population. Lancet 1985; 1:719–21.
180. Abd-Alla MD, Jackson TFHG, Gathiram V, El-Hawey AM, Ravdin JI. Differentiation of pathogenic and non-pathogenic Entamoeba histolytica infection by de-

tection of galactose-inhibitable adherence protein antigen in sera and feces. J Clin Microbiol 1993; 31:2845–50.
181. Ravdin JI. Intestinal disease caused by Entamoeba histolytica. In: Ravdin JI, ed. Amebiasis: human infection caused by Entamoeba histolytica. New York: Churchill Livingston, 1988:495–510.
182. Pillai S, Mohimen A. A solid-phase sandwich radioimmunoassay for Entamoeba histolytica proteins and the detection of circulating antigens in amoebiasis. Gastroenterology 1982; 83:1210–6.
183. Reed SL, Wessel DW, Davis CD. Entamoeba histolytica infection and AIDS. Am J Med 1991; 90:260–71.
184. Ravdin JI. Diagnosis of invasive amebiasis - time to end the morphology era. Gut 1994; 35:1018–21.
185. Krogstad DJ. Isoenzyme patterns and pathogenicity in amebic infection. N Engl J Med 1986; 315:390–1.
186. Gathiram V, Jackson TFHG. A longitudinal study of asymptomatic carriers of pathogenic zymodemes of Entamoeba histolytica. S Afr J Med 1987; 72:669–72.
187. Petri WA, Ravdin JI. Treatment of homosexual men infected with Entamoeba histolytica (letter). N Engl J Med 1986; 315:393.
188. Allason-Jones E, Mindel A, Sargeaunt PG, Katz D. Outcome of untreated infection with Entamoeba histolytica in homosexual men with and without HiV antibody. Br Med J 1988: 297:654–7.
189. Goldmeier D, Sargeaunt PG, Price AB, et al. Is Entamoeba histolytica in homosexual men a pathogen? Lancet 1986; 1:641–4.
190. Nanda R, Bevaja UK, Anand BS. Entamoeba histolytica cyst passers: Clinical features and outcome in untreated subjects. Lancet 1984; 2:301–3.
191. Anand BS, Tuteja MD, Kaur M, et al. Entamoeba histolytica cyst passers: Clinical profile and spontaneous eradication of infection. Dig Dis Sci 1993; 38:1825–30.
192. Kacker PP. A case of Giardia lamblia proctitis presenting to a V.D. clinic. Br J Venereal Dis 1973; 49:318–9.
193. Cook GC. Parasitic disease in clinical practice. London: Springer-Verlag, 1990.
194. Weller IVD. The gay bowel. Gut 1985; 26:869–75.
195. Cook GC. Enterobius vermicularis infection. Gut 1994; 35:1159–62.
196. Elford J, McDonald A, Kaldor JM. Kaposi's sarcoma as a sexually transmissible infection: an analysis of Australian AIDS surveillance data. The National HIV surveillance committee. AIDS 1993; 7:1667–71.
197. Beral V, Peterman TA, Berkelman RL, Jaffe HW. Kaposi's sarcoma among persons with AIDS: a sexually transmitted infection? Lancet 1990; 335:123–8.
198. Felman YM. Recent developments in sexually transmitted diseases: is Kaposi's sarcoma a sexually transmitted disease? Cutis 1990; 46:303–6.
199. Archiband CP, Schechter MT, Craib KJ, et al. Evidence for a sexually transmitted cofactor for Kaposi's sarcoma in a cohort of homosexual men. Int Conf AIDS 1990; 6:282.
200. Zampese M, Sander E, Rossi V, Reis M, Schwartsmann G. AIDS-associated

Kaposi's sarcoma (KS) in a couple: an additional evidence of KS as a sexually transmitted infection. Int Conf AIDS 1993; 9:401.

201. Albrecht H, Helm EB, Plettenberg A, Emminger C, Heise W, Stellbrink HJ. Kaposi's sarcoma in HIV infected women living in Germany—strong evidence for sexual transmission. Int Conf AIDS 1993; 9:395.
202. Endean ED, Ross CW, Strodel WE. Kaposi's sarcoma appearing as a rectal ulcer. Surgery 1987; 101:767–9.
203. Ensoli B, Barillari G, Giorelli V, et al. Biological mechanisms in the pathogenesis of AIDS associated Kaposi's sarcoma (meeting abstract). Proc Annu Meet Am Assoc Cancer Res 1994; 35:659.
204. Krown SE. AIDS-related Kaposi's sarcoma: clinical aspects (meeting abstract). Proc Annu Meet Am Assoc Cancer Res 1994; 35:659–60.
205. Lorenz HP, Wilson W, Leigh B, Schecter W. Kaposi's sarcoma of the rectum in patients with the acquired immunodeficiency syndrome. Am J Surg 1990; 160:681–3.
206. Volberding P. Clinical management of HIV-related malignancies. Annu Conf Australias Soc HIV Med 1993; 5:23.
207. Rabkin CS. Epidemiology of AIDS-related malignancies. Curr Opin Oncol 1994; 6:492–6.
208. Broder S. Overview of AIDS malignancies (meeting abstract). Proc Annu Meet Am Assoc Cancer Res 1994; 35:658.
209. Deans GT, McAleer JJA, Spence RAJ. Malignant anal tumors. Br J Surg 1994; 81:500–8.
210. Law CLH, Qassim M, Cunningham AL, Mulhall B, Grierson JM. Nonspecific proctitis: Association with human immunodeficiency virus infection in homosexual men. J Infect Dis 1992; 165:150–4.
211. Wilcox CM, Schwartz DA. Idiopathic anorectal ulceration in patients with human immunodeficiency virus infection. Am J Gastro 1994; 89:599–604.
212. Bach MC, Howell DA, Valenti AJ, et al. Aphthous ulceration of the gastrointestinal tract in patients with the acquired immunodeficiency syndrome (AIDS). Ann Intern Med 1990; 112:465–7.
213. Miles AJG, Connolly GM, Barton SE, et al. Persistent ulceration of the anal margin in homosexuals with HIV infection. J R Soc Med 1991; 84:87–8.
214. Nelson JA, Wiley Ca, Reynolds-Kohler C, Reese CE, Margaretten W, Levy JA. Human immunodeficiency virus in bowel epithelium from patients with gastrointestinal symptoms. Lancet 1988; 1:259–62.

15

Escherichia coli–Associated Diarrhea

PETER D. BLOOM, DAVID K. R. KARAOLIS, and EDGAR C. BOEDEKER
University of Maryland, Baltimore, Maryland

I. INTRODUCTION

Escherichia coli (*E. coli*) are gram negative rods which are the most prevalent facultative anaerobes in feces. *E. coli* is a diverse bacterial species comprising both commensal strains, which populate the mammalian colon, and pathogenic strains associated with systemic or mucosal (intestinal or urinary tract) disease. Pathogenic *E. coli*, which are associated with diarrheal disease, may be considered as clonal variants which have acquired the genetic information required for virulence encoded on extrachromosomal elements (plasmids), on bacteriophage which may be incorporated into the chromosome, or as large segments of inserted chromosomal DNA termed pathogenicity islands. Important aspects of virulence are the abilities to leave the colonic lumen; to colonize the small intestine; to colonize or invade epithelial cells; to translocate and survive systemically; and to produce toxins.

At present there are four major categories of *E. coli* recognized as causing diarrheal disease in humans which will be discussed here in detail: enteropathogenic *E. coli* (EPEC), enterotoxigenic *E. coli* (ETEC), enterohemorrhagic *E. coli* (EHEC) and enteroinvasive *E. coli* (EIEC). These four classes of *E. coli* have quite distinct modes of pathogenesis and they differ in their clinical presentation, epidemiology, and treatment recommendations. Other human pathogenic diarrheal clones of *E. coli* are continually emerging, and some of those which have begun to be defined include those with enteroaggregative (EAggEC) or diffusely adherent (DAEC) phenotypes. In addition, other pathogenic clones have emerged which distinctly target animal hosts, in a species-specific manner, but these are beyond the scope of the present chapter.

II. ENTEROPATHOGENIC *E. COLI* (EPEC)

The enteropathogenic *E. coli* strains isolated from infants with "summer diarrhea" and nosocomial nursery epidemics were the first *E. coli* recognized to cause diarrheal disease. Adam (1), in Germany in 1923, associated certain sorbitol-fermenting *E. coli* with infant infection and termed them "dyspepsiekoli". In 1933, Goldschmidt (2), well in advance of the serotyping scheme (1947) of Kauffman (3), showed that *E. coli* isolated from an epidemic were a serologically distinct group. In the 1940s, Bray isolated "*Bact. coli neapolitanum*" from the stools of 42 out of 44 cases of summer diarrhea, which the pediatrician Beavan noted to have a characteristic seminal odor. Antiserum raised in a pet rabbit to one of the isolates agglutinated *E. coli* from 95% of the infants with diarrhea, but only a few isolates from non-diarrheic infants.

Neter et al. (4) first proposed the term enteropathogenic *E. coli* (EPEC) to define, among epidemiologically unrelated clinical *E. coli* isolates, certain serotypes, with unique combinations of O (lipopolysaccharide), H (flagellar) and K (capsular) antigens, which were more often associated with diarrheal disease, than were the serotypes isolated from healthy controls. By Kauffman's methods, Adam's AI was serotype O55:K59, his AIV was O111:K58 and "*B. coli neapolitanum*" was O111:H-; all classical EPEC serotypes (5–8). From the 1950's until the 1970's serotyping remained the sole means of identifying this class of diarrhea-associated *E. coli*. As pathogenic mechanisms (including toxins and invasion) were defined for other classes of diarrhea-associated *E. coli*, but found to be absent in EPEC, the true virulence of these strains was questioned. Volunteer challenge studies conducted by Levine et al. (9) demonstrated that these strains were true pathogens, although their virulence mechanisms remained to be defined. Although EPEC now seldom cause disease in neonatal wards in industrialized nations (10), EPEC serotyping is still of some utility since EPEC of classical serotypes continue to cause disease in many parts of the world. However, definition of the genetically determined molecular pathogenic mechanisms of EPEC (16) has provided specific functional assays (18,30) and molecular probes (45–47) capable of identifying these disease related strains. It is now understood that EPEC pathogenesis is related to their unique association with, and alteration of, intestinal absorptive epithelial cells.

A. Presentation

EPEC infections may be prolonged and relapses are frequent. Stools are watery, but without blood or mucus. Fasting stool outputs of 100-200 ml/kg/day lead to dehydration in young infants. Vomiting often accompanies the diarrhea. Low grade fever is common; and anemia, weight loss, hypoalbuminemia and low serum bicarbonate are seen in protracted cases. Infants usually resume a normal growth curve after resolution of the illness. Delays of up to a month prior to initiation of effective therapy, as may occur in early cases during outbreaks, may lead to complications such as acrodermatitis-like skin rash requiring zinc replacement as high as 200-500 μg/kg/day. EPEC sepsis has not been documented. In early studies, overall mortality was around 30%, with fatality rates in epidemics as high as 50%, but more recent experience (11) suggests a much lower mortality rate (1 in 15) with the use of combined antibiotic and parenteral nutrition regimens.

B. Molecular Pathogenesis

EPEC produce a characteristic attaching and effacing (AE) lesion, best defined at the electron microscopic level (Fig. 1) in which the bacteria adhere intimately to the enterocyte surface in areas of localized destruction (effacement) of microvilli, and cytoskeletal rearrangement. These lesions were described in detail, and named, by Moon et al. (12) utilizing animal models. They had previously been observed by Staley (13) in O55 strains in newborn pigs, and by Polotsky (14), in the Soviet Union, in rabbit intestinal loops infected with EPEC strains. These lesions were not observed in human infections until the 1980's (11,15)

The development of these lesions can best be understood in terms of a three stage model (Fig. 2) of EPEC pathogenesis (16) in which initial attachment to intact epithelial cells (stage I) is mediated by type IV fimbriae. Microvillus effacement (stage II) accompanies a signal transduction cascade, leading to intimate attachment (stage III) with aggregation of filamentous F-actin in pedestals beneath adherent organisms. Stage I adherence is encoded by plasmid associated genes. Virulence genes sufficient for Stages II and III adherence are present in a 35 kilobase chromosomal "pathogenicity island" termed the locus of enterocyte effacement (LEE) (35).

Stage I Adherence

Cravioto et al. (17) demonstrated that 80% of EPEC isolates adhered to HEp-2 cells in tissue culture monolayers. This adherence was mannose resistant, therefore not mediated by common Type I fimbriae, and was rare in other *E. coli* isolates with only 14% of ETEC and 17% of normal flora *E. coli* isolates adhering. Scaletsky et al. (18) first reported that EPEC isolates have a distinctive pattern of adherence to HeLa cells termed "localized adherence" (LA), in which the bacteria aggregate in microcolonies on the surface of cultured cells. Baldini et al. (19) showed that this LA phenotype was encoded on a 70 MDa conjugative plasmid (pMAR2) in EPEC strain E2348/69 (serotype O127:H6), an isolate which caused diarrhea in volunteers (9). The name EPEC adherence factor (EAF) was given to a putative adhesin specified by the plasmid. Further volunteer challenge studies (20) showed that the EAF plasmid was necessary for full expression of pathogenicity, but its elimination did not completely eliminate virulence. Moreover, this plasmid was neither sufficient nor essential to produce the AE lesion in vitro (21). Giron detected plasmid-encoded Type IV fimbriae, which he termed "bundle forming pili" (BFP), after passage of an EPEC O111 strain on sheep blood (22). These BFP (Fig. 2,I) fimbriae tend to aggregate, forming bundles which induce the formation of microcolonies of bacteria, and are the best candidate for an EAF explaining the localized adherence phenotype.

Stage II Signaling

Donnenberg et al. (23) used transposon (TnPhoA) mutagenesis to identify a series of plasmid and chromosomal mutants of EPEC strain E2348/69 that were unable to invade HEp-2 cells. These mutants affected stage I (*bfp*), and stage III (*eae*) (vide infra), genes, as well as additional regions involved in signal transduction. It was demonstrated (24,25) that, after binding to epithelial cells, EPEC induce: elevation of intracellular calcium, generation of inositol phosphate, and tyrosine phosphorylation of eukaryotic proteins, the major phosphorylation substrate being a 90 kDa protein (Hp90)(Fig. 2,II). Hp90 phosphorylation, and AE lesion formation, requires the secretion of the products of genes *esp* (for *E. coli* secreted protein) *A* and *B* which lie just downstream of *eae*. Approximately 9Kb upstream from the *eae* gene lies a chromosomal region encoding a series of proteins characteristic of a Type III secretory apparatus, typically involved in the secretion and translocation of virulence determinants in both bacterial and plant pathogens. This family includes the products of Salmonella invA (26), Yersinia lcrD (27), and S. flexneri mxiA (28) secretory systems. These EPEC genes have been named *sep* (for secretion of *E. coli* proteins) by Jarvis et al. (29) and *sepA* and *sepB* are necessary for the secretion of signaling proteins.

Stage III Adherence

By electron microscopy (Fig. 1) EPEC are seen to be resting on a pedestal-like structures protruding from enterocytes which contain condensed aggregates of filamentous actin. Fluorescein isothiocyanate (FITC)-phalloidin, the fluorescein conjugate of a phallotoxin, binds specifically to polymerized F-actin (Fig. 2,III),

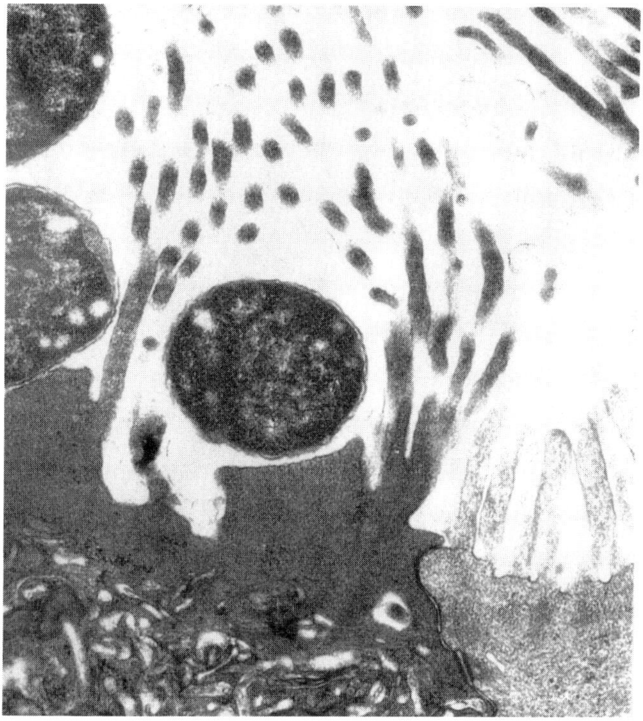

Figure 1 Enteropathogenic *E. coli* (EPEC) attaching/effacing (AE) lesion. Electron micrograph of an EPEC strain intimately adhering to an effaced intestinal epithelial cell. Note microvillus elongation and pedestal formation.

and is used to detect EPEC, at the light microscopic level, by the fluorescence of aggregated actin in epithelial cells underlying the attached bacteria. This forms the basis of the diagnostic fluorescent actin staining test (FAS) initially for EPEC (30). Jerse (31) used transposon mutagenesis, in conjunction with FAS testing, to identify a chromosomal gene *eae* (for *E. coli* attaching and effacing) required for the characteristic AE lesion. This gene was found to encode a 94-kDa outer membrane protein which was named intimin, and which shared homology with the integrin-binding invasin protein of *Yersinia*. Deletion of the *eae* gene was found to abolish AE activity in tissue culture and to significantly reduce the occurrence of diarrhea in volunteers (32,33). Moreover, full expression of intimin was shown to be under the control of a regulatory gene (*per*) in the EAF plasmid (34). Thus intimin has been shown to be the major determinant of Stage III attachment of EPEC to epithelial cells.

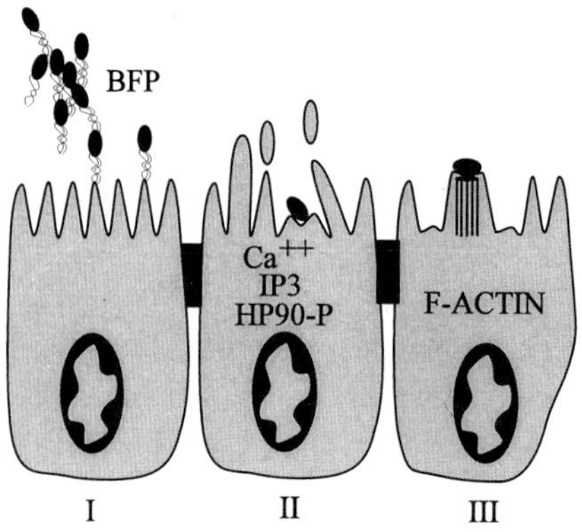

Figure 2 Three stages of the enteropathogenic *E. coli* (EPEC) attaching/effacing (AE) lesions. Stage I attachment is mediated by bundle-forming pili (BFP). Stage II (effacement) is associated with a signal transduction cascade of increased intracellular Ca++, inositol triphosphate (IP3) and tyrosine phosphorylation of a 90 kDa membrane protein (HP90-P). Stage III (intimate attachment) is mediated by bacterial intimin with the formation of condensed F-actin pedestals beneath closely adherent organisms.

Locus of Enterocyte Effacement (LEE)

Recently, McDaniel et al. (35) showed that a continuous 35-kb locus termed LEE (for locus of enterocyte effacement) contained genes sufficient for the formation of AE lesions including *eae*, *espB* and *sep* genes. This region was not found in normal flora, laboratory strains, or ETEC. In addition, probes spanning several regions within this locus were also found to be present in other bacterial pathogens that cause AE lesions including EHEC, *Citrobacter freundii*, and *Hafnia alvei*. This region is currently being investigated in several bacterial strains, but it appears to be a region of acquired DNA lying between typical insertion sequences, which is characteristic of a pathogenicity island.

C. Epidemiology

EPEC diarrhea is predominantly a disease of infants, however, there have been reports of sporadic outbreaks occurring in adults (36,37), including apparently healthy individuals (38,39). These outbreaks have usually been common-source outbreaks in which a large inoculum was presumably ingested. In the volunteer challenge studies performed by Levine et al (9,20) adults receiving inocula of 10^{10} organisms with bicarbonate to neutralize gastric acidity experienced diarrhea in 60-100% of cases depending on the strain administered. At times, this diarrhea was "cholera-like." Adult volunteers receiving inocula of 10^6 CFU, or fewer, rarely experienced diarrhea.

There is a strong age distribution of infection, the peak incidence occurring at about 6 months of age with the disease rarely occurring in children over 1 year of age (40). Large outbreaks of acute nosocomial diarrhea in developed countries are uncommon, but there have been reports of chronic diarrhea caused by EPEC in the U.S., including some child-care center outbreaks (41,42). Gurwith et al (43) compared the clinical course of EPEC diarrhea with that of non-bacterial gastroenteritis in hospitalized children in Winnipeg. Total duration was about 9 days in both groups, but the duration before hospitalization was twice as long in the EPEC group (4.6 vs. 2.4 days) and duration of diarrhea was longer in younger children. Most cases occurred in children under one year of age with the majority less than 6 months. EPEC disease was judged to be about as severe as that due to *Shigella sonnei*, and more severe than the nonbacterial cases.

D. Laboratory Diagnosis

The colonies of EPEC appear essentially identical to commensal *E. coli* on solid media containing lactose as a carbon source. Before the recognition of specific virulence factors, EPEC were traditionally identified by the presence of certain O:H:K antigen combinations. The serotypes with a worldwide predominance that have been shown to be associated with EPEC diarrheal disease are in serogroups O26, O55, O86, O111, O125, O126, O127, and O128. Thus, screening with pooled serotyping antisera has been important in differentiating EPEC from non-pathogenic commensal *E. coli* strains, but has largely been abandoned in the United States because of low incidence of EPEC infections, and the importance of other pathogenic types of *E. coli.* Full serotyping is only done in a few reference centers. Observation of characteristic localized adherence patterns in HeLa cells is still widely used in epidemiologic surveys (18). The fluorescent actin staining test (FAS), using FITC-phalloidin to identify AE lesions in Hep-2 cells, can be applied as a functional test (30). The plasmid from the EPEC plasmid pMAR2, encoding genes responsible for the localized adherence of EPEC to Hep-2 cells, has been used to provide a DNA probe capable of identifying the majority of classical EPEC isolates (44–46) in epidemiological studies. Other DNA probes have been prepared to identify *bfp*, and the *sep*, *esp*, and *eae* genes of the locus of enterocyte effacement, but their use remains largely a research tool.

E. Treatment and Prevention

Therapy is aimed at restoring hydration, administering effective antibiotics to eradicate the pathogens and then maintaining hydration and nutrition. The disease usually responds rapidly to administration of appropriate antibiotic therapy. This requires good in vitro sensitivity testing, particularly in epidemics, since the isolates are often multiply resistant, particularly to ampicillin, carbenicillin, cephalothin, kanamycin, sulfisoxazole and neomycin. They are often sensitive to chloramphenicol, gentamicin and tobramicin. Ampicillin has never been shown to be effective (47). Previous ampicillin therapy may favor infection, since a history of prior administration of ampicillin was frequent in protracted cases. Administration of oral, non-absorbable aminoglycosides, such as neomycin (100 mg/kg/day) may be initiated (48). Short courses of antibiotics may be used, since ten days of oral neomycin therapy was no better than three days of treatment (49). In Ethiopia (50), both trimethoprim-sulamethoxazole and mecillinam gave clinical and bacteriological cures at three days.

III. ENTEROTOXIGENIC *E. COLI* (ETEC)

The second major class of *E. coli* to be associated with diarrhea were the enterotoxin-producing ETEC, which were recognized in the late 1960s and early 1970s (51,52).

A. Presentation

ETEC are an important cause of diarrhea in infants and young children in developing countries, particularly in the tropics. They are also the most common cause of travelers diarrhea, which occurs in adult traveler's from industrialized countries who visit these endemic areas in the developing world. Similar disease were recognized earlier in neonatal herd animals including piglets, lambs, and calves (53). ETEC infection is characterized by watery diarrhea, often accompanied by low-grade fever, abdominal cramps, malaise, and vomiting. In its most severe clinical form, ETEC infection can cause cholera-like purging leading to dehydration, even in adults.

B. Molecular Pathogenesis

ETEC colonize the proximal small intestine where they can elaborate a heat-labile enterotoxin that is very similar to cholera toxin, a heat-stable enterotoxin, or they can elaborate both. The genes encoding these enterotoxins are found on transmissible plasmids (54). ETEC produce fimbrial adhesins, designated coli surface (CS) or colonization factors antigens (CFAs), which enable them to adhere to the small intestinal epithelium. By this mechanism they can overcome intestinal peristalsis them to colonize the small bowel (54). The fimbriae are encoded by plasmids that nearly always also encode ST and often LT. Thus the basic pathogenic mechanisms for ETEC infection are two: (Fig. 3) i. small intestinal colonization mediated by fimbrial adhesins and ii. the production of enterotoxins which induce intestinal secretion.

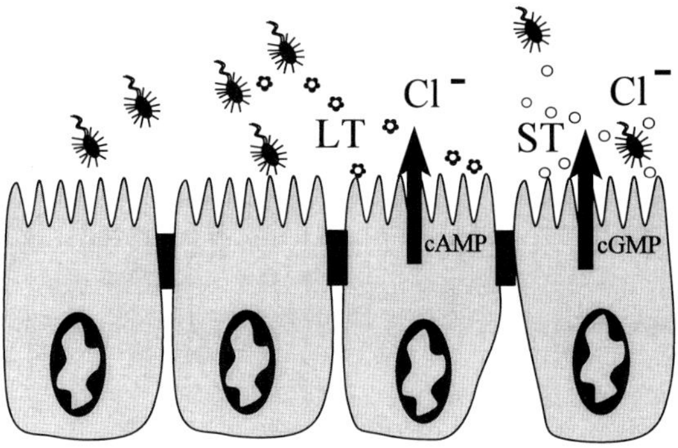

Figure 3 Enterotoxigenic *E. coli* (ETEC) pathogenesis. Motile ETEC organisms (upper left) adhere to normal small intestinal epithelial cells by their fimbrial colonization factor antigens (CFAs). They induce chloride secretion by the action of heat-labile toxin (LT) [pentamers] or heat stable toxin (ST) [circles].

1. Toxins

ETEC are characterized by the ability to synthesize the heat-labile toxin (LT) and/or the heat-stable toxin (ST). Genes encoding production of these enterotoxins are found on transferrable plasmids. Approximately 40% of ETEC strains isolated from cases of traveler's diarrhea and from non-hospitalized infants in endemic areas are of the LT+/ST+ phenotype, another 40% have LT–/ST+ strains, and the remainder yield LT+/ST– organisms (55). When village-based or outpatient studies are carried out in endemic areas, the most frequent isolates are LT–/ST+ (56). In contrast, in hospitalized patients (presumably the most severe cases), LT+/ST+ strains predominate (56).

a. LT is high-molecular-weight protein that resembles cholera toxin (CT) in structure, function, and mechanism of action. Both LT and CT are composed of one enzymatically active (ADP-ribosylating) A subunit joined to five receptor-binding B subunits. The receptors for LT B subunit found on enterocytes include GM1 ganglioside and a second glycoprotein (57). Following binding of LT to an enterocyte by its B subunits, the A subunit enters the cell. LT ADP-ribosylates the Gsá GTP-binding protein, leading to activation of adenylate cyclase in the enterocyte, and accumulation of cyclic AMP. The intracellular accumulation of cAMP elicits secretion by crypt cells and decreased absorption by villus tip cells. LT from human ETEC pathogens (LTh) is closely related to, but distinct from, LT found in porcine ETEC strains (LTp) (58). Both LTh and LTp are immunologically related to cholera toxin (59).

b. The heat-stable toxins represent a group of enterotoxigenic molecules which are found in many enteric pathogens. Two antigenically distinct types are found in ETEC: STa and STb. The former has been strongly linked to diarrheal disease. The latter has been shown to be associated with diarrhea in pigs, but its role in human disease is as yet unclear. ST is a small polypeptide. The active moiety is the common C-terminal 18-amino acid segment (60) containing six cysteines producing folding by internal disulfide bridges. The toxin binds to a membrane receptor located on a glycoprotein receptor/guanylate cyclase complex (61,62). ST thereby activates the particulate intestinal guanylate cyclase activity leading to an intracellular accumulation of cyclic GMP and inducing a net secretory state in the enterocyte (63). ST produced in vivo in the course of infection does not induce an antibody response.

2. *Fimbriae*

The adhesins of ETEC are non-flagellar hairlike appendages termed fimbriae (or pili) which mediate attachment to small bowel epithelium by lectin-like mechanisms involving host carbohydrate receptors (64). These diarrhea-associated *E. coli* appear to have adapted these adherence mechanisms to aid in colonization of the bowel (65), and the adhesins on ETEC of human origin have been designated colonization factor antigens (CFAs). In the presence of mannose, many fimbrial colonization factors mediate hemagglutination of certain erythrocytes, which distinguishes them from common type 1 fimbriae (64). There are three major groups of CFAs expressed by human ETEC strains, termed CFA/I, CFA/II and CFA/IV. Their structures are long filaments assembled from repeating protein subunits (subunit M.W.range 14-25Kd) which have been shown to exhibit several different morphologies at the electron microscopic level (66). The simplest case is CFA/I, whose morphology appears rigid and tubular with a diameter of approximately 7 nm, and which is made up a single repeating subunit. A second distinct morphology is that of thinner, flexible, wiry structures, often called fibrillae or fimbrillae (eg., CS3) (67). CFA/II and CFA/IV are complexes of surface structures consisting, in each case, of one of two antigenically distinct, but genetically related (68), types of fimbriae (CS1 and CS2 in CFA/II strains; CS4 and CS5 in CFA/IV strains) expressed together with the finer fibrillar structures (CS3 in CFA/II and CS6 in CFA/IV). Most ETEC so far studied possess one of these surface structures. From the point of view of antigen selection for vaccine development, approximately 80% of surveyed ETEC would express CFA/I, CS3 or CS6 (69). Recent studies using monoclonal antibodies suggest that diverse CFAs which appear to be antigenically distinct may share cross-reactive epitopes which might be exploited for vaccine design (70). More recently, structures (such as those named "longus" [71]) which do not fall easily into either group have also been identified; and new fimbriae are frequently identified in ETEC of novel serotypes (72).

The genetics of ETEC fimbriae frequently involve the interaction plasmid encoded and chromosomally encoded gene products. All are encoded by clusters of genes whose products are necessary for assembly and processing of the fimbrial proteins, in addition to the subunits constituting the physical structure of the fimbria itself. For most human ETEC, the major fimbrial subunit appears also to serve as the adhesin (in contrast to the case in urinary tract pathogens in which unique subunits serve as adhesins localized only at the tips of fimbriae). The expression of many ETEC fimbriae requires the presence of a DNA binding protein which activates transcription of fimbrial genes. These proteins are members of the AraC family of DNA binding proteins (73). There is a close correlation between presence of specific fimbrial adhesins and specific O serogroups. Thus, CFA/I is found in O15, O25, O63, O78, and O128 strains, whereas CFA/II is seen in O6, O8, O80, and O85 strains, and CFA/IV fimbriae are found in O25, O115, and O167 strains.

C. Epidemiology

When collections of ETEC from diverse geographic sources are serotyped, a limited number of O:H serotypes occur repeatedly throughout the world and account for the majority of the ETEC isolates (74–78). The most prevalent ETEC serotypes implicated in human diarrheal disease are O6, O8, O15, O20, O25, O27, O63, O80, O85, O115, O128, O128, and O159.

ETEC cause 30-72% of traveler's diarrhea (79). In industrialized countries, ETEC rarely cause infant or childhood diarrhea. The studies of Black et al in Bangladesh show that ETEC and rotavirus infection together are responsible for two-thirds of the cases of dehydrating infant diarrhea in that country (80). Prospective village-based studies carried out in a cohort of children in Bangladesh showed that in the first 2 years of life each child suffers an average of six to seven separate episodes of diarrhea per year (81). Approximately two episodes per child per year are due to ETEC. ETEC are the one enteropathogen that was significantly correlated with the development of clinical malnutrition.

In endemic areas, incidence rates diminish progressively after the first two years (82). Serological and epidemiological evidence strongly supports the notion that acquired immunity is responsible for low incidence rates in adults. The prevalence of LT antitoxin and of anti-CFA antibodies is high in older children and adults, as are mean titers. In contrast, when adult travelers from industrialized countries visit less developed areas, they are quite susceptible and attack rates for diarrhea are high.

D. Laboratory Diagnosis

Because of acute onset, and the self-limited nature, of ETEC infections, particularly in travelers, ETEC are seldom isolated from, and identified in, affected individuals prior to treatment. In contrast to the case with EHEC, no culture conditions help to screen ETEC from commensal *E. coli*. In epidemiologic surveys, *E. coli* isolated from diarrheal stools (usually 5–10 colonies/patient) are first screened for their ability to produce toxins (ST or LT), thereby defining them as ETEC. Subsequent study of the toxin+ colonies can then be undertaken to define their colonization factor antigens (by agglutination or colony blotting with specific antisera), or they can be serotyped. Unlike the case with EPEC serotyping, where pooled screening antisera were available, ETEC serotyping must be done in one of a few major reference centers. Definition of enterotoxin production in *E. coli* has traditionally involved the use of in vivo assays such as the suckling mouse assay (83) for ST and tissue culture assays for LT (84). Recently, PCR (85) and non-radioactive oligonucleotide probe technology (86) have permitted the direct assay of *E. coli* entertoxin DNA in stool samples, or in food (87).

E. Treatment and Prevention

For both main population groups affected by ETEC, children under 3 years of age living primarily in underdeveloped countries and adult travelers from developed countries who visit endemic areas of the third world, the main goals of prevention and treatment are the use of appropriate hygienic measures to prevent ingestion of the organism and oral rehydration once the illness has occurred. In both populations, with appropriate supportive therapy, illness is usually self-limited and of short duration. Nevertheless, especially in infants, dehydration may become life-threatening. Diarrheal illness due to ETEC must be differentiated, usually on clinical grounds, from diarrhea or dysentery due to other enteric pathogens in which the management may differ significantly. The presence of high grade fever, dysentery, or severe abdominal pain are not typical of diarrheal disease due to ETEC and should be obvious clues which indicate the presence of potentially more life threatening enteric pathogens.

1. Children Under 2-3 Years of Age in Developing Countries

a. Oral Rehydration Therapy. The mainstay of treatment for infants and children with mild to moderate dehydration, severe dehydration in facilities where fluids are not available for intravenous or intraosseous infusion, and maintenance volume replacement, is oral rehydration therapy (ORT)(88–90). The effectiveness of ORT, which depends upon the absorption of sodium and glucose across small bowel epithelium by a coupled transport mechanism, is based on the use of oral rehydration solution (ORS). The safety and efficacy of the ORS formulation recommended by the WHO and Unicef, which contains glucose (20g/L), sodium chloride (3.5 g/L), potassium chloride (1.5g/L), and either trisodium citrate (2.9g/L), or sodium bicarbonate (2.5g/L), has been well documented in numerous clinical trials (91). Although ORS has been responsible for saving millions of lives, its use does not shorten the duration of diarrhea and in rare cases has led to hypernatremia. Recent attempts to develop improved ORS in order to reduce the volume and duration of diarrhea have focused on rice based formulations (92–97), the early reintroduction of food (98), hypoosmolor solutions with reduced concentrations of glucose and sodium (99–102) and zinc supplementation (103). Further investigation is needed before these modifications can be recommended for routine use.

b. Antibiotics. Antibiotic treatment of ETEC infection is not recommended in this age group. However, in practice, it may be impossible to identify ETEC or other enteric pathogens as the causative agent of diarrhea if appropriate laboratory techniques are not available. Therefore, the decision to use antibiotics for diarrheal illness in this setting should be based on a clinical suspicion of illness due to other species of enteric pathogens which invade the gut mucosa, and spread locally or systemically in conjunction with epidemiologic surveillance and antibiotic resistance patterns.

c. Antimotility agents. The use of antimotility agents for acute diarrheal disease in this age group is not advised for two reasons: 1) diarrheal illness due to ETEC is usually self-limited and the expense is not warranted and 2) the possibility that in a patient infected with an invasive pathogen, antimotility agents may precipitate a more severe clinical illness by inhibiting clearance mechanisms in the gut which are dependent on normal motility.

2. *Travelers to Endemic Areas*

a. Avoidance of contaminated food and beverages. ETEC are the leading cause of traveler's diarrhea. Travelers should take precautions to avoid potentially contaminated food, beverages and ice in high risk areas. Uncooked food, unpasteurized milk products, fruits and vegetable that have not been peeled, and cooked food that has remained at room temperature for an extended period of time should be avoided. The oft-quoted advice, "If you can't boil it, cook it, or peel it, forget it," is generally sound. Nevertheless, as a practical matter, it is extremely difficult for travelers to prevent TD by dietary restriction. Drinking canned or bottled carbonated beverages, coffee or tea made with boiled water, beer or wine, may help to reduce the risk of ingestion of a contaminated product. If these types of beverages are not available water can be chemically disinfected with iodine. The germicidal activity of chlorine is more variable. Filters with a pore size of 2 microns or less should theoretically remove bacteria and parasite cysts but not viral pathogens.

b. Rehydration. Maintenance of adequate hydration is the only essential treatment for most diarrheal illnesses, yet many individuals still have an unfortunate tendency to stop oral intake when diarrhea occurs. Travelers should begin fluid replacement when diarrhea is recognized and oral intake should exceed stool losses. In most cases of TD, fluid replacement can be achieved with available safe liquids, preferably containing glucose sources, and a palatable source of salt. Alternately, "homemade" solutions can be formulated by adding a pinch of salt, a pinch of bicarbonate and a tablespoon of sugar to a liter of water. Packets of ORS containing glucose, NaCl, KCl and sodium citrate have been developed by the World Health Organization and are marketed by several commercial companies. These salts can be mixed with water to provide effective fluid replacement even in cases of severe purging. Such packets may be obtained before travel, but they are often more readily available in underdeveloped countries where they are effectively used as an alternative to intravenous therapy for cases of severe diarrheal disease (104).

c. Antibiotics. The use of antibiotics for the prevention of traveler's diarrhea due to bacterial pathogens has been advocated by some investigators for travelers making short term visits to underdeveloped countries. Several agents have been shown to provide effective prophylaxis against TD in clinical trials, however their routine use was not recommended at the most recent National Institutes of Health Consensus Development Conference (79,105) on TD because of concern over the strong probability of inducing severe, or even fatal, side effects in an attempt to prevent a nonfatal disease. Because many travelers are aware of studies demonstrating the effectiveness of prophylactic agents, they may request them from their physician or obtain them in the countries to which they travel. Travelers who seek to obtain the benefit of prophylactic agents should be clearly advised of the potential for severe adverse reactions and be willing to accept this risk/benefit ratio. Antimicrobial agents which have been demonstrated to be effective in reducing the incidence of travelers diarrhea include bismuth subsalicylate, doxycycline, trimethoprim sulfamethoxazole, trimethoprim, ciprofloxacin, and norfloxacin (106). The benefit of these agents also depends on constantly changing microbial resistance patterns in endemic areas. Currently the Centers for Disease Control and Prevention (CDC) does not recommend the routine use of prophylactic antibiotics although their use should be considered in certain high risk groups such as the immuno-compromised, Further information is available from the CDC on the world wide web at http://www.cdc.gov/cdc.html.

The average 3-5 day duration of TD due to ETEC may be shortened by 1-2 days in patients who take appropriate antimicrobial agents with the onset of illness. Commonly used antibiotics include trimethoprim/sulfamethoxazole and ciprofloxacin or other quinalone derivatives. Bismuth subsalicylate (BSS) given as 30 ml of the liquid Pepto-Bismol preparation every half hour for eight doses also shortens the course of TD (107). Prompt initiation of a 3-day course of empiric b.i.d. antibiotic therapy is recommended to shorten the duration of more severe cases of TD. Several regimens have been effective in field studies in shortening the duration of illness from 3, 4 or 5 days to 1.5 days or less. These include:

Ciprofloxacin (500 mg) b.i.d x 3 days. (108)
Trimethoprim/sulfamethoxazole (160 mg/800 mg) b.i.d. x three days. (109)
Trimethoprim alone (200 mg) b.i.d. x 3 days.
Doxycycline (100 mg) b.i.d. x 3 days.
Norfloxacin 400 mg b.i.d. x 3 days (110)

Ciprofloxacin has emerged as the treatment of choice. The older quinolone Norfloxacin at 400 mg b.i.d. may be used. The trimethoprim/sulfamethoxazole combination is still useful in the interior of Mexico. Doxycycline may be recommended for travelers sensitive to sulfonamides, but resistance to this drug is high in Southeast Asia and Central America. Photosensitivity reactions and fungal overgrowth are concerns with doxycycline and it should not be used in children because of permanent staining of teeth. Clinical trials are currently testing the efficacy of single, larger dose antibiotic therapy as an alternative to the three day courses currently recommended, and one published study (111) of single-dose ciprofloxacin (500mg) suggests that this is feasible.

d. Antimotility Agents. Synthetic opiates rapidly control diarrheal symptoms and cramping in mild to moderate cases of TD (112). They can be safely used for up to 3 days in cases of watery diarrhea. Because of concern that they can decrease clearance of invasive pathogens, such as Shigellae, synthetic opiates *should not* be used in the presence of bloody diarrhea, high fever (temperature greater than 101°F), or severe abdominal pain. The available synthetic opiates include diphenoxylate plus atropine (Lomotil) given initially (in adults) as 2 tablets q.i.d., then tapered over the next 2 days; and loperamide (Imodium) given (in adults) as 4 mg (two 2-mg capsules) initially, then 2 mg after each loose stool to a total of 16 mg/day (113). A liquid "over-the-counter" formulation of loperamide is available. None of the preparations should be given to children under the age of 2 years.

e. Combination Therapy. A recent study indicated a synergistic therapeutic effect of combining a 3-day course of antibiotics with an anti-diarrheal agent. In travelers to Mexico, 3 days of trimethoprim/sulfamethoxazole (160 mg/800 mg b.i.d.) together with loperamide (4-mg loading dose followed by 2 mg after each loose stool) was superior to either component alone in decreasing the duration of TD (114). The addition of loperamide to a 3 day regimen of ciprofloxacin appears to be safe, however, it did not have a significant clinical advantage over treatment with ciprofloxacin alone (115, 116)

f. Vaccines. No vaccines are currently available for any of the bacterial species responsible for traveler's diarrhea, although vaccine development is being actively pursued. Passive protection against ETEC disease has been achieved in volunteer challenge studies by the ingestion of immunoglobulins derived from the milk of hyperimmunized cows (117), but such products are not currently available nor have they been tested in field studies. Thus travelers must deal with this syndrome through a combination of preventive measures and self treatment once the characteristic symptoms occur.

IV. ENTEROHEMORRHAGIC *E. COLI* (EHEC)

EHEC are associated with foodborne epidemics of bloody diarrhea and hemorrhagic colitis (HC), which may progress to the development of hemolytic-uremic syndrome (HUS)(118,119). EHEC and HUS have been recognized since 1982 (120), but they received deserved, if delayed, national attention in 1993 when four died and over 600 became ill after eating contaminated hamburger from fast-food restaurants (121). Although there are several serotypes of EHEC that can cause disease, the predominant clone and most prevalent serotype is O157:H7. In 1994, seventeen independent outbreaks of EHEC disease, which resulted in ten deaths and involved over 1200 individuals, were reported to the Centers for Disease Control and Prevention (CDC). The CDC estimates that every year roughly 20,000 people in the U.S. become infected with EHEC and experience some form of clinical disease, and 200 deaths result from complications of EHEC. Outbreaks of infection with these agents are likely to continue, because of the capacity for wide distribution of infecting organisms provided by an efficient food distribution system. At present there is no established safe or effective therapy for EHEC infection.

A. Presentation

Enterohemorrhagic *Escherichia coli* cause a spectrum of diarrheal illness ranging from asymptomatic colonization, through mild diarrhea, to severe hemorrhagic colitis. The incubation period, following ingestion of as few as 100 organisms, ranges from 3-9 days, with a mean of 6.1 days (118,122). EHEC diarrhea is more prolonged in children, with an average duration of 9.1 days, than in adults (6.6 days average duration) (123). Hemorrhagic colitis manifests as severe abdominal cramping accompanied by bloody diarrhea. Blood usually appears in the stool between the second and fifth day of illness (124). Blood loss in stools ranges from less than one tablespoon per day to as much as 4 cups per day. The presenting physical examination may be remarkable for right lower quadrant pain and tenderness, abdominal distention, and rectal prolapse in children (125), but may be normal. Vomiting occurs in up to 75% of patients and ileus may be present in up to 24% of patients (123). Colonoscopy reveals mucosal edema with erosions and hemorrhage, and barium contrast studies confirm mucosal edema with "thumbprinting." A gradient of injury is present, with the most severe disease in the proximal colon and less severe disease distally in the rectum (125). Fever is not present in most patients, but when present, fever predicts a more severe clinical course (126).

While EHEC colitis is often self-limiting, EHEC infection can lead to severe complications including CNS disturbances and the hemolytic uremic syndrome (HUS) or post diarrheal thrombotic thrombocytopenic purpura (127,128). HUS (characterized by hemolytic anemia, thrombocytopenia and acute renal failure) is especially life-threatening for the young and elderly (129,130). The more severe the colitis, the higher the WBC count ($>$20,000), and the higher the initial fever, the more likely the patient is to have significant complications, including the development of HUS and central nervous system complications (131,132). Rare and unusual complications of EHEC have included rhabdomyolysis, pancreatic necrosis with subsequent diabetes mellitus, and acute intestinal obstruction from intestinal hematoma (82). Recurrent infection with the same EHEC serotype is unlikely, but has been reported and continues to place the patient at risk for developing HUS (133,134).

B. Molecular Pathogenesis

The clinical effects of EHEC infection depend upon the production of Shiga-like toxins (SLTs)(135,136,167), by bacteria that attach to the cells lining the intestinal tract in an intimate manner, known as attaching/effacing (AE) adherence (12,137). The relationship between these two virulence determinants needs to be better understood, but the delivery of SLTs to the systemic circulation results in vascular endothelial damage in many organs which is the hallmark of the disease.

1. *Shiga-like Toxins*

The essential characteristic of EHEC strains is their ability to produce Shiga-like toxins (SLTs), a family of bacterial cytotoxins structurally related to Shiga toxin produced by the dysentery bacillus *S. dysenteriae* (135,138–141). The relationship of these toxins to Shiga toxin was found by Konawalchuk et al. (142) when they showed this heat-labile toxin displayed a cytopathic effect on African green monkey kidney cells (Vero cells). This toxin became known as Verotoxin (143) The two major types of Shiga-like toxins are Shiga-like toxin-I (SLT-I) and Shiga-like toxin-II (SLT-II). Individual EHEC strains produce either or both toxins. Both toxins have been associated with hemorrhagic colitis and the development of HUS. Whereas Shiga toxin in *S. dysenteriae 1* is encoded by chromosomal genes, the genes encoding both SLT-I and SLT-II are carried on lysogenic bacteriophages (144–147) which infect EHEC strains. SLT-I is virtually identical to Shiga toxin, differing by a single amino acid, thus anti-Shiga toxin sera completely neutralizes SLT-I cytotoxic activity. SLT-II is functionally similar but antigenically distinct from Shiga toxin (135). SLT-II shares a 56% amino acid homology with SLT-I and is only partly neutralized by anti-Shiga toxin sera. Both SLT-I and SLT-II are multisubunit toxins (m.w. in range of 70,000) composed of one enzymatically active A subunit (approx m.w. 32,000) in noncovalent association with a pentamer of receptor-binding B subunits (approx m.w. 7,700)(18). The B-subunits of SLT-I and SLT-II recognize the same cellular glycolipid receptor, globotriaosylceramide (Gb_3)(148). The A subunits of both toxins are highly selective N-glycosidases that depurinate a specific adenine residue on the eukaryotic 60s ribosomal subunit (149). Following toxin binding, the A subunit is introduced into the cell where it inhibits ribosomal protein synthesis (150,151). EHEC-associated diarrheal and kidney diseases, including HC and HUS, result primarily from the action of SLT(s) on the microvasculature of the intestine and kidneys, where they target Gb_3 receptors on endothelial cells lining small vessels (165,166). These are extremely potent toxins with an in vitro cytotoxic dose for 50% of HeLa cells (CD_{50}) for SLT-I in the range of 1-2 ng/ml. The i.v. LD_{50} in rabbits is 100-200 ng/kg, and the i.v. dose inducing diarrhea and CNS lesions in 50% of rabbits is 10-20 ng/kg (152). Thus low levels of either reaching the circulation are able to induce profound vascular lesions in the endothelial cells expressing receptors in target organs including bowel, CNS and kidney. Recent evidence suggests that the toxins may be translocated across intact epithelium by a transcellular (rather than paracellular) pathway (153) (Fig. 4), but studies have not addressed the effect of adherence on toxin uptake. SLTs are poor immunogens and may not be recognized by immune competent cells in patients developing HUS (154).

2. *Attaching/Effacing (A/E) Adherence*

The second distinguishing characteristic of most EHEC strains is their ability to attach to the cells lining the intestinal tract in a particularly intimate manner, known as attaching/effacing (AE) (12) adherence. AE adherence is a property shared with enteropathogenic *E. coli* (EPEC) strains which are a leading cause of infantile diarrhea (155). The AE lesion is characterized (see Fig.1) by elongation and shedding of microvilli (12) and rearrangement of cytoskeletal elements, with an aggregation of filamentous actin beneath the areas of intimate bacterial attachment (30). The three stage model of pathogenesis formulated by Donnenberg and Kaper (16) for AE in EPEC (Fig. 2), also applies to EHEC strains (Fig. 4, I-III) with some minor differences i.e., a first stage of initial attachment mediated by fimbriae, followed by a second stage of signal transduction events (24) mediated by secreted proteins, and a third stage of intimate adherence with actin aggregation. EHEC strains have been shown to possess all the elements of the LEE region that was first found in EPEC (35). Like EPEC, EHEC strains have also been shown to produce AE lesions in rabbit and piglet models (156,157) and have been shown to be positive for FAS (30).

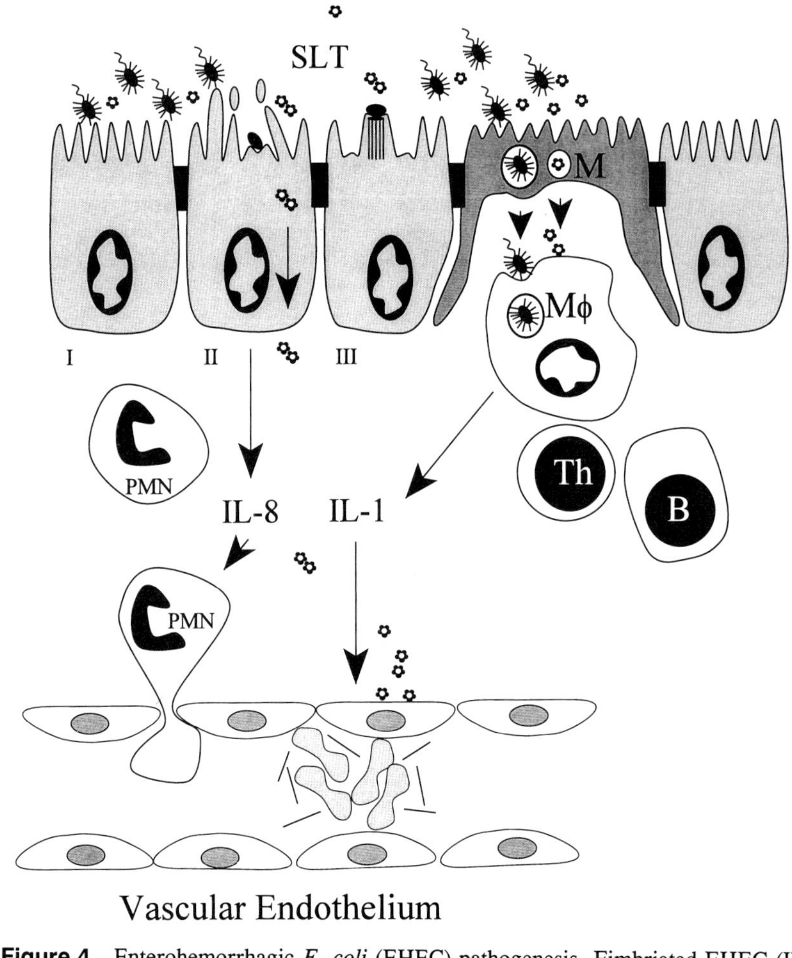

Figure 4 Enterohemorrhagic *E. coli* (EHEC) pathogenesis. Fimbriated EHEC (I) adhere to epithelial cells, then proceed to induce attaching/effacing (AE) lesions (II, III) as described in detail for EPEC (see Fig.2). They produce Shiga-like toxins (SLT) [pentamers] which cross epithelial cells by a transcellular pathway. The principle action of SLTs is on the vascular endothelium, which responds with increased permeability and diapedesis of inflammatory cells. Organisms sampled by M cells encounter macrophages (MΦ) and induce release of IL-1. This cytokine upregulates endothelial receptors for SLTs, thereby promoting toxin-induced vascular injury. Mucosal inflammation is enhanced by the release of chemokine IL-8 in response to AE adherence.

The *eae* gene of EHEC strain EDL 933 (O157:H7) has been cloned and sequenced with the homology between the EPEC and EHEC sequences being 86% and 83% at the nucleotide and amino acid levels, respectively (137). The O157:H7 *eae* gene, like the EPEC gene, is homologous to the invasin gene of

Yersinia pseudotuberculosis (51% similarity) with greatest at the C-terminal end implicated in integrin binding (137). Donnenberg et al. (158) constructed an *eae* mutant of an O157:H7 strain and showed that it was deficient in producing FAS+ lesions in HEp-2 cells in vitro, and did not produce AE lesions in vivo in newborn piglets. A second major gene shown to be involved in the AE process in EPEC (159,160), *espB*, which encodes a secreted protein, is also found in EHEC. There is controversy over the function of the EHEC *espB* gene product in signal transduction, specifically in the ability to induce tyrosine phopsphorylation of HSP-90 (Fig. 2).

Unlike EPEC, EHEC do not produce bundle forming pili, and the determinants of EHEC stage I (Fig. 4,I) adhesion to intestine are incompletely defined. Several candidates have been proposed. EHEC possess a 60- to 70 MDa plasmid (120,161) which codes for fimbriae. When EHEC isolates were cured of the 60- to 70 MDa plasmid, they failed to express fimbriae and lost the ability to adhere to intestinal cells (162). Recently, it has been shown that O157 strains adhere to HCT-8 human intestinal cells with a localized adherence phenotype, but also by a newly described phenotype termed "log jam" (163). This pattern was not seen on HEp-2 cells, was independent of *eae*, and was shared by pathogenic EHEC, EPEC, and EIEC. The determinant of the "log jam" phenotype has not been described.

3. *Role of Inflammatory Mediators in EHEC Disease* (164)

Endothelial cells are preferred targets for SLTs, endothelial alteration and injury is a major pathogenic mechanism in EHEC disease, and in vitro studies have demonstrated that SLT toxicity for endothelium is enhanced by proinflammatory cytokines. Importantly, in in vitro studies, IL-1 and TNFá induce, or upregulate, SLT receptors on endothelial surfaces (165). SLT receptor density correlates with the ability of SLTs to exert a direct cytotoxic effect on the endothelium. Pro-inflammatory cytokines also have direct actions on the endothelium, initiating endothelial alterations which promote inflammation. Moreover, these effectors, including IL-1 (166), TNFα (167), and LPS (endotoxin), act synergistically with SLT upon the endothelium to produce cytotoxic effects (Fig. 5). The process occurs not only in local mucosal vessels, but also in more distant sites, where toxin receptors are present on endothelium (serosal vessels, brain and kidney). Although SLTs bind to epithelial cells they seem to have little direct action on these cells as shown by studies demonstrating transcellular transport of SLTs across polarized epithelial cells without loss of barrier function (153).

C. Epidemiology

EHEC, in particular the O157:H7 strain, were first identified as being able to cause disease in humans in 1982 (120) and have become the leading cause of pediatric bloody diarrhea in North America (118). Since 1985, EHEC strains were found to be the predominant diarrhea-causing organism associated with HUS (168,169). The incidence of diarrhea associated with HUS has not changed significantly since 1971 and suggests that EHEC were pathogenic for humans prior to their recognition in 1982.

It has been estimated that EHEC strains such as O157:H7 may induce diarrheal disease in humans with an infectious dose of less than 100 ingested organisms (170). The majority of outbreaks due to EHEC have been traced back to a common source, in particular improperly cooked beef (169,171,172). Cattle, sheep, and goats are the most important animal reservoirs for EHEC organisms (173). Although a common food source is implicated in most outbreaks, transmission of EHEC has been documented from person to person in day care facilities, and in medical personnel caring for hospitalized patients (174,175). Transmission from asymptomatic patients may be a possible source of infection since asymptomatic patients have been reported with EHEC organisms recovered from their stool. This indicates that good hygiene is important in preventing the spread of EHEC disease (176).

EHEC disease has been documented in widely separated geographic regions such the U.S., Australia, Africa, Canada, Eastern Europe, Germany, England, Italy, Japan, Argentina, Chile and Mexico (169,177,178). Currently in the U.S, there are an estimated 10,000-20,000 cases of EHEC diarrhea per year with 200-500 deaths per year due to EHEC disease (170). At present this prevalence data is based on laboratory diagnosis of the O157:H7 serotype. This implies that the incidence figures are an underestimate of EHEC disease since, even today, some clinical and hospital laboratories do not culture bloody diarrhea for O157:H7; and those laboratories that do look for EHEC isolates only look for the O157:H7 serotype. Although reporting is improving, the true incidence of EHEC infection remains undetermined.

Whittam et al. have shown by multilocus enzyme electrophoresis that O157:H7 isolates represent a distinct clone (179) and that the O157:H7 clone was most closely related to a clone of O55:H7 strains (180). These investigators propose that O157:H7 strains emerged from an O55:H7 progenitor, already possessing a mechanism for adherence to intestinal cells, acquired secondary virulence factors (Shiga-like cytotoxins and plasmid-encoded adhesins) via horizontal transfer and recombination.

D. Laboratory Diagnosis

The laboratory features of EHEC colitis at presentation are nonspecific. Griffin et al. (124) reported 0-1 polymorphonuclear leukocytes per high power field in the stools of 68% of their patients with EHEC colitis and demonstrates that the relative scarcity of leukocytes in the bloody diarrhea of patients may be the most important clinical diagnostic feature.

The primary method to screen for *E. coli* O157:H7 in stools is growth on sorbitol-enriched MacConkey medium (SM Agar). O157:H7 strains do not ferment sorbitol and grows as colorless colonies after 24 hours incubation. Confirmatory tests for O157:H7 are conducted by agglutination with O157 antisera (118,170). Stool cultures need to be performed early, since it is often impossible to detect EHEC in stools after the onset of HUS (181,182,183).

Additional tests for the detection of EHEC are becoming available. Several promising methods to detect EHEC utilize ELISA techniques, based on rabbit or bovine anti-SLT-I and anti-SLT-II antibodies, to detect toxin in *E. coli* cultured from stool (184). Colony hybridization assays using specific DNA probes for SLT genes and their parent bacteriophages have also been used for detecting SLT in stool culture specimens (185). Polymerase chain reaction (PCR) primers for common regions of SLT-I, SLT-II, and SLT-II variants have been used to amplify SLT genes present in fecal filtrates (186,187).

E. Treatment and Prevention

At present, there are no specific therapies of proven benefit for the prevention or treatment of either hemorrhagic colitis caused by EHEC or the potentially fatal complications of EHEC infection, i.e. the hemolytic uremic syndrome (HUS) and thrombotic thrombocytopenic purpura (TTP)(170,170A). Only supportive care and sanitary measures to prevent the ingestion of EHEC in contaminated food and beverage products and person to person spread can be recommended with confidence.

1. Preventative Measures and Avoidance of Contaminated Foods

The main reservoir for *E. coli* 0157:H7 in the United States is the intestinal tract of cattle. Therefore, undercooked beef and food products which may be contaminated by bovine fecal matter present the greatest potential health risk. Outbreaks in the United States have been traced to undercooked hamburger and roast beef, vegetables grown using cow manure for fertilization, unpasteurized milk and apple cider, contaminated water and mayonnaise. The FDA has reported EHEC in samples of lamb, pork, and poultry taken from retail grocery stores however clinical illness has not been linked to meat other than beef. Thorough cooking of meat products to 160°F is recommended.

Elimination of the EHEC bacterial strain from the animal population is a desirable method for EHEC prevention. Although immunization or antibiotic treatment have been proposed, practical means for achieving this goal are not available (188). Since O157:H7 organisms do not casue recognizable disease in cattle, identification of the organisms in herd animals is dificult. Irradiation of food products is safe and effectively eliminates EHEC bacteria from food, but is not well received by consumers. Education of the general population to the benefits of an irradiated food supply, including information documenting the safety of food pasteurized in this way, may alleviate public fear of irradiation pasteurization (170A).

Patients with suspected EHEC infection should be considered highly contagious and appropriate precautions to prevent fecal-oral transmission should be taken. Early identification of index cases, and contaminated food sources will help reduce the size of outbreaks (169). In day care centers, health care facilities, and households, thorough hand-washing and good hygiene will prevent secondary infections.

2. *The Mainstay for Therapy for EHEC Colitis: Management of Fluid and Electrolytes, Monitoring Blood Loss and Observing for Signs of Progression to HUS* (170A)

a. Antibiotics. The use of antibiotics for the treatment of hemorrhagic colitis due to EHEC remains controversial, but cannot be recommended at the present time. A theoretical risk of treatment with bacteriocidal antibiotics is that the increased release of preformed SLT and endotoxin from bacteria may potentiate vascular endothelial injury. In vitro studies have shown increased production of SLT-I when EHEC bacteria are exposed to sub-inhibitory antibiotic concentrations (189). Antibiotics have been used in vitro to faciltiate detection of SLT in bacterial cultures (190). If this effect occurs in vivo, the patient would be exposed to larger doses of toxin and be at increased risk for progression into HUS. Furthermore, if inappropriate antibiotics are given, i.e. ones to which EHEC are resistant, EHEC may proliferate while the growth of normal competitive flora in the gut is inhibited. Antibiotics have provided no improvement in outcome for EHEC infected patients. They do not decrease the length or the severity of diarrhea. Two retrospective studies have implicated prior antibiotic usage as a risk factor for progression into HUS (126,130). Controlled studies investigating antibiotic use in EHEC colitis failed to confirm increased risk for HUS development, but also failed to demonstrate benefit of antibiotic therapy (191). There may be a risk from antibiotic treatment of EHEC colitis, but there is no clearly proven benefit from treatment (192). Individual studies are confounded by small numbers, differences in the time at which therapy was initiated, and the use of different antimicrobial agents which may have variable effects on SLT production and release by EHEC. Unless prospective controlled studies demonstrate improved outcomes without increased risk, there is no justification to use antibiotics for treatment of EHEC colitis.

b. Antimotility agents. Antimotility agents should **not** be given to patients with suspected EHEC infection as they may precipitate a more severe clinical illness by inhibiting mechanical clearance mechanisms in the gut.

c. Investigational therapies. Decreasing the toxin burden with the use of toxin binding agents, decreasing the delivery of toxin to endothelial receptors by systemic administration of SLT antibodies, and abrogating the resulting inflammatory response with cytokine antagonists are some of the treatment strategies currently being investigated. An ongoing study is using Synsorb-Pk (synthetic oligosaccharide Gb3 receptors attached to diatomaceous earth) in an effort to bind SLTs in the gut lumen and prevent the progression of EHEC colitis into HUS. This treatment is safe and presents only minor side effects in healthy volunteers, however there is no data concerning its efficacy in prevention of disease progression (193). In an animal model, systemic treatment with anti-CD18 antibody reduced the diarrhea rate in rabbits infected with *Escherichia coli* O157:H7 animals from 95% to 45%, and the treated animals displayed a marked reduction in tissue inflammation (194). Similar positive effects on HUS outcome from inhibition of leukocyte adhesion in humans have not been demonstrated.

3. *Therapies for HUS and TTP*

Appropriate supportive measures including dialysis and seizure control may be required for patients with renal or neurologic involvement. Patients with severe hemolysis may require blood transfusion. Experimental therapies include plasma exchange (195) and the intravenous administration of immune globulin.

V. ENTEROINVASIVE *E. COLI* (EIEC)

Shigella and *E. coli* are conventionally given separate species status, however, several studies have shown that *Shigella* and *E. coli* deserve to be considered one species (196–205). The different members of the *Shigella* species should best be thought of as pathogenic clonal lineages of *E. coli* that evolved through the acquisition of a virulence plasmid to become invasive pathogens of primates. This idea is only slowly being acknowledged, but the example of enteroinvasive *E. coli* (EIEC) serves to emphasize the point. In 1971, DuPont et al. (206) described *E. coli* strains that caused an invasive, dysenteric form of diarrhea. These strains were of distinct serogroups from ETEC and EPEC and were "*Shigella*-like" in their biochemical reactions, plasmid profiles, virulence properties, pathogenetic mechanisms, and the clinical illness produced. EIEC are lactose-negative, but many fall in O serogroups that cross-react with antisera directed against Shigella O antigens (207).

A. Presentation

EIEC characteristically cause both a dysenteric syndrome and watery diarrhea. The dysenteric nature of the stools (frequent, small volume with blood and pus) in some affected individuals reflects the severe inflammatory process associated with invasion of the colonic epithelium (Fig. 5) that can result from EIEC (and Shigella) infection. The watery diarrhea reflects the action of newly described enterotoxins.

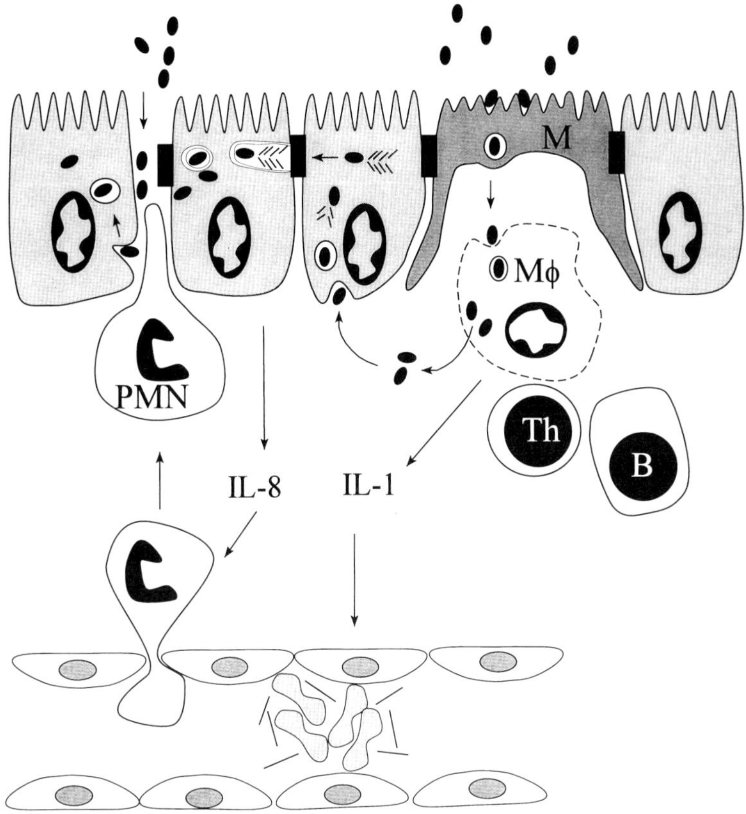

Figure 5 Enteroinvasive *E. coli* (EIEC) pathogenesis. Like shigella, EIEC enter the host via M cells over organized lymphoid tissue. They initiate mucosal inflammation by inducing macrophage (MΦ) apoptosis and release of IL-1. Released EIEC invade epithelial cells at the basolateral pole. They enter cells in cytoplasmic vacuoles, lyse the vacuoles to undergo cytoplasmic growth, then enter adjacent epithelial cells by propelling themselves on tails of aggregated actin. Invasion of epithelial cells by EIEC induces the secretion of the chemokine IL-8 which attracts inflammatory cells (PMNs). Ultimately, the host inflammatory response causing breakdown of cell-cell interactions which permits access of additional organisms to the basolateral poles of epithelial cells.

B. Molecular Pathogenesis

The pathognomonic feature of EIEC strains, which is shared with the Sonnei, Flexneri, Dysenteriae and Boydii clones of *Shigella*, is their ability to invade epithelial cells, particularly those in the colonic mucosa (206). This property can be assayed using the Sereny test for guinea pig keratoconjunctivitis (206).

Shigella and EIEC contain closely related 120- to 140-megadalton virulence plasmids that encode the genes required for epithelial cell invasiveness and cell to cell spread (208–211). Loss of these plasmids results in loss of invasiveness and pathogenicity. Many regions of the these plasmids have been characterized, including those encoding the invasion plasmid associated (Ipa) proteins, which are required for full invasiveness and (212), and those encoding *icsa* (*virG*) gene products essential for intercellular spread. (213). Ipa proteins enable the organisms to enter epithelial cells in endocytic vacuoles, then to lyse the vacuoles to undergo additional rounds of cytoplasmic proliferation (212,214). Invasion of adjacent cells is mediated by the plasmid encoded *icsA* virulence factor. EIEC and *Shigella* utilize the product of the *icsA* locus to mobilize host cell cytoskeletal components, thereby propelling themselves into adjacent epithelial cells on tails of polymerized actin (215,216,217) anchored to cadherin at tight junctions (218).

The inter-relationship of cellular invasion and cell-to-cell spread to the development of an inflammatory response can now be understood as a consequence of the shared ability of *Shigella* and EIEC to preferably enter the host via specialized lymphoepithelial cells over lymphoid follicles of the colon (Fig. 5) (related to M cells over the Peyer's patch) (219) and subsequently to invade epithelial cells from their basolateral aspect. This sequence of events was shown in experiments in which primates were infected with mutant *Shigella* organisms with intact genes for cellular invasion, but mutated only in the gene for cell-to-cell spread, *icsA* (*virG*). Thus the invading organisms were confined to the site of initial uptake, which proved to be scattered lesions located over lymphoid nodules, rather than generalized involvement of the absorptive epithelium. These results are entirely consistent with those of a careful clinical study of the rectal mucosa in shigellosis, which showed that epithelial cells over lymphoid follicles were the first to be damaged (220).

After gaining access to the subepithelial space in gut lymphoid tissue, EIEC organisms interact with, but are not killed by macrophages. To the contrary, infected macrophages undergo apoptotic death (221) (Fig. 5, MΦ) with the release of pro-inflammatory cytokines including IL-1 (222), IL-6 and TNF. These events may initiate the marked acute inflammatory response characterized by the transmigration of polymorphonuclear leukocytes (Fig. 5, PMN) and the resultant tissue destruction.

Organisms released from apoptotic macrophages can then invade colonic absorptive epithelial cells at the basolateral pole (Fig. 5). In vitro experiments by Sansonetti's group have demonstrated that invasion of human colonic Caco-2 cell lines by *S. flexneri* placed at the luminal surface is greatly enhanced by chemically disrupting the intracellular junctions allowing organisms access to the basolateral surface (223).

New evidence also suggests that invading organisms induce the synthesis and release of proinflammatory chemokines (such as IL-8) by epithelial cells (Fig. 5) (224). These cytokines are chemotactic for neutrophils which arrive in the lamina propria, transmigrating from vessels whose endothelium has been altered by the effect of IL-1. *S. flexneri* has been shown to induce PMN transmigration when placed on the luminal side of laboratory epithelial cell lines (Fig. 4, PMN)(225). Ultimate breakdown of the epithelial barrier, including transmigration of PMN into the lumen, may be a result of the acute inflammatory response which facilitates bacterial access to the basolateral pole of epithelial cells, additional rounds of bacterial invasion, and lysis of colonocytes.

Epidemiologic and clinical observation of EIEC disease reveals that a high proportion of EIEC infections result in watery diarrhea, without the dysentery syndrome so characteristic of *Shigella* infection (226, 227). Fasano et al have reported that when grown under iron-deprived conditions, EIEC secrete into the supernatant a 60-80 kDa enterotoxins which induce fluid accumulation in rabbit ileal loops, and increased short circuit current (Isc) in the Ussing chamber (228). These investigators showed that EIEC exhibited low level of Vero cell cytotoxins that are immunologically and genetically distinct from Shiga-like toxin I or II of EHEC. One moiety has been termed SHet (Shigella enterotoxin) II. It gene (designated *sen* and encoding a 63kDa protein) has been localized to the large virulence *inv* plasmid of both *Shigella* (83% of strains) and EIEC (75% of strains tested) (229).

C. Epidemiology

The predominant serogroups in which EIEC are found are O28, O112, O124, O136, O143, O144, O147, O152, and O164 (155). EIEC have been isolated from cases of diarrhea in both industrialized and less-developed countries, although with low frequency. Most cases in industrialized countries relate to foodborne outbreaks (230,231). Volunteer studies suggest that the typical inocula that occur in nature are probably 100-1000 times higher than those required for *Shigella* infection (206). These infections are usually self-limited indicating the eventual development of an effective IgA effector immune response. As for *Shigella*, this protective immunity is serogroup specific.

D. Laboratory Diagnosis

EIEC diagnosis depends on strong clinical suspicion, as in an outbreak setting, with investigation of lactose fermenting isolates. EIEC can be diagnosed by serotyping suspect *E. coli* isolates (232), by ELISA that detects outer membrane proteins associated with invasiveness (233) and by DNA probes that detect the genes needed for invasion (234), but these techniques are primarily applied in research laboratories in epidemiological investigations.

E. Treatment and Prevention

Recommendations for therapy and prevention parallel those for Shigellosis. Because of the invasive nature of these pathogens, antimotility agents should not be given to avoid lengthening the course of illness. As with non-shiga-toxin producing *Shigella*, antibiotic treatment may not be required. Administration of effective antibiotics, to which the organisms are sensitive, should shorten the course of illness, but no clinical trials of antibiotic treatment of EIEC have been reported. If organisms are identified in an outbreak setting, careful attention should be given to obtaining antibiotic sensitivities before administering antibiotic therapy.

VI. ENTEROAGGREGATIVE *E. COLI* (EAggEC)

A. Presentation and Epidemiology

Mannose-resistant adherence of *E. coli* to HEp-2 cells is characteristic of EPEC, of classical serotypes, when it occurs in a "localized" pattern which is now recognized as determined by the expression of bundle forming pili. Closer phenotypic analysis of patterns of Hep-2 adherence of *E. coli* strains isolated from patients (children and adult travelers) with diarrheal disease, and not of EPEC serotypes, yielded enteroadherent strains (235) which adhered in a "diffuse" manner, or in a pattern termed "aggregative adherence (AA)" (236), resembling stacked bricks. Moreover, the pathogenicity implied by the more frequent associations of strains with the AA adherence pattern with diarrheal cases than with controls. Epidemiological studies from diverse geographic areas, including Chile, Bangladesh (237), India (238), Mexico (239) and Brazil (240) implicated EAggEC as agents of diarrheal disease, particularly persistent disease, defined as lasting longer than 14 days. This impression was confirmed by studies in volunteers (241,242) for strains of some serotypes, notably O42:H18, in whom diarrhea occurred in 30-60% of those ingesting the strain. However other enteroaggregative *E. coli* (EAggEC) strains with the AA phenotype did not cause diarrhea in volunteers, thus it appears that properties other than those determining the adherence pattern are associated with virulence. This conclusion is also suggested by the frequent isolation of EAggEC from the stools of asymptomatic patients epidemiologic studies, although less frequently than from those of patients with diarrhea.

B. Pathogenesis

Studies of the pathogenesis of disease associated with the AA phenotype is complicated by the fact that strains sharing this phenotype are heterogeneous. In rabbit loops (243), and in gnotobiotic piglets (244), tested strains adhered to the epithelium and induced mucosal edema. Necrosis of villous tips was seen in the rabbit. In vitro adherence studies using a variety of EAggEC strains have demonstrated fimbriae of varied morphology ranging from rods to fibrillar bundles (245,246). These putative adhesins appear to confer a selective association with colonic rather than small bowel mucosa (243,247). Recent studies suggest that adherence may be less selective, but that cytotoxicity is localized to colon (248,249) A 65 MDa plasmid has been associated with the expression of fimbriae conferring an AA pattern of adherence (250). Savarino has described the encoding and expression of a cysteine containing-protein analogous to *E. coli* heat stable toxin, but even more closely related to the eukaryotic protein quanylin which is an endogenous ligand for membrane associated quanylate cyclase. He has designated this protein Enteroaggregative Stable toxin I (EASTI)(251), but its role in intestinal secretion is not defined, and it has now been found in ETEC and other *E. coli* (252). Other putative toxins present in some EAggEC strains induce increases in intracellular calcium, phosphorylation of host proteins (253) and necrosis in intestinal loops (254). Thus the enteroaggregative phenotype appears to be associated with a number of potential virulence determinants but a clear picture of the pathogenesis of these infections has not emerged.

C. Diagnosis and Treatment

Diagnosis depends on the recognition of the characteristic pattern of AA adherence to HEp-2 cells with careful attention to methodologic detail as described by Cravioto et al. (255). A DNA probe has been prepared from a 1kb fragment of the large plasmid from strain 17-2, which recognizes 40 to 90% of strains with the AA phenotype depending on their origin (256), but the genes specified by this probe have not been identified. Thus at this stage in our knowledge, EaggEC can be confidently associated with disease in outbreak settings, associated with common serotypes and stools consistently yield the same isolates in cases of persistent diarrhea (257). In such cases, antibiotic therapy based on sensitivity patterns could be recommended, but studies have not formally demonstrated the efficacy of antibiotics.

VI. DIFFUSELY ADHERENT *E. COLI* (DAEC)

Diffusely adherent *E. coli* (DAEC) have been recognized in surveys of diarrheal disease isolates by a unique pattern of adherence to cultured epithelial cells that can be distinguished from the localized adherence pattern of EPEC and the enteroaggregative pattern (258). Some of these surveys suggested a higher association of *E. coli* of this phenotype with diarrheal disease, particularly in children beyond infancy when results were stratified by age (259,260); but other studies did not demonstrate associations (261). Fimbriae (designated F1845) which confer the DA phenotype have been well-characterized (262) and their binding to decay accelerating factor on the surface of epithelial cells has been shown. A human volunteer challenge study, conducted in adults (263) with two strains given in doses of up to 1010 CFU, failed to demonstrate the ability of these strains to induce diarrheal disease.

VII. SUMMARY AND CONCLUSION

This chapter has reviewed the current knowledge of diarrhea-associated *E. coli* infections illustrating the multiple ways that commensal organisms have acquired genes encoding virulence mechanisms which permit them to leave the colonic lumen to colonize mucosal surfaces and intracellular locations and thereby to induce disease in the host. Recognition of these important infections is aided by understanding of pathogenic mechanisms which explain their characteristic clinical presentations. Since non-specific therapy is often the most important, definitive identification of these pathogens may not be required for successful treatment of individual cases of diarrheal disease. In outbreak settings, particularly in the case of EHEC infections which may have severe consequences, rapid, definitive identification of index cases may be of critical public health importance. One can anticipate that new classes of diarrhea associated *E. coli* will continue to emerge, representing clinical and scientific challenges to their recognition and identification.

REFERENCES

1. Adam A. Uber die biologie der dyspepsiekoli und ihre beziehungen zur pathologenesis de dyspepsie und intoxication. Jb Kinderheilk. 1923; 24:187–194.
2. Goldschmidt R. Untersuchungen zur aetiologie der durvhfallserkranktungen ser sauglings. Jb Kinderheilk. 1933; 139:318–358.
3. Kauffmann F. The serology of the coli group. J Immun. 1947; 57:71–100.
4. Neter E, Westphal O, Luderitz O, et al. Demonstration of antibodies against enteropathogenic *Escherichia coli* in sera of children of various ages. Pediatrics 1955; 16:801–807.
5. Bray J. Isolation of antigenically homogeneous strains of Bact. coli neapolitanum from summer diarrhea of infants. J Pathol Bacteriol 1945; 57:239–247.
6. Bray J, Beaven TED. Slide agglutination of Bact. coli va neapolitanum in summer diarrhea. J Pathol Bacteriol 1948; 60:395–401.

7. Giles C, and Sangster MB. An outbreak of infantile gastroenteritis in Aberdeen. J Hygiene 1948; 46:1–9.
8. Taylor J, Powell BW, Wright J. Infantile diarrhea and vomiting: a clinical and bacteriological investigation. Br Med 1949; 2:117–141.
9. Levine MM, Berquist EJ, et al. *E. coli* strains that cause diarrhea but do not produce heat-labile or heat-stable enterotoxins and are non-invasive. Lancet 1978; i:119–1122.
10. Toledo MRF, Alvariza MCB, Murahovschi J, Ramos SRT, Trabulsi, LR. Enteropathogenic *Escherichia coli* serotypes and endemic diarrhea in infants. Infect Immun 1983; 39:586–589.
11. Rothbaum R, McAdams AJ, Giannella R, Partin, JC. A clinicopathologic study of enterocyte-adherent *E. coli*: a cause of protracted diarrhea in infants. Gastroenterology 1982; 83:441–454.
12. Moon HW, Whipp SC, Argenzio RA, Levine MM, Giannella RA. Attaching and effacing activities of rabbit and human enteropathogenic Escherichia coli in pig and rabbit intestines. Infect Immun 1983; 41:1340–1351.
13. Staley TE, Jones EQ, Corley LD. Attachment and penetrationof *E. coli* into intestinal epithelium of the ileum in newborn pigs. Am J Path 1969; 56:371–392.
14. Polotsky YE, Dragunskaya EM, Seliverstova VG, et al. Pathogenic effect of enterotoxigenic *Escherichia coli* and *Escherichia coli* causing infantile diarrhea. Acta Microbiol Acad Sci Hung 1977; 24:221–236.
15. Clausen CR, Christie DL. Chronic diarrhea in infants caused by adherent enteropathogenic *Escherichia coli*. J Pediatr 1982; 100:358–361.
16. Donnenberg MS, Kaper JB. Enteropathogenic *Escherichia coli*. Infect Immun 1992; 60:3953–3961.
17. Cravioto A, Gross RJ, Scotland SM, Rowe B. An adhesive factor found in strains of *Escherichia coli* belonging to the traditional infantile enteropathogenic serotypes. Curr Microbiol 1979; 3:95–99.
18. Skaletsky ICA, Silva MLM, Trabulsi LR. Distinctive patterns of adherence of enteropathogenic *Escherichia coli* to HeLa cells. Infect Immun 1984; 45:534–536.
19. Baldini MM, Kaper JB, Levine MM, et al. Plasmid-mediated adhesion in enteropathogenic *Escherichia coli*. J Pediatr Gastroenterol Nutr 1983; 2:534–538.
20. Levine MM, Nataro JP, Karch H, et al. The diarrheal response of humans to some classic serotypes of enteropathogenic *Escherichia coli* is dependent on a plasmid encoding an enteroadhesiveness factor. J Infect Dis 1985; 152:550–559.
21. Knutton S, Baldini MM, Kaper JB, McNeish AS. Role of plasmid-encoded adherence factors in adhesion of enteropathogenic *Escherichia coli* to HEp-2 cells. Infect Immun 1987; 5:78–85.
22. Giron JA, Ho ASY, Schoolnick GK. An inducible bundle-forming pilus of enteropathogenic *Escherichia coli*. Science 1991; 254:710–713.
23. Donnenberg MS, Calderwood SB, Donohue-Rolfe A, et al. Construction and analysis of TnphoA mutants of enteropathogenic *Escherichia coli* unable to invade HEp-2 cells. Infect Immun 1990; 58:1565–1571.
24. Rosenshine I, Donnenberg MS, Kaper JB, Finlay BB. Signal transduction between enteropathogenic *Escherichia coli* (EPEC) and epithelial cells: EPEC induces

tyrosine phosphorylation of host cell proteins to initiate cytoskeletal rearrangement and bacterial uptake. EMBO J 1992; 11:3551–3560.
25. Baldwin TJ, Ward W, Aitken A, et al. Elevation of intracellular calcium levels in HEp-2 cells infected with enteropathogenic *Escherichia coli*. Infect Immun 1991; 59:1599–1604.
26. Galan JE, Ginocchio C, Costeas, P. Molecular and functional characterization of the Salmonella invasion gene invA: homology of InvA to members of a new protein family. J Bacteriol 1992; 174:4338–4349.
27. Plano GV, Barve SS, Straley SC. LcrD, a membrane-bound regulator of the Yersinia pestis low-calcium response. J Bacteriol 1991; 173:7293–7303.
28. Andrews GP, Maurelli AT. mxiA of Shigella flexneri 2a, which facilitates export of invasion plasmid antigens, encodes a homolog of the low-calcium-response protein, LcrD, of Yersinia pestis. Infect Immun 1992; 60:3287–3295.
29. Jarvis KG, Giron JA, Jerse AE, et al. Enteropathogenic *Escherichia coli* contains a putative type III secretion system necessary for the export of proteins involved in attaching and effacing lesion formation. Proc Natl Acad Sci USA 1995; 92:7996–8000.
30. Knutton S, Baldwin T, Williams PH, McNeish AS. Actin accumulation at sites of bacterial adhesion to tissue culture cells: basis of a new diagnostic test for enteropathogenic and enterohemorrhagic *Escherichia coli*. Infect Immun 1989; 57:1290–1298.
31. Jerse AE, Yu J, Tall BD, Kaper JB. A genetic locus of enteropathogenic E*scherichia coli* necessary for the production of attaching and effacing lesions on tissue culture cells. Proc Natl Acad Sci USA USA. 1990; 87:7839–7843.
32. Donnenberg MS, Kaper JB. Construction of an eae deletion mutant of enteropathogenic *Escherichia coli* by using a positive-selection suicide vector. Infect Immun 1991; 59:4310–4317.
33. Donnenberg MS, Tacket CO, James SP, et al. Role of the eaeA gene in experimental enteropathogenic *Escherichia coli* infection. Journal of Clinical Investigation 1993; 92:1412–1417.
34. Jerse AE, Kaper JB. The eae gene of enteropathogenic *Escherichia coli* encodes a 94-kilodalton membrane protein, the expression of which is influenced by the EAF plasmid. Infect Immun 1991; 59:4302–4309.
35. McDaniel TK, Jarvis KG, Donnenberg MS, Kaper JB. A genetic locus of enterocyte effacement conserved among diverse enterobacterial pathogens. Proc Natl Acad Sci USA 1995; 92:1664–1668.
36. Stevenson JS. Bact. coli D433 in cases of diarrhoea in adults. British Medical Journal 1950; 2:195–196.
37. Stevenson JS. Further observations on the occurrence of Bact. coli D433 in adult faeces. British Medical Journal 1952; 2:123–124.
38. Costin ID, Voiculescu D, Gorcea, V. An outbreak of food poisoning in adults associated with Escherichia coli serotype 86:B7:H34. Pathol Microbiol 1964; 27:68–78.
39. Schroeder SA, Caldwell JR, Vernon TM, et al. A waterborne outbreak of gastroenteritis in adults associated with *Escherichia coli*. Lancet 1968; 1:737–740.

40. Levine MM, Edelman R. Enteropathogenic *Escherichia coli* of classic serotypes associated with infant diarrhea: epidemiology and pathogenesis. Epidemiologic Reviews 1984; 6:31–51.
41. Paulozzi LJ, Johnson KE, Kamahele LM, et al. Diarrhea associated with adherent enteropathogenic *Escherichia coli* in an infant and toddler center, Seattle, Washington. Pediatrics 1986; 77:296–300.
42. Bower JR, Congeni BL, Cleary TG, et al. *Escherichia coli* O114:nonmotile as a pathogen in an outbreak of severe diarrhea associated with a day care center. J Infect Dis 1989; 160:243–247.
43. Gurwith MJ, Wiseman DA, chow, P. Clinical and laboratory assessment of the pathogenicity of serotyped enteropathogenic *E. coli*. J Infect Dis 1977; 135: 736–743.
44. Baldini MM, Nataro JP, Kaper JB. Localization of a determinant for HEp-2 cell adherence by enteropathogenic *Escherichia coli*. Infect Immun 1986; 52:334–336.
45. Nataro JP, Maher KO, Mackie P, Kaper JB. Characterization of plasmids encoding the adherence factor of enteropathogenic *Escherichia coli*. Infect Immun 1987; 55:2370–2377.
46. Jerse AE, Martin WC, Galen JE, Kaper JB. Oligonucleotide probe for detection of the enteropathogenic *Escherichia coli* (EPEC) adherence factor of localized adherent EPEC. J Clin Microbiol 1990; 28:2842–2844.
47. Garcia del Olarte D, Trujillo H, Agudedo N, et al. Treatment of diarrhea in malnourished infants and children. A double blind study comparing ampicillin and placebo. Am J Dis Child 1974: 127:379–388.
48. Levine MM, Antimicrobial therapy for infectious diarrhea. Rev Infect Dis 1986; 8:S207–S216.
49. Nelson JD. Duraiton of meomycin therapy therapy for enteropathogenic *E. coli* diarrheal disease: a comparative study of 113 cases. Pediatrics 1971; 48; 248–258.
50. Thoren A, Wolde-Mariam T, Stintzig G, et al. Antibiotics in the treatment of gastroenteritis caused by enteropathogenic *E. coli*. J Infect Dis 1980; 141:27–31.
51. Gorbach SL, Banwell JG, Chatterjee BD, et al. Acute undifferentiated human diarrhea in the tropics. I. Alterations in intestinal microflora. J Clin Invest.1971; 50:881–889.
52. Sack RB. Enterotoxigenic *Escherichia coli*: identification and characterization. J Infect Dis 1980; 142:279–286.
53. Gaastra W, de Graaf, FK. Host-specific fimbrial adhesins of noninvasive enterotoxigenic *E. coli* strains. Microbiol Rev 1982; 46:129–161.
54. Levine MM, Kaper JB, Black RE, et al. New knowledge on pathogenesis of bacterial enteric infections as applied to vaccine development. Microbiol Rev 1983; 47:510–550.
55. Levine MM, Ferreccio C, Prado V, et al. Epidemiologic studies of *Escherichia coli* diarrheal infections in a low socioeconomic level peri-urban community in Santiago, Chile. Amer J Epidemiol 138:849–869.
56. Black RE, Merson MH, Rowe B, et al. Enterotoxigenic *E. coli* diarrhea: acquired immunity and transmission in an endemic area. Bull WHO 1981;59:263–268.

57. Holmgren J, Fredman P, Lindbald M, et al. 1982. Rabbit intestinal glycoprotein receptor for Escherichia coli heat-labile enterotoxin lacking affinity for cholera toxin. Infect Immun 1982; 38:424–433.
58. Geary S.J, Marchlewicz BA, Finkelstein RA. 1982. Comparison of heat-labile enterotoxins from porcine and human strains of *E. coli*. Infect Immun 1982; 36:215–220.
59. Clemens J D, Finkelstein RA. Demonstration of shared and unique immunologic determinants in enterotoxins from *V. cholerae* and *E. coli*. Infect Immun 1978; 22:709–713.
60. Chan S-K, Giannella RA. Amino acid sequences of heat stable enterotoxin produced by *E. coli* pathogenic for man. J Biol chem 1981; 26:7744–7746.
61. Hirayama T, Wada A, Iwata N, et al. Glycoprotein receptors for a heat-stable enterotoxin (STh) produced by enterotoxigenic *Escherichia coli*. Infect Immun 1992; 60:4213–4220.
62. Rudner XL, Nicchitta C, Almenoff JS. Biogenesis, cellular localization, and functional activation of the heat-stable enterotoxin receptor (guanylyl cyclase C). Biochemistry 1996;35:10680–6.
63. Field M, Graf LH, Laird WJ, Smith PL. Heat-stable enterotoxin of *Esherichia coli*: in vitro effects on guanylate cyclase activity, cyclic GMP concentration and ion transport in the small intestine. Proc Natl Acad Sci 1978; 75:2800–2804.
64. Cassels FJ, Wolf MK. Colonization factors of diarrheagenic *E. coli* and their intestinal receptors. J Ind Microbiol 1995; 15:214–226.
65. Klemm P. FImbrial adhesins of *Escherichia coli*. Rev Infect Dis 1985; 7:321–340.
66. Mol O, Oudega B. Molecular and structural aspects of fimbriae biosynthesis and assembly in *Escherichia coli*. FEMS Microbiol Rev 1996;19:25–52.
67. Levine MM, Ristaino P, Marley G, et al. Coli surface antigens 1 and 3 of colonization factor antigen II-positive enterotoxigenic *Escherichia coli*: morphology, purification, and immune responses in humans. Infect Immun 1985; 44:409–420.
68. Froehlich BJ, Karakashian A, Sakellaris H, Scott JR. Genes for CS2 pili of enterotoxigenic Escherichia coli and their interchangeability with those for CS1 pili. Infect Immun 1995;63:4849–56.
69. Wolf M, Taylor D, Boedeker E, et al. Characterization of Enterotoxigenic Escherichia coli (ETEC) isolated from soldiers in the Middle East in 1989 and 1990. J Clin Micro 1993; 31:851–856.
70. Rudin A, McConnell MM, Svennerholm AM. Monoclonal antibodies against enterotoxigenic Escherichia coli colonization factor antigen I (CFA/I) that cross-react immunologically with heterologous CFAs. Infect Immun 1994;62:4339–46
71. Giron JA, Levine MM, Kaper JB. Longus: a long pilus ultrastructure produced by human enterotoxigenic *Escherichia coli*. Mol Microbiol 1994;12:71–82.
72. Valvatne H, Sommerfelt H, Gaastra W, et al. Identification and characterization of CS20, a new putative colonization factor of enterotoxigenic *Escherichia coli*. Infect Immun 1996;64:2635–42.
73. Caron J, Coffield LM, Scott JR. A plasmid-encoded regulatory gene, *rns*, required for expression of the CS1 and CS2 adhesins of enterotoxigenic *Escherichia-coli*. Proc Natl Acad Sci USA 1989; 86:963–967.

74. Echeverria P, Ørskov F, Ørskov I, Plianbangchang D. Serotypes of enterotoxigenic *Escherichia coli* in Thailand and the Philippines. Infect Immun 1982; 36:851–856.
75. Merson MH, Ørskov F, Ørskov I, et al. Relationship between toxin production and serotype in enterotoxigenic *Escherichia coli*. Infect Immun 1979; 23:325–329.
76. Merson MH, Rowe B, Black R., et al. Use of antisera for identification of enterotoxigenic *Escherichia coli*. Lancet 1980; 2:222–224.
77. Ørskov F, Ørskov I. Special *Escherichia coli* serotypes among enterotoxigenic strains from diarrhoea in adults and children. Med Microbiol Immunol 1976; 162:73–80.
78. Reis MHL, Matos DP, Pestana de Castro, et al. Relationship among enterotoxigenic phenotypes, serotypes, and sources of strains in enterotoxigenic *Escherichia coli*. Infect Immun 1980; 28:24–27.
79. NIH Consensus Conference Traveller's Diarrhea. A balanced critical appraisal of the epidemiology, etiologies, presentation and treatment of traveller's diarrhea. J. Amer. Med. Assoc. 1985; 253:2700–2704.
80. Black RE, Merson MH, Huq I, et al. Incidence and severity of rotavirus and *E. coli* diarrhea in rural Bangladesh. Implications for vaccines development. Lancet 1981; i:141–143.
81. Black RE, Brown KH, Becker S, et al. Longitudinal studies of infectious diseases and physical growth of children in rural Bangladesh. II. Incidence of diarrhea and association with known pathogens. Am. J. Epidemiol. 1982; 115:315–324.
82. Edelman R, Levine MM. Summary of an international workshop on typhoid fever. Rev Infect Dis 1986; 8:329–349.
83. Dean AG, Ching Y-C, Williams RG, Harden LB. Test for *E. coli* enterotoxin using infant mice: application in a study of diarrhea in children in Honolulu. J Infect Dis 1972; 125:407–411.
84. Sack DA, Sack RB. Test for enterotoxigenic *E. coli* using Y-1 adrenal cells in miniculture. Infect Immun 1975; 11:334–6.
85. Stacy-Phipps S, Mecca JJ, Weiss JB. Multiplex PCR assay and simple preparation method for stool specimens detect enterotoxigenic Escherichia coli DNA during course of infection. J Clin Microbiol 1995;33:1054–9.
86. Schultsz C, Pool GJ, van Ketel R, et al. Detection of enterotoxigenic Escherichia coli in stool samples by using nonradioactively labeled oligonucleotide DNA probes and PCR. J Clin Microbiol 1994;32:2393–7.
87. Deng MY, Cliver DO, Day SP, et al. Enterotoxigenic *Escherichia coli* detected in foods by PCR and an enzyme-linked oligonucleotide probe. Int J Food Microbiol 1996;30:217–29.
88. Avery ME, Snyder JD. Oral Rehydration Therapy for Acute Diarrhea: The Underused Simple Solution. NEJM 1990;323:891–894.
89. Mahalanbis D. Current Status of Oral Rehydration as a Strategy for Control of Diarrheal Diseases. Indian J Med Res, 1996;104:115–24.
90. Casteel HB, Foedorek SC. Oral rehydration therapy. Ped Clinic North Amer 1990:37;295–311.
91. Hischhorn N, Greenough WB III. Progress in Oral Rehydration Therapy. Sci Am 1991;264:50–56.

92. Guiraldes E, Trivino ., Hodgson MI, et al. Treatment of acute infantile diarrhoea with a commercial rice-based oral rehydration solution. J Diarrhoeal Dis Res 1995:13;207–211.
93. Jirapinyo P, Moran JR. Comparison of oral rehydration solutions made with rice syrup solids or glucose in the treatment of acute diarrhea in infants. J Med Assoc Thai 1996;79:154–60.
94. Pizarro D, Posada G, Sandi L, Moran RJ. Rice-based oral electrolyte solutions for the management of infantile diarrhea. NEJM 1991;324:517–21
95. Molina S, Vettorazzi C, Peerson JM, et al. Clinical trial of glucose-oral rehydration solution (ORS), rice dextrin-ORS, and rice flour-ORS for the management of children with acute diarrhea and mild or moderate dehydration. Pediatrics 1995;95:191–7.
96. Cohen MB, Mezoff AG, Laney DW Jr, et al. Use of a single solution for oral rehydration and maintenance therapy of infants with diarrhea and mild to moderate dehydration [see comments]. Pediatrics 1995;95:639–45.
97. Maulen-Radovan I, Fernandez-Varela H, Acosta-Bastidas M, Frenk S. Safety and efficacy of a rice-based oral rehydration salt solution in the treatment of diarrhea in infants less than 6 months of age. J Pediatr Gastroenterol Nutr 1994;19:78–82.
98. Fayad IM, Hasnem M, Duggan C, et al. Comparative efficacy of rice-based and glucose-based oral rehydration salts plus early reintroduction of food. Lancet 1993; 342:772–75.
99. Santosham M, Fayad I, Abu Zikri M, et al. A double-blind clinical trial comparing World Health Organization oral rehydration solution with a reduced osmolarity solution containing equal amounts of sodium and glucose. J Pediatr 1996;128:45–51.
100. Anonymous. Multicentre evaluation of reduced-osmolarity oral rehydration salts solution. International Study Group on Reduced-osmolarity ORS solutions. Lancet 1995;345:282–5.
101. Mahalanabis D, Faruque AS, Hoque SS, Faruque SM. Hypotonic oral rehydration solution in acute diarrhoea: a controlled clinical trial. Acta Paediatr 1995;84:289–93.
102. el-Mougi M, el-Akkad N, Hendawi A, et al. Is a low-osmolarity ORS solution more efficacious than standard WHO ORS solution? J Pediatr Gastroenterol Nutr 1994;19:83–6.
103. Sazawal S, Black RE, Bhan MK, et al. Zinc supplementation in young children with acute diarrhea in India. NEJM 1995;333:839–44.
104. Santosham, M., Daum, R.S., Dillman, L., et al. Oral Rehydration Therapy of Infantile Diarrhea. NEJM 1982; 306:1070–1076.
105. Gorbach SL, Edelman R, eds. Traveler's Diarrhea, NIH Consensus Development Conference. Rev. Infect. Dis. 1986; 8:S109–S227.
106. DuPont HL, Ericcson CD. Prevention and Treatment of Traveler's Diarrhea. NEJM 1993;328:1821–1827.
107. DuPont HL, Sullivan, P, Pickering LK, Ackerman MS. Symptomatic Treatment of Diarrhea with Bismuth Subsalicylate among Students Attending a Mexican University. Gastroenterology 1977; 73:715–718.

108. Ericsson CD, Johnson PC, DuPont HL, et al. Ciprofloxacin or Trimethoprim-Sulfamethoxazole as Initial Therapy for Traveler's Diarrhea. Ann Int Med.1987; 106:216–220.
109. DuPont HL, Reves RR, Galindo E, et al. Treatment of Travelers' Diarrhea with Trimethoprim/Sulfamethoxazole and with Trimethoprim Alone. NEJM 1982; 307: 841–844.
110. Mattila L, Peltola H, Siitonen A, et al. Short-term treatment of traveler's diarrhea with norfloxacin: a double-blind, placebo-controlled study during two seasons. Clin Infect Dis 1993; 17:779–782.
111. Salam I, Katelaris P, Leigh-Smith S, Farthing MJG. Randomised trial of single-dose ciprofloaxacin for traveler's diarrhoea. Lancet 1994;334:1537–39.
112. Van Loon FPL, Bennish ML, Speelman P, Butler C. Double blind trial of loperamide for treating acute water diarrhoea in expatriates in Bangladesh. Gut 1989;30:492–495.
113. Steffen R, Heusser R, Tschopp A, DuPont HL. Efficacy and Side-Effects of Six Agents in the Self-Treatment of Traveller's Diarrhoea. Travel Medicine International 1988; 153–157.
114. Erricsson CD, DuPont HL, Mathewson JJ, et al.. Treatment of Traveler's Diarrhea with Sulfamethoxazole and Trimethoprim and Loperamide. JAMA 1990; 263:2578–261.
115. Taylor DN, Sanchez JL, Candler W, et al. Treatmet of traveler's diarrhea: Ciprofloxacin plus loperamide compared with ciprofloxacin alone. Annals of Internal Med 1991;114:731–734.
116. Petruccelli BP, Murphy GS, Sanchez JL, et al. Treatment of Traveler's Diarrhea with ciprofloxacin and loperamide. J Inf Dis. 1992; 165:557–560.
117. Tacket CO, Losonsky G, Link H, et al. Protection by Milk Immunoglobulin Concentrate Against Oral Challenge with Enterotoxigenic *Escherichia coli*. NEJM 1988; 318: 1240–1243.
118. Griffin PM, Tauxe RV. The epidemiology of infections caused by *E. coli* 0157:H7 and other enterohemorrhagic *E. coli*, and the associated hemolytic-uremic syndrome. Epidemiol Rev 1991; 13:60–98.
119. Boyce TG, Swerdlow DI, Griffin PM. *E. coli* 0157:H7 and the hemolytic-uremic syndrome. New Engl J Med 1995; 333:364–368.
120. Riley LW, Remis RS, Helgerson SD, et al. hemorrhagic colitis associated with a rare *e. coli* serotype. N Engl J Med 1983; 308:681–685.
121. Bell BP, Goldoft M, Griffin PM, et al. A multistate outbreak of *E. coli* 0157:H7-associated bloody diarrhea and hemolytic uremic syndrome from hamburgers: the Washington experience JAMA 1994; 272:1349–1352.
122. Rosenweig JN, Gourley GR. Verotoxic *Escherichia coli* in human disease. J Pediatr Gastroenterol Nutr 1991; 12:295–304.
123. Remis RS, MacDonald KL, Riley LW, et al. Sporadic cases of hemorrhagic colitis associated with Escherichia coli O157:H7-clinical, epidemiologic, and bacteriologic features. Ann Intern Med 1984;101:624–626.
124. Griffin PM, Ostroff SM, Tauxe RV, et al. Illness associated with *Escherichia coli* O157:H7 Infections. A broad clinical spectrum. Ann Intern Med 1988;109:705–712.

125. Lopez EL, Devoto S, Fayad A, et al. Association between severity of gastrointestinal prodrome and long-term-prognosis in classic hemolytic-uremic syndrome. J Pediatr 1992;120:210–215.
126. Pavia AT, Nichols CR, Green DP, et al. Hemolytic-uremic syndrome during an outbreak of *Escherichia coli* O157:H7 Infections in institutions for mentally retarded persons: Clinical and epidemiologic observations. J Pediatr 1990;116:544–551.
127. Pickering LK, Obrig TG, Stapleton B. Hemolytic-Uremic Syndrome and enterohemorrhagic *Escherichia coli.* Pediatr Infect Dis J 1994;13:459–476
128. Martin DL, MacDonald KL, White KE, et al. The epidemiology and clinical aspects of the hemolytic uremic syndrome in Minnesota. N Engl J Med 1990; 323:1161–1167.
129. Ryan CA, Tauxe RV, Hosek GW, et al. *E. coli* O157:H7 diarrhea in a nursing home: clinical, epidemiological and pathogical findings. J Infect Dis 154:631–638, 1986.
130. Carter AO, Borcyyk AA, Carlson JAK, et al. A severe outbreak of *E. coli* O157:H7-associated hemorrhagic colitis in a nursing home. N Engl J Med 317:1496–1500, 1987.
131. Hamano S, Nakanishi Y, Nara T, et al. Neurologic manifestations of hemorrhagic colitis in the outbreak of *Escherichia coli* O157:H7 Infection in Japan. Acta Paediatr 1993;82:454–458.
132. Rowe PC, Orrbine E, Wells GA, et al. Epidemiology of hemolytic-uremic syndrome in Canadian children from 1986 to 1988. J Pediatr 1991;119:218–224.
133. Robson WLM, Leung AKC, Miller-Hughes DJ. Recurrent hemorrhagic colitis caused by *Escherichia coli* O157:H7. Pediatr Inf Dis J 1993;12:699–701.
134. Siegler RL, Griffin PM, Barrett TJ, Strockbine NA. Recurrent hemolytic uremic syndrome secondary to *Escherichia coli* O157:H7 infection. Pediatrics 1993;81:666–668.
135. Tesh VL, O'Brien AD, Microreview: The pathogenic mechanisms of Shiga toxin and the Shiga-like toxins. Molec Microbiol 1991; 5:1817–1822.
136. Ostroff S M, Tarr PI, Neill MA,et al. Toxin genotypes and plasmid profiles as determinants of systemic sequelae in *E. coli* O157:H7 infection. J Infect Dis 1989; 160:994–998
137. Yu J, Kaper JB. Cloning and characterization of the eae gene of enterohemorrhagic *Escherichia coli* O157:H7. Mol Microbiol 1992; 6:411–417.
138. O'Brien AD, Holmes RK. Shiga and Shiga-like toxins. Microbiol Rev 1987; 51:206–220.
139. O'Brien AD, Lively TA, Chen ME, et al. *Escherichia coli* O157:H7 strains associated with hemorrhagic colitis in the United States produces a Shigella dysenteriae 1 (Shiga)-like cytotoxin. Lancet 1983; i:702
140. Jackson MP, Structure-function analyses of Shiga toxin and the Shiga-like toxins. Microb. Pathogen 8:235–242, 1990.
141. O'Brien AD, Lively TA, Chang TW, Gorbach SL. Purification of Shigella dysenteriae 1 (Shiga)-like toxin from *Escherichia coli* O157:H7 strain associated with hemorrhagic colitis. Lancet 1983, ii:573.

142. Konawalchuk J, Speirs JI, Stavric S. Vero response to a cytotoxin of *E. coli*. Infect Immun 1977; 18:
143. Cantey JR. Shiga toxin: an expanding role in the pathogenesis of infectious diseases. J Infect Dis 1985; 151:766–779.
144. Strockbine NA, Marques LRM, Holmes RK, O'Brien AD. Two toxin-converting phages from Escherichia coli O157:H7 strain 933 encode antigenically distinct toxins with similar biological activities. Infect Immun 1986; 53:135–140.
145. Smith WH, Green P, Parsell Z. Vero cell toxin in *E. coli* and related bacteria: transfer by phage and conjugation and toxic action in laboratory animals, chickens and pigs. J Gen Microbiol 129:3121–7, 1983.
146. Newland JW, Strockbine NA, Miller SF, et al. Cloning of Shiga-like toxin structural genes from a toxin converting phage of *E. coli*. Science 1985;230:179–81
147. O'Brien AD, Newland JW, Miller SF, et al. Shiga-like toxin-converting phages from Escherichia coli strains that cause hemorrhagic colitis or infantile diarrhea. Science 1984; 226:694–696.
148. Donohue-Rolfe A, Jacewicz M, et al. Pathogenesis of Shigella diarrhea: evidence for a developmentally regulated glycolipid receptor of Shigella toxin involved in the fluid secretory response of rabbit small intestine. J Infect Dis 1988;157:1023–31.
149. Hovde CJ, Calderwood SB, Mekalanos JJ, Collier RJ. Evidence that glutamic acid 167 is an active-site residue of Shiga-like toxin I. Proc Nat Acad Sci USA 1988;85:2568–72.
150. Endo Y, Tsurugi K, Yutsudo T, Takeda Y, Ogasawara T, Igarashi K. Site of action of a Vero toxin (VT2) from *Escherichia coli* O157:H7 and of Shiga toxin on eukaryotic ribosomes: RNA N-glycosidase activity of the toxins. Eur. J. Biochem. 1988; 171:45–50.
151. Obrig T, Moran T, Brown J. The mode of action of Shiga toxin on peptide elongation of eukaryotic protein synthesis. Biochem J 1987; 244:287–294.
152. Gyles CL. VT Toxemia in Animal Models. pp 233–240 in Karmali MA & Goglio AG eds. Recent Advances in Verocytotoxin-producing *E. coli* infections. Elsevier Science, 1994.
153. Acheson DWK, Moore R, Jackewicz M, et al. Translocation of Shiga-like toxin across intact epithelial cell monolayers in tissue culture. Pp 205–208 in Karmali MA & Goglio AG. Recent Advances in Verocytotoxin-producing *Escherichia coli* infections. Elsevier Science, Amsterdam, 1994.
154. Chart H, Law D, Rowe B, Acheson DWK. Patients with haemolytic uraemic syndrome caused by Escherichia coli O157: absence of antibodies to Verocytotoxin VT1 or VT2. J Clin Pathol 1993; 46:1053–1054.
155. Levine MM. *E. coli* that cause diarrhea: enterotoxigenic, enteropathogenic, enteroinvasive, ennterohemorrhagic and enteroadherent. J Infect Dis 155: 377–389, 1987.
156. Sherman P, Soni R, Karmali M. Attaching and effacing adherence of Vero cytotoxn-producing Escherichia coli to rabbit intestinal epithelium in vivo. Infect Immun 1988; 56:756–761.
157. Tzipori S, Wachsmuth IK, Chapman C, et al. The pathogenesis of hemorrhagic

colitis caused by Escherichia coli O157:H7 in gnotobiotic piglets. J Infect Dis 1986; 154:712–716.
158. Donnenberg MS, Tzipori S, McKee ML, et al. The role of the eae gene of enterohemorrhagic Escherichia coli in intimate attachment in vitro and in a porcine model. J Clin Invest 1993; 92:1418–1424.
159. Donnenberg MS, Yu J, Kaper JB. A second chromosomal gene necessary for intimate attachment of enteropathogenic Escherichia coli to epithelial cells. J Bacteriol 1993, 175:4670–4680.
160. Foubister V, Rosenshine I, Donnenberg, MS, Finlay BB. The eaeB gene of enteropathogenic Escherichia coli is necessary for signal transduction in epithelial cells. Infect Immun 1994; 62:3038–3040.
161. Wells JG, Davis BR, Wachsmuth IK, et al. Laboratory investigation of hemorrhagic colitis outbreaks associated with a rare Escherichia coli serotype. J Clin Microbiol 1983; 18:512–520.
162. Karch H, Heeseman J, Laufs R, et al. A plasmid of enterohemorrhagic Escherichia coli O157:H7 is required for expression of a new fimbrial antigen and for adhesion to epithelial cells. Infect Immun 1987; 55:455–461.
163. McKee,ML, O'Brien AD. Investigation of enterohemorrhagic Escherichia coli O157:H7 adherence characteristics and invasion potential reveals a new attachment pattern shared by intestinal *E. coli*. Infect Immun 1995; 63:2070–2074.
164. Remuzzi G, Zoja C. Endothelial Cell Physiology. In Karmali MA and Goglio AG, eds. Recent Advances in Verocytotoxin-producing *E. coli* infections. Elsevier Science, 1994:309–316.
165. van der Kar NCAJ, Monnens LAH, Karmali MA, van Hinsbergh VVM. Tumor necrosis factor and interleukin-1 induce expression of the verocytotoxin receptor Globotriasoylceramide on human endothelial cells: implications for the pathogenesis of the hemolytic uremic syndrome. Blood 80:2755–2764, 1993.
166. Kaye SA, Louise CB, Boyd B, et al. Shiga toxin-associated hemolytic uremic syndrome: Interleukin-1 beta enhancement of shiga toxin cytotoxicity toward human vascular endothelial cells in vitro. Infect Immun 61:3886–3891, 1993.
167. Tesh VL, Samuel JE, Perera LP, et al. Evaluation of the role of shiga and shiga-like toxins in mediating direct damage to human vascular endothelial cells. J Infect Dis 164:344–352, 1991.
168. Karmali M, Petric M, Lim C, et al. The association between idiopathic hemolytic uremic syndrome and infection by Verotoxin-producing *Escherichia coli*. J Infect Dis 1985; 151:775–789.
169. Kaplan BS, McGowan KL. Hemolytic uremic syndrome. Curr Op Infect Dis 1994; 7:351–357.
170. Brotma, M, Giannella RA, Alm PF, et al. Consensus conference statement: Escherichia coli O157:H7 infections—an emerging national health crisis, July 11-13, 1994. Gastroenterology 1995; 108:1923–1934.
170A. Tarr PI. *E. coli* O157:H7: Clinical, Diagnostic, and Epidemiological Aspects of Human Infection. Clin Infect Dis.1995;20:1–10.
171. Marsh J, MacLeod AF. A restaurant-associated outbreak of *E. coli* O157 infection. J Pub Hlth Med 1992; 14:78–83.

172. Spika JS, Parsons JE. HUS and diarrhoea associated with *E. coli* O157:H7 in a day care center. J Pediatr 1986; 109:287–291.
173. Beutin L, Aleksic S, Zimmerman S, Gleier K. Virulence factors and phenotypic traits of verotoxigenic strains of Escherichia coli isolated from human patients in Germany. Medical Microbiology and Immunology (Belg.). 1994; 183:13–21.
174. Belongia EA, Osterholm MT, Soler JT, et al. Transmission of Escherichia coli O157:H7 infection in Minnesota day-care facilities. JAMA 1993; 269:883–888.
175. Karmali MA, Arbus G, Petric M, et al. Hospital-acquired Escherichia coli O157:H7 associated hemolytic uraemic syndrome in a nurse (letter). Lancet 1988; i:526.
176. Rowe PC, Orrbine E, Lior H, et al. Diarrhoea in close contacts as a risk factor for childhood hemolytic uraemic syndrome. Epidemiol Infect 1993; 10:9–16.
177. Bitzan M, Ludwig K, Klemt M, et al. The role of Escherichia coli O157 infections in the classical (enteropathic) hemolytic uraemic syndrome: results of a Central European, multicenter study. Epidemiol Infect 1993; 110:183–196.
178. Cordovez A, Prado V, Maggi L, et al. Enterohemorrhagic *Escherichia coli* associated with hemolytic-uremic syndrome in Chilean children. J Clin Microbiol 1992; 30:2153–2157.
179. Whittam TS, Wilson RA. Genetic relationships among pathogenic *Escherichia coli* of serogroup O157. Infect Immun 1988; 56:2467–2473.
180. Whittam TS, Wolfe ML, Wachsmuth IK, et al. Clonal relationships among Escherichia coli strains that cause hemorrhagic colitis and infantile diarrhea. Infect Immun 1993; 61:1619–1629.
181. Cordovez A, Prado V, Maggi L, et al. Enterohemorrhagic Escherichia coli associated with hemolytic-uremic syndrome in Chilean children. J Clin Microbiol 1992; 30:2153–2157.
182. Luzzi I, Minelli F, Gianviti A, Caprioli A. Impaired detection of faecal verocytotoxin in the presence of Clostridium difficile cytotoxin in patients with hemolytic-uremic syndrome. Eur J Clin Microbiol Infect Dis 1992; 11:934–936.
183. Tarr PI, Neill MA, Clausen CR, et al. *Escherichia coli* O157:H7 and the hemolytic-uremic syndrome: importance of early cultures in establishing the etiology. J Infect Dis 1990; 162:553–556.
184. Law D, Harmour AA, Acheson DWK, et al. Diagnosis of infections with Shiga-like toxin-producing *Escherichia coli* by the use of enzyme-linked immunosorbent assays for Shiga-like toxins on cultured stool samples. J Med Microbiol 1994; 40:241–245.
185. Newland JW, Neil RJ. DNA probes for Shiga-like toxins I and II for toxin converting bacteriophages. J Clin Microbiol 1988; 26:1292–1297.
186. Brian M, Frosolono M, Murray BE, et al. Polymerase chain reaction for diagnosis of enterohemorrhagic Escherichia coli infection and hemolytic-uremic syndrome. J Clin Microbiol 1992; 30:1801–1806.
187. Paton AW, Paton JC, Goldwater PN, Manning PA. Direct detection of *Escherichia coli* Shiga-like toxin genes in primary fecal cultures by polymerase chain reaction. J Clin Microbiol 1993; 31:3063-3067.
188. Voelker R. New strategies aimed at *E. coli* O157:H7. JAMA 1994; 272–503.

189. Walterspiel JN, Ashkenazi S, Morrow AL, Cleary TG. Effect of sub-inhibitory concentrations of antibiotics on extracellular Shiga-Like Toxin I. Infection 1992; 20:25–29.
190. Karch H, Strockbine, NA, O'Brien AD. Groweth of *E. coli* in the presence of trimethoprim-sulfamethoxasole facilitates detection of Shiga-like toxin-producing strains by colony blot assay. FEMS Micriol. Lett 1986; 35:141–145.
191. Proulx F, Turgeon JP, Delage G, et al. Randomized, controlled trial of antibiotic therapy for *Escherichia coli* O157:H7 enteritis. J Pediatr 1992; 121:299–303.
192. Center for Disease Control. 1993 Update: Multistate outbreak of *E. coli* O157:H7. MMWR 1993;42:258–263.
193. Armstrong GD, Rowe PC, Orrbine E, et al. Results of a phase 1 study into the use of Synsorb-Pk for preventing hemolytic uremic syndrome (HUS). Second International Symposium on Verocytotoxin (Shiga-Like toxin) Producing *Escherichia coli* infection, Bergamo, Italy, June 1994;AO4.8.
194. Elliott E, Li Z, Stiel D, et al. Modulation of host response to *Escherichia coli* O157:H7 Infection by anti-CD18 antibody in rabbits. Gastroenterology 1994;106:1554–1561.
195. Loirat C, Sonsino E, Hinglais N, et al. Treatment of the childhood hemolytic uraemic syndrome with plasma. A multicentre randomized controlled trial. The French Society of Paediatric Nephrology. Pediatr Nephrol 1988;2:279–85.
196. Ewing WH. Serological relationships between shigella and coliform cultures. J Bacteriol 1953; 66:333–340.
197. Brenner DJ, Fanning GR, Steigerwalt AG, et al. Polynucleotide sequence relatedness among three groups of pathogenic *Escherichia coli* strains. Infect Immun 1972; 6:308–315.
198. Brenner DJ, Fanning, GR, Skerman FJ, Falkow, S. Polynucleotide sequence divergence among strains of *Escherichia coli* and closely related organisms. J Bacteriol 1972; 109:953–965.
199. Brenner DJ, Fanning GR, Miklos GV, Steigerwalt AG. Polynucleotide sequence relatedness among Shigella species. Int J Syst Bacteriol 1973; 23:1–7.
200. Goullet P. Esterase electrophoretic pattern between Shigella species and *Escherichia coli*. J Gen Microbiol 1980; 117:493–500.
201. Ochman H, Whittam TS, Caugant DA, Selander RK. Enzyme polymorphism and genetic population structure in *Escherichia coli* and Shigella. J Gen Microbiol 1983; 129:2715–2726.
202. Hartl DL, Dykhuizen DE. The population genetics of Escherichia coli. Annu Rev Genet 1984; 18:31–68.
203. Whittam TS, Ochman H, Selander RK. Multilocus genetic structure in natural populations of Escherichia coli. Proc Natl Acad Sci USA 1983; 80:1751–1755.
204. Karaolis DKR, Lan R, Reeves PR. Sequence variation in *Shigella sonnei* (Sonnei), a pathogenic clone of *Escherichia coli*, over four continents and 41 years. J. Clin. Microbiol. 1994; 32:796–802.
205. Stevenson G, Neal B, Liu D, et al. Structure of the O-antigen of E. coli K-12 and the sequence of its rfb gene cluster. J Bacteriol 1994; 176:4144–4156.
206. DuPont HL, Formal SB, Hornick RB, et al. Pathogenesis of *Escherichia coli* diarrhea. N Engl J Med 1971; 285:1–9.

207. Pai T, Pacsa S, Emody L, Voros S. Antigenic relationship among virulent enteroinvasive *E. coli*, *Shigella flexneri*, and *Shigella sonnei* detected by ELISA. Lancet 1983;ii:102 (letter).
208. Sansonetti PJ, Kopecko DJ, Formal SB. 1982. Involvement of a plasmid in the invasive ability of *Shigella flexneri*. Infect Immun 35:852–860.
209. Harris JR, Wachsmuth IK, Davis BR, Cohen ML. High-molecular weight plasmid correlates with *Escherichia coli* enteroinvasiveness. Infect Immun 1982; 37:1295–1298.
210. Hale TL, Sansonetti PJ, Schad PA, et al. Characterization of virulence plasmids and plasmid-associated outer membrane proteins in Shigella flexneri, Shigella sonnei, and *Escherichia coli*. Infect Immun 1983; 40:340–350.
211. Gomes TA, Toledo MRF, Trabulsi LR, et al. DNA probes for identification of enteroinvasive *Escherichia coli*. J Clin Microbiol 1987; 25:2025–2027.
212. Hale TL. 1991. Genetic basis of virulence in *Shigella* species. Microbiol Rev. 55:206–224.
213. Hale TL, Formal SB. In: Roth JA, ed. Virulence mechanisms of bacterial pathogens. Washington, DC: American Society for Microbiology; 1988:61–9.
214. Sansonetti P, Ryter A, Clers P, et al. Multiplication of *Shigella flexneri* within HeLa cells: lysis of the phagocytic vacuole and plasmid-mediated contact hemolysis. Infect Immun 1986;51:41–49.
215. Sansonetti PJ. In: Sansonetti PJ, ed. Pathogenesis of shigellosis. Berlin: Springer-Verlage; 1992:1–19.
216. Kadurugamuwa JL, Rohde M, Wehland J, Timmis KN. Intercellular spread of *Shigella flexneri* through a monolayer mediated by membranous protrusions and associated with reorganization of the cytoskeletal protein vinculin. Infect Immun 1991;59:3463–71.
217. Bernardini ML, Mounier J, D'Hauteville H, et al. 1989. Identification of *icsA*, a plasmid locus of *Shigella flexneri* that governs bacterial intra- and intercellular spread through interaction with F-actin. Proc Natl Acad Sci USA 86:3867–3871.
218 . Sansonetti PJ, Mounier J, Prevost MC, Mege M. Cadherin expression is required for the spread of *Shigella flexneri* between epithelial cells. Cell 1994;76:829–839.
219. Sansonetti PJ. Genetic molecular basis of epithelial cell invasion by *Shigella* species. Rev Inf Dis 1991;13:S285–292.
220. Methan MM, Mathan VI. Morphology of rectal mucosa of patients with shigellosis. Rev Infect Dis 1991;13:S314–318.
221. Zychlinsky A, Prevost MC, Sansonetti PJ. *Shigella flexneri* induces apoptosis in infected macrophages. Nature 1992;358:167–169.
222. Zychlinsky A, Fitting C, Cavaillon J, Sansonnetti PJ. Interleukin 1 is released by murine macrophages during apoptosis induced by Shigella flexneri. J Clin Invest 1994;94:1328–1332.
223. Munier J, Vasselon T, Hellio R, et al. *Shigella flexneri* enters human colonic Caco-2 epithelial cells through the basolateral pole. Infect Immun 1992;60:237–248.
224. Jung HC, Eckmann L, Yang S, et al.. A distinct array of proinflammatory

cytokines is expressed in human colon epithelial cells in response to bacterial invasion. J Clin Invest 1995;95:55–65.

225. Perdomo OJJ, Cavaillon JM, Heurre M, et al. Acute inflammation causes epithelial invasion and mucosal destruction in experimental shigellosis. J Exp Med 1994;10:1307–1319.

226. Tulloch FE, Ryan KE, Formal SB, Franklin FA. Invasive enteropathic *E. coli* dysentery. Ann Int Med 1973; 79:13–17.

227. Echeverria P, Sethabutr O, Pitarangsi C. 1991. Microbiology and diagnosis of infections with *Shigella* and enteroinvasive *Escherichia coli*. Rev Infect Dis 13(supplement 4):S220–S225.

228. Fasano A, Kay BA, Russell RG, et al. 1990. Enterotoxin and cytotoxin production by enteroinvasive *Escherichia coli*. Infect Immun 58:3717–3723.

229. Natatro JP, Seriwatama J, Fasano A, et al. Identification and cloning of a novel plasmid-encoded enterotoxin of enteroinvasive *E. coli* and *Shigella* strains. Infect Immun 1995; 63:4721–4728.

230. Lanyi B, Szita J, Ringelhann M, Kovack K. A waterborne outbreak of enteritis associated with *Escherichia coli* serotype O124:72:32. Acta Microbiologica Hungaricae 1959; 6:77.

231. Marier R, Wells JG, Swanson RC, et al. An outbreak of enteropathogenic *Escherichia coli* foodborne disease traced to imported French cheese. Lancet 1973; ii:1376–1378.

232. Toledo MRF, Trabulsi LR. Correlation between biochemical characteristics of Escherichia coli and results of the Sereny test. J Clin Microbiol 1983; 17:419–421.

233. Pal T, Pacsa AS, Emody L, et al. Modified enzyme-linked immunosorbent assay for detecting enteroinvasive Escherichia coli and virulent Shigella strains. J Clin Microbiol 1985; 21:415–418.

234. Wood PK, Morris Jr, JG, Small PLC, et al. Comparison of DNA probes with the Sereny test for identification of invasive Shigella and Escherichia coli strains. J Clin Microbiol.1986; 24:498–500.

235. Matthewson JJ, Oberhleman RA, DuPont HL, et al. Enteroadherent *E. coli* as a cause of diarrhea among children in Mexico. J Clin Microbiol 1987; 25:1917–1919.

236. Nataro JP, Kaper JB, Robins-Browne R, Pet al. Patterns of adherence of diarrheagenic *E. coli* to HEp-2 Cells. Pediatric Infect Dis J 1987; 6:829–831.

237. Henry FJ, Udoy AS, Wanke CA, Aziz KMA. Epidemiology of persistent diarrhea and etiologic agents in Mirzapur, Bangladesh. Acta Pediatr Scand 1992; 81 Suppl. 381:39–44.

238. Bhan MK, Raj, P, Levine MM, et al. Enteroaggregative *E. coli* associated with persistent diarrhea in a cohort of rural children in India. J Infect Dis 1989; 159:1061–1064.

239. Cravioto A, Tello A, Navarro A, et al. Association of *E. coli* HEp-2 adherence patterns with type and duration of diarhea. Lancet 1991; 337:262–264.

240. Wanke CA, Schorling JB, Barfrett LJ, et al. Potential role of adherence traits of *E. coli* from persistent diarrhea in an urban Brazilian slum. Pediatric Infect Dis J. 1991; 10:746–751.

241. Methewson JJ, Johnson PC, DuPont, HL, Pathogenecity of enteroadherent *E. coli* in adult volunteers. J Infect Dis 1986; 154:524–527.
242. Nataro JP, Deng Y, Cookson S, et al.. Heterogeneity of enteroaggregative Escherichia coli virulence demonstrated in volunteers. J Infect Dis 1995; 171:465–8.
243. Vial PA, Robins Browne R, Lior H, et al. Characterization of enteroadherent-aggregative *E. coli*, a putative agent of diarrheal disease. J Infect Dis 1988;158:70–79.
244. Tzipori S, Montanaro J, Robins-Browne R, et al. Studies with enteroaggregative *E. coli* in the gnotobiotic piglet gastroenteritis model. Infect Immun 1992; 60:5302–5306.
245. Knutton S, Shaw RK, Bhan MK, et al. Ability of enteroaggregative *E. coli* strains to adhere in vitro to human intestinal mucosa. Infect Immun 1991; 59:3722–3739.
246. Nataro JP, Yikang D, Giron JA, et al. Aggregative adherence fimbria I expression in enteroaggregative *E. coli* requires two unlinked plasmid regions. Infect Immun 1993; 61: 1126–1131.
247. Yamamoto T, Endo S, Yokota T, Echeverria P. Characteristics of adherence of enteroaggregative *E. coli* to human and animal mucosa. Infect Immun 1991; 59:3722–3739.
248. Nataro JP, Hicks S, Phillips AD, Vial PA, Sears CL. T84 cells in culture as a model for enteroaggregative *Escherichia coli* pathogenesis. Infect Immun 1996; 11:4761–8.
249. Hicks S, Candy DC, Phillips AD. Adhesion of enteroaggregative *Escherichia coli* to pediatric intestinal mucosa in vitro. Infect Immun 1996;11:4751–60.
250. Savarino SJ, Fox P, Deng Y, Nataro JP. Identification and characterization of a gene cluster mediating enteroaggregative *Escherichia coli* aggregative adherence fimbria I biogenesis. J Bacteriol 1994;176:4949–57.
251. Savarino, SJ, Fasano A, Watson J, et al. Enteroaggregative *E. coli* heat-stable enterotoxin I represents another subfamily of *E. coli* heat-stable toxin. Proc Nat Acad Sci USA 1993; 90:3093–3097.
252. Savarino SJ, McVeigh A, Watson J, et al. Enteroaggregative *Escherichia coli* heat-stable enterotoxin is not restricted to enteroaggregative *E. coli*. J Infect Dis 1996;173:1019–22.
253. Baldwin TJ, Knutton S, Sellers L, et al. Enteroaggregative *E. coli* strains secrete a heat-labile toxin antigenically related to *E. coli* hemolysin. Infect Immun 1992; 60; 2092–2095.
254. Eslava C, Villaseca J, Morales R, et al. Identification of a protein with toxigenic activity produced by enteroaggregative *E. coli*. Abstr Gen Mtg Am Soc Microbiol. 1993; B105:44 (abstract).
255. Cravioto A, Gross RJ, Scotland SM, Row B. An adhesive factor found in strains of *E. coli* belonging to the traditional infantile enteropathogenic serotypes. Curr Microbiol 1979;3:95–99.
256. Debroy C, Bright BD, Wilson RA, Yealy J, Kumar R, Bhan MK. Plasmid-coded DNA fragment developed as a specific gene probe for the identification of enteroaggregative *Escherichia coli*. J Med Microbiol 1994;41:393–8.

257. Nataro JP, Enteroaggregative and diffusely adherent *E. coli*. In: Blaser MJ et al eds. Infections of the Gastrointestinal Tract. Raven Press, NY, 1995;727–737.
258. Nataro JP, Kaper JB, Robins-Browne R, et al. Patterns of adherence of diarrheagenic *E. coli* to HEp-2 cells. Pediatr Infect Dis 1987;6:829–831.
259. Giron JA, Jones T, Millan Velasco F, et al. Diffuse-adhering *E. coli* (DAEC) as a putative cause of diarrhea in Mayan children in Mexico. J Infect Dis 1991;35:278–283.
260. Jallat C, Livrelli V, Darfeuille-Michaud A, Rich C, Joly B. *E. coli* strains involved in diarrhea in France: high prevalence and heterogeneity of diffusely adhering strains. J Clin Microbiol 1993;31:2031–2037.
261. Cravioto, A, et al. Association of *E. coli* HEp-2 adherence patterns with type and duration of diarrhea. Lancet 1991;337:262–64.
262. Bilge SS, Clausen CR, Lau W, Moseley SL. Molecular characterization of a fimbrial adhesin, F1845, mediating diffuse adherence of diarrhea-associated *E. coli* to HEp-2 cells. J Bacteriol 1989;171:4281–4289.
263. Tacket CO, Moseley SL, Kay B, et al. Challenge studies in volunteers using *E. coli* strains with diffuse adherence to HEp-2 cells. J Infect Dis 1990;162:550–552.

16

Chronic Small Intestinal Infections

PHILLIP P. TOSKES
University of Florida, Gainesville, Florida

I. INTRODUCTION

Chronic small intestinal infections discussed in this chapter include small intestine bacterial overgrowth, tropical sprue, Whipple's disease, tuberculosis, and histoplasmosis. Special emphasis will be given to the bacterial overgrowth syndrome because it is a relatively common condition and indeed may be the most frequent cause of malabsorption in the elderly (1). Bacterial overgrowth also takes on special importance because it may be a treatable component of the malabsorption seen in patients with other diseases such as Crohn's disease, intestinal lymphoma, or radiation enteritis. Bacterial overgrowth is also associated with conditions that are chronic, such as motility disturbances or previous surgery to the intestinal tract. Therefore, management of small intestine bacterial overgrowth is a life-long endeavor. On the other hand, tropical sprue, Whipple's disease, and enteric histoplasmosis and tuberculosis are chronic infections of the small bowel that cause intestinal abnormalities that persist until the bacteria are eradicated by appropriate therapy.

II. BACTERIAL OVERGROWTH

Small intestine bacterial overgrowth is an under-appreciated condition associated with excessive numbers of bacteria within the proximal small intestine. In this condition, the flora within the small intestine resemble the flora in the colon. The bacteria then in the proximal small intestine compete with the human host for ingested nutrients. This leads to intraluminal bacterial catabolism of nutrients, often with production of toxic metabolites and direct injury to the enterocyte. A complex array of clinical symptoms result which then bring the patient to the attention of clinicians. Traditionally, small intestine bacterial overgrowth has been linked to patients with anatomical abnormalities of the small intestine such as occur in patients who have undergone gastrojejunal anastomoses. However, such aggressive surgeries are not as often encountered today. Instead, dysmotility syndromes such as gastroparesis and irritable bowel syndrome and chronic pancreatitis account for a large part of the associated conditions observed in patients with bacterial overgrowth. Thus, bacterial overgrowth should be strongly considered in patients with these clinical conditions who have compatible symptoms or who do not respond to standard therapies. Since bacterial overgrowth is poorly recognized and is often not suspected by the clinician, an extensive, expensive, and often fruitless investigation is pursued, which is frustrating to both the patient and the clinician.

A. Normal Enteric Flora

The stomach and small intestine usually contain few bacteria. These bacteria are mainly gram-positive aerobes or facultative anaerobes in concentrations of up to 10^4 organisms per ml of jejunal secretions. There may be an occasional coliform in the upper intestine, but the healthy subject does not harbor anaerobic bacteroides. Table 1 details the qualitative and quantitative aspects of normal bacterial flora within the gastrointestinal tract. A zone of transition occurs at the ileum demarking the sparse populations of aerobic flora present in the proximal small intestine and the very dense bacterial populations of anaerobic microorganisms present in the colon. In the ileum, the concentrations of microorganisms increases to the levels of 10^5 to 10^9 organisms per gram of contents.

Table 1 Normal Bacterial Flora Within the Gastrointestinal Tract

	Stomach	Jejunum	Ileum	Cecum
Total bacterial counts[a]	0–3	0–4	5–8	10–12
Aerobes and facultative anaerobes	0–3	0–4	2–5	2–9
Anaerobes	0	0	3–7	9–12

[a]Log 10 of the number of viable micro-organisms per gram of contents.
Source: Toskes PP, Bacterial overgrowth of the gastrointestinal tract. Adv Intern Med 1993; 38:387–407.

While enterobacteria occur only transiently in small numbers in the proximal small intestine, such organisms are regularly found in large numbers in the ileum. Strict anaerobes, which normally cannot survive in the jejunum, frequently colonize the ileum.

However, it is in the colon that dramatic changes in the intestinal flora are seen. The total number of micro-organisms increases up to one millionfold and approximately 10^9 to 10^{12} micro-organisms per gram of colonic contents are found. The colon is inhabited by fastidious anaerobic organisms, such as bacteroides, anaerobic lactobacilli, and clostridia. Following a resection of the ileocecal valve, the populations of the most distal portions of the ileum tend to resemble those of the cecum. Bacterial overgrowth within the small intestine is usually prevented by a series of endogenous defense mechanisms. In order of decreasing importance, these factors are listed in Table 2. Of all of these factors, the most important is the cleansing action of the normal motility of the small intestine. In the relatively stagnant contents of the colon, bacterial growth is abundant, whereas bacteria are rapidly cleared from the small intestine. Mucus may assist in this removable of bacteria. The crucial importance of normal small-bowel motility is emphasized by the observation that whenever normal motility is interrupted, bacterial overgrowth rapidly results.

Interactions between bacteria within the lumen of the small intestine represent important but poorly understood controlling factors influencing the bacterial populations within the intestine. Without the oxygen-utilizing aerobic bacteria, such as coliforms and enterococci, the colon would not be sufficiently anaerobic to maintain the large populations of fastidious anaerobes such as bacteroides. In the bacterial overgrowth syndrome, the flora of the small intestine closely resembles that of the normal colon. Bacterial counts may reach 10^{10} bacteria per ml secretions. Bacteroides and anaerobic lactobacilli usually are the major organisms present but enterobacteria enterococci, clostridia, and diphtheroids may also be present in high concentrations (2,3).

Table 2 Endogenous Defense Mechanisms for Preventing Bacterial Overgrowth

Intestinal motility
gastric-acid secretion
intact ileocecal sphincter
immunoglobulins within intestinal secretions
ill-defined mucosal factors
bacteriostatic properties of pancreatic/biliary secretion

B. Clinical Conditions Associated With Bacterial Overgrowth

Table 3 lists some of the conditions associated with bacterial overgrowth of the small intestine. Anatomic abnormalities such as Billroth II anastomosis, surgery for Crohn's disease, and intestinal strictures are the most frequent causes of clinically important bacterial overgrowth. For example, following a partial gastrectomy and a Billroth II anastomosis, stasis in the afferent loop results in marked bacterial overgrowth within the small intestine and consequent seeding of the remainder of the small intestine (4). Overgrowth also was noted in patients with diverticula of the small intestine (Fig. 1) especially if the patient had an associated decrease in acid secretion (5). Intestinal obstruction from Crohn's disease, adhesions, radiation damage, lymphoma, or tuberculosis may cause bacterial overgrowth (6-9). Severe malabsorption from bacterial overgrowth can occur in patients with gastrocolic or gastrojejunocolic fistulae, with colonic contents passing into the stomach and small intestine. Patients with Kock distal ileal pouches may experience malabsorption secondary to bacterial overgrowth (10).

Table 3 Clinical Conditions Associated With Bacterial Overgrowth

Gastric proliferation
Hypo- or achlorhydria, especially when combined with motor or anatomic disturbances
Sustained hypochlorhydria induced by omeprazole
Small Intestinal Stagnation
Anatomic
Afferent loop of Billroth II partial gastrectomy
Duodenal–jejunal diverticulosis
Surgical blind loop (end-to-side anastomosis)
Surgical recirculating loop (end-to-side anastomosis)
Obstruction (stricture, adhesion, inflammation, neoplasm)
Motor
Scleroderma
Idiopathic intestinal pseudo-obstruction
Absent or disordered migrating motor complex (MMC)
Diabetic autonomic neuropathy
Abnormal communication between proxmial and distal gastrointestinal tract
Gastrocolic or jejunocolic fistula
Resection of diseased ileocecal valve
Miscellaneous
Chronic pancreatitis
Immunodeficiency syndromes
Cirrhosis

Source: Ref. 2. Gastrointestinal Disease, Sleisenger MH, and Fordtran JS, editors, WB Saunders, Philadelphia, 5th ed., 1994 (pp. 1106-1118).

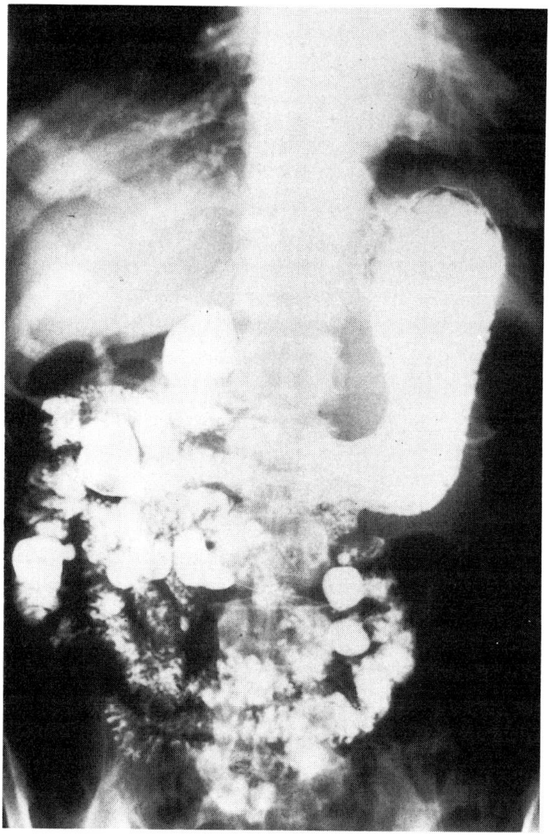

Figure 1 Multiple duodenal and jejunal diverticula in a patient with malabsorption secondary to bacterial overgrowth. (From Toskes PP. Bacterial overgrowth of the gastrointestinal tract. Adv Intern Med 1993; 38:387–407).

Patients with scleroderma (11) (Fig. 2), intestinal pseudo-obstruction (12), and diabetic autonomic neuropathy (13) are examples of dysmotility syndromes associated with bacterial overgrowth. Bacterial overgrowth is particularly apt to develop if the motility disorder is combined with decreased gastric-acid secretion. Some patients with an absent or abnormal migrating motor complex (MMC) may develop bacterial overgrowth and have no radiographic abnormalities (14).

In older individuals, bacterial overgrowth is the most common cause of clinically significant malabsorption (1,15,16). The elderly often have motor disorders of the small intestine, a history of prior gastrointestinal surgery, and decreased acid secretion. While some studies show correction of failure to thrive

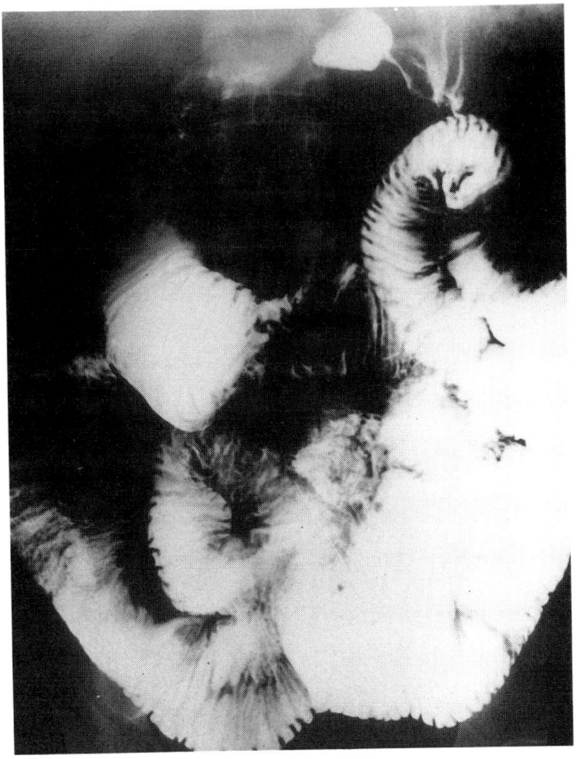

Figure 2 Diffusely dilated small intestine in a patient with scleroderma and malabsorption due to bacterial overgrowth. (From Toskes PP. Bacterial overgrowth syndromes. In: Bockus Gastroenterology, 5th ed., 1995; 1174–1182).

in elderly subjects following treatment with antibiotics, suggesting bacterial overgrowth as a significant cause of malabsorption, other studies in healthy elderly subjects demonstrate bacterial overgrowth to be present, but it appeared to be of little, if any, clinical significance (17,18). These latter studies reported normal absorption of nutrients despite significant overgrowth in the proximal small intestine, a condition that has been called "simple colonization." The difference may be that in those with simple colonization, the intestinal function is relatively normal, but in those with true bacterial overgrowth and malabsorption, there is an associated hypomotility of the small intestine or the presence of anatomical abnormalities.

A recent report demonstrated bacterial overgrowth in outpatients with reflux esophagitis or peptic ulcer disease who were being treated with omeprazole for approximately five weeks (19). Whether bacterial overgrowth following omeprazole therapy will have any clinical consequences is yet to be defined. It appears that the bacterial overgrowth related to omeprazole treatment is similar to the simple colonization observed in the healthy elderly subject. Perhaps the long-term use of omeprazole might lead to clinically-significant overgrowth, especially if there is an associated abnormality such as a dysmotility syndrome of the small intestine. Recent clinical experiences with scleroderma and reflux esophagitis patients point to the importance of both normal intestinal motility and normal gastric-acid secretion in preventing clinically-significant bacterial overgrowth. These patients were doing relatively well on antacids and H_2 receptor antagonists, but some developed severe malabsorption following initiation of omeprazole therapy.

Patients with chronic pancreatitis may have concomitant bacterial overgrowth (20) and may require treatment with both antibiotics and pancreatic enzymes in order to gain weight and cease having diarrhea. Although the mechanism whereby these patients develop bacterial overgrowth is speculative, it is interesting to point out that canine pancreatic secretions have antibacterial activity (21) and that culture-proven bacterial overgrowth has been documented in dogs with pancreatic insufficiency (22). Bacterial overgrowth in these pancreatitis patients may result from the decreased motility associated with abdominal pain, the use of narcotics, and previous pancreatic surgery. As Table 3 points out, patients with immunodeficiency syndromes and cirrhosis have also been shown to have concomitant bacterial overgrowth (23-25). The immunodeficient subjects were demonstrated to have an increase intestinal permeability but the relevance of the overgrowth in patients with cirrhosis is still ill-defined.

C. Clinical Features of Bacterial Overgrowth

As Table 4 points out, the signs and symptoms of bacterial overgrowth are varied and some patients may manifest all or some of these signs and symptoms.

Although in the past, when structural abnormalities of the small intestine often associated with bacterial overgrowth, steatorrhea, and vitamin B_{12} mal-

Table 4 Clinical Features of Bacterial Overgrowth

Diarrhea
Weight loss
Bloating and flatulence
Abdominal pain
Nausea
Steatorrhea
Vitamin B_{12} deficiency

absorption and deficiency were key clinical features, it now appears that the other symptoms detailed Table 4 predominate. In a recent evaluation of 100 consecutive symptomatic patients demonstrated to have bacterial overgrowth by the C^{14}-xylose breath test, the most common clinical features, in decreasing order of frequency, were diarrhea, weight loss, bloating and flatulence, abdominal pain, and nausea. Steatorrhea was much less common and vitamin B_{12} deficiency was not noted (26).

In patients with strictures or fistulae caused by Crohn's disease, or hypomotility caused by scleroderma or intestinal pseudo-obstruction, the clinical features of the primary disease may completely overshadow the manifestations of bacterial overgrowth. It may be difficult to determine in these patients the extent to which the malabsorption is related to the primary intestinal disease or to the secondary bacterial overgrowth.

D. Pathogenesis of Malabsorption Secondary to Bacterial Overgrowth

The anemia noted in most patients with bacterial overgrowth, particularly in those with overgrowth due to structural abnormalities of the small intestine, is related to vitamin B_{12} deficiency. The anemia is macrocytic and serum levels of vitamin B_{12} are decreased. Some of these patients have developed neurological abnormalities and the anemia can be corrected by small doses of vitamin B_{12}. If the B_{12} malabsorption cannot be corrected by the exogenous administration of intrinsic factor, but can be corrected by antibiotic therapy, this points strongly to bacterial overgrowth as the cause. Vitamin B_{12} malabsorption occurs in this setting because of competitive uptake of the vitamin by gram-negative aerobes and various anaerobes that are part of the overgrowth flora. Intrinsic factor effectively inhibits the aerobic microbial uptake of the vitamin B_{12} but has no effect on the vitamin B_{12} uptake by gram-negative anaerobes such as bacteroides (27). These observations point to the gram-negative anaerobes as the likely cause for the vitamin B_{12} malabsorption in the overgrowth state. Some patients may also develop iron deficiency, since there may be blood loss through the gastrointestinal tract in the overgrowth state, perhaps from ulcerated areas within the stagnant loops. Thus,under these circumstances, the patient may manifest a mixed type of anemia. In contrast, folic-acid deficiency is not a problem in the overgrowth state. The micro-organisms in the overgrowth flora synthesize folic acid which is absorbed by the host. For this reason, patients with small-intestine bacterial overgrowth tend to have high folate levels in the blood.

Bloating and abdominal pain may result from the metabolism of fat and carbohydrates within the lumen of the small intestine by the overgrowth flora. A number of toxic metabolites may be produced by these bacteria, which then impair transport of nutrients, including water, across the damaged small intestine. This leads to abdominal distension, pain, diarrhea and/or steatorrhea.

Steatorrhea in the overgrowth state results from several defects. First, the bacteria in the overgrowth state deconjugate bile salts to form free bile acids that are readily reabsorbed from the jejunum. The free bile acids, therefore, do not remain in the lumen of the intestine and do not solubilize lipids. Micelle formation is impaired because of this and fat may be poorly absorbed (28). Accumulation of toxic concentrations of free bile acids may also contribute to the steatorrhea (29). In addition, these toxic substances may lead to a patchy intestinal mucosal damage that may also play a role in fat malabsorption (30).

Diarrhea in the overgrowth state comes about because of bacterial production of organic acids, thereby increasing the osmolarity of the intestinal contents and decreasing the intraluminal pH. These bacterial metabolites such as free bile acids, hydroxylated fatty acids, and organic acids stimulate secretion of water and electrolytes into the lumen (28, 29).

It has long been appreciated that a decreased urinary xylose excretion in the overgrowth state may be demonstrated. This decreased xylose excretion results due to intraluminal bacterial catabolism of the xylose and to diminished absorption of the xylose through the damaged small intestine (31). Decreased serum levels of protein may occur in the overgrowth state and may lead to edema. The etiology of the hypoproteinemia is multifactorial and may result from decreased uptake of amino acids by the damaged small intestine, intraluminal breakdown of protein and protein precursors by bacteria, and antibiotic reversible protein losing enteropathy (30,32,33).

It has also been noted that in the experimental overgrowth state small intestinal motility disturbances are present that can be reversed with antibiotic therapy (34). Thus, the malabsorption in the bacterial overgrowth condition is a dual defect relating to intraluminal abnormalities and damage to the enterocyte.

E. Diagnosis

It is crucial that the clinician have a low threshold for suspecting bacterial overgrowth of the small intestine as the cause of malabsorption in a given patient. Indeed, it is one of the more common forms of malabsorption and certainly deserves consideration since it is a rather easily treatable condition. Patients who manifest gastroparesis, irritable bowel syndrome or chronic pancreatitis, whose condition is not responding to the usual therapy, should be considered as candidates for associated bacterial overgrowth. Likewise, the elderly who may have decreased acid secretion in association with a motility disturbance or a previous surgery on the gastrointestinal tract should be considered as candidates for bacterial overgrowth, should they demonstrate signs or symptoms of malabsorption. Clues to the presence of this condition may be an increased serum folate level or a decreased urinary xylose excretion as well as vitamin B_{12} malabsorption and steatorrhea.

The gold-standard for diagnosing bacterial overgrowth is a properly collected and appropriately cultured aspirate from the proximal small intestine. However, intestinal cultures should be attained under anaerobic conditions, serially diluted, and cultured on selective media. In patients with malabsorption associated with bacterial overgrowth, the total concentration of bacteria usually exceeds 10^5 organisms per ml of jejunal secretions. Bacteroides anaerobic lactobacilli, coliforms, and enterococci are all likely to be present. An intestinal culture requires intubation of the small intestine which is not comfortable for the patient, is time-consuming, and expensive.

A number of breath tests to detect bacterial overgrowth have been developed and utilized for a number of years. The two breath tests that are most commonly employed throughout the world are a 1-gram C^{14}-xylose breath test and a hydrogen breath test. The 1-gram C^{14}-xylose breath test appears to be sensitive and specific enough to detect the presence of bacterial overgrowth in the great majority of patients (35-38). Elevated $14CO_2$ levels appear within the breath in 85% of patients within the first 60 minutes of the test with a 30 minute breath sample being the most reliable. Xylose is attractive as a substrate because: a) xylose is catabolized by gram negative aerobes which are always part of the overgrowth flora, b) xylose is predominantly absorbed in the proximal small bowel as contrasted to the predominant ileal absorption of bile salts leading to virtually no dumping of xylose into the colon, and c) xylose is metabolized substantially less than other proximally absorbed substrates such as glucose. A number of laboratories throughout the world have evaluated the C^{14}-xylose breath test and have documented its reliability in detecting small-intestine bacterial overgrowth. In those studies that utilize the intestinal culture as the gold-standard and evaluated shorter sampling intervals, particularly the 30-minute time point, the sensitivity and specificity approximates 90%.

The other breath test that has been used relatively frequently throughout the world is the breath hydrogen analysis following the administration of a carbohydrate. The basis for this test is that hydrogen production does not occur in mammalian tissues. Therefore, following carbohydrate administration, any hydrogen production in the exhaled breath must come from the activity of the enteric flora upon the substrate. Excessive breath hydrogen production has been noted in patients with bacterial overgrowth following the administration of 50 to 80 grams of glucose or 10 to 12 grams of lactulose (39–41). Fasting levels of breath hydrogen in a patient suspected of having overgrowth are also helpful since about one-third of patients with culture-proven overgrowth will have elevated fasting levels of breath hydrogen before a substrate is administered to the patient (42).

The hydrogen breath test does not involve radiation exposure to the human host, but the test suffers from a lack of sensitivity and specificity. A recent study comparing the lactulose and glucose hydrogen breath test to small-intestinal culture found a sensitivity of 68% for lactulose and 62% for glucose and a specificity of 44% and 83% respectively (43).

Another recent study compared the 1-gram ^{14}C-xylose breath test to a 10-gram lactulose H_2 breath test and a 80-gram glucose H_2 breath test in 20 subjects with culture-proven overgrowth and 10 control subjects (40). The ^{14}C-xylose breath test was abnormal in 19 of 20 subjects with overgrowth and none of the 10 control subjects. In contrast, the H_2 breath test demonstrated quite mixed results giving inadequate sensitivity and specificity.

It should also be appreciated that a number of factors affect hydrogen production by the intestinal bacteria. Recent studies have demonstrated that up to 27% of normal subjects failed to show any rise in breath hydrogen following the administration of lactulose (40,44,45).

Although the C^{14}-xylose breath test involves trivial radiation exposure, the test has not been recommended for children. A carbon-13 labeled xylose breath test is on the horizon and has been shown to be successful in diagnosing overgrowth in pilot studies to date. The clinical efficacy committee of the American College of Physicians suggested that the 1-gram C^{14}-xylose breath test is an appropriate test for routine clinical use.

F. Treatment

Clinicians must recognize that bacterial overgrowth is often a life-long condition and therefore medical therapy must be administered to patients at intermittent intervals. It is often not possible to correct the underlying lesion in the intestine leading to the overgrowth, such as multiple diverticula, scleroderma, and diabetes. It is important also to remember that the bacterial overgrowth may be a treatable component of the malabsorption seen in patients with other diseases of the intestine, such as Crohn's disease, intestinal lymphoma, or radiation enteritis. Of course, bacterial overgrowth may be present in a patient without causing any disease. An abnormal breath test or a pathological culture must be put in perspective by the clinician and appropriate decisions made.

Selection of an antimicrobial agent based on the sensitivities of the microorganisms within the lumen of the intestine seems to be a logical step to take but is not practical because so many different bacterial species are present within the intestine. What is needed is an antimicrobial agent that will be active against both main groups of bacteria in the overgrowth state that lead to malabsorption—gram-negative aerobes and gram-negative anaerobes. If appropriate microbial therapy is given and the bacteria are responsive to the therapy, there should be a noticeable improvement in diarrhea or steatorrhea within a week of therapy. One of the first agents utilized was tetracycline but a large percentage of bacteroides, often the bacteria responsible for causing the malabsorption, are resistant to the tetracycline therapy.

The clavulonic acid derivative, Augmentin, in a dose of 875 mg twice a day, is effective in suppressing both aerobic and anaerobic flora. An alternative choice would be a cephalosporin (e.g., Keflex), 250 mg four times a day, and metronidazole, 250 mg three times a day. If these agents are not effective, chloramphenicol (50 mg/kg in four divided doses) may be employed and is quite effective. Single anaerobic agents such as metronidazole and clindamycin do not appear to be as effective in clinical practice as agents effective against both aerobes and anaerobes.

Antimicrobial agents with poor activity against anaerobes should not be used in treating bacterial overgrowth. These include penicillin, ampicillin, the oral aminoglycosides, kanamycin, and neomycin. In many patients, a single course of therapy for 10 days will suffice and a patient may remain symptom-free for months. Some patients seem to be recurring more quickly than in the past and they must be put on cyclic therapy one week out of every four. A minority of patients seem to need continuous therapy for one to two months. A recent retrospective review of 54 patients with bacterial overgrowth reveals that those with gastroparesis, irritable bowel syndrome, or chronic pancreatitis in association with bacterial overgrowth usually responded to the first trial of antibiotics and developed few recurrences (46). In contrast, patients who have previously undergone intestinal surgery, who had scleroderma and had associated bacterial overgrowth were more refractory and seemed to require multiple courses of antibiotics. There are no adequately controlled clinical trials in regard to choice of antimicrobial agents, duration of therapy, or appropriate management of recurrences.

Prolonged antibiotic therapy is not without potential problems, especially the development of bacterial resistance. Patients may also develop diarrhea, intolerance of the medication, and, rarely, enterocolitis. Thus it is important to establish a solid diagnosis rather than employ empirical therapy. Because of these problems, it has been hoped that a prokinetic agent might be developed that can clear the small intestine of the overgrowth flora and avoid the need for frequent antimicrobial therapy. A recent provocative study in five patients with intestinal scleroderma and bacterial overgrowth is noteworthy in that regard (47). Octreotide (Sandostatin) stimulated the motor activity in these patients evoking Phase III motor complexes that propagated at the same velocity as spontaneous complexes in normal subjects. This treatment also decreased nausea, vomiting, bloating, and abdominal pain in these patients and cleared bacterial overgrowth, as demonstrated by complete normalization of abnormal breath hydrogen tests. A small dose of octreotide was used, 25 to 50 micrograms, and only at bedtime so not to impair the motor response to feeding. It should be cautioned that larger doses of octreotide, such as those used to treat the carcinoid syndrome, could lead to hypomotility and more bacterial overgrowth. Whether this salutary effect of low-dose octreotide will be confirmed remains to be determined.

Nutritional support should not be neglected as an important part of the therapy program for people with bacterial overgrowth. To reduce diarrhea and steatorrhea, a lactose-free diet and substitution of a large part of dietary fat by medium chain triglycerides may be necessary. The medium chain triglyceride formulation may be in the form of a liquid diet (Lipisorb) which has recently been introduced into the market. Patients with vitamin B_{12} deficiency should receive parental injections of vitamin B_{12} to replete their stores. Deficiencies of other nutrients such as calcium and vitamin K should also be corrected. Finally, it should be stressed again that clinicians should have a low threshold for suspecting bacterial overgrowth as the cause of malabsorption in a given patient because the entity is rather common and readily treatable. Figure 3 presents a cost-effective, efficient algorithm for evaluating patients with malabsorption. The algorithm emphasizes the performance of noninvasive tests (breath tests for bacterial overgrowth, serum trypsin levels for pancreatic exocrine insufficiency) for the more common etiologies of malabsorption in contrast to an intestinal biopsy to document nontropical sprue, a somewhat rare cause of malabsorption in the United States.

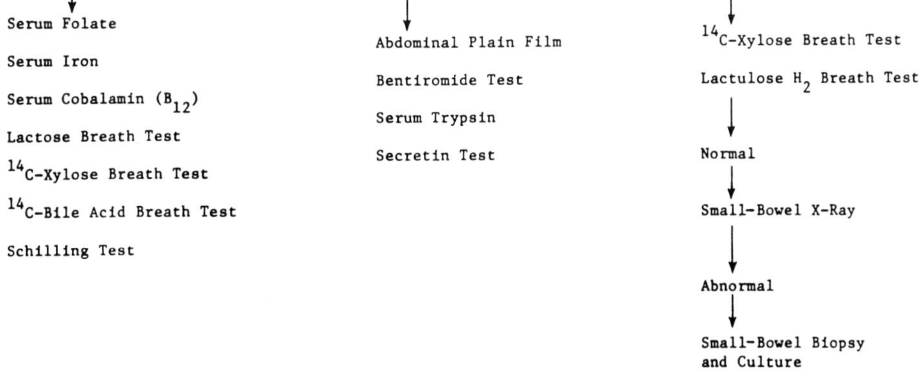

Figure 3 Algorithm for evaluation of malabsorption. (From Ref. 48.)

III. TROPICAL SPRUE

Although the pathogenesis of tropical sprue is still not clearly defined, it appears that overgrowth of the small intestine by toxigenic strains of coliform bacteria are responsible for the abnormality. Unlike bacterial overgrowth of the small intestine as described above, there is no overgrowth of bacteroides in the patients with tropical sprue. Eradication of the coliforms in the patient with tropical sprue results in cure of the intestinal abnormalities. The coliforms isolated from patients with tropical sprue contain toxins that cause abnormalities in the small intestine (52,53). Although tropical sprue seems to be an infectious disease that leads to malabsorption, the possible role of folic-acid deficiency in this disease is unclear. Large doses of folic acid or vitamin B_{12} lead to improvement of both the structure and function of the small intestine in patients with tropical sprue. Tropical sprue affects people who visit or become residents of certain tropical areas. It has been found in Europeans, working or staying in India and Southeast Asia, Americans living in Puerto Rico and the Philippines, and natives of Puerto Rico, Cuba, Haiti, and the Dominican Republic.

A. Clinical Features

Most patients complain initially of acute watery diarrhea, abdominal cramps, and excessive gas. Months later, patients develop severe malabsorption and depletion of body folic-acid stores. Some may develop vitamin B_{12} deficiency and severe megaloblastic anemia. Malabsorption of xylose is common and steatorrhea is present in up to 90% of patients. Tropical sprue should be considered in any person returning from the countries or areas mentioned above who has experienced diarrhea for more than one month, particularly if weight loss is significant. Although the histological abnormalities are more prominent in the jejunum early in the course of tropical sprue, the entire small bowel soon becomes equally affected. The villi are abnormal but a completely flat biopsy as found in non-tropical sprue is decidedly uncommon.

B. Treatment

The administration of large doses of folic acid or vitamin B_{12} without antibiotic therapy produces a prompt correction of the megaloblastic anemia and a return of appetite and weight gain. Although there may be dramatic improvement with folic-acid administration, this kind of therapy usually fails to completely reverse the intestinal abnormalities, and chronic symptoms will persist. Treatment with tetracycline and nonabsorbable sulfonamides is usually effective in eradicating the contaminating coliform bacteria. If given alone, antimicrobial therapy is effective within weeks. Thus, it would appear reasonable to give both folic acid (5 mg) orally per day together with vitamin B_{12} (1000 μg) parenterally once a week for several weeks, in order to replace tissue stores, and tetracycline 250 mg four times a day. This combination therapy will result in complete healing of the intestinal abnormalities within months. Although native residents who have been treated in this way may get recurrences within several years after stopping therapy, this does not appear to be the case with visitors who have been treated and who have returned to temperate climates.

III. WHIPPLE'S DISEASE

Whipple's disease is a systemic bacterial disease of middle-aged white men caused by a bacillus, which was identified in 1992 and named *Tropheryma whippelii* (54). Involved tissues are infiltrated with macrophages that stain with periodic acid-shift reaction (Figs. 4 and 5).

A. Clinical Features

Diarrhea, arthralgias, malabsorption, pericarditis or endocarditis, dementia, fever of undetermined cause, or a wasting syndrome may be parts of the presenting manifestations. The organism has not been cultured but has been identified by polymerase chain reaction. Clinicians should have a high index of suspicion for this disease in patients who present with weight loss, diarrhea, arthralgias, and abdominal pain. It is particularly important to consider this disease if there is increased skin pigmentation and the arthralgias came before the other symptoms (55). The disease is best diagnosed by an intestinal biopsy (Figs. 4 and 5).

B. Treatment

Antibiotics are the treatment of choice. It is appropriate to continue treatment for one year. Careful, long-term follow-up of all treated patients is necessary. Repeat biopsy should be done only if the patient fails to respond or relapses. The PAS positive macrophages persist in the lamina propria of the intestine for many years after successful treatment. The initial recommendation for treatment is the oral administration of double-strength Trimethoprin-sulfamethoxazole twice daily for one year. If the patient is extremely ill and cannot take oral medications, then parenteral penicillin is helpful.

IV. TUBERCULOSIS

In the western hemisphere, abdominal tuberculosis is a disease of immunocompromised hosts. Intestinal tuberculosis may develop as a primary focus of infection or secondary to pulmonary involvement. The ileocecal area and the

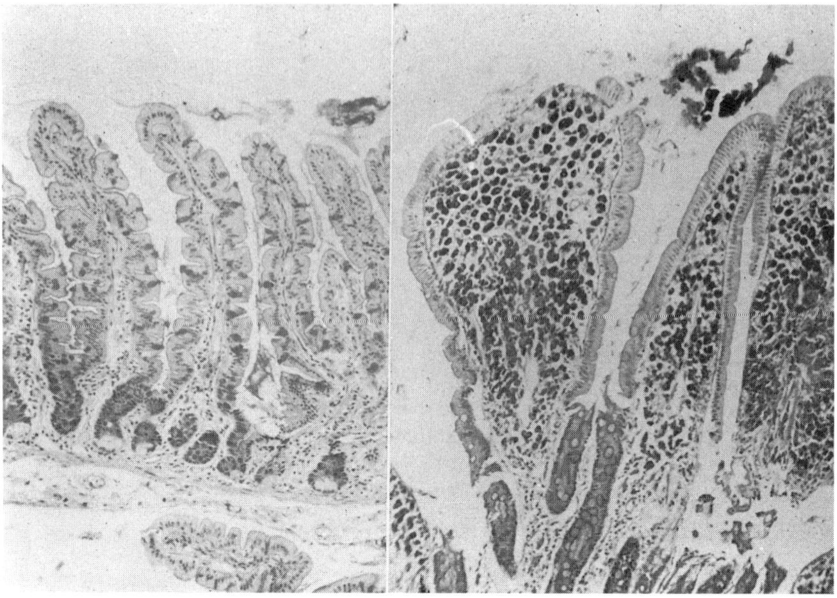

Figure 4 PAS stain of intestinal biopsy. The left is normal, the right is positive for Whipple's disease. Note the PAS positive macrophages within the lamina propria of the intestine.

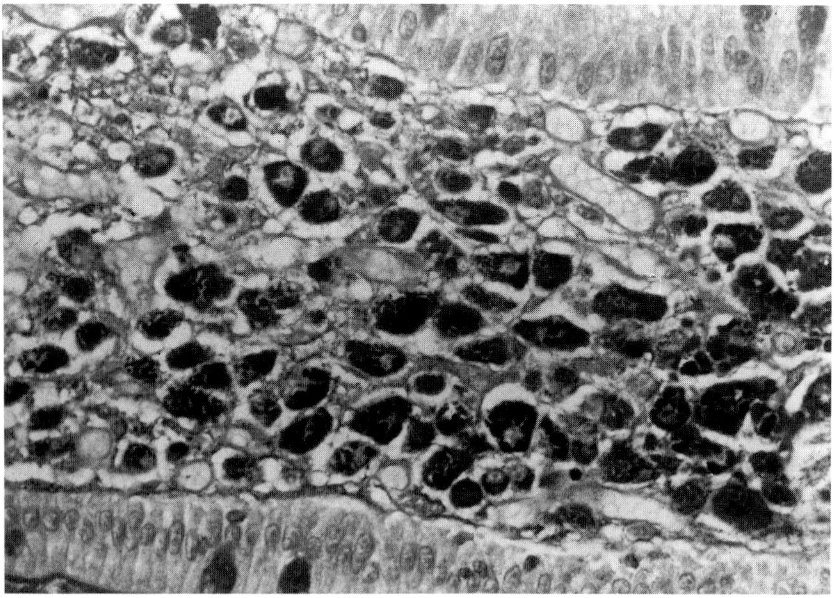

Figure 5 High-power view of intestinal lamina propria filled with PAS positive macrophages.

colon are most commonly involved and can be confused with Crohn's disease or carcinoma. Patients have nonspecific symptoms which include fever, night sweats, anorexia, nausea, abdominal pain, diarrhea, and weight loss. Strictures in the intestine are usually shorter than that of Crohn's and are found in multiple areas. The ulcerations that are found in these areas are not longitudinal, as seenin Crohn's, but are often circumferential. Complications seen include obstruction, hemorrhage, and malabsorption, often due to bacterial overgrowth on top of the obstruction caused by the tuberculosis (56).

Treatment mandates three antibacterial agents initially usually isoniazid (300 mg per day), ethambutol (15 mg/kg/day) and rifampicin (600 mg per day).

V. HISTOPLASMOSIS

Patients with disseminated histoplasmosis present with multiple system involvement including the liver, gastrointestinal tract, or central nervous system. Initial symptoms usually include fever, chills, malaise, anorexia, and weight loss. The patients may demonstrate an ulcerative enteritis in the terminal ileum or colon (57). Patients often have simultaneous involvement of various levels of the gastrointestinal tract. Rarely, the disease can present as a protein-losing enteropathy with a large intestinal villi mimicking Whipple's disease (58). Diagnosis is best made by biopsy of the rectum or involved parts of the gastrointestinal tract. The *Histoplasma capsulatum* can be demonstrated in the tissue. Skin tests for histoplasmin are not helpful. Treatment includes amphotericin B (two over 10 weeks for adults) or ketoconazole (200 to 400 mg daily for six months).

REFERENCES

1. Haboudi N, Montgomery R. Small bowel bacterial overgrowth in elderly people: clinical significance and response to treatment. Age Ageing 1992: 21:13–19.
2. Toskes PP, Donaldson R: Enteric bacterial flora and bacterial overgrowth syndrome. In: Sleisenger MH, Fordtran JS, eds. Gastroinetesinal Disease, 5th Ed. Philadelphia: WB Saunders, 1994; 1106–1118.
3. Simon GL and Gorbach SL. The intestinal flora in health and disease. A review. Gastroenterology 1984; 86:174–193.
4. Goldstein F, Wirts CW, Kramer S. The relationship of afferent limb stasis and bacterial flora to the production of post-gastrectomy steatorrhea. Gastroenterology 1961; 40:47–55.
5. Doig A and Girdwood RG. The absorption of folic acid and labeled cyanocobalamine in intestinal malabsorption with observations on the fecal excretion of fat and nitrogen and the absorption of glucose and xylose. QJ Med 1960; 29:333–374.
6. Beeken WL and Kanish RE. Microbial flora of the upper small bowel in Crohn's

disease. Gastroenterology 1973; 65:390–397.
7. Bishop RF and Anderson CM. Bacterial flora of stomach and small intestine in children with intestinal obstruction. Arch Dis Child 1960; 35:487–492.
8. Swan RW. Stagnant loop syndrome resulting from small bowel irradiation injury and intestinal bypass. Gyn Oncol 1974; 8:441–445.
9. Russell RM, Abadi P, Ismail-Beigi F. Role of bacterial overgrowth on the malabsorption syndrome of the primary small intestinal lymphoma. Cancer 1977; 89:8579–8583.
10. Kelly DG, Phillips SF, Kelly KA, et. al. Dysfunction of the continent ileostomy: Clinical features and bacteriology. Gut 1983; 24:193–198.
11. Kahn I, Jeffries GH, Sleisenger MH. Malabsorption in intestinal scleroderma. Correction by antibiotics. N Engl J Med 1966; 274:1339–1344.
12. Pearson AJ, Brzechwa-Adjukiewicz A, McCarthy CF. Intestinal pseudo-obstruction with bacterial overgrowth in the small intestine. Am J Dig Dis 1969; 14:200–205.
13. Goldstein F, Wirts EC, Kowlessar OD. Diabetic diarrhea and steatorrhea. Microbiologic and clinical observations. Ann Intern Med 1970; 72:215–218.
14. Vantrappen G, Janssens J, Hellemans J, et.al. The interdigestive motor complex of normal subjects and patients with bacterial overgrowth of the small intestine. J Clin Invest 1977; 59:1158–1166.
15. Roberts SH, James O, Jarvis EH. Bacterial overgrowth syndrome without "blind loop": a cause for malnutrition in the elderly. Lancet 1977; 2:1193–95.
16. McEvoy A, Dutton J, James OF. Bacterial contamination of the small intestine is an important cause of occult malabsorption in the elderly. Br Med J 1983; 287:789–793.
17. Lipski P, Kelly P, James F. Bacterial comtamination of the small bowel in elderly people: Is it necessarily pathological. Age Ageing 1992; 21:13–19.
18. Saltzman J, Kowdley K, Pedrosa M, et al. Bacterial overgrowth without clinical malabsorption in elderly hypochlorhydric subjects. Gastroenterology 1994; 106:615–623.
19. Fried M, Slegrish H, Frei R, et al. Duodenal bacterial overgrowth during treatment with omeprazole in outpatients. Gut 1996; 35:23–29.
20. Lembeke B, Kraus B, Lankisch PG. Small intestinal function in chronic relapsing pancreatitis. Hepatogastroenterology 1985; 32:149–155.
21. Rubinstein E, Mark Z, Haspel J, et al. Antibacterial activity of the pancreatic fluid. Gastroenterology 1985; 88:927–932.
22. Williams DA, Batt RM, McLean L. Bacterial overgrowth in the duodenum of dogs with exocrine pancreatic insufficiency. J Am Vet Med Assoc 1987; 191:201–206.
23. Piqnata C, Budillon G, Monaco G, et.a. Jejunal bacterial overgrowth and intestinal permeability in children with immunodeficiency syndromes. Gut 1990; 31:879–882.
24. Martini GA, Phear EA, Ruebner E, et al: The bacterial content of the small intestine in normal and cirrhotic subjects: Relation to the methionine toxicity. Clin Sci 1956; 16:35–51.
25. Correia JP, Garnel M, Monteiro E, et al: Bacteriology of the small intestine in cirrhotic subjects and its relation to malabsorption. Am J of Gastroenterol 1971;

56:428–435.
26. Kumar A, Forsmark CE, Toskes PP. Small bowel bacterial overgrowth: The changing face of an old disease. Gastroenterology 1996; 110:A340.
27. Welkos SA, Toskes PP, Baer H, et al. Importance of anaerobic bacteria in the cobalamin malabsorption of experimental rat blind loop syndrome. Gastroenterology 1981; 80:313–320.
28. Kim YS, Spritz N, Blum M, et al. The role of altered bile acid metabolism in the steatorrhea of experimental blind loop. J Clin Invest 1966; 45:956–962.
29. Wanitschke R and Ammon HV. Effects of dihydroxy bile acids and hydroxy fatty acids on the absorption of oleic acid in the human jejunum. J Clin Invest 1978; 61:178–186.
30. Giannella RA, Rout WR, Toskes PP. Jejunal brush border injury and impaired sugar and amino acid uptake in the blind loop syndrome. Gastroenterology 1974; 67:965–974.
31. Toskes PP, King CE, Spivey JC, et al. Xylose catabolism in experimental rat blind loop syndrome: Studies including newly developed d-(^{14}C) xylose breath test. Gastroenterology 1978; 74:691–697.
32. Varcoe R, Holliday D, Tavill A. Utilization of urea nitrogen for albumin synthesis in the stagnant loop syndrome. Gut 1974; 15:898–902.
33. King CE and Toskes PP. Protein-losing enteropathy in the human and experimental rat blind loop syndrome. Gastroenterology 1981; 80:504–509.
34. Justus PG, Fernandez A, Martin JL, et al. Altered myoelectric activity in the experimental blind loop syndrome. J Clin Invest 1983; 72:1064–1071.
35. King CE, Toskes PP, Spivey JC, et. al. Detection of small intestine overgrowth by means of a ^{14}C-D-xylose breath test. Gastroenterology 1979; 79:75–82.
36. Schneider A, Novis B, Chen V, et. al. Value of the ^{14}C-D-xylose breath test in patients with intestinal bacterial overgrowth. Digestion 1985; 32:86–91.
37. Rumessen JJ, Gudmand-Hoyer E, Bachmann E, et al. Diagnosis of bacterial overgrowth of the small intestine. Scand J Gastroenterol 1985; 20:1267–75.
38. Pruthi HS, Mehta SK, Pathak CM. Evaluation of ^{14}C-D-xylose breath test in the diagnosis of small intestinal bacterial overgrowth. Indian J Med Res 1984; 80:598–600.
39. Metz G, Cassull MA, Drasar BS, et al. Breath-hydrogen test for small intestinal bacterial colonization. Lancet 1976; 1:688–689.
40. King CE and Toskes PP. Comparison of the 1-gram ^{14}C-Dxylose, 10-gram lactulose-H_2 and 80 gram glucose H_2 breath tests in patients with small intestine bacterial overgrowth. Gastro 1986; 91:1447–1451.
41. Rhodes JM, Middleton P and Jewell DP. The lactulose hydrogen breath test as a diagnostic test for small-bowel bacterial overgrowth. Scand J Gastroenterol 1979; 4:333–336.
42. Perman JA, Modler S, Barr RG, et al. Fasting breath hydrogen concentration: normal values and clinical application. Gastroenterology 1984; 87:1358–1363.
43. Corazza GR, Menozzi MG, Strocchi A, et al. The diagnosis of small bowel bacterial overgrowth. Gastroenterology 1990; 98:302–305.
44. Strocchi A, Sorge M, Pranzo L, et al. Intraindividual variability in H_2 production capacity. Gastroenterol Internat 1:593, 1988 (Suppl 1).
45. Gilat T, Ben Hur H, Gelman-Malachi E, et al. Alterations of the colonic flora and

their effect on the hydrogen breath test. Gut 1978; 19:602–605.
46. Kumar A, Forsmark CF, Toskes PP. The response of small bowel bacterial overgrowth to treatment: Effects of coexisting conditions. Gastroenterology 1996; 110:A340.
47. Soudah HC, Hasler WL, Owyang C. Effect of Octreotide on intestinal motility and bacterial overgrowth in scleroderma. N Engl J Med 1991; 325:1461–1467.
48. Toskes P. Malabsorption. In: Wyngaarden J, Smith L, Bennett J, eds. Cecil's Textbook of Medicine. 19th Ed. Philadelphia: WB Saunders, 1992:687–699.
49. Gorbach SL, Mitra R, Jacobs B, et al. Bacterial contamination of the upper small bowel in tropical sprue. Lancet 1969; 1:74.
50. Klipstein FA, Holdeman LV, Corcino JJ, Moore WEC. Enterotoxigenic intestinal bacteria in tropical sprue. Ann Intern Med 1973; 79:632.
51. Tomkins AM, Drasar BS, James WPT. Bacterial colonisation of jejunal mucosa in acute tropical sprue. Lancet 1975; 1:59.
52. Klipstein FA, Engert RF, Short HB. Enterotoxigenicity of colonising coliform bacteria in tropical sprue and blind-loop syndrome. Lancet 1978; 2:342.
53. Klipstein FA, Horowitz IR, Engert RF, Shenk EA. Effect of *Klebsiella pneumoniae* enterotoxin on intestinal transport in the rat. J Clin Invest 1975; 56:799.
54. Relman DA, Schmidt TM, MacDermott RA, Falkow S. Identification of the uncultured bacillus of Whipple's disease. New Engl J Med 1992; 327:293.
55. Dobbins WO III. Whipple's disease. Springfield, IL: Charles C Thomas, 1987.
56. Sherman S, Rohwedder JJ, Ravikrishnan KP, Weg JG. Tuberculosis enteritis and peritonitis: report of 36 general hospital cases. Arch Intern Med 1980; 140:506.
57. Cappell MS, Mandell W, Grimes MM, Neu HC. Gastrointestinal histoplasmosis. A review. Dig Dis Sci 1988; 33:353.
58. Banks S, Trey C, Gans I, et al. Histoplasmosis of the small bowel with "giant" intestinal villi and secondary protein losing enteropathy. Am J Med 1965; 39:492.

Index